Thomson Delmar Learning's

ADMINISTRATIVE MEDICAL ASSISTING

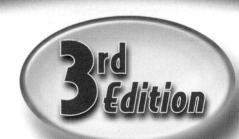
3rd Edition

Wilburta Q. Lindh, MA

Marilyn S. Pooler, RN, MA, MEd

Carol D. Tamparo, CMA, PhD

Barbara M. Dahl, CMA, CPC

THOMSON
DELMAR LEARNING

Australia Canada Mexico Singapore Spain United Kingdom United States

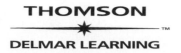

Thomson Delmar Learning's Administrative Medical Assisting, Third Edition
by Wilburta Q. Lindh, Marilyn S. Pooler, Carol D. Tamparo, and Barbara M. Dahl

Vice President, Health Care Business Unit:
William Brottmiller

Editorial Director:
Matthew Kane

Acquisitions Editor:
Rhonda Dearborn

Developmental Editor:
Sarah Duncan

Editorial Assistant:
Debra Gorgos

Marketing Director:
Jennifer McAvey

Marketing Coordinator:
Kimberly Duffy

Technology Director:
Laurie K. Davis

Technology Project Manager:
Mary Colleen Liburdi

Technology Project Coordinator:
Carolyn Fox

Production Director:
Carolyn Miller

Production Manager:
Barbara A. Bullock

Production Editor:
Jack Pendleton

Project Editor:
Natalie Pashoukos

For permission to use material from this text or product, contact us by
Tel (800) 730-2214
Fax (800) 730-2215
www.thomsonrights.com

Library of Congress Cataloging-in-Publication Data
ISBN 1-4018-8135-1

Notice to the Reader

Publisher does not warrant or guarantee any of the products described herein or perform any independent analysis in connection with any of the product information contained herein. Publisher does not assume, and expressly disclaims, any obligation to obtain and include information other than that provided to it by the manufacturer.

The reader is expressly warned to consider and adopt all safety precautions that might be indicated by the activities described herein and to avoid all potential hazards. By following the instructions contained herein, the reader willingly assumes all risks in connection with such instructions.

The publisher makes no representations or warranties of any kind, including but not limited to, the warranties of fitness for particular purpose or merchantability, nor are any such representations implied with respect to the material set forth herein, and the publisher takes no responsibility with respect to such material. The publisher shall not be liable for any special, consequential, or exemplary damages resulting, in whole or part, from the reader's use of, or reliance upon, this material.

CONTENTS

ABOUT THE AUTHORS

Wilburta (Billie) Q. Lindh, MA, holds professor emerita status at Highline Community College, Des Moines, Washington. She is the former program director and consultant to the Medical Assistant Program at Highline Community College and the 2000 Outstanding Faculty Member of the year. Lindh is a member of the SeaTac Chapter of the American Association of Medical Assistants (AAMA) and has lectured at AAMA seminars on the importance of communication. She is coauthor of *Therapeutic Communications for Allied Health Professions* published by Thomson Delmar Learning. She also coauthored *The Radiology Word Book* and *The Ophthalmology Word Book*, texts frequently used by transcriptionisrs, and is the medical assistant chapter author for *Guide to Careers in the Health Professions*.

Marilyn S. Pooler, RN, MA, MEd, is a professor in medical assisting. She taught for more than 25 years at Springfield Technical Community College in Springfield, Massachusetts, and served as Department Chairperson for several years. She has served on the Certifying Board of the AAMA Task Force for test construction and was a site surveyor for the AAMA for many years. Pooler has been a speaker at numerous local and state medical assisting meetings and seminars, emphasizing the importance of education, certification, and recertification of medical assistants. For a number of years, Pooler was a member of the executive board of the Northeast Association of Allied Health Educators. Pooler presently works in Health Services at Baypath College, Longmeadow, Massachusetts, at Baystate Medical Associates in Springfield, Massachusetts, in the gastroenterology clinic and for the Center for Business and Technology at Springfield Technical Community College, where she teaches refresher courses to medical assistants, licensed practical nurses, and registered nurses.

Carol D. Tamparo, CMA, PhD, served as a medical assistant instructor for 24 years and as program director for medical assisting for 15 years at Highline Community College in Des Moines, Washington. She was the Dean of Business and Allied Health programs at Lake Washington Technical College in Kirkland, Washington, for 4 years and currently is president of the Lake Washington College Foundation. She is the coauthor of *Therapeutic Communications for Health Professionals; Medical Law, Ethics, & Bioethics for Ambulatory Care;* and *Diseases of the Human Body.* She is a member of the SeaTac Chapter of AAMA and volunteers as a CASA advocate *(guardian ad litum)* in the King County Court System. She resides in Des Moines, Washington, with her husband, Tom.

Barbara M. Dahl, CMA, CPC, has dedicated her professional life to the recognition and advancement of medical assisting through quality education, increased public awareness, legislative compliance, and positive professional enhancement. She is a tenured faculty member at Whatcom Community College in Bellingham, Washington, and has been the Medical Assisting Program Coordinator and Department Chair since 1991. She is an active member of the Whatcom County Chapter of Medical Assistants, Washington State Society of Medical Assistants, AAMA, and the Washington State Medical Assisting Educators. She is a former chapter and state president and has served on and chaired many committees on the chapter, state, and national levels. She was instrumental in designing the AAMA Excel award-winning WSSMA Web site and continues to serve as the state Web master. Through the years she has acquired a wealth of knowledge and understanding about the professional and legal aspects of medical assisting, particularly in relation to the Washington State HCA law. She is also a member of the American Association of Professional Coders and is a founding member of the Whatcom Professional Coders, for which she has served as president. She proctors both the AAMA and the AAPC examinations. She has been an educational presenter/speaker at both Washington and Oregon state conferences and at Oregon State's Leadership Retreat.

ACKNOWLEDGMENTS

The authors personally acknowledge the following people:

To my husband, who continually supports and assists in so many ways, thank you. To my family for support and encouragement, and to Laura Lindh, who provided expertise for some chapters, thank you. To the students, graduates, and fellow colleagues who challenge me to stay current with skills and up-to-date with technology, thank you.

Billie Q. Lindh, MA

Thanks to my friends who were very supportive of my efforts, and a special thanks to my husband, Jud, for his patience and understanding during this endeavor.

Marilyn S. Pooler, RN, MA, MEd

Many thanks to those who believed that this edition was necessary and who recognized the abilities of each of its authors. Thanks to my husband, Tom, who was very patient during this undertaking and helped in numerous ways. To Billie, Marilyn, and Barbara, thanks for being such supportive and top-notch authors. Thanks to Barbara Murray for input and suggestions. Thanks to all the Delmar staff who make this text what it is.

Carol D. Tamparo, CMA, PhD

This writing experience has been exciting and humbling at the same time. I most definitely have received more than I have given. Mostly I have learned about myself. Having spent so many years educating and training medical assisting students, I am so astounded that I have helped produce a product that will serve as a learning tool for medical assisting students everywhere. I thank my students for all their patience and assistance; they are an absolute wealth of ideas! Much thanks to my college administrators for their endorsements. I thank my family for all their support, especially my husband, Ed, for his faith in my abilities and for fixing me breakfast, lunch, and dinner on those many Saturdays while I was glued to the computer; my son, Nik, for his amazing work on the workbook competencies; my former student, Sheila Atwater, and colleague, Sheri Greimes, for their generosity in sharing their laboratory expertise; my good friend and colleague, Lisa Carter, for her emotional support, excellent medical business acumen, and friendship. I thank the other authors, Billie, Carol, and Marilyn, for listening to my ideas and mentoring me through my first real writing experience. I also thank Sarah Duncan, my developmental editor, for her wise and calming nature that kept me reasonable and grounded during this writing experience. Most of all, though, I thank God that this project is finished! (And for blessing me with this unique and never-to-be-forgotten opportunity.)

Barbara M. Dahl, CMA, CPC

A sincere thank you to Joanne Cerrato, former coauthor, for her many invaluable contributions to the formation of the first edition of this text.

Special thanks to Janice Payne, CPC, for reviewing and editing Chapters 18 and 19. For the last 17 years Janice has worked as a CPC for insurance companies that were Medicare carriers, as well as carriers for large physician groups. Janice was primary caregiver for her dad the last 7 years. He passed away late October 2004. Thank you for your help during your time of mourning.

A sincere thank you to the medical assisting students at Whatcom Community College and at the following facilities for their assistance with the art program in this book: Madrona Medical Group and Bellingham Walk-in Clinic.

REVIEWERS

Julie L. Akason, RN, BSN
Department Head of Medical Assisting
Argosy University/Twin Cities
Eagan, MN

Diana E. Alagna, RN
Certified Phlebotomy Instructor
Medical Assisting Program Director
Branford Hall Career Institute
Southington, CT

Carole Berube, MA, MSN, BSN, RN
Professor Emerita in Nursing
Medical Assisting Program Faculty
Bristol Community College
Fall River, MA

Norma Bird, MEd, CMA
Medical Assisting Program Director/
 Instructor
Idaho State University College of
 Technology
Pocatella, ID

Michelle Blesi, CMA
Medical Assisting Program Director/
 Instructor
Century College
White Bear Lake, MN

Cheryl H. Bordwine, BS, HCA
 NCICS
Medical and Business Instructor
Texas School of Business
Friendswood, TX

David Bruce Drumm, PCMA, ASB,
 AE
Medical Department Coordinator
Computer Learning Network
Mechanicsburg, PA

George Fakhoury, MD, DORCP,
 CMA
Academic Program Manager,
 Healthcare
Heald College
San Francisco, CA

Deborah Fox, CAHI/CMA
Medical Assisting Program Supervisor
Porter and Chester Institute
Wethersfield, CT

Jeanette Goodwin, BSN CMA
Medical Assisting Program Chair
Southeast Community College
Lincoln, NE

Michaelea Holten, CRTT, NCMA
Medical Assisting Program Director
Pioneer Pacific College
Portland, OR

Diane M. Klieger, RN, MBA, CMA
Medical Assisting Program Director
Pinellas Technical Education
 Centers-SP
St. Petersburg, FL

Gerry Landes, CMA
Medical Assisting Department Chair
Bryman College
Everett, WA

Renee Levert, MA
Allied Health Manager
Kaplan Higher Education
Roswell, GA

Claire E. Maday-Travis, MA, MBA,
CPHQ
Allied Health Program Director
The Salter School
Wooster, MA

Joseph E. McCann, BA, LVN (Ret)
Instructor
San Antonio College
San Antonio, TX

Tanya Mercer, BS, RN, RMA
Allied Health Curriculum Developer
KAPLAN Higher Education
Roswell, GA

Brigitte Niedzwiecki, RN, MSN
Medical Assistant Program Director
Chippewa Valley Technical College
Eau Claire, WI

Margaret O. Noirjean, RN, BSN
Instructor
Dakota County Technical College
Rosemount, MN

Deborah Odegaard, BS, CMA
Instructor, Medical Assistant
Program
Des Moines Area Community
College
Ankeny, IA

D. J. Overbey, RN, CCRC
Medical Assisting Program Director
Virginia College at Austin
Austin, TX

Nanciann Rosier, MEd, BSEd
Medical Assisting Technology
Instructor
Ohio University Lancaster Campus
Lancaster, OH

Trevor Smith, DC, DAHom, FASA
Instructor
National College of Business &
Technology
Nashville, TN

Stephanie J. Suddendorf, CMA,
AAS
Medical Assistant Program Director
Minnesota School of Business/Globe
College
Minneapolis, MN

Lori Warren, MA, RN, CPC, CCP,
CLNC
Medical Department Co-Director
Spencerian College
Louisville, KY

Prior Edition Reviewers

Kaye Acton
Director of Medical Assisting Program
Alamance Community College
Graham, NC

Magdalena Andrasevits, NRCMA
Medical Assistant Program Director
Sanford-Brown College
North Kansas City, MO

Joseph DeSapio, RMA
Director of Facility and Library
Resources
Medical Assisting Instructor
Ultrasound Diagnostic School
New York, NY

Eleanor K. Flores, RN, BSN, MEd
Briarwood College
Southington, CT

Tova Green
IVTC Fort Wayne
Fort Wayne, IN

Karen Jackson, NR-CMA
Medical Program Chair
Education America, Dallas Campus
Garland, TX

Barbara G. Kalfin, BS, AAS,
CMA-C
Medical Assisting Extern Coordinator
Instructor, Medical Assisting Program
City College
Ft. Lauderdale, FL

Theresa Offenberger, PhD
Professor of Medical Assisting
Cuyahoga Community College
Cleveland, OH

Agnes Pucillo, LPN
Medical Assisting Program Director
Ultrasound Diagnostic School
Iselin, NJ

Patricia Schrull, RN, MBA, MEd,
CMA
Program Director, Medical Assisting
Program
Lorain County Community College
Elyria, OH

Janet Sesser, BS Ed. Admin., RMA,
CMA
Corporate Director of Education,
Allied Health
High-Tech Institute, Inc.
Phoenix, AZ

LIST OF PROCEDURES

PREFACE

The world of health care has changed rapidly over the past few years, and as medical assistants, you will be called on to do more and respond to an increasing number of administrative responsibilities, especially in this age of managed care. Now is the time to equip yourself with the skills you will need to excel in the field. Now is the time to maximize your potential, expand your base of knowledge, and dedicate yourself to becoming the best multifaceted, multiskilled medical assistant that you can be.

The new edition of *Thomson Delmar Learning's Administrative Medical Assisting* will guide you on this journey. This text is part of a dynamic learning system that also includes a student software CD, workbook, and online materials. Together, this learning package maps to the entry-level competencies identified by the Accrediting Bureau of Health Education Schools (ABHES) and the Commission on Accreditation of Allied Health Education Programs (CAAHEP), as well as the standards defined by American Association of Medical Assistants' (AAMA's) Role Delineation Study and American Medical Technologists' (AMT's) Registered Medical Assistant Competency Inventory.

You will find that this edition provides you with more opportunities to use your critical thinking skills, through case studies, question boxes, scenarios, and features that tie directly to *Thomson Delmar Learning's Skills and Procedures and Critical Thinking for Medical Assistants DVD Series*. You will also see that the text responds to the growing need to learn about softer skills such as professionalism, as well as practical skills, including how to comply with Health Insurance Portability and Accountability Act (HIPAA) regulations and deal with privacy issues on the job.

How the Text Is Organized

Thomson Delmar Learning's Administrative Medical Assisting, 3rd edition, presents a logical, in-depth review of all administrative competencies required of today's multiskilled medical assistants—*in full color!*

- **Section I, General Procedures (Chapters 1 through 9),** provides the groundwork for understanding the role and responsibilities of the medical assistant. Topics include the medical assisting profession, the health care team, history of medicine, therapeutic communications, coping skills for the medical assistant, legal and ethical issues, and emergency procedures and first aid. New in Section I: Additional information about AMT, RMA,

CMAS, and ABHES; Introduction of Integrative Medicine and Alternative Therapies; Mechanisms for making ethical decisions; Provider level CPR; New procedure: Identifying Community Resources.

- **Section II, Administrative Procedures (Chapters 10 through 21),** provides up-to-date information on all administrative competencies required of medical assistants. Topics include creation of the facility environment, computer use, telecommunications, patient scheduling, medical records management, written communications, transcription, insurance and coding, management of facility finances, billing and collections, and accounting practices. New in Section II: Emphasis on the use of computers for all aspects of financial management; Electronic and online scheduling; Electronic medical records; Accounts receivable ratio and collection ratio; New procedures, including: recording a NSF check, software installation, CPT and ICD-9-CM coding, and software installation.

- **Section III, Professional Procedures (Chapters 22 through 25),** examines the role of the medical assistant as office and human resources manager and provides tools and techniques to use when preparing for externship, medical assisting credentials, and employment. New in Section III: Management styles; Risk Management; CMA and RMA certification process; E-résumés.

- **Glossary** includes definitions of all key terms, with related chapter numbers indicated.

- **Student Software CD** includes StudyWARE with quizzes and activities, as well as the Critical Thinking Challenge, which presents real-life scenarios in which you must use your critical thinking skills to choose the most correct action in response to the situation.

How Each Chapter Is Organized

All chapters include similar features and presentation and function as building blocks to a comprehensive medical assisting education. However, each chapter is also a self-contained module and can be studied in any order or independently of other chapters in the text.

Features include:

- **Key terms, chapter outline,** and **objectives** to help identify important concepts and provide direction for the chapter

- **Featured Competencies,** which map the chapter material to ABHES and CAAHEP competencies

- An **introduction** with a real-life **scenario**
- **Spotlight on Certification** for CMA, RMA, and CMAS examinations
- **Graphic icons, photographs,** and **figures** in full-color to illustrate the text discussion
- **Procedures** with step-by-step instructions, rationales, and **charting examples**
- **Patient Education, HIPAA,** and **Critical Thinking** boxes
- **Case Studies** with critical thinking questions
- **Study for Success** checklist to provide a track for learning and reviewing the material
- **Summary** to assess and reinforce concepts learned in the chapter
- **Review Questions,** in multiple choice and critical thinking short answer formats
- **Web Activities** for exploration and research using the Internet
- **The DVD Hook-Up,** tying the chapter material to *Thomson Delmar Learning's Critical Thinking and Skills and Procedures DVD Series*
- **References/Bibliography** for further study

EXTENSIVE TEACHING/ LEARNING PACKAGE

The complete supplements package helps instructors efficiently manage time and resources and helps students to develop the necessary skills and competencies required by the demanding profession of medical assisting.

Student Workbook

The workbook helps you learn and reinforce the essential competencies needed to become a successful, multiskilled medical assistant. Medical Office Simulation Software is included with the workbook on CD-ROM. Each chapter includes:

- Pre-test and post-test
- Vocabulary builder exercises and word games
- Learning review in true/false, matching, and fill-in-the-blank style questions
- Certification review
- Case studies
- Competency Assessment checklists

Student Workbook, ISBN 1-4018-8136-X

Instructor's Resource Manual

The Instructor's Resource Manual is a dynamic teaching tool to help you plan the course and implement activities by chapter. It contains the following features:

- Instructor Tips and Strategies for teaching, lesson planning, and evaluation
- How to incorporate the book in your classroom
- Chapter Overviews, Lesson Plans, Activities
- Printed Test Bank and Answers
- Answers to Review Questions and Case Studies
- Answers to Workbook Questions
- Grids mapping the text content to ABHES and CAAHEP competencies and certification exams

    Instructor's Resource Manual, ISBN 1-4018-8137-8

WebTutor Advantage

Designed to complement the book, WebTutor is an online classroom management tool that takes your course beyond the classroom wall. WebTutor is a content-rich, Web-based teaching and learning aid that reinforces and helps clarify complex concepts; it is available on WebCT and Blackboard platforms. WebTutor provides rich communication and course management tools, including a Course Calendar, Chat, E-Mail, Threaded Discussions, Web Links, and a White Board. It also includes additional content, including:

- Learning Links explore health care topics through research on the Internet
- Critical Thinking Questions and Case Studies with DVD clips
- Discussion Questions and Quizzes for each chapter
- Unit Tests, Section Tests, and a comprehensive Final Exam
- PowerPoint presentation with DVD clips

WebTutor Advantage on WebCT, ISBN 1-4018-8129-7

WebTutor Advantage on Blackboard, ISBN 1-4018-8130-0

WebTutor Toolbox

With WebTutor Toolbox, you get the same rich communication tools and funcionality of this Web-based teaching and learning aid. Chapter components include objectives, advance preparation, and FAQs.

WebTutor Toolbox on WebCT, ISBN 1-4180-3104-6

WebTutor Toolbox on Blackboard, ISBN 1-4180-3103-8

HOW TO USE THIS BOOK

Thomson Delmar Learning's **Administrative Medical Assisting**, 3rd edition, contains many features that make it an easy-to-use learning system. They include:

Chapter Outline

At the beginning of each chapter, you will find an outline of all major headings. Review these headings of topic areas before you study the chapter. They are a road map to your understanding.

Key Terms

All key terms are listed at the beginning of each chapter. Within the text, the term is always bold-faced at its first occurrence for easy identification. Turn to the glossary for definitions of all key terms.

Spotlight on Certification

This feature maps the chapter material to the content outlines of the RMA, CMA, and CMAS certifying examinations to help you prepare to obtain medical assistant credentials.

Objectives

Performance objectives test your knowledge of the key facts presented in the chapter. Use these objectives, together with review questions, to test your understanding of the chapter's content.

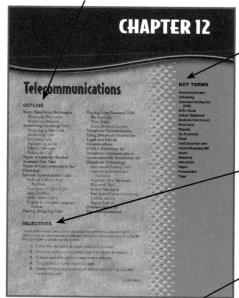

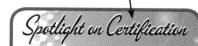

Spotlight on Certification

RMA Content Outline
- Patient relations
- Other personal relations
- Patient resource materials

CMA Content Outline
- Basic principles (Psychology)
- Hereditary, cultural, and environmental influences on behavior
- Adapting communication to individual's ability to understand
- Professional communication and behavior
- Patient advocate

CMAS Content Outline
- Professionalism

Featured Competencies

Entry-Level Competencies defined by ABHES and CAAHEP are listed at the beginning of each chapter to focus on the skills and functions that medical assistants will need to perform on the job.

FEATURED COMPETENCIES

CAAHEP—ENTRY-LEVEL COMPETENCIES

Legal Concepts
- Identify and respond to issues of confidentiality
- Demonstrate knowledge of federal and state health care legislation and regulations

Patient Instruction
- Instruct individuals according to their needs

ABHES—ENTRY-LEVEL COMPETENCIES

Professionalism
- Project a positive attitude
- Maintain confidentiality at all times
- Be courteous and diplomatic

Patient Education

This feature helps all current and future medical assistants anticipate patient concerns and provides sound suggestions for effective patient communication.

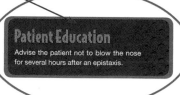

Patient Education
Advise the patient not to blow the nose for several hours after an epistaxis.

Real-Life Scenarios

The introduction in each chapter includes an overview of the material *and* a real-life scenario. Through these scenarios you will come to understand some of the stimulating challenges faced by medical assistants and gain insight into how these challenges are overcome.

Procedures

Step-by-step procedures are conveniently grouped together at the end of each chapter. They give step-by-step instruction on all important administrative, clinical, and general competencies as defined by AAMA and AMT.

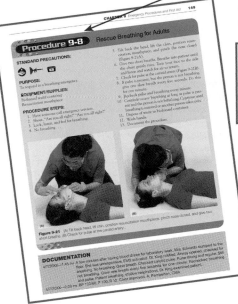

Critical Thinking

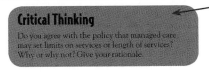

Topical questions sprinkled throughout the chapter are designed to stimulate critical thinking for discussion and emphasize skills necessary for medical assissting.

HIPAA

These boxes highlight important information relating to the Health Insurance Portability and Accounting Act of 1996 to help you comply with regulations and deal with privacy issues on the job.

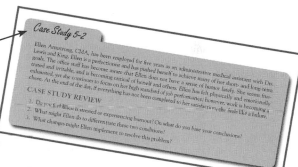

Case Studies

The case studies with accompanying review questions encourage a problem/solution approach. Use the case studies to put your knowledge into practice and arrive at a deeper understanding of the profession.

Study for Success

Before the activities at the end of each chapter, use this feature as a checklist to help focus and track your study of the material.

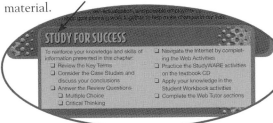

Review Questions

Test your comprehension of the chapter with structured multiple choice questions and open-ended critical thinking questions that require you to combine an understanding of chapter material with your personal insight and judgment.

The DVD Hook-Up

This tool provides synopses and scene references for *Thomson Delmar Learning's Critical Thinking and Skills and Procedures for Medical Assisting DVD Series* to show real-world application of the chapter material. Critical thinking questions can facilitate thought-provoking discussion and the DVD journal summary encourages you to share your ideas and grasp important issues that come up in the medical office.

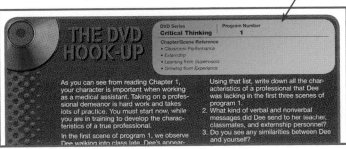

Web Activities

This feature at the end of each chapter gives you practice navigating the Internet and using it as a research tool by suggesting online activities.

xxi

HOW TO USE THE STUDENT SOFTWARE CD

The Critical Thinking Challenge

You are on a three-month externship in a medical office. You will be confronted with a series of situations in which you must use your critical thinking skills to choose the most appropriate action in response to the situation.

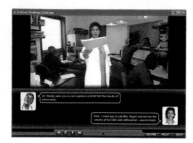

You may consult with members of the office staff and document resources to help you choose the best action, but not all of these resources will be available at all times or always offer helpful advice.

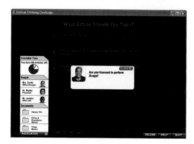

Your decisions will be evaluated in three categories: how your decisions affect the practice, the patient, and your career.

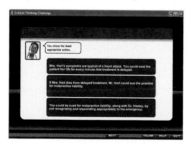

Your goal is to be hired by Dr. Healey's office as a full-time medical assistant. However, if you show a lack of critical thinking skills that threatens the well-being of the practice and the patients, Dr. Healey will terminate your externship and you will have to start over.

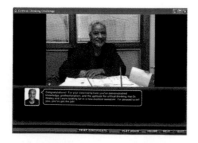

StudyWARE™

StudyWARE™ is interactive software with learning activities and quizzes to help you study key concepts and test your comprehension. The activity and quiz content corresponds with each unit in the book.

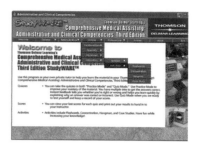

Each unit contains Multiple Choice, True/False, and Fill-in-the-Blank quizzes that can be taken in practice mode, which gives immediate feedback after each question, or in quiz mode, which allows your score for each quiz to be stored or printed.

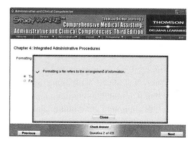

The activities within each unit include Flash Cards, Concentration, Hangman, Case Studies, and Championship Games.

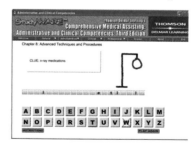

Medical Terminology Audio Library

Practice your pronunciation and recognition of medical terms using the Audio Library. You may search for terms by word or body system. Once you've selected a word, it is pronounced correctly and defined on the screen.

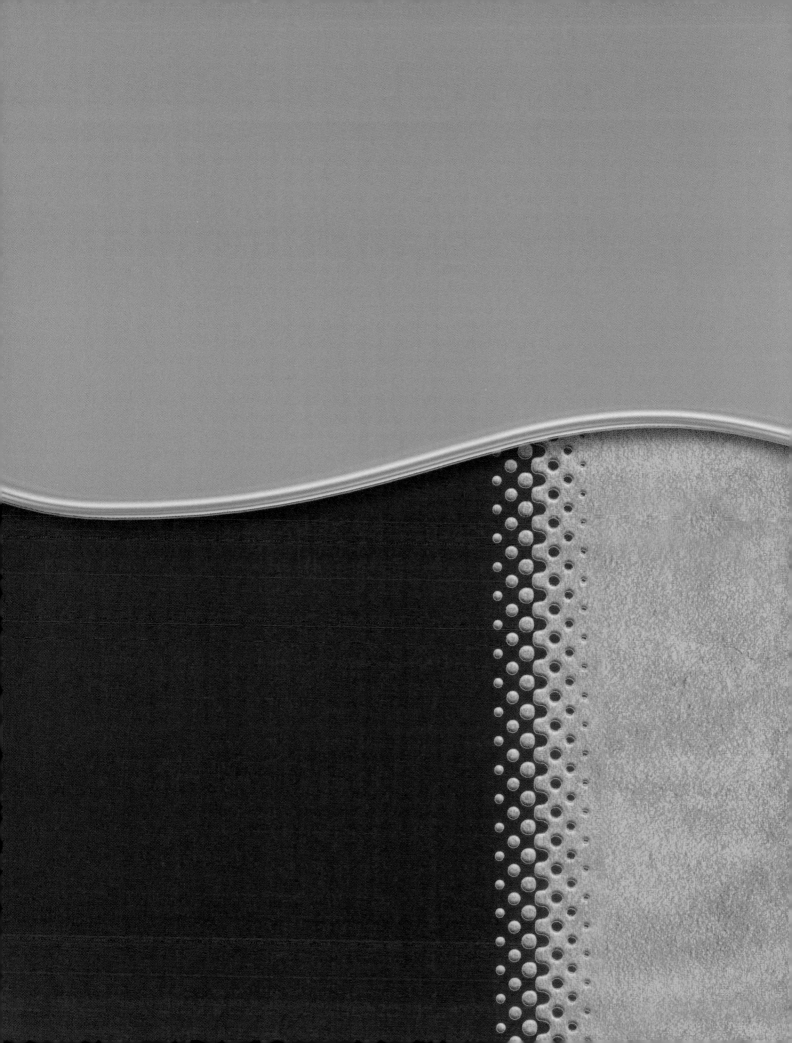

UNIT 1

Introduction to Medical Assisting and Health Professions

CHAPTER 1

Medical Assisting as a Profession

OUTLINE

OBJECTIVES

The student should strive to meet the following performance objectives and demonstrate an understanding of the facts and principles presented in this chapter through written and oral communication.

1. Define the key terms as presented in the glossary.
2. Identify and discuss nine personal attributes that are important for a professional medical assistant to possess.
3. Discuss the history of medical assisting.
4. Describe the American Association of Medical Assistants and list its three major functions.
5. Discuss the role of the American Medical Technologists Association in credentialing of Medical Assistants.

(continues)

KEY TERMS

Accreditation
Ambulatory Care Setting
Attribute
Bachelor's Degree
Certification
Certified Medical Assistant
  (CMA)
Competency
Compliance
Credentialed
Cultivate
Dexterity
Diploma
Disposition
Empathy
Externship
Facilitate
Improvise
Integrate
Internship
License
Licensure
Litigious
Practicum
Professionalism
Proprietary
Registered Medical
  Assistant (RMA)
Scope of Practice

FEATURED COMPETENCIES

CAAHEP—ENTRY-LEVEL COMPETENCIES

Professionalism

- Project a professional manner and image
- Demonstrate initiative and responsibility
- Work as a member of a health care team
- Prioritize and perform multiple tasks
- Adapt to change
- Promote the CMA credential
- Enhance skills through continuing education

Legal Concepts

- Perform within legal and ethical boundaries
- Recognize professional credentialing criteria

ABHES—ENTRY-LEVEL COMPETENCIES

Professionalism

- Project a positive attitude
- Maintain confidentiality at all times
- Be a "team player"
- Be cognizant of ethical boundaries
- Exhibit initiative
- Adapt to change
- Evidence a responsible attitude
- Conduct work within scope of education, training and ability

Communication

- Be attentive, listen and learn
- Professional components
- Allied health professions and credentialing

OBJECTIVES (continued)

6. Explain accreditation, certification, and continuing education as they pertain to the professional medical assistant.
7. Identify the importance of the accreditation process to an educational institution.
8. Recall two methods to obtain recertification.
9. List five means of obtaining continuing education units.
10. Describe the certifying agency that certifies medical assistants as registered medical assistants.
11. Describe the externship experience.
12. Recall two criteria for the selection of externship sites.
13. List three benefits of externship to student and site.
14. Describe the profession of medical assisting and analyze its career opportunities in relationship to your interests.
15. Differentiate among certification, licensure, and registration.
16. State the importance of understanding the scope of practice for the medical assistant.

SCENARIO

A group of high school freshmen have come to tour the medical assisting class and laboratory areas. The Program Director of Medical Assisting is showing the students around the department. The Program Director then takes them into the medical assisting laboratory where the senior medical assistant students are there practicing their clinical skills. Each senior student pairs up with a high school freshman, and each pair talks about medical assisting, with the medical assistant students answering questions the others may have. The medical assistant students are in uniform as part of their preparation to go into various health care agencies to do their externship or practicum. The medical assistant students look professional, clean, fresh, and motivated. They tell the high school students about medical assisting and describe the personal and physical attributes desirable for those who want to become medical assistants. They explain the importance of these attributes, as well as what duties a professional medical assistant performs and what education is needed to pursue a career in medical assisting.

Throughout the question and answer discussions, the senior medical assistant students and the program director stress the importance of ethics, empathy, attitude, dependability, and teamwork as favorable attributes. Individuals seeking a career in medical assisting should develop and maintain these attributes.

INTRODUCTION

Historically, medical science has been fascinating to most people. Perhaps you have been drawn to medical assisting because you too are intrigued by medicine and want to learn about advances in health care and become involved in providing care to patients. More than likely you have a desire to help others.

Medical assistants have always played an integral role in physicians' offices and **ambulatory care settings** *such as clinics and urgent care facilities, where health care services are offered on an outpatient basis. And now more than ever, because of the explosion of knowledge and high technology in medicine, medical assistants are involved in an ever-widening scope of clinical and administrative duties. With the medical assistant's expanded role has come the responsibility to become a well-educated and highly competent professional dedicated to providing the highest quality of health care.*

Consumers of health care have become increasingly aware, primarily through the media, of the availability of the latest advances, techniques, and discoveries in medicine. They realize that they have a right to have health care provided to them by educated, skilled, and competent professionals.

As you study to become a medical assistant, it is important for you to understand what a professional is. According to Merriam-Webster's Collegiate Dictionary, 10th edition, it is "one who has acquired a specialized body of knowledge, skills, and attitudes." You will practice **professionalism** *as you learn the technical and ethical standards of this profession.*

You will learn to **integrate,** *or unify, your desire and need to help others with the knowledge, skills, and attitudes you acquire through your studies. By blending all of these, you will be able to provide patients with the best health care possible and will learn what it means to be a professional medical assistant.*

PERSONAL ATTRIBUTES OF THE PROFESSIONAL

There are certain characteristics or personal qualities that medical assistants should strive to cultivate. These are the **attributes** that identify a true professional; when caring for patients, these qualities should come from the heart. They will enable the patient to trust you, the caregiver.

Empathy

To have **empathy** means to consider the patient's welfare and to be kind. It means stepping into the patient's place, discovering what the patient is experiencing, and then recognizing and identifying with those feelings.

Medical assistants should treat patients as they themselves would want to be treated. A visit to the doctor's office is often a time of fear and anxiety. Apprehension can be allayed tremendously when patients realize that their caregiver understands their feelings and desires to make their lives more pleasant and comfortable. See Figure 1-1.

It is important to realize that patients' health problems can have a profound effect on you, the medical assistant. By maintaining a balanced outlook, medical assistants can safeguard themselves from becoming too emotionally involved with patients' problems. Empathy is extremely important in the health care profession; however, emotionalism can cloud one's judgment.

Attitude

A friendly, warm **disposition** and a sense of humor will help patients feel more at ease. A sincere affection for people can be conveyed by actions that **facilitate** open and honest communication. Your attitude should radiate genuine interest.

On occasion, difficult patients can test the tolerance level of the most experienced medical assistant because they seldom seem to be content with the care or services received. But no matter what the circumstances, patients should never be treated with disinterest or in an unfriendly manner. The medical assistant should always be pleasant and courteous.

 When giving care to patients, do so unrestricted by your concerns about their attitudes, disease, race, religion, economic status, or sexual orientation.

As a member of the health care delivery team, the medical assistant needs to be cooperative and supportive

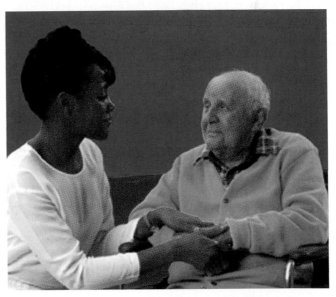

Figure 1-1 The medical assistant should have a friendly disposition and communicate empathy for the patient.

of all other members, working with the team in an honest, open manner while keeping in mind the patient's right to privacy and confidentiality.

Dependability

When providing for a patient's well-being, it is important to focus attention on activities in the office or clinic environment that will demonstrate that you are well-organized, accurate, and responsive to patients' needs.

Being dependable means that employer and coworkers rely on the medical assistant to be respectful of them, of patients, and of equipment and materials. Other members of the health care team will expect you to be accountable for the duties and responsibilities you undertake. A dependable person interacts with coworkers in a supportive manner, is punctual, and limits absences from work.

Initiative

The willingness and ability to work independently shows initiative. A person with initiative is observant, notices work that needs to be done, and then takes action to complete those tasks without being told to do them. Employer and coworkers must be able to count on one another to anticipate patients' needs and be attentive to work that needs to be accomplished. The successful medical assistant will be ready to pitch in and recognize when others need assistance.

By asking appropriate questions and seeking information that will improve performance, medical assistants will demonstrate that they have the foresight and the "get up and go" needed to complete the numerous and varied tasks of the ambulatory care environment.

Flexibility

The ability to be adaptable is a trait that serves all professionals well. When caring for ill people, unexpected situations arise daily, and medical assistants must be able to respond to a variety of situations (many of them emergencies and unanticipated) without losing a sense of equilibrium. Finding solutions to problems and developing alternative action plans demonstrates flexibility. To **improvise,** or solve problems that arise either routinely or spontaneously, is a characteristic worth nurturing.

Desire to Learn

A willingness to continually learn and grow is the mark of a true professional. With the growing technology in medicine, there is an ongoing necessity for constant learning.

Medical assistants must be dedicated to high standards of performance, which can be accomplished by showing a desire to acquire information and by constantly updating their knowledge and skills. Keeping abreast of the latest diseases, treatments, procedures, and techniques can be achieved in a variety of ways, such as college courses, seminars, workshops, reading, and simply by being observant. The sharper the power of observation, the more the medical assistant will learn from physician, employer, and coworkers.

Physical Attributes

Appearance is important in patients' perceptions of the delivery of their care. Imparting the look of a professional requires an appearance that is clean and fresh and wholesome; in general, an appearance that reflects good health habits (Figure 1-2). Good personal hygiene practices (daily shower, deodorant), weight control, and healthy-looking skin, hair, teeth, and nails all contribute to a professional appearance. Rest, good nutrition, regular exercise, and recreation all promote good health.

Female medical assistants should wear only appropriate light daytime makeup. For the safety of both the professional and the patient, no necklaces or dangling earrings should be worn. The only jewelry worn should be single earposts or wedding rings. Hair should be neat and off the collar. Fingernails should be short and manicured. Male medical assistants should be clean-shaven and have short hair. The only jewelry worn should be a wedding ring. Colognes, perfumes, and aftershave should

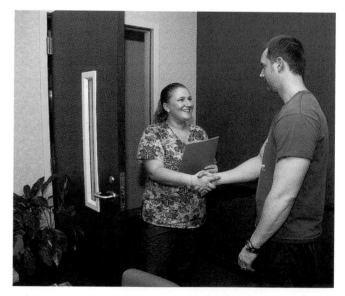

Figure 1-2 A professional, neat appearance makes patients feel at ease with their health care provider.

not be worn at work. Body piercings and tattoos should not be visible.

Patient care can place physical demands on medical assistants. Lifting and moving patients is often required, and the use of correct body mechanics will help minimize injuries to the back. Although every reasonable accommodation is made for physically challenged medical assistants, to be mobile without assistance is important because medical assistants move about throughout the day while performing tasks and procedures. It is frequently necessary to bend, stoop, kneel, and crouch, especially when filing and retrieving patients' records, and for other tasks as well. Most procedures require that medical assistants have the ability to hear and see well for the accurate completion of tasks (Figure 1-3). Listening to blood pressures, taking a medical history, observing patients, performing phlebotomy, and identifying microorganisms under a microscope are some of the routine tasks and procedures performed daily in a medical facility.

Manual **dexterity** is also needed for manipulating certain instruments and for entering data using a computer.

Ability to Communicate

It is important that medical assistants learn to develop the ability to communicate well verbally and nonverbally with patients, staff, and other professionals.

Compliance with the physician's treatment plan is important for a positive outcome of patients' illnesses (Figure 1-4). Also, patients will feel more comfortable

and less threatened in a medical office or ambulatory center that encourages staff to keep them informed.

Ethical Behavior

No discussion about personal attributes is complete without the mention of ethics. Ethics is a system of values each individual has that determines perceptions of right and wrong. Our life experiences mold this set of values, which is considered a personal code of ethics.

Medical ethics govern medical conduct or that behavior practiced as health care providers. These ethics involve relationships with patients, their families, fellow professionals, and society in general. Good ethical behavior will have a positive impact on the profession of medical assisting and on the medical community as well. By adhering to the medical assistants' Code of Ethics, we endeavor to elevate the profession to a position of dignity and respect. (A more in-depth discussion of this Code of Ethics can be found in Chapter 8.)

The personal qualities of empathy, healthy attitude, dependability, initiative, flexibility, the desire to learn, a wholesome physical presence, the ability to communicate well, and ethical behavior are some of the characteristics that most professionals have and that medical assistants

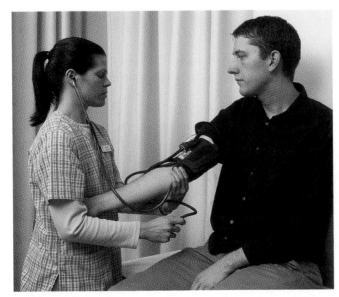

Figure 1-3 Measuring blood pressure is a task that requires the medical assistant to see and hear well.

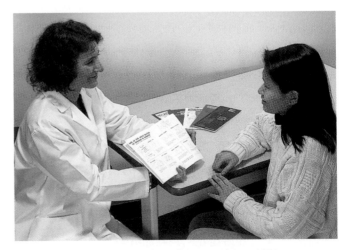

Figure 1-4 Patient education requires skill in communicating instructions to patients in language appropriate to their needs.

should strive to develop. When entering into the profession of medical assisting, it is important to learn more about these and other qualities and to begin to **cultivate** and refine them.

HISTORICAL PERSPECTIVE OF MEDICAL ASSISTING

Historically, when physicians began their practices, it was common for them to hire individuals and train them on the job. Physicians originally hired nurses, but eventually they came to realize that nurses alone could not perform the variety of duties that are required in medical offices and ambulatory care centers. The nurse's role was limited to assisting the physician with clinical procedures, whereas the medical assistant's role was and is much broader and includes a large number of activities, procedures, and responsibilities, both administrative and clinical.

Today, with a much more informed patient comes the need for educated and credentialed medical assistants. In addition, in today's **litigious** atmosphere, which makes health care providers vulnerable to malpractice suits, most employers recognize the importance of employing medical assistants who are professionally prepared through formal education. Physicians want knowledgeable and dependable medical assistants so they can focus their time and attention on the medical decisions, treatments, and techniques for which they have been educated and licensed. This leaves the medical assistant to assist the physician in the operation and management of the practice.

It was in 1978 that the profession of medical assisting was formally recognized by the United States Department of Education. Twenty-four years before this official recognition of the profession, a group of medical assistants gathered to establish a professional organization. With support, encouragement, and guidance from the

American Medical Association (AMA), the American Association of Medical Assistants (AAMA) was founded in 1956 (Figure 1-5). The first president of the organization was Maxine Williams.

In 1991, the AAMA's board of trustees approved the current definition of medical assisting:

> Medical Assisting is an allied health profession whose practitioners function as members of the health care delivery team and perform administrative and clinical procedures.

AMERICAN ASSOCIATION OF MEDICAL ASSISTANTS

The AAMA has three major purposes:

1. Accreditation
2. Certification
3. Continuing education

Accreditation and certification standards were developed by the AMA and the AAMA through the Commission on Accreditation of Allied Health Education Programs (CAAHEP) for schools wishing assurance that their medical assistant programs are of the highest quality and satisfy CAAHEP criteria.

Accreditation

The AAMA works jointly with the AMA to define the essential components and appropriate standards of quality that educational institutions offer in their medical assistant curriculum. The United States Department of Education has approved the AAMA/AMA as an **accreditation,** or approving, body for educational programs for medical assistants. A medical assisting program that is accredited meets the standards as outlined in the *Standards and Guidelines for an Accredited Education Program for the Medical Assistant. Standards* are the minimum standards of quality used in accrediting programs that prepare individuals to enter the medical assisting profession. On-site review teams evaluate the program's **compliance** with, or adherence to, the standards. All aspects of programs seeking accreditation status undergo scrutiny to ascertain the program's quality and to ensure continued compliance with the standards.

Certification

As the profession grew and developed, some states came to require special licensure or certification to perform certain tasks; in other states, health professionals were

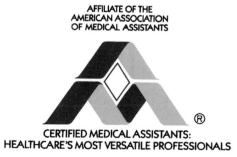

AFFILIATE OF THE
AMERICAN ASSOCIATION
OF MEDICAL ASSISTANTS

CERTIFIED MEDICAL ASSISTANTS:
HEALTHCARE'S MOST VERSATILE PROFESSIONALS

Figure 1-5 Logo of the American Association of Medical Assistants, a professional organization founded in 1956. (Courtesy of the American Association of Medical Assistants.)

challenged by the skill and broad spectrum of the medical assistant's ability. To defend medical assistants whose right to practice clinical procedures was being challenged, the AAMA responded at their 1995 convention with the following policy, which became effective February 1, 1998:

> that any candidate for the AAMA Certification Examination be a graduate of a CAAHEP-accredited medical assisting program. This requirement would become effective February 1, 1998. Anticipated benefits of the recommendation are to: (1) safeguard the quality of care to the consumer; (2) ensure the CMA's role in the rapidly evolving health care delivery system; and (3) continue to promote the identity and stature of the profession.

Certification is voluntary, not mandatory, for medical assistants to practice, although the AAMA strongly urges those who are eligible to take the national certification examination. The examination measures professional **competency** at job entry level. Successful completion of the examination earns the individual the status of being certified and of being known as a **certified medical assistant (CMA).** The initials follow the individual's name. Conferring of the CMA status is referred to as being **credentialed** (Figure 1-6). It signifies recognition of competency by having attained a certain level of knowledge and skill.

The examination is offered twice yearly simultaneously at more than 200 test sites across the United States. In October 2004, a third examination was added on a trial basis. If, as anticipated, there is a demonstrated need for the third examination, the AAMA will consider making it permanent.

Recertification of the credential must be undertaken within five years from the date of certification to maintain current status as a CMA. Two routes are available to recertify. One is by accumulating approved continuing education units, and the other is by taking the certification examination again.

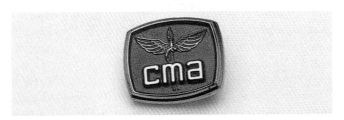

Figure 1-6 Certified medical assistant (CMA) pin awarded by the American Association of Medical Assistants on successful completion of the national certification examination.

The status of a medical assistant's credentials (whether current or not current) is a public record available at the AAMA executive office, 20 N. Wacker Dr., Suite 1575, Chicago, IL 60606-2963; 1-800-228-2262, www.AAMA-WTL.org. The AAMA Board of Trustees approved a policy change at the association's 1999 annual convention in Nashville. Effective January 1, 2003, all certified medical assistants who are employed or seeking employment *must* have current status as a CMA to use the credential. The mandatory current status for use of the CMA designation protects patients, employers, and the medical assistant's right to practice. Certification and recertification attest to the medical assistant's desire for professional development.

At one time, the credentials CMA-A (Certified Medical Assistant, Administrative), CMA-C (Certified Medical Assistant, Clinical), CMA-AC (Certified Medical Assistant, Administrative and Clinical), and CMA-Ped (Certified Medical Assistant, Pediatrics) were awarded to candidates who successfully passed specialty examinations in addition to the basic CMA examination.

Although these specialty examinations have been phased out for newly graduated medical assistants, current medical assistants who have already earned these specialty credentials can maintain them and continue to be recertified through the Continuing Education Hours method. Currently, there are approximately 95,000 CMAs in the United States.

Continuing Education

The AAMA vigorously encourages continuing education for all medical assistants. This can be accomplished through various means such as educational meetings, seminars, workshops, conventions, and the "Quest for Excellence," AAMA's series of home study courses for continuing education credit.

Membership in the AAMA is tri-level: local, state, and national. Educational meetings are held regularly at local and state meetings and conventions. The annual AAMA national convention provides an excellent forum for attaining knowledge through its educational offerings and for networking with other medical assistants.

Continuing an education is a lifelong process and serves as testimony to a commitment to professionalism.

AMERICAN MEDICAL TECHNOLOGIST

Founded in 1939, the American Medical Technologist (AMT) is a national certification and professional membership association that represents 27,000 allied health care individuals. Its purpose is to certify and credential medical assistants, clinical laboratory personnel, allied health instructors, dental assistants, medical administrative specialists, and others. In 1972, the AMT established the certification examination for medical assistants. The designation of **registered medical assistant (RMA)** is conferred on those individuals who successfully pass the examination (Figures 1-7A and B).

The Accrediting Bureau of Health Education Schools (ABHES) accredits private postsecondary institutions and programs that prepare individuals for entry into the profession of medical assisting. In 1991, ABHES spun off from the AMT and became a separate entity.

Certification

The AMT has its own committees, conventions, bylaws, state chapters, officers, registrations, and certification examinations.

RMA is a voluntary credential for the profession of medical assisting. RMA credentials are national, and examinations are given throughout the United States in both computerized and paper and pencil format. The exam consists of 200–210 multiple choice questions, covering general, administrative, and clinical areas. Voluntary means that neither the federal government nor most states require a medical assistant to be either certified or registered to practice the profession. Most employers, however, prefer to employ credentialed medical assistants. Most physicians desire hiring employees with the credentials because they recognize that doing so safeguards the quality of patient care and reduces the risk for liability issues for themselves.

RMAs have been active in legislation to protect medical assistants, assuring improvement in medical assistant education and providing for continuing education opportunities.

Another profession that the AMT certifies is the Medical Administrative Specialist (MAS). Individuals who successfully pass the AMT certification examination are conferred with the credential of Certified Medical Administrative Specialist (CMAS). The CMAS exam is given in both computerized and paper and pencil format. The exam consists of 200–210 multiple choice questions.

An MAS serves an important role in the hospital, clinic, or medical office. The MAS is competent in a multitude of skills such as medical records management, coding and billing for insurance, practice finance management, information processing, and fundamental management practices. The MAS also is familiar with the clinical and administrative concepts that are required to coordinate office functions in the health care setting.

Graduating from a program accredited by either CAAHEP or ABHES has significant benefits, such as proof that the student has completed a program that meets national standards, recognition of their education by their professional peers, and eligibility for AMT credentialing exams.

Some medical assistants may choose to attain both RMA and CMAS credentials.

It is important to remember that credentialing, whether through the AAMA (CMA) or AMT (RMA), is evidence to employers and patients alike that you want the profession of medical assisting to be recognized and promoted. Also, credentials safeguard patients, because you will deliver health care at the highest quality with the most current techniques and procedures. Credentials help secure the medical assistant's role in the health care field.

For more information, call 1-800-275-1268 or write to AMT, 710 Higgins Rd., Park Ridge, IL 60068, or access their Web site, at: www.amt1.com.

EDUCATION OF THE PROFESSIONAL MEDICAL ASSISTANT

Formal education of medical assistants takes place in community and junior colleges, as well as in **proprietary** schools. The AAMA has established educational requirements for program directors to follow for their programs to be considered accredited. These requirements were previously known as the Developing A CUrriculuM (DACUM) Analysis. In 1997, in coordination with the National Board of Medical Examiners, educators, and practicing CMAs, the AAMA developed

Figure 1-7 (A) Logo of the American Medical Technologists. (B) Logo of Registered Medical Assistant. (Courtesy of American Medical Technologists.)

the Medical Assistant Role Delineation Chart, which is the occupational analysis of the medical assisting profession, (see Appendix B to review this chart). In addition, the entry-level competencies that must be mastered by students in academic programs and the *Standards* (formerly "Essentials") *and Guidelines for an Accredited Education Program for the Medical Assistant* are revised to reflect the findings of the Role Delineation Study. On graduation, the student will receive a **diploma** or certificate of completion.

Educational institutions seeking accreditation for a medical assisting program must develop the curricula to these *Standards and Guidelines* to ensure the highest quality medical assistant education and employment preparedness.

Although not a complete list, some of the administrative, general (transdisciplinary), and clinical courses include those shown in Table 1-1.

Another aspect of an educational medical assisting program is the **externship,** a period when students participate in a **practicum.** This provides an excellent opportunity to apply theory to practice.

Preparation for Externship

Externship, practicum, and **internship** are all terms used to define the transition period between the classroom and actual employment. An externship is planned and supervised by a coordinator from the medical assisting program and the health care facility that agrees to become a partner in the education and employability of the student.

Externship Sites. Sites for externship are chosen carefully to ensure that a variety of experiences is available for the student. The sites should provide the student with adequate administrative, clinical, and general experiences. The staff at the various sites must be willing to make a commitment to the medical assistant's education by spending appropriate time observing and instructing the student.

Benefits of Externship. The externship experience is mutually beneficial to the student and staff at the health care facility that is providing the educational experiences.

Some of the benefits to the student are the opportunity to:

- Apply classroom knowledge and skill in a real-world medical setting

TABLE 1-1	TYPICAL ADMINISTRATIVE, GENERAL, AND CLINICAL COURSES IN AN ACCREDITED MEDICAL ASSISTING PROGRAM

Administrative Courses

Computer Applications
Manual Recording of Patients' Data
Scheduling Appointments
Maintaining Medical Records
Word Processing/Keyboarding
Billing/Collections/Managing Patients' Accounts
Coding/Insurance Claims
Telephone Triage
Personnel Management

General Courses

Anatomy and Physiology
Medical Terminology
Human Diseases
Patient Education
Medical Law and Ethics

Clinical Courses

Infection Control
Pharmacology/Administration of Medications
Assisting Techniques/Physical Examination
Assisting with Minor Surgery
Basic Laboratory Procedures/Routine Blood and Urine Testing
Cardiopulmonary Resuscitation and First Aid

- Recognize improvement in performance and knowledge

- Understand that there may be more than one acceptable method of performance

- Begin to establish a network of support through colleagues

Some of the benefits to the externship site are:

- Greater alertness of staff because of their educational responsibilities to the student

- Opportunity for staff to observe students who will soon be seeking employment

- Possibility that staff will learn more about the profession of medical assisting

Critical Thinking

Patients and physicians desire professional medical assistants who have had the benefit of a formal education to work for them. Discuss the impact of this education on patients and employers. Why is it important to both groups?

Educational Institutions

Educational institutions that confer associate or bachelor degrees require general education courses for graduation in addition to the administration and clinical courses.

There are four-year institutions of higher learning that offer a **bachelor's degree** to medical assistants who have graduated with an associate's degree from a community or junior college. The graduate is accepted as a third-year student and can obtain a bachelor's degree in such areas as health care management or health care facility administrator.

Because there is a demand for medical assistant educators, some experienced medical assistants take education courses to become allied health educators.

CAREER OPPORTUNITIES

Medical assistants have been described as health care's most versatile, multifaceted professionals. That medical assistants possess a broad scope of knowledge and skills makes them ideal professionals for any ambulatory care setting. Indeed, because of such versatility, medical assistants find employment in a variety of settings: offices, clinics, hospitals, medical laboratories, insurance companies, government agencies, pharmaceutical companies, and educational institutions. Although the range of employment opportunities continues to grow, in the past decade, about four of five medical assistants were employed in physicians' offices and clinics. About one in five worked in offices of other health care practitioners, such as chiropractors, optometrists, and podiatrists. There are other career opportunities available to the medical assistant. Some medical assistants work as phlebotomists, coding specialists, medical laboratory assistants, and CMASs. The outlook for employment for medical assistants is promising. According to the AAMA, there are currently 1.3 million medical assistants in the work force. The United States Department of Labor Bureau of Statistics listed medical assisting as one of the fastest growing allied health professions for the years 1998–2012.

Increased employment opportunities for medical assistants result from the increased medical needs of an aging population, growth in the number of health care practitioners and their desire to hire the most qualified person for the task, increased diagnostic testing, greater volume and complexity of paperwork and computer information, managed care's emphasis on ambulatory care, and the insurance-mandated shorter stay of patients in hospitals.

REGULATION OF HEALTH CARE PROVIDERS

One way health care providers can be regulated is through the process of credentialing. Credentialing recognizes health care providers who are professionally and technically competent. Recognition comes from professional associations, certifying agencies, and the state or federal government. Regulation ensures:

- Competence of health care providers
- A minimum standard of knowledge, training, and skill
- The limiting of the performance of certain procedures to a specific occupation

Licensure, certification, and registration are three kinds of regulations/credentialing. See Table 1-2.

Scope of Practice

Medical assisting is not licensed as a profession; however, some states require that medical assistants be graduates of an accredited medical assisting program to work as medical assistants.

Two examples of licensed professions are medicine and nursing. A **license** regulates the activities of these

TABLE 1-2 COMPARISON OF REQUIREMENTS FOR CERTIFICATION, LICENSURE, AND REGISTRATION

	Certification	Licensure	Registration
Practice Requirement	Voluntary	Mandatory	Voluntary
Conferred by	Nongovernmental agency or professional association	Legislated by each state	Professional association
	If qualified and meets requirements	If qualified and meets requirements	Listed on an official roster
	Must pass national examination	Must pass state examination	Passing examination not always required
How restrictive	Used by most professional associations	Most restrictive	Least restrictive

professions by enacting laws that specify educational requirements and by defining the **scope of practice.** A license is conferred on an individual who successfully completes specialized educational requirements and successfully passes an examination administered by the state in which the individual resides. The state grants a license to that individual to practice medicine or nursing. Licensure forbids anyone who is not licensed from performing activities that are designated by that particular license. For example, the law states that the physician's license allows diagnosing and prescribing treatment. If someone were to diagnose or prescribe without a license, that individual would be committing an illegal act and would be practicing medicine without a license, which is considered a felony.

There are state laws that govern the practice of medicine and nursing (medical practice acts, nursing practice acts), and many states have acts that give physicians the right to delegate certain clinical procedures to qualified allied health professionals. Because medical assistants are not required to be licensed, they are allowed to perform clinical procedures only under the supervision of the physician or other licensed health care professional who is granted the right and who delegates the specific clinical procedures to them.

In some states, including California, Washington, and others, unlicensed health care providers are required to have authorization from the state to perform allergy testing and venipuncture and to give injections. A regis-

tration fee and mandatory training are required. In such circumstances, medical assistants or other health care providers would be breaking the law if they performed these procedures without registration and training.

In some states, authorization is required for unlicensed health care providers to expose patients to X-rays.

Medical assistants do not perform procedures for which they have not been educated and trained. The AAMA's Role Delineation Chart (see Appendix B) is an excellent reference source that identifies which clinical, administrative, and general (transdisciplinary) procedures medical assistants are educated to perform. However, because of the variability of state statutes, the medical assistant would be wise to check with the AAMA or AMT if in doubt about the legality of certain clinical procedures.

Critical Thinking

A medical assistant relates to a patient on the telephone that her symptoms are "probably the flu" and to "take over-the-counter cough syrup" for her cough. Is this an appropriate or inappropriate action for the medical assistant to take? Discuss your answer and explain why you came to your decision.

SUMMARY

Progress has been made in the advancement of the profession of medical assisting since the first group of medical assistants gathered to become organized and formed the AAMA. For example, the number of certified medical assistants has exceeded 95,000 and continues to grow since certification began in 1963. The total number of medical assistants in the work force is approximately 1.3 million, and employment opportunities continue to grow. Educational requirements have become increasingly important. The AAMA and the AMT continue to promote standards of excellence for its members, encouraging continuing education and awarding continuing education credits to members of AAMA and AMT via various means.

All of these factors are evidence of a strong professional perspective and should offer encouragement and support to any student or graduate of medical assisting.

Becoming a professional is a gradual process and cannot be learned in its entirety from a textbook. The challenge of becoming a professional medical assistant will require open-mindedness and a desire for continued learning and education, certification and recertification of the CMA or RMA credential, and professional involvement through organizational participation.

As the scope of work done by medical assistants broadens and medical assistants seek and require formal education, the professional medical assistant will gain additional respect and be in even greater demand. Medical assistants must continuously pursue excellence, which is the hallmark of all professional behavior.

STUDY FOR SUCCESS

To reinforce your knowledge and skills of information presented in this chapter:

❏ Review the Key Terms
❏ Answer the Review Questions
  ❏ Multiple Choice
  ❏ Critical Thinking
❏ Navigate the Internet and complete the Web Activities

❏ Practice the StudyWARE activities on the textbook CD
❏ Apply your knowledge in the Student Workbook activities
❏ Complete the Web Tutor sections
❏ View and discuss the DVD situations

Multiple Choice

1. Medical assisting has been recognized by the United States Department of Education as a profession since what year?
   a. 1956
   b. 1964
   c. 1978
   d. 1995
2. The AAMA was established as a professional organization in what year?
   a. 1945
   b. 1956
   c. 1962
   d. 1967
3. The "Quest for Excellence" is:
   a. a professional publication for medical assistants
   b. a code of professional behavior for medical assistants
   c. otherwise known as ethical behavior
   d. the AAMA's series of home study courses
4. The designation RMA is awarded by the:
   a. AAMA
   b. ABHES
   c. AMA
   d. AMT
5. Increased employment opportunities for medical assistants result from:
   a. decreases in diagnostic testing
   b. computers decreasing volume of paperwork
   c. managed care's emphasis on ambulatory care
   d. longer hospital stays for patients
6. Ethics is:
   a. a system of values each individual has that determine perceptions of right and wrong
   b. a code established by an agency that has nothing to do with the medical assistant's belief in right or wrong
   c. making patients more comfortable
   d. willingness to work as a team member
7. Accreditation means:
   a. meeting appropriate standards
   b. obtaining the CMA or RMA credential
   c. being listed on an official roster
   d. having a curriculum with courses that are unrestricted
8. Licensure is:
   a. voluntary and up to the individual practitioner
   b. unrestrictive in scope
   c. conferred on an individual through a nongovernment agency
   d. legislated by each state

9. Manual dexterity refers to the ability to:
   a. lift and move patients
   b. bend, stoop, and crouch
   c. see and hear well
   d. manipulate instruments

Critical Thinking

1. For each personal attribute used in this textbook to describe a professional, identify individuals from your family, friends, church, or community who possess one or more of these traits. Give examples.
2. Discuss the importance of certification and recertification.
3. Differentiate among certification, licensure, and registration.
4. Explain what is meant by the scope of practice for the medical assistant. Are there legal implications that could occur? Give an example of what might become a legal issue with regard to the medical assistant and scope of practice of the profession.
5. Describe the profession of medical assisting and look carefully at its career opportunities. How do these opportunities relate to your interests in the profession?
6. Examine several physical attributes that are important for a medical assistant to have and explain why each is important.
7. Explain the importance of continuing education for all health care providers, but particularly for the medical assistant.

1. Visit the American Medical Technologist (AMT) Web site at www. amt1.com
   • What allied health professions other than medical assistants and medical laboratory technicians are credentialed by AMT?
   • Does AMT have a code of ethics for the medical assistant?
   • What are the eligibility requirements for individuals to take the RMA examination? The CMA's examination?
2. Visit the American Association of Medical Assistants Web site at http://www.aama-ntl.org
   • What allied health profession(s) does the AAMA sponsor?
   • What resources are available on the Web for medical assistants interested in continuing education?

THE DVD HOOK-UP

DVD Series	Program Number
Critical Thinking	1

Chapter/Scene Reference
• *Classroom Performance*
• *Externship*
• *Learning from Supervisors*
• *Growing from Experience*

As you can see from reading Chapter 1, your character is important when working as a medical assistant. Taking on a professional demeanor is hard work and takes lots of practice. You must start now, while you are in training to develop the characteristics of a true professional.

In the first scene of program 1, we observe Dee walking into class late. Dee's appearance is in total disarray and her attitude is poor. Even though Dee promised her teacher that she would work on her professional characteristics, Dee enters her externship with the same attitude that she possessed in school. After Dee speaks with her externship supervisor, she starts to realize that her teacher is right, and that she does need to develop her professional skills if she is going to succeed as a medical assistant.

1. This chapter lists characteristics that are important to possess as a professional. Using that list, write down all the characteristics of a professional that Dee was lacking in the first three scenes of program 1.
2. What kind of verbal and nonverbal messages did Dee send to her teacher, classmates, and externship personnel?
3. Do you see any similarities between Dee and yourself?

DVD Journal Summary

After watching the designated scenes from program 1, write a paragraph in your journal that summarizes what you learned from watching these scenes. What kind of verbal and nonverbal messages do you typically send to your classmates? What will you do to improve other people's impressions of your professional characteristics?

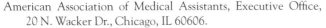

REFERENCES/BIBLIOGRAPHY

American Association of Medical Assistants, Executive Office, 20 N. Wacker Dr., Chicago, IL 60606.

American Medical Technologists, Allied Health Professions, · 710 Higgins Rd., Park Ridge, IL 60068.

Balasa, D. (2000). Securing the future for medical assistants to practice. *Professional medical assistant*, January/February 2000, 6–7.

Merriam-Webster (2002). *Merriam-Webster's collegiate dictionary* (11th ed.). Springfield, MA: Author.

CHAPTER 2

Health Care Settings and the Health Care Team

KEY TERMS

Acupuncture
Ambulatory Care Setting
Fringe Benefits
Health Maintenance
  Organization (HMO)
Homeopathy
Independent Physician
  Association (IPA)
Integrative Medicine
Managed Care Operation
Preferred Provider
  Organization (PPO)
Triage

OBJECTIVES

The student should strive to meet the following performance objectives and demonstrate an understanding of the facts and principles presented in this chapter through written and oral communication.

1. Define the key terms as presented in the glossary.
2. Analyze the benefits and limitations of working in the different health care settings.
3. Assess the role and impact of managed care in the health care environment.
4. Identify and describe the three primary medical management models.
5. Describe the function of the health care team.

(continues)

FEATURED COMPETENCIES

CAAHEP—ENTRY-LEVEL COMPETENCIES

Legal Concepts

- Perform within legal and ethical boundaries
- Demonstrate knowledge of federal and state health care legislation and regulations

ABHES—ENTRY-LEVEL COMPETENCIES

- Be a "team player"
- Be impartial and show empathy when dealing with patients
- Serve as liaison between physician and others
- Allied health professions and credentialing

OBJECTIVES (continued)

6. Discuss the role of the medical assistant in the health care team.
7. List and describe a minimum of 12 physician specialists.
8. List and describe a minimum of three alternative health care specialists.
9. List and describe a minimum of 12 allied health professionals.
10. Compare and contrast the types of nurses.
11. Critique alternative therapies and discuss their role in today's health care setting.

SCENARIO

You always had thought you wanted to be a medical assistant and work in a clinic where you would see a variety of patients. But after discussing this chapter in class, you are really intrigued with becoming an emegency medical technician. What kind of research can you do to make certain you have chosen the right path? Consider working hours, rate of pay, patient contact, required schooling, and job availability.

INTRODUCTION

There are few professions in our society as rich and complex as the health care profession. Particularly in recent years, the health care environment has been very much in flux as the profession seeks ways to provide quality care while containing costs. This effort to curtail costs has resulted in the rise of managed care, which, in turn, has spawned a number of medical models such as health maintenance organizations (HMOs) and preferred provider organizations (PPOs), two well-known managed care entities.

Many other types of physician networks and alliances are also being established as providers merge to give patients the best of care whereas controlling their costs. Ambulatory care settings, where services are provided on an outpatient basis, have become increasingly pivotal to consumer health care as insurers direct dollars away from hospitals and toward outpatient care.

Just as the medical setting continues to evolve to meet new societal needs, health care technology is ever-changing. Health care is a dynamic, stimulating industry that requires the medical assistant and other professionals to constantly develop new skills if they are to contribute to the team effort. The range

of skills within the health care team is astonishing, and includes physicians, or medical doctors, in more than 25 specialties, an increasing number of nontraditional alternative practitioners licensed to practice, and more than 20 kinds of allied health professionals.

AMBULATORY HEALTH CARE SETTINGS

Although medical assistants may work in a number of different environments, including laboratories or hospitals, most are employed in an **ambulatory care setting** such as a medical office (either a solo-physician or group practice), an urgent or primary care center, or a managed care organization such as an HMO.

Often, the medical assistant will choose to work in one setting rather than another based on interests, personality, and work preferences. For instance, the individual practice may provide medical assistants with the opportunity to use their full array of skills, whereas in urgent care centers, the work of the medical assistant may be more specialized in nature.

FORMS OF MEDICAL PRACTICE MANAGEMENT

Medical assistants employed in ambulatory care settings or medical offices and clinics are likely to see three major forms of medical practice management: sole proprietorships, partnerships, and corporations.

Whatever form of management is chosen by physicians, they are responsible for the employees that serve with them. (Refer to the discussion of *respondeat superior* in Chapter 7.) Physician–employers and their medical assistants must have the kind of healthy working relationship where mutual trust and respect are apparent. The physician must understand the skill level of the medical assistant, and the medical assistant must feel secure enough to ask any necessary questions or admit any errors. Critical errors are often made when this trust does not exist between employer and employee. This causes a breakdown in the delivery of the best health care for patients.

Sole Proprietorships

In the past, many physicians preferred a solo practice. A solo practice entitles the physician or sole proprietor to hold exclusive right to all aspects of the medical practice or sole proprietorship, including profits and debts. If the business fails, the sole proprietor's personal property may also be attached.

A sole proprietorship may employ other physicians to participate in the practice. The employed physician(s) would be entitled to any employee **fringe benefits** such as health insurance and paid vacation, but the solo practitioner is not so entitled.

Partnerships

When two or more physicians join together under a legal agreement to share in the total business operations of the practice, a partnership is formed. Several physicians who share a facility and practice medicine are often referred to as a group. Partners share income, expenses, debt, equipment, records, and personnel according to a predetermined agreement. Partners are liable for only their own actions, but may be liable for the whole amount of the partnership debts.

Corporations

Physicians may form a corporation, usually referred to as a professional service corporation. The physician shareholders are considered employees of the corporation. A corporation allows income and tax advantages to all employees. A variety of fringe benefits can be offered to the employees, which may include pension, profit-sharing plans, medical expense reimbursement, and life, health, and disability insurance. These benefits are separate from salary. Another advantage is that professional employees of a corporation are liable only for their own acts, and personal property cannot be attached in litigation. A sole proprietor may incorporate if the practice is large enough.

The health maintenance organization (HMO) is one type of corporation in which physicians often practice. Basically, physicians are employees of the HMO and are paid by various methods; physicians in the HMO usually serve as the primary care physician (PCP). In this situation, a referral from the PCP may be necessary before a patient can see a specialist or allied health professional.

Figure 2-1 Different forms of medical practice management.

Medical assistants should also recognize the three major forms of medical practice management and how they affect salary, benefits, and liability issues (Figure 2-1).

Individual and Group Medical Practices

For years, the most common form of medical office was the individual physician or group practice. This model competes with a variety of other models such as urgent care centers and HMOs, but many medical assistants still find the individual or group practice a challenging place of employment.

Individual Practices. In the individual practice, also called the solo practice, one primary physician sees and treats all patients. Although this type of arrangement is

limited in the number of people it can serve, many patients feel secure in this kind of health care setting because they come to know and trust their doctor. Because they always see the same doctor, they feel their health care is being managed in a personal way. The solo-physician practice, however, can be an expensive arrangement, because one doctor must undertake the costs of office space, equipment, and personnel.

Group Practices. Group practices are attractive arrangements where two or more physicians can share the costs of space, equipment, and personnel. The advantages of a group practice are not solely economic, however; physicians learn from and consult one another, and patients receive the benefit of this exchange of information and knowledge. Often, a group practice may have more than one office and some employees may be asked to travel between sites to cut overhead. Group practices may also be formed to offer specialized care, such as oncology or women's health care.

In most group practices, patients may request that they see the same physician for all appointments, although sometimes patients are assigned to the next available doctor. For emergencies, group practices have the staff and flexibility to ensure that there is always a doctor on call.

Most medical practices are still groups of three or four doctors, but in the most recent past a trend shows a return to one- and two-doctor practices. Merritt, Hawkins, and Associates, a staffing and recruiting firm in Texas, reports that physicians in two-person partnerships increased from 9% in 1998 to 22% in 2002. In the same period, physicians placed in group settings decreased from 53% to 41%. A consulting firm in California, Professional Management and Marketing, reports that solo start-ups have increased fivefold in the last three years.

This trend seems to be led by some primary care physicians who learned firsthand that a bigger practice may not always be better. Many physicians in small groups allowed large practice management firms to acquire their assets and manage the business side of their practice. In some cases, these practice management firms were sold to even larger practice management companies that eventually went bankrupt, forcing them to shed all their practices. This dilemma left physicians with no recourse except to start over. Therefore, a number of physicians are returning to the **preferred provider organization (PPO)**, where physicians network to offer discounts to employers and other purchasers of health insurance and agree to discounted fees for services.

Urgent Care Centers

Urgent care centers are usually private, for-profit centers that provide services for primary care, routine injuries and illnesses, and minor surgery. Sometimes laboratory services and a radiology department are located on the premises. Physicians and other health care professionals in the center are often salaried employees, not owners who share in the profits, and often are associated with other medical facilities.

The pace in most urgent care centers is brisk, and typically a number of doctors are working at one time. Patients are usually requested to make appointments, but drop-ins are accepted in some centers, especially for emergencies.

Because these centers often see a higher volume of patients, usually for a lower cost than the traditional solo-physician or small group practice, some experts predict that urgent care centers will continue to grow in popularity.

Managed Care Operations

 Health maintenance organizations, or **HMOs,** are probably the most familiar **managed care operation.** Originally, HMOs were designed to provide a full range of health care services under one roof. More recently, the HMO without walls has become established, which is typically a network of participating physicians within a defined geographic area.

Originally, the HMO with walls was conceived to provide patients with comprehensive health care services at one facility. Today, as managed care and managed competition sweep the health care industry, other arrangements include the preferred provider organization (PPO), where physicians network to offer discounts to employers and other purchasers of health insurance, and the **Independent Physician Association (IPA),** of which the members agree to treat patients for an agreed-upon fee.

The Impact of Managed Care in the Health Care Setting

 The emergence of managed care in today's society provides new administrative and clinical challenges to members of the health care team as they struggle to provide the best health care while working within limitations often imposed by insurance carriers. Virtually all health care settings, whether they are individual practices or urgent care centers, are experiencing the impact of managed care, where physicians network and compete to serve patients better and more cost-efficiently.

Under managed care, critics charge, health care dollars have grown scarce, physicians must strive to provide the same quality for reduced reimbursement, preapprovals must be obtained for many services, and some services may be denied because they are not considered cost-effective.

Critical Thinking

Do you agree with the policy that managed care may set limits on services or length of services? Why or why not? Give your rationale.

Clinically, managed care may set limits on services or length of services. Second opinions are encouraged and sometimes required. In some systems, the patient selects a primary care physician, who is considered the gatekeeper and who must provide a referral for specialist care. Critics of managed care point out that restricting or denying services may lead to an increase in professional liability.

Administratively, paperwork and documentation have become increasingly important to ensure proper reimbursement. Although it is the patient's responsibility to understand the conditions of the insurance policy, these are often difficult to understand or interpret. The medical staff must be fully aware of when a preapproval or treatment plan is required, when a second opinion is necessary for reimbursement, and of other clauses and restrictions that affect care and reimbursement for care.

At the same time, although managed care is challenging even the most resilient of providers, the very real need to keep costs down has also generated considerable creativity and energy among the health care profession as physicians seek to use technology more efficiently; as they collaborate on new, cost-effective delivery methods; and as everyone involved in health care—insurers, providers, and patients—works together to contain costs by emphasizing prevention and lifestyle changes.

THE HEALTH CARE TEAM

In every kind of health care setting, the team concept is critical to the quality of patient care. A primary care physician is most likely the main source of health care for patients. From time to time, however, a specialist will be sought or recommended. A number of different allied health professionals, including the medical assistant, will supply additional health care as ordered by the physician. Increasingly, patients are looking outside traditional medicine for portions of their health care. A study published by the *New England Journal of Medicine* in 1993 indicated that more than one third of the adult population chose alternative over conventional forms of medical treatment. In 2001, the World Health Organization (WHO) estimated that between 65% and 80% of the world's population relied on alternative medicine as their primary health care source. One third of all medical schools in the United States now have courses in alternative medicine, and many people in the United States seem to desire a more "natural" approach to health care whenever possible. Although alternative care may not be covered by medical insurance, traditional and nontraditional health care practices are nonetheless blending in many areas.

In whatever manner health care is sought, all members of the health care team must communicate, sometimes in person and sometimes just through the medical history and record, with one another to ensure quality patient care. Note Patient Education box for another major member of the health care team.

The Role of the Medical Assistant

In the ambulatory care setting, a critical allied health professional is the medical assistant. The medical assistant, performing both administrative and clinical tasks under the direction of the physician, is an important link between patient and physician. The medical assistant serves in many capacities—receptionist, secretary, office manager, bookkeeper, insurance coder and biller, sometimes transcriptionist, patient educator, and clinical assistant. The latter requires the medical assistant to be able to administer injections and perform venipuncture, prepare patients for examinations, assist the physician with examinations and special procedures, and perform electrocardiography and various laboratory tests. Medical assistants **triage** and assess patient needs when scheduling appointments and tests. However, although medical assistants have a broad range of responsibilities, it is critical that they perform only within the scope of their training and personal capabilities and always function within ethical and legal boundaries and state statutes.

Because medical assistants are often the patient's first contact with the facility and its physicians, a positive attitude is important. They must be excellent communicators, both verbally and nonverbally, and project a professional image of themselves and their physician-employer. Medical assistants who believe in their work, who are proud of their career, and who convey compassion and caring provide a positive experience for patients who may be ill or in a great deal of discomfort.

The Title "Doctor"

The public is often confused by the title *doctor*. The term implies an earned academic degree of the highest level in a particular area of study. Physicians have earned the MD, or Doctor of Medicine, degree. In the medical field, the abbreviation *Dr.* is used and the title *doctor* is addressed to the person qualified by education, training, and licensure to practice medicine.

Other medical degrees include the Doctor of Osteopathy (DO), Doctor of Dentistry (DDS), Doctor of Optometry (OD), Doctor of Podiatric Medicine (DPM),

Patient Education

Continually remind your patients of the important role they carry in their own health care. *Only your patients* know exactly what happens to their bodies and minds in any particular illness. *Only your patients* know if their pain is too much to bear. *Only your patients* know whether they will remain on any treatment regimen established. *Only your patients* know if they are already embracing some alternative form of treatment. *Only your patients* know how much financial burden they can handle for health care. In initial interviews and pre-physician preparations, ask your patients questions that encourage them to tell you what is happening, whether they are coping, and how their particular problem affects their daily lives. Listen to them carefully. Do not rush or second-guess their responses. Be mindful of the special needs of elderly patients and individuals for whom English is their second language. They are likely unfamiliar with taking a major role in their own health care. Always remember to be therapeutic and observe nonverbal cues. Empower your patients to be a member of their own health care team.

CRITICAL THINKING: Discuss with a peer what action might be taken when patients refuse all opportunities to be a member of their own health care team. How might you encourage patients to take even a small part in their own health care? How would major decisions be made?

Doctor of Chiropracty (DC), and Doctor of Naturopathy (ND).

In nonmedical disciplines, the persons who have achieved a doctorate conferred by a college or university include the Doctor of Education (EdD) and the Doctor of Philosophy (PhD). Both the EdD and PhD have several areas of specialty.

Health Care Professionals and Their Roles

Medical Doctors. A doctorate degree in medicine and a license to practice allows a person to diagnose and treat medical conditions. The doctor of medicine candidate will attend four years of medical school after receiving a bachelor's degree. Newly graduated MDs enter into a residency program that is three to seven years of additional training and education depending on the specialty chosen. This residency comes under the direct supervision of senior physician educators. Family practice, internal medicine, and pediatrics require a three-year residency; general surgery requires a five-year residency. Some refer to the first year of residency as an internship; the American Medical Association (AMA) no longer uses this term, however. At this point, many physicians choose to be board certified, which is optional and voluntary. Certification assures the public that the doctor's knowledge, experience, and skills in a particular specialty have been tested and deemed qualified to provide care in that specialty. Doctors can be certified through 24 specialty medical boards and in 88 subspecialty fields. See Table 2-1 for a partial listing of these fields.

Physicians must still obtain a license to practice medicine from a state or jurisdiction of the United States in which they are planning to practice. They apply for the permanent license after completing a series of examinations and completing a minimum number of years of graduate medical education. Doctors must continue to receive a certain number of continuing medical education (CME) requirements per year to ensure that the doctor's knowledge and skills are current. CME requirements vary by state, professional organizations, and hospital staff organizations.

Osteopathy. Osteopaths are generally recognized as equal to medical doctors in all respects. The Doctor of Osteopathy, or DO, is a fully qualified physician licensed to perform surgery and prescribe medication. The training and education is quite similar to that of the MD. Osteopathic medicine was established in 1874 by Dr. Andrew Taylor Still, who was one of the first physicians to study the attributes of good health to better understand the process of disease. He identified the musculoskeletal system as a key element of health, and encouraged preventive medicine, eating properly, and keeping fit. The education of an osteopath includes a four-year undergraduate degree plus four years of medical school. After graduation from

TABLE 2-1   SELECTED MEDICAL AND SURGICAL SPECIALTIES

Specialties	Title of Doctor	Description
Allergy and Immunology	Allergist and Immunologist	Evaluates diseases/disorders of the immune system and problems related to asthma and allergy
Dermatology	Dermatologist	Evaluates disorders/diseases of skin, hair, nails, and related tissues
Family Practice	Family Practitioner	Treats the whole family from infancy to death
Internal Medicine	Internist	Provides comprehensive care, practices preventive care, treats long-term and chronic conditions
Obstetrics and Gynecology	Obstetrician and Gynecologist	Provides care to pregnant women, delivers babies, treats disorders/diseases of reproductive system
Ophthalmology	Ophthalmologist	Provides comprehensive care of the eye and its structures and offers vision services
Otolaryngology	Otolaryngologist	Treats diseases/disorders of the ears, nose, and throat
Pediatrics	Pediatrician	Treats diseases/disorders of children and adolescents; monitors growth and development of children
Psychiatry and Neurology	Psychiatrist and Neurologist	Diagnoses and treats patients with mental, emotional, or behavioral disorders
General Surgery	Surgeon	Operates to repair or remove diseased or injured parts of the body
Colon and Rectal	Colorectal Surgeon	Operates to remove or repair diseased colon and rectal areas of the body
Neurological	Neurosurgeon	Treats conditions of the nervous systems, often through surgery
Plastic	Plastic Surgeon	Repairs and reconstructs physical defects; provides cosmetic enhancements
Thoracic	Thoracic Surgeon	Performs surgery on the respiratory system, chest, heart, and cardiovascular system
Urology	Urologist	Treats diseases/disorders of the urinary tract

medical school, a DO can choose to practice in any of the 18 American Osteopathic Association specialty areas, requiring from two to six years of additional training. Approximately 65% of all osteopathic physicians practice in primary care areas such as family practice, pediatrics, obstetrics/gynecology, and internal medicine. DOs must pass a state licensure examination and maintain currency in their education. Most patients will find little difference between an MD and a DO. However, doctors of osteopathy also will be able to incorporate osteopathic manipulative treatment (OMT) in their treatment of patients as deemed helpful.

Integrative Medicine and Alternative Health Care Practitioners

Many **integrative medicine** and alternative health care practitioners also carry the title *doctor*, but they have a different training regimen than required for the MD or DO. The training is highly specialized and specific; and when licensed, these professionals are allowed to diagnose and treat medical conditions.

As mentioned earlier, alternative therapies are increasingly being perceived as complements to traditional health care in a form of integrative medicine. In this text, three broad disciplines are identified: chiropractic, naturopathy, and Oriental medicine/acupuncture.

Chiropractic. Chiropractic is a branch of the healing arts that gives special attention to the physiological and biochemical aspects of the body's structure and includes procedures for the adjustment and manipulation of the articulations and adjacent tissues of the human body, particularly of the spinal column. Chiropractic is a drug-free, nonsurgical science that does not include pharmaceuticals or surgery.

The roots of chiropractic care may be traced back to the beginning of recorded time. Writings from China and Greece written in 2700 B.C. and 1500 B.C. mention spinal manipulation and maneuvering of the lower extremities to ease lower back pain. Daniel David Palmer founded the chiropractic profession in the United States in 1895. Throughout the twentieth century, doctors of chiropractic gained legal recognition and licensure in all 50 states.

Doctors of chiropractic (DC) complete four to five years of study at an accredited chiropractic college. The curriculum includes a minimum of 4,200 hours of classroom, laboratory, and clinical experience. About 555 hours are devoted to adjustive techniques and spinal analysis. This specialized education must be preceded by a minimum of 90 hours of undergraduate courses focusing on science. On successful completion of their education and training, doctors of chiropractic must also pass the national board examination and all examinations or licensure requirements identified by the particular state in which the individual wishes to practice.

Doctors of chiropractic frequently treat patients with neuromusculoskeletal conditions, such as headaches, joint pain, neck pain, lower back pain, and sciatica. Chiropractors also treat patients with osteoarthritis, spinal disk conditions, carpal tunnel syndrome, tendonitis, sprains, and strains. Chiropractors also may be found treating a variety of other conditions such as allergies, asthma, and digestive disorders. There are obstacles to chiropractors in some areas, however, because states vary in what they authorize chiropractors to practice and may limit their ability to practice **homeopathy** or **acupuncture** or to dispense or sell dietary supplements.

Naturopathy.

Naturopathy, often referred to as "natural medicine," is based on the belief that the cause of disease is violation of nature's laws. The goal of the naturopath is to remove the underlying causes of disease and to stimulate the body's natural healing processes. Naturopathic treatments may include fasting, adhering to natural food diets, taking vitamins and herbs, tissue minerals, counseling, homeopathic remedies, manipulation of the spine and extremities, massage, exercise, naturopathic hygienic remedies, acupuncture, and applications of water, heat, cold, air, sunlight, and electricity. Most of these treatment methods are used to detoxify the body and strengthen the immune system.

In the United States, a Doctor of Naturopathy (ND) or Doctor of Naturopathic Medicine (NMD) will receive education, training, and credentials from a full-time naturopathy college. The full-time education includes two years of science courses and two years of clinical work. Naturopaths are currently licensed to practice in 11 states, and other states are considering licensure. In many states, naturopaths practice independently and unlicensed, or they practice under the direction of a physician.

Oriental Medicine and Acupuncture.

Oriental medicine is a comprehensive system of health care with a history of more than 3,000 years. Oriental medicine includes acupuncture, Chinese herbology and bodywork, dietary therapy, and exercise based on traditional Oriental medicine principles. This form of health care is used extensively in Asia and is rapidly growing in popularity in the West.

Oriental medicine is based on an energetic model rather than the biochemical model of Western medicine. The ancient Chinese recognized a vital energy behind all life-forms and processes called *qi* (pronounced "chee"). Oriental healing practitioners believe that energy flows along specific pathways called meridians. Each pathway is associated with a particular physiological system and internal organ. Disease is the result of deficiency or imbalance of energy in the meridians and their associated physiological systems. Acupuncture points are specific sites along the meridians. Each point has a predictable effect on the vital energy passing through it. Modern science has measured the electrical charge at these points, corroborating the locations of the meridians. Traditional Oriental medicine uses an intricate system of pulse and tongue diagnosis, palpation of points and meridians, medical history, and other signs and symptoms to create a composite diagnosis. A treatment plan then is formulated to induce the body to a balanced state of health.

The World Health Organization (WHO) recognizes acupuncture and traditional Oriental medicine's ability to treat many common disorders, including the following disorders:

- *Gastrointestinal disorders:* food allergies, peptic ulcer, chronic diarrhea, constipation, indigestion, anorexia, gastritis

- *Urogenital disorders:* stress incontinence, urinary tract infections, and sexual dysfunction

- *Gynecological disorders:* irregular, heavy, or painful menstruation; premenstrual syndrome (PMS); and infertility

- *Respiratory disorders:* emphysema, sinusitis, asthma, allergies, and bronchitis

- *Neuromusculoskeletal disorders:* arthritis; migraine headaches; neuralgia; insomnia; dizziness; and low back, neck, and shoulder pain

- *Circulatory disorders:* hypertension, angina pectoris, arteriosclerosis, and anemia

- *Eye, ear, nose, and throat disorders:* otitis media, sinusitis, and sore throats

- *Emotional and psychological disorders:* depression; anxiety; and addictions to alcohol, nicotine, and drugs

- *Pain:* elimination or control of pain for chronic and painful debilitating disorders

In the hands of a comprehensively trained acupuncturist, patients will not find acupuncture painful. Sterile, very fine, flexible needles about the diameter of a human hair are used in treatment. Practitioners may also recommend herbs, dietary changes, and exercise together with lifestyle changes.

Training for acupuncture and Oriental medicine may be obtained in schools and colleges accredited by the Accreditation Commission for Acupuncture and Oriental Medicine. There is a minimum of two years of undergraduate study required, and some colleges prefer applicants to have a bachelor's degree. Most of these specialized programs are three years and on completion graduates are conferred with a Masters in Acupuncture and Oriental Medicine (MAOM) or a Masters in Acupuncture (MA) degree. Nearly all states regulate the practice of acupuncture and Oriental medicine, either through licensure or a ruling by the Board of Medical Examiners. It is likely that passing a national certification examination or other testing procedure is required before licensure. Many doctors (MDs, DOs, DCs, and NDs) have become qualified to perform acupuncture and to use Oriental medicine in their practices through additional education and training.

Future of Integrative Medicine

There was a time when chiropractors were not accepted by the medical establishment and had difficulty with licensure. Naturopaths, acupuncturists, and Oriental medicine practitioners face similar challenges, and states vary greatly in their regulations of any form of alternative medicine.

The road may be bumpy for alternative practitioners, but their numbers are increasing rapidly. By 2010, the number of chiropractors is projected to double, and the number of naturopaths is expected to triple. Oriental medicine practitioners, including acupuncturists already licensed in 42 states and in the District of Columbia, are likely to grow even more. This latter fact is partially attributed to the Asian American population that is expected to increase by as much as 95% by 2010. Managed care health plans are offering increased access to alternative medicine clinicians, mostly because of the ability to expand patient choices at a lower cost. It is expected that states will broaden their licensure to increased numbers of well-educated and trained alternative practitioners.

Neither the growth in the number of alternative medicine practitioners nor the laws and insurance practices that facilitate their access by patients likely would have occurred without broad public acceptance of alternative and complementary medicine. Americans seem quite willing to pay out-of-pocket expenses for alternative forms of treatment such as massage therapy, aromatherapy, biofeedback, guided imagery, hydrotherapy, hypnotherapy, and homeopathy. Furthermore, there are many patients seeking a more integrated form of medicine that occurs when primary care physicians are willing to refer to an alternative practitioner and vice versa. See Table 2-2 for a brief description of a few alternative modalities that fairly easily integrate with traditional medical practices.

ALLIED HEALTH PROFESSIONALS AND THEIR ROLES

In the health care team, allied health professionals bring specific educational backgrounds and a broad array of skills to the medical environment. Medical assistants are considered allied health professionals. Table 2-3 lists some of the allied health professionals recognized by the Commission on Accreditation of Allied Health Education Programs (CAAHEP) and the Accrediting Bureau of Health Education Schools (ABHES).

As a medical assistant, you may not work directly with all the identified allied health care professionals, but you are likely to have contact with many of them by telephone and written or electronic communication. Knowledge of the roles these health professionals play enables you to interact more intelligently with all members of the health care team.

In addition to the professionals listed in Table 2-3, you may encounter some or all of the following health care professionals in daily patient care.

TABLE 2-2   SELECTED ALTERNATIVE MEDICINE MODALITIES

Acupressure: A massage technique that applies pressure to specific acupuncture-like points on the body; pressure encourages the flow of vital energy *(qi)* along the meridian pathways. It is used to control chronic pain, migraine headaches, and backaches.

Aromatherapy: The inhalation and bodily application of essential oils from aromatic plants to relax, balance, rejuvenate, restore, or enhance the body's mind and spirit. It strengthens the self-healing process by indirect stimulation of the immune system.

Biofeedback: Biofeedback machines gauge internal bodily functions and help patients tune in to these functions and identify the triggers that evoke symptoms. Relaxation can be taught to relieve the symptoms.

Guided Imagery: Uses images or symbols to train the mind to create a definitive physiological or psychological effect; relieves stress and anxiety and reduces pain.

Homeopathy: Healing that claims highly diluted doses of certain substances can leave an energy imprint in the body and bring about a cure. Homeopathic remedies are made from naturally occurring plant, animal, or mineral substances and are manufactured by pharmaceutical companies under strict guidelines.

Hydrotherapy: Hydrotherapy uses the buoyancy, warmth, and effects of water and its turbulence to speed recovery after surgery and to reduce pain and stress, spasm and discomfort. It is especially beneficial for work- or sports-related injuries and arthritis.

Hypnotherapy: Hypnotherapy facilitates communication between the right and left sides of the brain with the patient in a state of focused relaxation when the subconscious mind is open to suggestions. It is currently used to help people lose weight, stop smoking, reduce stress, and relieve pain, anxiety, and phobias.

Massage: Massage reduces stress, manages chronic pain, promotes relaxation, and increases circulation of the blood and lymph. Hand stroking on the body helps patients become more familiar with their pain.

TABLE 2-3 SELECTED ALLIED HEALTH PROFESSIONS

Occupation	Abbreviations	Job Description
Anesthesiologist Assistant	AA	Performs preoperative tasks, performs airway management and drug administration for induction and maintenance of anesthesia during surgery under direction of a licensed and qualified anesthesiologist
Athletic Trainer	AT	Provides a variety of services including injury prevention, recognition, immediate care, treatment, and rehabilitation after athletic trauma
Clinical Laboratory Technician *Associate Degree*	CLT	Performs all routine tests in a medical laboratory and is able to discriminate and recognize factors that directly affect procedures and results. Works under direction of pathologist, physician, medical technologist, or scientist
Diagnostic Medical Sonographer	DMS	Provides patient services using medical ultrasound under the supervision of a physician
Electroneurodiagnostic Technologist	EEG-T	Possesses the knowledge, attributes, and skills to obtain interpretable recordings of a patient's nervous system functions
Emergency Medical Technician—Paramedic	EMT-P	Recognizes, assesses, and manages medical emergencies of acutely ill or injured patients in prehospital care settings, working under the direction of a physician (often through radio communication)
Health Information Administrator	RRA	Manages health information systems consistent with the medical, administrative, ethical, and legal requirements of the health care delivery system
Health Information Technician	ART	Possesses the technical knowledge and skills necessary to process, maintain, compile, and report patient data
Medical Assistant	MA	Functions under the supervision of licensed medical professionals and is competent in both administrative/office and clinical/laboratory procedures
Medical Illustrator	MI	Creates visual material designed to facilitate the recording and dissemination of medical, biological, and related knowledge through communication media
Occupational Therapist	OT	Educates and trains individuals in the application of purposeful, goal-oriented activity in the evaluation, diagnosis, and treatment of loss of ability to cope with the tasks of daily living and impairment caused by physical injury, illness, or emotional disorder, congenital or developmental disability; or the aging process
Ophthalmic Medical Technician or Technologist	OMT	Assists ophthalmologists to perform diagnostic and therapeutic procedures
Personal Trainer	PT	Develops activity plans for each individual that integrates a complete approach to fitness and wellness through exercise, strength training, and proper diet
Physician Assistant (includes Surgeon's Assistant)	PA	Practices medicine under the direction and responsible supervision of a Doctor of Medicine or Osteopathy; performs diagnostic, therapeutic, preventive, and health maintenance services in any setting in which the physician renders care
Radiographer	RT(R)	Provides patient services using imaging modalities, as directed by physicians qualified to order and perform radiologic procedures
Respiratory Therapist	RRT	Applies scientific knowledge and theory to practical clinical problems of respiratory care
Surgical Technologist	ST	Works as an integral member of the surgical team, which includes surgeons, anesthesiologists, registered nurses, and other surgical personnel delivering patient care and assuming appropriate responsibilities before, during, and after surgery

Health Unit Coordinator

Health unit coordinators (HUCs) perform nonclinical patient care tasks for the nursing unit of a hospital. This profession requires a self-motivated, mature individual who can handle the stress and hectic pace of coordinating personnel and their duties at the nurses' station. Also called unit secretary, administrative specialist, ward clerk, or ward secretary, a health unit coordinator receives on-the-job training with an emphasis on administrative office skills.

Medical Laboratory Technologist

Medical laboratory technologists (MLTs) physically and chemically analyze, as well as culture, urine, blood, and other body fluids and tissues. They work closely with physician specialists such as oncologists, pathologists, and hematologists. Knowledge of specimen collection, anatomy and physiology, biochemistry, laboratory equipment, asepsis, and quality control is essential. The American Society of Clinical Pathology (ASCP) is a professional organization that oversees credentialing

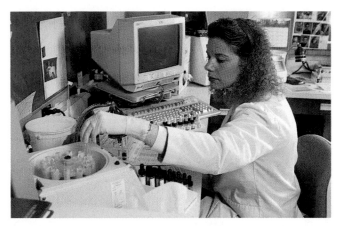

Figure 2-2 Medical laboratory personnel performing blood analysis. (Courtesy of Foote Health Systems.)

and education in the medical laboratory professions. See Figure 2-2.

Nurses

Neither ABHES nor CAAHEP is responsible for nurse education or accreditation, but they are listed here as a major participant in health care. Nurses are licensed by the state in which they practice. Although nurses' education and training are oriented to bedside care, some are employed in medical offices as clinical assistants, especially in offices where surgery is performed. Nurses play a number of roles on the health care team.

Registered Nurse. In the United States, registered nurses (RNs) are professionals who have completed at a minimum, a two-year course of study at a state-approved school of nursing and passed the National Council Licensure Examination (NCLEX-RN). Employment settings most often include hospitals, convalescent homes, clinics, and home health care.

Licensed Practical Nurse. A licensed practical nurse (LPN) is a professional trained in basic nursing techniques and direct patient care. LPNs practice under the direct supervision of an RN or physician and are employed in similar settings to RNs. Training includes completion of a state-approved program in practical nursing and successful completion of a national licensure examination.

Nurse Practitioner. Sometimes referred to as an Advanced Registered Nurse Practitioner (ARNP), a nurse practitioner (NP) is an RN who, by advanced education (usually a master's degree) and clinical experience in a branch of nursing, has acquired expert knowledge in a specific medical specialty. Nurse practitioners are employed by physicians in private practice or in clinics, and sometimes practice independently, especially in rural areas. ARNPs may or may not be licensed to prescribe medications.

Registered Dietitian

Registered dietitians (RDs) have specialized training in the nutritional care of groups and individuals and have successfully completed an examination of the Commission on Dietetic Registration. Dietitians assist patients in regulating their diets. Although they are typically employed in hospitals and clinics, they can also be found working with the public in personal nutritional counseling. Education includes a bachlor's degree with a major in dietetics, food and nutrition, or food service systems management in addition to completion of an approved internship.

Pharmacist

Pharmacists (RPh) are licensed by each state to prepare and dispense all types of medications, as well as medical supplies related to medication administration. They may practice in hospitals, medical centers, and pharmacies. The minimum training for a pharmacist is a five-year bachelor's degree; some pharmacists pursue a Doctor of Pharmacy degree (PharmD), which is offered by major universities in the United States.

Pharmacy Technician

Pharmacy technicians assist the pharmacist with preparation and administration of medications, as well as perform receptionist and billing duties. In hospitals, nursing homes, and assisted living facilities, their responsibilities may include reading patient charts and preparing and delivering medications to patients. Pharmacists must check all orders before delivery. The technician can copy the information about the prescribed medication onto the patient's profile. Professional certification of pharmacy technicians varies from state to state and is administered by state pharmacy associations. See Figure 2-3.

Phlebotomist

Phlebotomists (LPTs) are trained in the art of drawing blood for diagnostic laboratory testing. Phlebotomists are also referred to as laboratory liaison technicians. Phlebotomists may be nationally certified and are employed in medical clinics, hospitals, and laboratories. Training consists of one to two semesters in a community college program or on-the-job training.

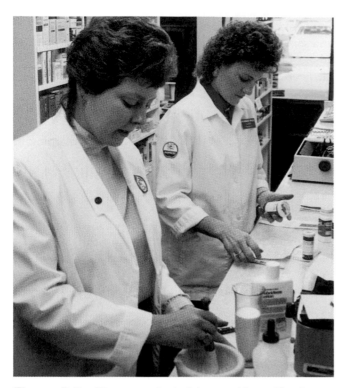

Figure 2-3 Pharmacy technician working with pharmacist in preparing medications. (Courtesy of the Michigan Pharmacists Association and the Michigan Society of Pharmacy Technicians.)

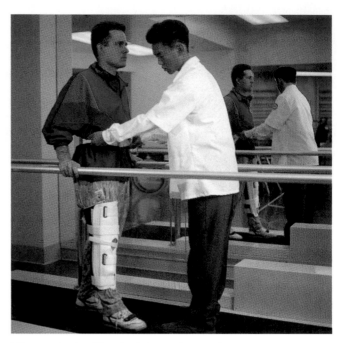

Figure 2-4 Physical therapist working with a patient requiring physical rehabilitation.

Physical Therapist

Physical therapists (PTs) are licensed professionals who assist in the examination, testing, and treatment of physically disabled or challenged people. They also assist in physical rehabilitation of patients after an accident, injury, or serious illness using special exercises, application of heat or cold, *ultrasound* therapy, and other techniques. Educational requirements for a PT are a minimum of a four-year bachelor's degree (Bachelor of Science) or a special certificate course after obtaining the Bachelor of Science in a related field. PTs must also successfully complete a state licensure examination. See Figure 2-4.

Physical Therapy Assistant

Physical therapy assistants (PTAs) are trained to use and apply physical therapy procedures, such as exercise, and physical agents under the supervision of a physical therapist. The PTA has earned an Associate of Science degree from an accredited program and must pass a licensure or registry examination in selected states.

THE VALUE OF THE MEDICAL ASSISTANT TO THE HEALTH CARE TEAM

With their broad range of competencies in both administrative and clinical areas, medical assistants are increasingly valued as health care team members. Medical assistants are the great communicators, serving as liaison between physician and hospital staff and between physician and any number of allied and other health professionals. Because they are the first providers to see or speak with patients, they undertake responsibility for directing, informing, and guiding patient care while establishing a professional and caring tone for the entire health care team. The value of a competent, professional, compassionate medical assistant is immeasurable in today's fast-paced and challenging health care environment.

Case Study 2-1

The number of sole proprietors and small partnerships may be increasing.

CASE STUDY REVIEW

1. What role has managed care had in this event?
2. Describe the impact, if any, this fact has on quality health care.

Case Study 2-2

You are the medical assistant for a family practice physician, Bill Claredon, who is close to retirement. He is much adored by all his patients, but he thinks alternative medicine is outright quackery. Marjorie Johns, a patient with debilitating back pain, tells you she is seeing an acupuncturist and is taking less and less of her prescribed medications. You quietly mention that to Dr. Claredon before he enters the examination room to see Marjorie. He glares at you with disgust at the information and is quite agitated when he enters the examination room. Describe the discussion that you think will occur between Dr. Claredon and Marjorie. If Marjorie is unhappy when she is ready to leave the facility, is there anything you can do or say to help her? Can you do anything to help Dr. Claredon?

SUMMARY

The health care environment is a dynamic service that changes rapidly in response to new technology and societal needs. In an effort to reduce the cost of health care, managed care will continue to have a profound impact on all health care settings. A strong health care team is critical in the health care setting, as primary care physicians, specialists of all disciplines, alternative care practitioners, and allied and other health professionals collaborate on the best way to provide integrative medicine and quality patient care. In almost any health care environment, but especially the ambulatory care setting, the medical assistant is a vital link in the team and is responsible for a range of responsibilities, both clinical and administrative.

STUDY FOR SUCCESS

To reinforce your knowledge and skills of information presented in this chapter:

- ❑ Review the Key Terms
- ❑ Consider the Case Studies and discuss your conclusions
- ❑ Answer the Review Questions
  - ❑ Multiple Choice
  - ❑ Critical Thinking
- ❑ Navigate the Internet and complete the Web Activities
- ❑ Practice the StudyWARE activities on the textbook CD
- ❑ Apply your knowledge in the Student Workbook activities
- ❑ Complete the Web Tutor sections
- ❑ View and discuss the DVD situations

REVIEW QUESTIONS

Multiple Choice

1. Medical assistants are mostly employed in:
   a. hospitals
   b. nursing facilities
   c. ambulatory care settings
   d. insurance companies
2. A health maintenance organization is one kind of:
   a. managed care operation
   b. individual practice
   c. sole proprietorship
   d. hospital
3. With its emphasis on controlling costs, managed care is likely to affect:
   a. only hospitals
   b. all health care settings
   c. only physicians in private practice
   d. only patients
4. The health care team:
   a. should exclude the patient as part of the team
   b. is only important in the hospital setting
   c. is made up of physicians and nurses
   d. includes physicians, nurses, allied health care professionals, patients, and integrative medicine practitioners
5. Integrative health care approaches:
   a. are increasingly accepted as complementary to traditional health care
   b. are always covered by insurance
   c. are seldom approved for licensure
   d. are not important to understand
6. A medical assistant permitted by law to draw blood for diagnostic laboratory testing performs a procedure similar to those performed by a:
   a. health unit coordinator
   b. health information technician
   c. phlebotomist
   d. respiratory therapist
7. The distinct difference between the PA and the MA is that the PA:
   a. draws blood and gives injections
   b. practices medicine
   c. performs diagnostic services
   d. both b and c
8. Physicians just establishing their practice often seek to work with another physician in the same field. When expenses and profits are shared, this form of management is called a/an:
   a. HMO
   b. corporation
   c. sole proprietor
   d. group or partnership

9. Managed care may be identified as care that:
   a. offers unlimited services
   b. forbids second opinions
   c. establishes a primary care physician as gatekeeper
   d. offers protection to physicians against liability
10. An alternative approach to medicine that treats patients using thin, flexible needles is called:
    a. acupuncture
    b. naturopathy
    c. chiropractic
    d. homeopathy

Critical Thinking

1. Evaluate the different health care settings and discuss the pros and cons of working in each setting.
2. From a patient's point of view, which health care setting do you think offers the most benefits? Why?
3. Review the three forms of medical management models. Which is probably the most advantageous from the physician's point of view? From the medical assistant's point of view? Justify your responses.
4. Recall a few types of allied health professionals and, working in small groups, create scenarios in which the medical assistant needs to coordinate patient care with two or three allied professionals.
5. Identify as many reasons as you can for why patients might be seeking alternative approaches to traditional medicine. Explain your choices.
6. Compare Doctors of Osteopathy and Chiropractic. When and why might one be selected over the other?
7. Discuss the validity of licensure or national certification for health care practitioners.

WEB ACTIVITIES

1. American Board of Medical Specialties (http://www.abms.org): Use this site to review details of the specialties. What does board certified mean? Identify those for whom you would most enjoy working and give your reasons.
2. Natural Healers (http://www.naturalhealers.com): Scan this Web site for a listing of most alternative therapy modalities. Select one modality and identify the schools/colleges where education is available and what kind of credentialing is necessary to practice the modality.

3. http://www.integrativemedicine.org identifies a Web site that may prove helpful for health care professionals. It is a membership site, but access is available for introduction and explanation of services. Identify two or three reasons that make this site beneficial to anyone embracing integrative medicine.

4. American Osteopathic Association (http://www. osteopathic.org): After you visit this Web site, discuss the role of the osteopath as a primary care physician in today's health care structure.

5. American Medical News (http://www.amednews. com): This is a newspaper for American's physicians. Find and identify as many articles as you can that discuss how physicians and alternative therapy practitioners identify their roles, where they merge, and where they conflict.

6. American Chiropractic Association (http://www. amerchiro.org): Locate two colleges that educate and train chiropractors. Determine the tuition and cost of each.

7. If you have doubts about alternative medicine, you might want to view the following Web site: http://www.quackwatch.org. It is helpful to research as many thoughts on a subject as possible. Examine the validity of the Web site and whether any biases are evident.

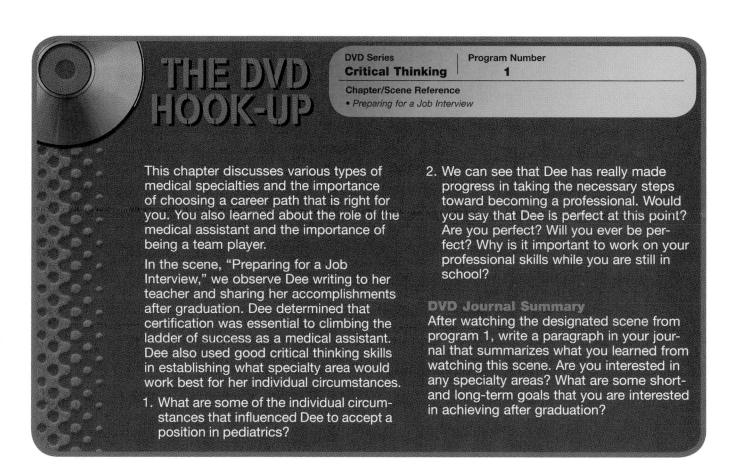

THE DVD HOOK-UP

DVD Series	Program Number
Critical Thinking	**1**

Chapter/Scene Reference
• *Preparing for a Job Interview*

This chapter discusses various types of medical specialties and the importance of choosing a career path that is right for you. You also learned about the role of the medical assistant and the importance of being a team player.

In the scene, "Preparing for a Job Interview," we observe Dee writing to her teacher and sharing her accomplishments after graduation. Dee determined that certification was essential to climbing the ladder of success as a medical assistant. Dee also used good critical thinking skills in establishing what specialty area would work best for her individual circumstances.

1. What are some of the individual circumstances that influenced Dee to accept a position in pediatrics?

2. We can see that Dee has really made progress in taking the necessary steps toward becoming a professional. Would you say that Dee is perfect at this point? Are you perfect? Will you ever be perfect? Why is it important to work on your professional skills while you are still in school?

DVD Journal Summary
After watching the designated scene from program 1, write a paragraph in your journal that summarizes what you learned from watching this scene. Are you interested in any specialty areas? What are some short- and long-term goals that you are interested in achieving after graduation?

REFERENCES/BIBLIOGRAPHY

Adams, K. E., Cohen, M. H., Eisenberg, D., & Jonsen, A. R. (2002). Ethical considerations of complementary and alternative medical therapies in conventional medical settings. *Annals of Internal Medicine, 137*(8), 660–664.

American Board of Medical Specialties. (2000). *Approved ABMS specialty boards & certificate categories*. Evanston, IL: Author.

Eisenberg, D. M., Cohen, M. H., Hrbek, A., Grayzel, J., Van Rompay, M. I., & Cooper, R. A. (2002). Credentialing comple-mentary and alternative medical providers. *Annals of Internal Medicine, 137*(12), 965–973.

Frenkel, M. A., & Borkan, J. M. (2003). An approach for integrating complementary-alternative medicine into primary care. *Family Practice, 20*(3), 324–332.

Health professions career & education directory (2004–2005). (2004). Chicago, IL: American Medical Association.

Tamparo, C. D., & Lewis, M.A. (2005). *Diseases of the human body* (4th ed.). Philadelphia: F.A. Davis Publishers.

Triveri, Jr., L., & Anderson, J. W. (2002). *Alternative medicine. The definitive guide* (2nd ed.). Berkeley, CA: Celestial Arts.

CHAPTER 3

History of Medicine

OUTLINE

Cultural Heritage in Medicine
Medical Specialists in History
History of Medical Education
History of Attitudes toward
Illness

Historical Medical Treatments
Significant Contributions to
Medicine
Frontiers in Medicine

OBJECTIVES

The student should strive to meet the following performance objectives and demonstrate an understanding of the facts and principles presented in this chapter through written and oral communication.

1. Define the key terms as presented in the glossary.
2. Discuss the effects of culture on medicine.
3. Identify the role of religion, magic, and science in medicine's history.
4. Describe how attitudes toward illness are manifested today.
5. Identify a minimum of three previously used common medical treatments.
6. Recall a minimum of three theories/practices of ancient medicine that are still prevalent today.
7. Name and describe the historical roles of medical specialists.
8. Discuss the role of women in medicine.
9. Trace the progression of medical education.
10. Name at least five significant contributions to medicine.
11. Identify a minimum of three recent developments in medicine.

You may recall your mom putting a mentholated salve on your chest when you had a cold. Your cousins had to take a spoonful of cod-liver oil each night before they went to bed. Grandma made chicken soup with homemade noodles when you had the flu. An apple a day, mustard plaster for the chest, hot or cold steam in a room, and many more are medical practices of years gone by. Many still stand, however, and from them others have developed. Interestingly, medicine has a rich history, and every culture exhibits that history differently. The more you know and understand of that history and its various cultural influences, the more effective and therapeutic will be your communication with patients.

INTRODUCTION

*A historical overview of medicine must do more than identify a series of contributions by physicians. It must remind us that more than one discipline and more than one philosophy have contributed to medicine. This is perhaps more true now than ever as our world becomes smaller and our society becomes increasingly **pluralistic,** ethnically, culturally, and religiously.*

CULTURAL HERITAGE IN MEDICINE

Today's health professional will give care to individuals of varied cultures who hold differing philosophical beliefs toward medicine. The informed and caring health professional will recognize that a person's culture and ethnic heritage play an enormous role in any kind of health care. For example, if the patient's cultural experience leans toward a more natural, nonmedical form of health care, treating the patient with prescription drugs will necessitate an explanation and rationale for the use of medications. Otherwise, the patient may refuse to take all or part of the medications, thus hindering recovery. It would be better to seek a treatment for the patient that embraces both the health care professional's desire to heal and the individual's wish to respect cultural tradition.

In every society, medicine has been an important element for its people. From the earliest time, culture was an important influence on medicine, and modern day medicine is in many ways a reflection of this diverse and rich heritage.

It is certain that religion, magic, and science all played a vital part in the history of medicine. Religion was important because it was perceived that certain gods were to be called on for a cure through ceremonies, prayers, and sacrifices. Magic was practiced because it was such an important part of many societies and was seen as an essential ingredient to chase away evil spirits. The importance of science was demonstrated in the use of plants and minerals for medicinal purposes. The use of plants and minerals is found throughout medicine's history. Unearthed clay tablets reveal hundreds of plants, minerals, and animal substances used for medicinal purposes in ancient Mesopotamia and Babylon. The Chinese **pharmacopoeia** was rich in the use of herbs.

Skeletal remains of prehistoric cultures show advanced stages of arthritis, a nearly toothless jaw, and only a 20- to 40-year life span for humans. Skull bones reveal round holes referred to as trephination, believed necessary to release the evil spirits thought to be causing a person's illness. Mesopotamian cultures believed that illness was a punishment by the gods for violation of a moral code. Ancient Egyptians believed the body was a system of channels for air, tears, blood, urine, sperm, and feces. All the channels were thought to come together in the rectum, and were believed to become easily clogged. Thus, emetics, enemas, and purges of the anus were common treatments. In ancient India, plastic surgery was practiced. Punishment for adultery was cutting off the nose, therefore allowing physicians many opportunities to practice and refine the art of nose reconstruction.

The ancient Chinese cultures examined and carefully monitored the pulse in each wrist. It was believed that the pulse had hundreds of characteristics important in medical treatment. There were five methods of treatment to bring a person back to the right track. They were:

1. Cure the spirit.
2. Nourish the body.

Critical Thinking

Are there any indications today that moral behavior, or lack of it, may be the cause of disease and illness? Give examples.

3. Give medications.
4. Treat the whole body.
5. Use acupuncture and moxibustion.

Acupuncture is the piercing of the skin by very thin, flexible needles into any of 365 points along 12 meridians that transverse the body and transmit the active life force called "qi" (pronounced "chee") (Figure 3-1). Each of these spots is related to a particular organ. **Moxibustion** requires the use of a powdered plant substance that is made into a small mound on the person's skin and then burned, usually raising a blister.

Even today's **allopathic,** or traditional, physicians would agree that the first four methods of treatment from Chinese culture are excellent guidelines for health care.

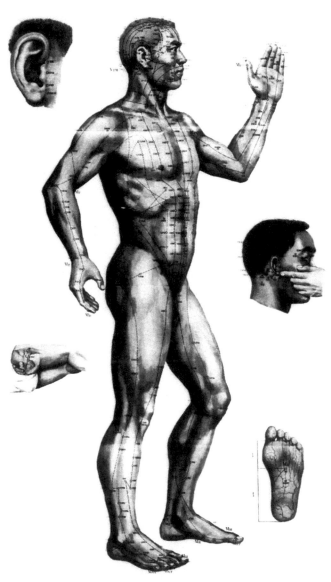

Figure 3-1 Chinese acupuncture points and meridians. (Courtesy of the World Health Organization.)

There also is an increasing awareness that acupuncture has a valid place in allopathic medicine, especially for the control of some types of pain.

MEDICAL SPECIALISTS IN HISTORY

Medicine's history gives early evidence of many "specialists" in the healing arts. They were known by various names—witch doctors, medicine men and women, shamans or healing priests, and physicians. These healers were more than ancestors of the modern physician, however, for they performed many functions that involved the welfare of the entire community or village. By today's standards, they were considered to be equivalent to spiritual advisers, social workers, counselors, and teachers.

Whereas women were accepted as healers in primitive societies, later cultures reduced their status to that of being allowed to care only for women and to assist in childbirth. In any culture that granted women only secondary status, women were also considered unqualified to become physicians. In Chinese culture, the first reference to a female physician mentioned by name is in documents from the Han dynasty (206 B.C.–A.D. 220). In Muslim society, the reluctance of Arabic physicians to violate social taboo and touch the genitals of female strangers further encouraged relegating the practice of obstetrics and gynecology to midwives.

Women were not accepted as medical doctors in Western culture until the nineteenth and twentieth centuries. Italy granted women the status earlier than other cultures. In the United States, the first female physician was Elizabeth Blackwell, who was awarded her degree in 1849. Although she was snubbed by the public, she soon earned the respect of her colleagues. When she refused to be absent from class when the male reproductive system was discussed, her fellow male students supported her actions.

From the earliest times, it appears that some payment was expected for medical services rendered. In many instances, the payment was dependent on the status of the physician, as well as the patient. At the same time, some cultures punished a physician who was not successful in treatment by forcing that physician to treat only those too poor to pay.

HISTORY OF MEDICAL EDUCATION

During the rise of Christianity, emphasis was placed on the soul rather than the body; therefore, early Christian monks held great control over medicine. This is evidenced by St. Benedict of Nursia (480–554), who forbade the study of medicine. The care of the sick was encouraged, but only through prayer and divine intervention. Thus, Christ's healing mission was institutionalized in a fashion that was to control medical care almost completely for the next 500 years, until the seventh century.

At that time, however, the religion of Islam moved to preserve the classical learning that had been achieved in medicine, and practitioners were not only able to return to the same methods as those practiced by earlier Greek and Roman cultures, but medical study was now encouraged.

Medical education in established universities began in the ninth century. These universities included Salerno in southern Italy, the University of Montpelier in southern France, and the University of Paris. By the time the Renaissance was at its height in the midfifteenth century, the physician had become licensed, was receiving great status, and was attending the ill in a velvet bonnet and fur-trimmed cloak.

Art and science were more closely related during the Renaissance than at any other period. Michelangelo (1475–1564) spent years on careful human dissection, and this anatomical detail is evident in his paintings in the Sistine Chapel in the Vatican in Rome. Leonardo da Vinci (1452–1519) made anatomical preparations from which he produced drawings representing the skeletal, muscular, nervous, and vascular systems. His accurate sketch of the spinal vertebrae went undiscovered for more than 100 years.

HISTORY OF ATTITUDES TOWARD ILLNESS

Various attitudes prevailed toward the ill person. A sick person might be excused from daily activity, but was likely to be shunned if the disease was believed to be a punishment by the gods for mortal sin. This forced isolation may well have been beneficial to the community. In contrast, touching by Jesus was an important component of healing, as was the faith of the individual involved. The New Testament parable of the Good Samaritan helped establish a nexus between the early church and a concern for the sick. It was believed that though the body might be wasted and foul with disease, the purity of the soul guaranteed life everlasting. This was unlike the pagan religions that tended to abandon individuals thought to be ill because they were in disfavor with the gods.

 Native Americans had various feelings about illness. The ill were treated with kindness among the Navaho and Cherokee, and some who recovered from serious illness were considered to have extraordinary powers. However, if a tribe was faced with famine, suicide by the aged and infirm was considered the highest form of bravery. The Eskimos put their older

adults unprotected onto ice floes. Neither the Romans nor the Greeks treated the hopelessly ill or deformed, and unwanted infants were disposed of quickly or left to die.

 Some of these attitudes are seen even today. The Western medical community and the consumers it serves are heatedly debating the right to choose life or death and the ethics and legality of physician-assisted suicide, which is acceptable in many other cultures. Even with our vast knowledge of medicine and the disease process, many individuals are still fearful of any illness they do not understand or that they perceive as threatening their health—AIDS is a good example. This fear is often accompanied by public ill treatment of the individuals suffering from certain diseases. For example, Cuba quarantines everyone who tests positive for human immunodeficiency virus (HIV) infection, even if they show no signs of illness.

HISTORICAL MEDICAL TREATMENTS

The writings of ancient Egypt reveal that when a woman suspected she was pregnant, she urinated over a mixture of wheat and barley seeds combined with dates and sand. If any of the grains sprouted, she was surely pregnant. If the wheat grew, she would have a boy. If the barley grew, it would be a girl. Urine is still used in modern tests to determine pregnancy.

During the Ming dynasty (1368–1644), Chinese medicine seemed to reach its peak. This is the time that Li Shih-chen wrote his Pen ts'ao kang mu, "The Great Herbal." This pharmacopoeia summarizes what was known of herbal medicine up to the late sixteenth century, describing in detail more than 1,800 plants, animal substances, minerals, and metals, together with their medicinal properties and applications.

Early medical treatments were often crude. For a sore throat, a physician might mix barley water, vinegar, and mulberry syrup for a gargle. Someone suffering with rheumatism might be given a prescription of chopped mice, lynx claws, and elk hooves. Rhubarb, senna, bitter apple, turpentine, camphor, and mercury were among the physicians' staples. Some physicians washed the instruments used in treating the ill; others scoffed at such a practice. **Malaria,** diphtheria, tuberculosis, **typhoid,** and dysentery were commonplace. Leprosy was prevalent; and venereal diseases were rife. Smallpox was frequent in villages; sometimes the sufferer would be placed in a meat pickling vat and fumigated. The death toll from such diseases was particularly high among children. Finally, in the eighteenth century, Edward Jenner made a great contribution to the prevention of disease by discovering a method of vaccination against smallpox.

Critical Thinking

What steps are taken today in hospitals and in ambulatory care settings to prevent the spread of harmful bacteria and viruses? What steps do you personally take?

Medicine progressed rapidly during the nineteenth century. Two important discoveries occurred: anesthesia to alleviate pain during surgery, and the realization that some bacteria cause disease. Once it had been proved that certain bacteria were causes of diseases and were transmissible agents responsible for contagion, greater care was taken to prevent that transmission. **Asepsis** became important to reduce the risk for infection. The Hungarian physician and obstetrician Ignaz Philipp Semmelweis (1818–1865) was able to prove that physicians who came from an autopsy directly to the care of postpartum women, without scrubbing their hands and washing instruments, carried infection with them that often caused puerperal fever (**septicemia** after childbirth) and death to the new mothers.

The names of Louis Pasteur (1822–1895), Joseph Lister (1827–1912), and Robert Koch (1843–1910) are familiar to all bacteriologists. Louis Pasteur has sometimes been referred to as the father of preventive medicine as the result of his work in recognizing the relationship between bacteria and infectious disease (Figure 3-2). Joseph Lister revolutionized surgery because of his belief in Pasteur's theory of using carbolic acid as an antiseptic spray. He insisted that all instruments and physicians' hands be washed with the solution. Robert Koch used the culture-plate method for isolating bacteria and demonstrated how cholera was transmitted by food and water. His discovery changed the way health departments cared for persons with infectious disease.

Fortunately, early in the twentieth century, society was finally liberated from many of the infectious and epidemic diseases that had scourged the human race for millennia. Smallpox vaccinations became common, and causes of **yellow fever, typhus,** and **bubonic plague** were determined. Life expectancy increased. Tuberculosis became less frequent. In 1922, Frederick G. Banting and a medical student, Charles Best, were able to isolate and inject insulin into a 14-year-old boy who was dying of diabetes. Two weeks later, the boy was alive and alert. By 1923, insulin was available for general sale in pharmacies throughout the world. Antibiotics were discovered and the Salk and Sabin vaccines were found for poliomyelitis.

The first electrocardiogram machine was invented in 1903. George Papanicolaou discovered cancer cells in 1928, the same year penicillin was discovered by

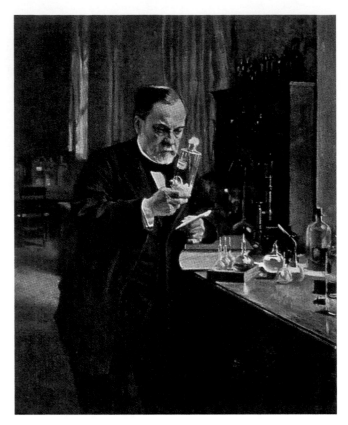

Figure 3-2 Louis Pasteur, the father of preventive medicine.

Alexander Fleming. Penicillin, however, required further development, which was accomplished by Howard Florey and Ernst Chain, and was finally brought into production in 1945. C. Walton Lillehei performed the first successful open-heart surgery in 1952. Dr. Christian Barnard performed the first human heart transplant in 1967. Advancing technology enabled medicine to march steadily forward.

Yet, as we enter the twenty-first century, we are quite aware of the limitations of modern medicine. AIDS is a reminder that plagues are still possible. In developing countries torn with war and strife, cholera causes the deaths of thousands simply because there is no proper sanitation. In the microbial world, there are new, drug-resistant strains of malaria, tuberculosis, and other diseases that are not responding to known treatments. The challenge of medicine is as strong today as it was 100 years ago.

Critical Thinking

Do you agree with the statement: "The challenge of medicine is as strong today as it was 100 years ago"? Identify your reasoning and give examples.

SIGNIFICANT CONTRIBUTIONS TO MEDICINE

Hippocrates (c. 460–c. 377 B.C.) is the physician most frequently recalled from the Greek culture. It is not known why his name surfaces above all other Greek physicians, for some were surely just as prominent. His writings, however, have contributed much to today's medical culture. Hippocrates is remembered by many for his well-known Hippocratic Oath, which established guidelines for a physician's practice of medicine. Although few physicians swear to this oath today when they embark on their medical career, it is still recognized for its validity and wisdom.

There are various translations of the Hippocratic Oath, but all communicate the same fundamental message.

It would be impossible to identify all the other individuals who made significant contributions to medicine in this text. However, Table 3-1 lists several notable individuals in the history of medicine.

FRONTIERS IN MEDICINE

There has been phenomenal growth in medicine in the past two decades. Only a few advances are mentioned here. Much better imaging leading to much better diagnosis is now available. Where exploratory surgery might have been

TABLE 3-1　IMPORTANT PERSONS AND EVENTS IN THE HISTORY OF MEDICINE

Moses (1205 B.C.)	Advocate of health rules in Hebrew religion
1000 B.C.	Beginnings of Ancient Chinese medicine
Hippocrates (460–377 B.C.)	Greek physician; "father of medicine"
Chang Chung-ching (168–196)	Chinese physician; called the Hippocrates of China
1368–1644	Chinese medicine reaches its peak
Andreas Vesalius (1514–1564)	Brussels physician; wrote first anatomical studies
Anton van Leeuwenhoek (1632–1723)	Dutch lens grinder; discovered lens magnification
John Hunter (1728–1793)	Founder of scientific surgery
Edward Jenner (1749–1823)	Developed smallpox vaccine
Rene Laennec (1781–1826)	Invented the stethoscope
Samuel Hahnemann (1755–1843)	German physician; established homeopathy
Ignaz Semmelweis (1818–1865)	Introduced hand washing to prevent childbed fever
W. T. G. Morton (1819–1868)	U.S. physician; introduced ether as anesthetic
Louis Pasteur (1822–1895)	"Father of bacteriology"
Florence Nightingale (1820–1910)	Founder of modern nursing
Elizabeth Blackwell (1821–1910)	First female physician in the United States
Clara Barton (1821–1912)	Started the American Red Cross in 1881
Joseph Lister (1827–1912)	Laid the groundwork on asepsis
Andrew Taylor (1828–1917)	Established the first school of osteopathy in 1892
Daniel David Palmer (1845–1913)	Founded chiropractic profession in Iowa in 1895
Elizabeth G. Anderson (1836–1917)	First female physician in Great Britain
Frederick G. Banting (1891–1941)	Isolated and injected insulin for diabetes treatment in 1922
1903	First electrocardiogram machine invented
Robert Koch (1843–1910)	Bacteriologist; developed culture-plate method
Wilhelm Roentgen (1845–1923)	Discovered X-rays (roentgenograms)
George Papanicolaou (1883–1962)	Discovered cancer cells in 1928
Sir Alexander Fleming (1881–1955)	Discovered penicillin in 1928
Albert Schatz (1920–2005)	Discovered streptomycin in 1943; cure for tuberculosis
1945	Penicillin brought into production
Paul Zoll (1911–1999)	Created the first heart pacemaker in 1952
C. Walton Lillehei (1918–1999)	Performed first successful open-heart surgery in 1952
John Gibbon (1903–1973)	First heart–lung machine used for surgery (1953)
Joseph Murray (1919–)	First person-to-person kidney transplant in 1954
Christian Barnard (1922–2001)	First human heart transplant performed in 1967
Ian Wilmut (1944–)	Cloned a Finn Dorset sheep called Dolly in 1996
1990–2000	Human genome map created by team of scientists
2000–present	Adult stem cells used in treatment of disease

THE OATH OF HIPPOCRATES

I swear by Apollo Physician and Aesculapius and Hygeia and Panacea and all the gods and goddesses, making them my witnesses, that I will fulfill according to my ability and judgment this oath and this covenant:

To hold him who has taught me this art as equal to my parents and to live my life in partnership with him, and if he is in need of money to give him a share of mine, and to regard his offspring as equal to my brothers in male lineage and to teach them this art—if they desire to learn it—without fee and covenant; to give a share of precepts and oral instruction and all the other learning to my sons and to the sons of him who has instructed me and to pupils who have signed the covenant and have taken an oath according to the medical law, but to no one else.

I will apply dietetic measures for the benefit of the sick according to my ability and judgment; I will keep them from harm and injustice.

I will neither give a deadly drug to anybody if asked for it nor will I make a suggestion to this effect. Similarly, I will not give to a woman an abortive remedy. In purity and holiness I will guard my life and my art.

I will not use the knife, not even on sufferers from stone, but will withdraw in favor of such men as are engaged in this work.

Whatever houses I may visit, I will come for the benefit of the sick, remaining free of all intentional injustice, of all mischief, and in particular of sexual relations with both female and male persons, be they free or slaves.

performed in the past to determine a diagnosis, noninvasive ultrasound, CT scans, and MRIs assist in diagnosis now. People who have worn glasses or contact lenses for many years are turning to laser eye surgery and implantable lenses.

Recently, surgeons performed the first successful human larynx transplant. Consider the implications of the AIDS saliva test that creates a needle-free way to test for HIV. Needleless injections are now possible. There is a flu prevention inhaler and an osteoporosis pill.

Since 2000 there has been successful use of adult stem cells in the treatment of some diseases. Adult bone marrow stem cells are able to produce multiple tissues, and adult stem cells from various organs of the body have shown amazing abilities to develop into healthy tissue. Adult stem cells can be stimulated to form insulin-secreting pancreatic cells, to repair eye retina damage, and to stimulate growth in children with bone disease. There is the possibility that the adult stem cells will also be able to treat Parkinson's disease and other degenerating neural disorders. In the meantime, the political debate continues over the use of human embryonic stem cells.

Experimentation with aromatherapy indicates that some aromas actually improve brain function. Research has shown that individuals suffering from dementia often respond favorably to the odor of freshly roasted coffee and bread baking. Inhaling the scents of green apple, banana, and peppermint stimulates positive feelings. It is thought that with aromatherapy we will soon accelerate learning and speed up rehabilitation for people who have had a stroke.

Who can possibly predict what the future will bring in medicine?

Case Study 3-1

You are a male physician on call in your hospital's emergency department when a woman, five months pregnant, is brought in. She is hemorrhaging. Her husband shuns you and demands a female physician. You quickly realize this couple is Muslim. Role-play this scenario with a classmate. How can you solve the dilemma? Consider the possibility that your only female physician is out of the country on vacation.

Case Study 3-2

Your physician–employer, Dr. Anne Shea, an internist in Southern California, is considering renting office space to an acupuncturist and a naturopath, because many of her patients often seek treatment from both. Dr. Shea believes her practice can be integrated, therefore allowing patients one-stop treatment for their illnesses. As the medical assistant and office manager, you are asked to participate in a meeting of all three practitioners to discuss guidelines for the clinic. What questions will you ask the group?

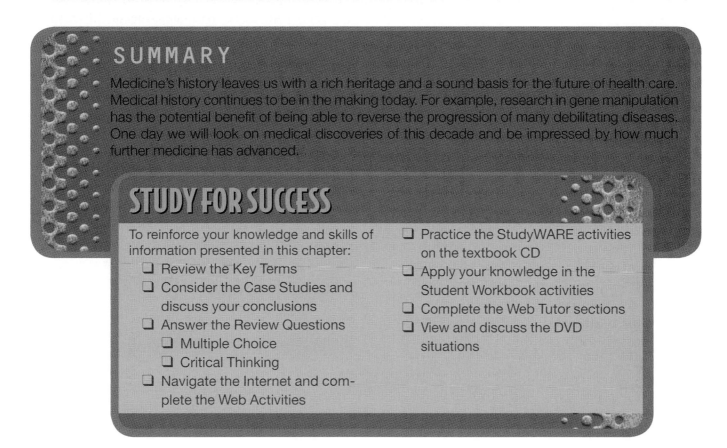

SUMMARY

Medicine's history leaves us with a rich heritage and a sound basis for the future of health care. Medical history continues to be in the making today. For example, research in gene manipulation has the potential benefit of being able to reverse the progression of many debilitating diseases. One day we will look on medical discoveries of this decade and be impressed by how much further medicine has advanced.

STUDY FOR SUCCESS

To reinforce your knowledge and skills of information presented in this chapter:

❏ Review the Key Terms
❏ Consider the Case Studies and discuss your conclusions
❏ Answer the Review Questions
   ❏ Multiple Choice
   ❏ Critical Thinking
❏ Navigate the Internet and complete the Web Activities

❏ Practice the StudyWARE activities on the textbook CD
❏ Apply your knowledge in the Student Workbook activities
❏ Complete the Web Tutor sections
❏ View and discuss the DVD situations

REVIEW QUESTIONS

Multiple Choice

1. A pharmacopoeia is:
   a. a book describing drugs and their preparation
   b. an ancient religious rite used in medicine
   c. a source of magic
   d. used only by twentieth-century physicians

2. At one time, women were typically allowed to use their health care skills to:
   a. cure everyone in society
   b. care only for women and to assist in childbirth
   c. become physicians
   d. care only for older adults

3. An accurate sketch of the spinal vertebrae was created during the Renaissance by:
   a. Leonardo da Vinci
   b. Michelangelo
   c. early Christian monks
   d. Louis Pasteur

4. Hippocrates is a Greek physician often called:
   a. the founder of scientific surgery
   b. the inventor of the smallpox vaccine
   c. the father of medicine
   d. the father of preventive medicine

5. The first woman physician in the United States was:
   a. Florence Nightingale
   b. Clara Barton
   c. Elizabeth Anderson
   d. Elizabeth Blackwell
6. The physician who introduced hand washing to prevent childbed fever was:
   a. Joseph Lister
   b. John Hunter
   c. Ignaz Semmelweis
   d. Edward Jenner
7. Medicine was greatly influenced by:
   a. Greek and Chinese physicians
   b. Culture and science
   c. Religion and magic
   d. b and c

Critical Thinking

1. With a group of peers, identify the effects of culture on today's medicine.
2. How does the role of a medical specialist today compare to the role of a medical specialist in the past? Consider both similarities and dissimilarities.
3. You are the medical assistant. Your physician–employer has just prescribed opiates for a young Asian woman suffering from migraine headaches. You overhear the young woman arguing with her mother who thinks that she should take non-addictive Chinese herbs. What, if anything, would you do?
4. Discuss with a peer the role of women in medicine today. What difficulties, if any, might a female physician face today? Compare today's difficulties with those of female health care practitioners 100 years ago.
5. Using the example of aromatherapy use in Frontiers in Medicine, identify any new frontiers using integrative medicine that you know about or have seen used in patient treatment.
6. Breakthroughs in medicine often have been realized through accident or a number of trial and error experiments. Human experimentation is also often necessary. Discuss the need for continued research, funding for research and experimentation, and how patients might often be involved.
7. From your personal experience and observations, identify ways in which physicians (both nontraditional and traditional) have been paid for their services. What major changes in the payment process have been evidenced in the last decade?

WEB ACTIVITIES

The World Wide Web is an ideal place to seek evidence of new and emerging technologies in medicine. One such avenue is "Medical Breakthroughs" reported by Ivanhoe Broadcast News, Inc. Identify at least two or three recent discoveries you find particularly interesting from your research on the Web.

1. Do an Internet search using the keywords "penicillin discovered" to find some interesting sites. Determine the reasons it took so long to put penicillin into production. What kind of hurdles do new medications face today before they are available on the market to consumers and patients?
2. Two physicians reviewed many medical discoveries to determine the 10 greatest discoveries in the history of Western medicine. Using the keywords "medicine's ten greatest discoveries," identify the names of the two physicians. How many discoveries were researched? What do these physicians name as the "greatest medical achievement of all time"? Are all 10 of the discoveries listed in this text? The two physicians are betting on cures for two ailments in the future. Name them. Have the cures been found?
3. Access the Internet to compare/contrast medical schools and universities in the United States with medical universities in China. What major differences do you note? Are there any similarities?

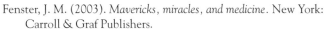

REFERENCES/BIBLIOGRAPHY

Fenster, J. M. (2003). *Mavericks, miracles, and medicine*. New York: Carroll & Graf Publishers.

Lewis, M. A., & Tamparo, C. D. (2002). *Medical law, ethics, and bioethics for ambulatory care* (5th ed.). Philadelphia: F.A. Davis.

Lyons, A. S., & Petrucelli II, J. R. (1978). *Medicine: An illustrated history*. New York: Harry N. Abrams, Inc.

Warden, C. D. (1986). *Health care in the 1980s from a consumer's perspective*. Unpublished doctoral dissertation, Union Graduate School, Seattle, WA.

UNIT 2
The Therapeutic Approach

Therapeutic Communication Skills

OUTLINE

OBJECTIVES

The student should strive to meet the following performance objectives and demonstrate an understanding of the facts and principles presented in this chapter through written and oral communication.

1. Define the key terms as presented in the glossary.
2. Identify the importance of communication.
3. List and define the four basic elements of the communication cycle.
4. Identify the four modes or channels of communication most pertinent in our everyday exchange.
5. Discuss the importance of active listening in therapeutic communication.

(continues)

KEY TERMS

Active Listening
Bias
Body Language
Buffer Words
Closed Questions
Clustering
Compensation
Congruency
Cultural Brokering
Decode
Defense Mechanism
Denial
Displacement
Encoding
Hierarchy of Needs
Indirect Statements
Interview Techniques
Kinesics
Masking
Open-Ended Questions
Perception
Prejudice
Projection
Rationalization
Regression
Repression
Roadblocks
Sublimation
Therapeutic
   Communication
Undoing

Patient Care

• Perform telephone and in-person screening

Professional Communications

• Recognize and respond to verbal communications

• Recognize and respond to nonverbal communications

• Demonstrate telephone techniques

Patient Instruction

• Instruct individuals according to their needs

• Identify community resources

ABHES—ENTRY-LEVEL COMPETENCIES

Communication

• Be attentive, listen, and learn

• Be impartial and show empathy when dealing with patients

• Adapt what is said to the recipient's level of comprehension

• Serve as liaison between physician and others

• Use proper telephone techniques

• Interview effectively

• Use appropriate medical terminology

• Recognize and respond to verbal and non-verbal communication

• Principles of verbal and nonverbal communication

• Adaptation for individualized needs

Administrative Duties

• Locate resources and information for patients and employers

OBJECTIVES (continued)

6. Differentiate between the terms *verbal* and *nonverbal communication.*

7. Analyze the five Cs of communication, and describe their effectiveness in the communication cycle.

8. Demonstrate the following body language or nonverbal communication behaviors: facial expressions, territoriality, position, posture, gestures/mannerisms, and touch.

9. Identify and explain congruency in communication.

10. Discuss the use of Maslow's hierarchy of needs in therapeutic communication.

11. Recall at least four influences on therapeutic communication related to culture, and describe four common biases/prejudices in today's society.

12. Recall at least three steps to building trust with culturally diverse patients.

13. Discuss cultural brokering and its use in medical facilities.

14. Discuss communication modification for electronically transmitted messages.

15. Recall eight significant roadblocks to therapeutic communication.

16. List and describe seven common defense mechanisms.

17. Compare/contrast closed questions, open-ended questions, and indirect statements.

18. List four tools or considerations when communicating on the telephone.

19. Demonstrate the correct way to speak into the mouthpiece of a telephone by answering an incoming call and closing a telephone conversation.

SCENARIO

In the two-doctor office of Drs. Lewis and King, four medical assistants constantly interact with patients, allaying their concerns, scheduling their appointments, instructing them on medications, and helping them understand their insurance coverage. On any given day, office manager Marilyn Johnson, CMA, is greeting patients warmly as they arrive for their appointments. Some patients, such as Anna and Joseph Ortiz, are new to the practice. Marilyn's warm manner puts them at ease. Other patients, such as Martin Gordon, who has prostate cancer, may be depressed and anxious. Marilyn tries to create an environment where they feel free to share their concerns and anxieties.

While Marilyn is busy with patients, administrative medical assistant Ellen Armstrong, CMA, is on the telephone, scheduling appointments, answering patient questions, and making decisions about what calls need priority attention. Ellen projects a warm, courteous presence over the telephone; she maintains her composure, even when faced with difficult calls, and tries always to ask the right questions of callers in a nonthreatening manner.

INTRODUCTION

Of all the tasks and skills required of the medical assistant in the ambulatory care setting, none is quite so important as communication. Communication is the foundation for every action taken by health care professionals in the care of their patients. Because medical assistants are often the liaison between patient and physician, it is critical to be aware of all the complexities of the communication process.

Everyday, Marilyn, Ellen, and the two clinical medical assistants at the offices of Drs. Lewis and King face many communication challenges. This chapter describes effective communication principles, applies those principles to face-to-face communication, as well as telephone communication, and describes the basic roadblocks to communication. The key word to all communication in the medical setting is therapeutic. In all conversations with patients, the more therapeutic the conversation, the more satisfied the patient will be with the care provided.

IMPORTANCE OF COMMUNICATION

Therapeutic communication differs from normal communication in that it introduces an element of empathy into what can be a traumatic experience for the patient. It imparts a feeling of comfort in the face of even the most horrific news about the patient's prognosis. The patient is made to feel validated and respected. Therapeutic communication uses specific and well-defined professional skills.

Communication in the health care setting is the foundation of all patient care and is of the utmost importance. Communication must be in nontechnical language the patient can understand, delivered with feeling for the patient's emotional situation and state of mind, yet it still must be technically accurate. The medical staff must be alert to the patient's state of stress and whether defense mechanisms have taken over to the extent that the patient has "tuned out" and is no longer communicating with the staff.

Patients seeking an ambulatory care service look for medical professionals with technical skills and a clinical staff capable of communicating with them. Questions frequently asked by individuals seeking a new physician and clinic include: "Will the doctor talk with me so that I understand?" "Will the doctor listen to what I have to say?" and "Can I talk to the doctor honestly and openly?" The answer to all of these questions needs to be "yes." This chapter discusses these issues and presents some specific techniques for therapeutic communication.

BIASES AND PREJUDICES

Personal preferences, biases, and prejudices will enter into many physician–patient relationships. Such biases affect the types of communication possible. When individuals are not aware of their biases or prejudices, hostile attitudes may prevail.

For therapeutic communication to take place, biases must be examined, a person's comfort level with each bias determined, and measures taken to ensure that a hostile attitude is not present. **Bias** is defined as a slant toward a particular belief. **Prejudice** is defined as an opinion or judgment that is formed before all the facts are known; prejudice is a preconceived and unfavorable concept. Common biases and prejudices in today's society include:

1. A preference for Western style medicine
2. Choosing physicians according to gender
3. Prejudice related to a person's sexual preference
4. Discrimination based on race or religion
5. Hostile attitudes toward people with different value systems than one's own

Critical Thinking

Define in your own words the terms *bias* and *prejudice*. Now identify one bias and one prejudice that you have. How will these impact your ability to respond therapeutically in the medical setting? What steps can you take to become more accepting of the uniqueness of others, thereby improving therapeutic communication?

6. A belief that people who cannot afford health care should receive less care than someone who can pay for full services

 Medical assistants must recognize such biases and prejudices so that their own culture with its biases does not prevent them from responding therapeutically in communications with patients. Such recognition requires being aware of the differences among human beings and willingly accepting the uniqueness of each person.

THE COMMUNICATION CYCLE

All communication, whether social or therapeutic, involves two or more individuals participating in an exchange of information. The communication cycle involves sending and receiving messages even when unconsciously aware of them.

Four basic elements are included in the communication cycle. They are: (1) the sender, (2) the message and a channel or mode of communication, (3) the receiver, and (4) feedback (Figure 4-1).

The Sender

The sender begins the communication cycle by **encoding** or creating the message to be sent. This is an important step, and much care should be taken in formulating the message. Before creating the message, the sender must observe the receiver to determine the complexity of the words to be used within the message, the receiver's ability to interpret the message, and the best channel by which to send the message.

The Message

The message is the content being communicated. The message must be understood clearly by the receiver. Various levels of complexity in communication are used depending on the ability of the receiver to recognize and

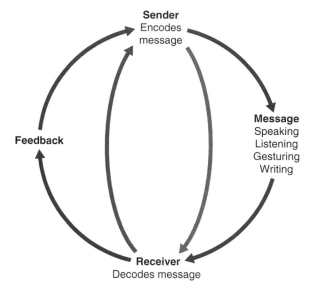

Figure 4-1   The communication cycle and channels of communication.

understand the words contained within the message. Children do not have the vocabulary base or the cognitive skills to communicate and understand at the same level as adults. The health of the receiver also must be considered. A patient who is experiencing stress or in pain may find it difficult to concentrate on the message. If the patient is of a different nationality or culture from the sender, verbal communication may require special skill. When visual or hearing acuity is impaired, another challenge must be surmounted.

The four modes of communication, also called channels of communication, most pertinent in our everyday exchange include: (1) speaking, (2) listening, (3) gestures or body language, and (4) writing. These modes or channels are affected by our physical and mental development, our culture, our education and life experiences, our impressions from models and mentors, and in general by how we feel and accept ourselves as individuals. Each mode or channel of communication has its appropriateness and must be considered when formulating the message.

The Receiver

The receiver is the recipient of the sender's message. The receiver must **decode,** or interpret, the meaning of the message. The primary sensory skill used in verbal communication is listening. It is hard work to concentrate and listen. When decoding the message, the receiver must be aware that not only the spoken words, but the tone and pitch of the voice and the speed at which the words are spoken carry meaning and must be evaluated.

The idea of minimum necessary access to protected health information (PHI) is important to job performance. HIPAA requires that a reasonable effort be made to limit access to PHI to only what is necessary to accomplish the intended purposes of the use, disclosure, or request. The information accessed must fit the needs of the job description and nothing more. Employees must be careful to not discuss PHI with those outside the scope of their work. For example, a Certified Medical Administrative Specialist scheduling appointments does not need to know the diagnosis after the patient has been seen by the physician.

Feedback

Feedback takes place after the receiver has decoded the message sent by the sender. Feedback is the receiver's way of ensuring that the message that is understood is the same as the message that was sent. Feedback also provides an opportunity for the receiver to clarify any misunderstanding regarding the original message and to ask for additional information.

LISTENING SKILLS

A vital part of feedback in the communication cycle is listening. A good listener is alert to all aspects of the communication cycle—the verbal and nonverbal message, as well as verification of the message through appropriate feedback.

Active listening is one method used in therapeutic communication. In this technique, the received message is sent back to the sender, worded a little differently, for verification from the sender.

Sender: "How can I possibly pay this fee when I have no insurance?"
Receiver: "You're worried about paying your bill?"

The preceding example illustrates how the receiver is able to validate the sender's concerns at the same time the message is checked for accuracy. The door is then left open for a therapeutic response, such as:

Sender: "Our bookkeeper will be glad to work out a payment plan with you that will fit your resources."

Active listening involves listening with a "third ear," that is, being aware of what the patient is *not* saying or

picking up on hints to the real message by observing body language. The health care professional should have three listening goals:

- To improve listening skills sufficiently so that patients are heard accurately

- To listen either for what is *not* being said or for information transmitted only by hints

- To determine how accurately the message has been received

So many health professionals try to "fix" everything with a recommendation, a prescription, even advice. Sometimes, none of those things is necessary. The patient simply needs someone to listen, to acknowledge the difficulty, and to remember that the patient is not helpless in finding a solution to the problem.

Skill in communication takes years of practice and frequent review. It will never become perfect; we can only hope that we will become better at it with each passing day. Communication is and always will be the basis for any therapeutic relationship (Tamparo & Lindh, 2000).

TYPES OF COMMUNICATION

We communicate by what we say, and also by our tone of voice, body movements, and facial expressions. The following paragraphs present the aspects of verbal and nonverbal communication. The importance of maintaining consistency between verbal and nonverbal messages also is stressed.

VERBAL COMMUNICATION

Verbal communication takes place when the message is spoken. However, one must keep in mind that unless the words have meaning, and unless the sender and the receiver apply the same meaning to the spoken words, verbal communication may be misunderstood. If, for example, you overhear a conversation in a language foreign to you, you are indeed a witness to verbal communication, but you may not understand the message. To have any meaning, the spoken word must be understood by all parties of the communication (Tamparo & Lindh, 2000).

The Five Cs of Communication

In the book *Professional Development*, Mary Wilkes and C. Bruce Crosswait (1995) identify the five Cs of Communication in business. They are: (1) complete, (2) clear, (3) concise, (4) courteous, and (5) cohesive. These five Cs apply equally well in health care professions.

Complete. The message must be complete, with all the necessary information given. The medical assistant cannot expect the patient to be compliant if all the instructions are not given and understood.

Clear. The information given in the message must also be clear. The use of eye contact enhances clarity. Health care professionals must be able to articulate by using good diction and by enunciating each word distinctly. The patient must be allowed time to process the message and verify its meaning. The message must also be heard to promote understanding.

Concise. A concise message is one that does not include any unnecessary information. It should be brief and to the point (Figure 4-2). Patients must not be overloaded with technical terms that may not be understood or that tend to distract them by diverting their attention away from the balance of the message.

Courteous. Courtesy is important in all aspects of communication. It only takes a moment to acknowledge a patient with a smile or by name. Knocking on the examination room door before entering validates the patient's right to privacy and builds self-esteem.

When a patient must be placed on hold on the telephone, thank the patient for waiting. Try not to keep the patient waiting too long if you must find information.

Remember to be courteous to colleagues in the office. Good working relationships and professionalism are always enhanced by simple courtesy.

Cohesive. A cohesive message is organized and logical in its progression. The cohesive message does not ramble and does not jump from one subject to another. The patient should be able to follow the message easily. The medical assistant should always allow time to summarize

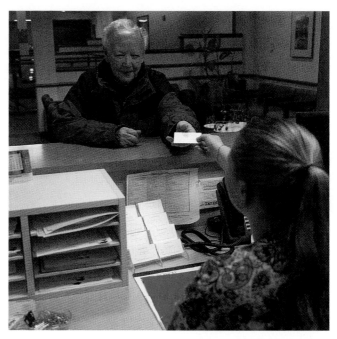

Figure 4-2 To say to the patient after greeting her by name, "I've completed an appointment card to remind you of your next appointment, Tuesday at 2:00 PM," is an example of a concise message that is brief and to the point.

detailed messages and use responding skills to verify that the patient fully understands the message.

When communicating within the health professions, keep in mind the following:

1. Good communication skills are necessary in establishing rapport with patients.
2. Patients feel respected and validated when called by their full name, such as Mary O'Keefe or Mrs. O'Keefe.
3. Patients should be encouraged to verbalize their feelings.
4. Patients should be given technical information in a manner that they can understand.
5. Patients should be allowed to make practical application to their personal health needs.

NONVERBAL COMMUNICATION

Verbal communication alone is not always adequate in conveying the message being sent. In most instances, more than one mode or channel of communication is used. Nonverbal communication, often referred to as **body language,** includes the unconscious body movements, gestures, and facial expressions that accompany speech. The study of body language is known as **kinesics** (Figure 4-3).

Patient Education

Sensitive medical assistants will encourage patients to verbalize their concerns. The ability to ask questions in a nonprobing way and to elicit patient response is an important function in any ambulatory care setting, because it is critical to know a patient's history, current medications, and other relevant data.

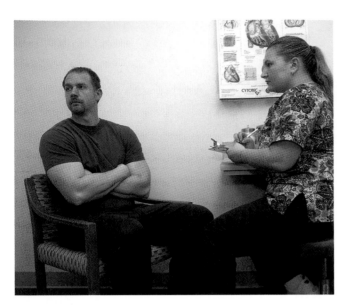

Figure 4-3 Body language can communicate more than spoken words.

Nonverbal communication is the language we learn first. It is learned seemingly automatically when infants learn to return a smile or respond to touches on the cheek. Much of our body language is a learned behavior and is greatly influenced by the primary caregivers and the culture in which we are raised.

Feelings and emotions are communicated most often through nonverbal means. The body expresses its true repressed feelings using body language. Most of the negative messages we communicate are also expressed nonverbally and usually are unintentional. Experts tell us that 70% of communication is nonverbal. The tone of voice communicates 23% of the message—only 7% of the message is actually communicated by the spoken word (Wilkes & Crosswait, 1995).

Facial Expression

Facial expression is considered one of the most important and observed nonverbal communicators. Each facet or aspect of the anatomy of the face sends a nonverbal message.

Often expressions of joy and happiness or sorrow and grief are reflected through the eyes. The anatomy of the eyes does not change, but the movements of the structures surrounding the eyes enhance or magnify the message being communicated.

Children are told it is not polite to stare at people. It is acceptable to stare at animals in the zoo or art objects in the museum, but not at humans. Staring is dehumanizing and is often interpreted as an invasion of privacy.

The medical assistant must learn not to stare when patients present with ailments that make them "look" different. Patients such as these are individuals who have needs, who perhaps feel pain and discomfort, and who have decreased self-esteem and value. These feelings will only be amplified if the medical assistant and other health professionals are unable to "see" them as humans. A lack of eye contact may also be viewed as avoidance or disinterest in being involved.

The movements of the eyebrow indicate many non-verbal cues as well. Surprise, puzzlement, worry, amusement, and questioning are often nonverbal messages reflected by the position of the eyebrow. Wrinkling of the forehead sends similar messages.

 Cultural influences affect customs and different forms of facial expressions. It is important to remember that there are many cross-cultural similarities in body language, but there are also many differences. Various cultures denote different meanings to various gestures. If your patient is from another culture, never assume that gestures used hold the same meaning for the patient as they do for you. For example, some cultures believe that prolonged eye contact is rude and an invasion of privacy, whereas others consider it a sign of intimacy. Some people stare at the floor when concentrating or thinking through a process. Other cultures avoid eye contact to display modesty, whereas others feel eye contact expresses hostility or aggression. It is important to understand the cultures of the patients treated in the facility in which you are employed.

Territoriality

Territoriality is the distance at which we feel comfortable with others while communicating. In the classroom, for example, students claim their territory the first day of class. The area is well defined by using books and papers, or by placing the arm, hand, or chair on boundary lines. When another invades the territory, a shift in body position or the use of eye contact sends the message, "This is my area." Individuals may feel threatened when others invade their personal space without permission. Some examples of comfortable personal space for U.S. culture are as follows:

- Intimate: touching to 6 inches

- Personal: 1½ to 4 feet

- Social: 4 to 12 feet

- Public: 12 to 15 feet

As with facial expressions, territoriality or personal space will be handled differently by various cultures. For example, there is no word for privacy in the Japanese language. Population numbers require crowding together publicly, as well as privately. Public crowding is often viewed as a sign of warmth and pleasant intimacy in Japan. In the private home, several generations may live together; however, each considers this space to be his own and resents intrusion into it.

 Arabs like to touch their companions, to feel and to smell them. To deny a friend your breath is to be ashamed. When two Arabs talk to each other, they look each other in the eyes with great intensity. U.S. businessmen often end a business arrangement with a handshake; however, American Indians may view a handshake as an act of aggression or an offensive behavior. Each culture has its own distinct nonverbal communication cues.

The medical assistant may perform many invasive tasks during the course of an office visit. Examples include taking vital signs or giving injections, both of which require touching the patient. It is beneficial to explain procedures that invade another's space before beginning the procedure so that it will not be perceived as threatening. This helps to empower the patient by involving the patient in the decision-making process and builds a sense of trust in the medical assistant.

Posture

Like territoriality, posture is important to allied health care professionals. Posture relates to the position of the body or parts of the body. It is the manner in which we carry ourselves, or pose in situations. We tend to tighten up in threatening or unknown situations and to relax in nonthreatening environments. Those who study kinesics believe that a posture involves at least half the body, and that the position can last for nearly five minutes.

When the patient is seated with the arms and legs crossed, the message of closure or being opinionated may be relayed. In contrast, sitting in a chair relaxed with the hands clasped behind the head indicates an attitude of being open to suggestions. Slumped shoulders may signal depression, discouragement, or, in some cases, even pain.

Position

Position, the physical stance of two individuals while communicating, is a key factor to consider while communicating with the patient. Most physician–patient relationships use the face-to-face communication arrangement. When speaking with a patient, the physician or medical assistant will want to maintain a close but comfortable position, enabling observation of all cues being sent, both verbal and nonverbal (Figure 4-4).

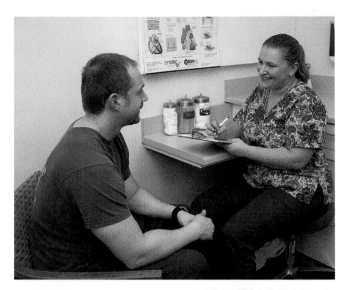

Figure 4-4 Positive posture and position encourage therapeutic communication.

Standing over a patient can convey a message of superiority, and too much distance between the two parties may be interpreted as avoidance or exclusivity. Generally, leaning toward the patient expresses warmth, caring, interest, acceptance, and trust. Moving away from the patient may be interpreted as dislike, disinterest, boredom, indifference, suspicion, or impatience.

Whenever possible, it is best to have a chair in the examination room and to have the patient seated comfortably in the chair to begin the communication cycle. The medical assistant or physician can sit on a stool that can be moved easily toward the patient. This arrangement aids the patient in feeling valued, listened to, and cared for as a fellow human being.

Gestures and Mannerisms

Most of us use gestures and mannerisms when we "talk" with our hands. This form of body language may be useful in enhancing the spoken word by emphasizing ideas, thus creating and holding the attention of others.

Touch

Touch is a powerful tool that communicates what cannot be expressed in words. Its appropriateness in the patient/health professional relationship has well-defined boundaries and requires the use of good judgment on the part of the professional. Infants who are not touched, cuddled, and loved do not grow and develop as those who receive these reassuring gestures. Children of Vietnamese, Cambodian, Hmong, or Thai families traditionally consider the head to be the site of the soul. During conversation and patient assessment, avoid touching the patient's head unless it is necessary for the examination. Southeast Asian clients may fear bodily intrusion; therefore, physical examination and treatment procedures should be explained carefully and completely before they are performed. The touch that communicates caring, sincerity, understanding, and reassurance is usually welcomed and considered to be a therapeutic response. Most patients will understand and accept the touching behavior as it relates to the medical setting; however, we must remember that not all patients are comfortable with touch. Whenever the patient is not comfortable with touch, ask permission and create as safe and reassuring an environment as possible.

CONGRUENCY IN COMMUNICATION

Using some keys to successful communication promotes effective communication. There must be **congruency** between the verbal and nonverbal communication. Shaking your head NO while saying YES verbally sends a mixed message. In most cases, the nonverbal messages will be accepted as the intended message.

It is also important to remember that most nonverbal messages are sent in groups of various forms of body language. The grouping of nonverbal messages into statements or conclusions is known as **clustering. Masking** involves an attempt to conceal or repress the true feeling or message. The perceptive professional will be aware of all these messages.

Perception as it relates to communication is the conscious awareness of one's own feelings and the feelings of others. To be most useful and therapeutic as health professionals, we must first explore our own feelings and appreciate and accept ourselves.

Learning to use perception involves the ability to sense another's attitudes, moods, and feelings. It takes practice and experience to develop and use this skill effectively. Being attentive to other professionals and observing their use of perception will yield insight into its usefulness and provide an example to emulate. A word of caution—the use of perception may easily be misinterpreted, especially when going with your feeling or assessment of what is happening regarding the patient. Always follow perceived assessments with verbal validation before assuming your perception of the circumstance is correct.

Nonverbal communication is easily misinterpreted. Careful observation for congruency between verbal and nonverbal communication, and clustering nonverbal cues being sent into nonverbal statements will strengthen our ability to interpret the message accurately.

CULTURAL INFLUENCE ON THERAPEUTIC COMMUNICATION

 For true therapeutic communication to take place, the influence of culture must be considered. Cultural influences include one's ethnic heritage, geographic location and background, genetics, age, sex, economics, educational experiences, life experiences, and value systems.

Any or all of these influences may exhibit themselves when health care is sought by patients. A patient's ethnic heritage may indicate a slant toward the Eastern influence in medicine as opposed to the traditional Western style more commonly taught in the United States today. Geographic location and background may indicate that a person is more comfortable with a family physician in a small clinic than one in a large metropolitan multispecialty practice.

Age and sex are factors with a strong influence on communication. How and when do you communicate with a young child? What do you communicate to that child? How do you impress upon an older gentleman who has taken little medications throughout his lifetime that he now must take his pill everyday? In a culture where the husband is the authority, how does the doctor discuss with the female patient the inadvisability of another pregnancy at this time?

The influence of economics may reveal a discomfort if the office staff and patients have a different perception about how billing is managed and when and how payment is expected. A discussion of billing and payment procedures at the first office visit or before a major procedure will be beneficial to all concerned parties.

Educational and life experiences will, in part, determine how patients react to their care. Patients with family members being treated for a chronic illness will have more knowledge and understanding of that illness in their own lives. Individuals who have already suffered a great deal of loss and grief in their lives may handle the information of a life-threatening illness more calmly than someone who has experienced little grief.

Establishing Cross-Cultural Communication

Before cross-cultural communication or any therapeutic communication can begin, the patient must first be willing to discuss his or her health care issues, listen to the professional's questions, and give honest answers to those questions. The patient must trust the professional. Several steps to building trust include:

- Risk/Trust: The need for the helping professional to build an atmosphere of trust, making it easier for the patient to risk expressing feelings and attitudes about the problem, is essential. Trust has to be earned. Remember to promise no more than you can deliver, be honest, and carefully and thoroughly explain procedures and policies. Answer all questions truthfully and honestly.

- Empathy: Empathy is the ability to accept another's private world as if it were your own. Empathy communicates identification with and understanding of another's situation. It states, "I'm available to walk this road with you."

- Respect: Respect values another person and considers him or her as a special individual. It is important to respect the patient's personal space, to provide privacy, and to use his or her full name and title when appropriate.

- Genuineness: This means being real and honest with others. The health care professional must be able to communicate honestly with others, while being careful not to blame or condemn.

- Active listening: Active listening involves verbal and nonverbal clues that send the message you are completely involved in the communication. Sit facing the patient with no barriers, such as a desk, between you. Lean toward the patient slightly to convey genuine concern and interest. Establish and maintain appropriate eye contact to elicit interest and concern. Maintain an open, relaxed posture to establish a nonthreatening environment for the patient. Listen carefully to the words the patient uses to describe problems, and use those terms rather than medical terminology when discussing symptoms.

Cultural Brokering

Cultural brokering is "the act of bridging, linking, or mediating between groups or persons through the process of reducing conflict or producing change" (National Center for Cultural Competence, Georgetown University Center for Child and Human Development, Georgetown University Medical Center, 2004). A cultural broker serves as a go-between, or one who advocates on behalf of another individual or group within the health care community. The 2000 Census indicates the projected demographic trends in the United States are more complex than ever measured previously. The belief systems related to health, healing, and wellness are diverse, with many cultural variations in the perception of illness and disease and their causes. Cultural brokers respect the values of diverse cultures and health care systems and are knowledgeable of both. They are able to overcome any existing language barriers, so that everyone understands each other clearly. The goal of the Cultural Broker Project is to increase the capacity of health care and mental health programs to design, implement, and evaluate culturally and linguistically competent service delivery systems. Cultural and linguistic competence have been determined to be fundamental in the goal of eliminating racial and ethnic disparities in health care. The project also defines the values, characteristics, areas of awareness, knowledge, and skills required of a cultural broker. The Cultural Broker Project is tailored to the needs and preferences of health care settings of the communities served by the program.

Cultural brokers may assume the role of medical interpreter. An interpreter is one who takes the spoken message in one language and converts it to another language. Interpreters do not provide word-to-word equivalence, but rather focus on the accurate expression of equivalent meaning. They serve as communicators and liaisons between the patient and the provider in health care facilities. If an interpreter is necessary, it is important to remember to speak directly to the patient, not the interpreter. If English is the second language or a heavy accent is involved, speaking clearly and slowly can greatly enhance communication.

In some cases, a family member may serve as the interpreter. This may not be the best solution, because the family member may not understand the medical terminology. It would also be difficult for a family member to be the one to share a life-threatening diagnosis or a poor prognosis.

Patient Education

Do not assume that a patient who does not speak English, or does not speak it fluently, is stupid, does not understand, and cannot pay.

Maslow's Hierarchy of Needs

Abraham Maslow is considered the founder of humanistic psychology and is most well known for his **hierarchy of needs** (Figure 4-5). *Webster's Dictionary* defines hierarchy as "a group of persons or things arranged in order of rank, grade, class etc." According to Maslow's theory, human needs could be grouped into five levels. He also theorized that each level of need must be satisfied before one could move on to the next level.

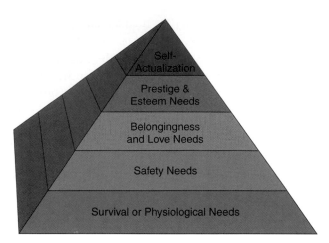

Figure 4-5 Maslow's hierarchy of needs.

The needs in the first level include physiologic or survival needs. These needs include food, water, and air to breathe—homeostasis for the body. The second level includes needs of safety and security; that is, the need for security, stability, and protection. Everyone has the desire to be free from fear and anxiety. Safety needs also include the need for structure, law and order, and limits.

The third level involves belonging and love needs. This level of need involves both giving and receiving affection. Additional words that express our connectedness are roots, origins, peers, friends, family, neighborhood, territory, clan, class, and gang. We have a basic animal tendency to herd, flock, join, and belong.

The fourth level, prestige and esteem needs, come from a basic need for a stable, healthy self-respect for ourselves and others. There is the desire for achievement, strength, and confidence. Also, there is the need for recognition, prestige, reputation, status, and even fame. Satisfaction of these needs leads to feelings of self-confidence and worth. The final level is self-actualization. In this stage, we are at our peak, doing what truly fits us. It is an achievement of potential.

Individuals may move back and forth from one need to another depending on circumstances.

Critical Thinking

An established patient arrives 20 minutes early for his appointment. He is in obvious pain and discomfort and tells the receptionist, "I can't sleep, I can't eat, and I can't go to work today." Which of Maslow's stages most accurately describes this patient? What actions should the medical assistant take to assist this patient?

Understanding this hierarchy helps to assess a patient's needs. If the most basic of needs are not met, it is highly unlikely that a patient can be successful with any treatment protocol. Keeping this hierarchy in mind will help to facilitate therapeutic communication.

COMMUNITY RESOURCES

There may be circumstances in which a patient will need a referral to a community resource. These resources range from the more simple acts of arranging with Meals on Wheels to deliver a hot meal daily to making complex arrangements for skilled nursing facilities or hospice care. The medical assistant will need to know the patient's name, address, and telephone number, as well as the particular resource needed, the diagnosis, and the reason for the service.

It is helpful to have a list of community resources readily available. The list may be computerized, or hardcopy information may be filed in a notebook. The information should be put into categories for ease in locating it quickly. See Procedure 4-1 for steps in developing a Community Resource Reference.

TECHNOLOGY AND COMMUNICATION

Face-to-face communication is the mode of choice in most physician offices today. However, technological devices are becoming more and more accepted as a means of communication. Technology-mediated communication and a greater reliance on cyberspace technology will greatly affect communication in the twenty-first century. Examples of new technologies in medical offices include interactive videoconferencing, clinical e-mail, automated routing units, instant messaging, paging systems (see Chapter 12), and physician digital assistants (PDAs) (see Chapters 11 and 12).

Do these new communication methods change the communication cycle? There is still a message, a sender, a receiver, and feedback. What changes is the way in which the message is encoded and decoded. The content of the message will be examined for credibility rather than one's dress, eye contact, facial expression, vocal inflection, and posture. Technology does not convey emotions nearly as well as face-to-face or even telephone conversations. Another factor to consider is that your composed message may not look like what your reader sees. The software and hardware that you use for composing, sending, sorting, downloading, and reading may be completely different from what your recipient uses. Modifications to the format may change the intended emphasis or meaning of the message.

There are several advantages for the use of e-mail rather than postal mail (commonly referred to as "snail mail"). E-mail is less expensive and faster than mailing a letter. Because the turnaround time can be so fast, e-mail is more conversational than traditional paper-based media. An e-mail transmission is less intrusive than a telephone call and less bother than a fax. When one uses e-mail transmissions, differences in location and time zone are less of a problem. See Chapters 11 and 15 for additional information regarding e-mail.

ROADBLOCKS TO THERAPEUTIC COMMUNICATION

Being sensitive to patients' unique personalities and needs will enable the health care professional to avoid **roadblocks** to communication (Table 4-1).

It must be the concern of each health care professional to facilitate communication by encouraging and enabling patients to express themselves honestly without fear. Roadblocks close communication and prevent quality care of the total person.

DEFENSE MECHANISMS

When patients are frightened, ashamed, guilty, or threatened, they often will resort to defense mechanisms as a means of avoiding injury to their ego. We all use them to some limited extent, but they become harmful when they result in a breakdown in therapeutic communication. Failure by the patient to face problems often results in inability to provide satisfactory treatment on the part of the medical practitioner. Recognizing common defense mechanisms enables the medical staff to minimize the triggering event and to communicate more effectively.

Defense mechanisms are defined as behavior that is used to protect the ego from guilt, anxiety, or loss of esteem. Employment of defense mechanisms is most often unconscious to the person using them. It is the body's way of seeking relief from uncomfortable or painful reality. A mentally healthy person uses defense mechanisms to put a problem on hold until sufficient time has passed to permit him or her to address it without unacceptable emotional pain. Excessive use of defense mechanisms or failure to address a problem even after sufficient time has elapsed is a sign of a mental health issue.

Defense mechanisms are usually readily apparent to the disaffected observer; however, they are difficult to analyze without knowledge of the motive behind the behavior. The following paragraphs describe some commonly observed defense mechanisms.

Regression is an attempt to withdraw from an unpleasant circumstance by retreating to an earlier, more secure stage of life. It is usually used when the person feels powerless to affect the events causing the pain; it can be thought of as a desperation move. A toddler's regression to bed-wetting or soiling himself or herself shortly after a new baby arrives in the family is an example of this defense mechanism. Use of a security blanket by an adult or child when faced with something that disrupts his or her life is another example.

Denial is refusal to accept painful information that is readily apparent to others. This defense mechanism commonly is encountered in the case of a person being diagnosed with a disease such as cancer or experiencing the death of a close family member or associate. Denial has a devastating effect on communication. The person will not hear what you say, but will quite frequently acknowledge what you are saying. Careful attention to what the person is saying will reveal that he or she does not accept his or her situation and is not mentally conscious that it is happening. Denial is often the first stage of an emotional response after a traumatic event. The next stage is anger toward the event, the medical staff,

TABLE 4-1 ROADBLOCKS TO COMMUNICATION

Roadblock	Example
Reassuring clichés	"Don't worry, Mr. McKay, about not having a job; you'll find another one really soon."
Moralizing/lecturing	"If you were smart, Mrs. Johnson, you'd lose fifty pounds and you wouldn't have such a problem with your diabetes and hypertension."
Requiring explanations	"Why would you not want to have chemotherapy, Mr. Gordon? Seeing your wife die of cancer should surely make you want to seek treatment."
Ridiculing/shaming	"Ha, ha, Mr. Gordon! It's not *prostrate*—it's prostate cancer."
Defending/contradicting	"Mr. Marshal, I assure you the physician is *very busy*. He will not see you until he has finished with his other patients."
Shifting subjects	"Yes, Mrs. Jover, your work is very interesting, but I must ask you to sign this permission form to test for HIV."
Criticizing	"Mrs. O'Keefe, why in the world would you stay with an abusive husband?"
Threatening	"There is no way you will get rid of this cough if you do not stop smoking, Mr. Fowler."

God, or others. The stage after anger is frequently depression. A mentally healthy person eventually reaches the final stage of acceptance.

Repression is similar to denial, but it is a totally unconscious reaction. In the case of repression, the person seems to experience temporary amnesia. It is the mind's way of defending itself from mental trauma by forgetting or wiping things out of the conscious memory. A child unconsciously forgetting to tell parents that he or she got into trouble at school is an example. The fear associated with the event becomes overwhelming, causing the mind to forget. Repression should not be confused with outright lying. In severe cases, repression can be related to mental illness.

Projection is attributing unacceptable desires, impulses, and thoughts falsely to others to avoid acknowledging they are actually the person's own experiences. It is a means of defending against feelings or urges the person does not want to admit they are experiencing. A mother who abuses her child might accuse the medical assistant of being rough with the child while performing patient assessment to conceal her feelings of wanting to throttle the child. Projection is an indication of mental illness.

Sublimation is the channeling of a socially unacceptable behavior into a socially acceptable behavior. An overly aggressive person directed to play football to relieve their aggression is an example. Constructive behavior is substituted for destructive behavior.

Displacement is the unconscious transfer of unacceptable emotions, thoughts, or feelings from one's self to a more acceptable external substitute. A patient who is angry with the doctor for some reason slams the door as he or she leaves the clinic.

Compensation is a conscious or unconscious overemphasizing of a characteristic to offset a real or imagined deficiency. This defense mechanism involves substituting strength for a weakness and may be viewed as healthy. An example is the young boy whose physical stature keeps him from being a football star, so he compensates by achieving an academic award.

Rationalization is the mind's way of making unacceptable behavior or events acceptable by devising a rational reason. The purpose of rationalization is to avoid embarrassment or guilt, or to avoid obeying a directive. The rational reason is usually a stretch of the truth and can be quite apparent to disinterested individuals. An example is the patient who tells the doctor that he or she did not take his or her blood pressure medication because he or she did not have enough time before leaving for work. The medication easily could have been taken at home or at work. Most people rationalize things to some extent, but excessive rationalization may be construed as unhealthy.

Undoing is actions designed to make amends or to cancel out inappropriate behavior. Showering the abused person with gifts to compensate for unacceptable actions that took place in the past is an example.

THERAPEUTIC COMMUNICATION IN ACTION

The following sections identify the proper communication techniques that the medical assistant should use as part of the two most important communication functions they perform: patient interview techniques and telephone techniques.

Interview Techniques

 All health professionals must be adept at **interview techniques**—knowing how to encourage the best communication between themselves and the patient. It is important to remember that an unequal relationship exists between the health professional and the patient. The health professional, whether it be the physician or the medical assistant, is in the power position and has a great deal of control over the patient. Therefore, it is important to equalize the relationship as much as possible. That is the reason why some professionals use the term *client* rather than *patient*.

Early in the interview, the patient must feel comfortable enough to risk being honest with the health professional. The health professional must build an atmosphere of trust by showing concern for the patient. A gentle touch and a warm, caring facial expression may be all that is necessary. Always be honest and genuine in your responses to patients. Be sympathetic and empathic and create an environment that is free of hypocrisy.

When the medical assistant is interviewing the patient for the chief complaint, it is important to listen with a "third" ear. Listen to what the patient is not saying but is apt to exhibit through nonverbal communication.

You might choose to share your observation of the nonverbal message with the patient, thus encouraging the patient to verbalize more freely. When feelings are shared, validate and acknowledge those feelings through such statements as "I understand your distress." You can verify the communication by reflecting or paraphrasing what the patient has said.

You will be asking **closed questions** during the interview. Closed questions can be answered with a simple yes or no.

"Are you still taking your medication?"
"Are you in pain now?"

You will also use **open-ended questions** with the patient. These questions encourage therapeutic communication because the patient is required to verbalize more information.

"What kind of help will you have at home during your recovery?"

"How are you coming along on this diet?"

Indirect statements will also prove helpful in facilitating therapeutic communication. An indirect statement will elicit a response from a patient without the patient feeling questioned.

"Tell me what you've been doing since you retired."

"I'd like to know more about your exercise program."

Telephone Techniques

 It often has been said that the telephone is the lifeline of the physician's office. Communication over the telephone requires understanding on the part of each communicator (Figure 4-6).

Each medium uses the proper tools to get the job done. Speaking on the telephone is much like a conversation between two blindfolded individuals. The facial expressions cannot be seen, there is no eye contact, and there is no visual feedback. The listener will interpret mood by the tone, the pacing of voice, and the words spoken. When speaking on the telephone, quick conclusions are drawn. Often, we jump to conclusions, and the communication is misinterpreted.

The old, cold, aloof, formal business greeting comes across like frostbite in the medical office setting. It sounds curt, bored, and uncaring. Think of welcoming a new acquaintance into your home, then practice the same characteristics when speaking on the telephone. Speak clearly, use words that will be easily understood, and ask questions to verify that the patient has understood the message being conveyed.

Concentrate on enunciating and being understood. If you hear, "What? I didn't understand you. I can't hear you," slow down and speak a little louder with distinct enunciation directly into the mouthpiece. The mouthpiece should be held one to two inches away from the mouth. Project your voice at the mouthpiece, and then project another foot further. Your voice is the delivery system for your words and thoughts. Speak with confidence and conviction.

Have you ever called an office and had the firm name clipped off? The name of the office is important. To avoid clipping off the office name, practice using buffer words. **Buffer words** are expendable; if you clip them off, at least the office name remains intact. Use buffer words before the

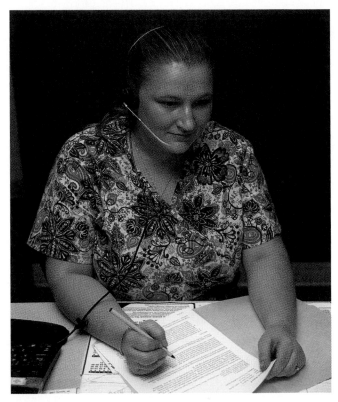

Figure 4-6 When communicating over the telephone, listen with full attention to make certain the message sent and received is correct.

office name and before you identify yourself. "Good morning, this is Inner City Health Care. This is Walter, how may I help you?" *Good morning* and *this is* are buffer words.

All the techniques for effective face-to-face communication must be more intentionally observed when the communication is over the telephone because you cannot see the person with whom you are speaking. You must listen with full attention to make certain that the message sent and received is correct.

To close a telephone conversation to schedule an appointment, for example, consider the following:

1. Use the patient's name if it can be done without announcing the name to persons in the reception area.
2. Confirm the date and time of the appointment.
3. Identify the physician if there is more than one physician in the office.
4. Give any specific instructions that may be necessary.
5. Say good-bye.

For more information on telephone techniques, see Chapter 12.

The following Health Insurance Portability and Accountability Act (HIPAA) guidelines should be followed when communicating information to patients by telephone:

- Determine whether the patient has requested confidential communications. The office policy and procedure manual should provide guidelines for making this determination.
- If the patient has not requested protected health information (PHI), the patient should simply be called at the normal phone number contained in their records. If the patient has requested PHI and has provided an alternate telephone number, care must be taken to ensure that only the alternate number is called.

- The caller should identify himself or herself by name, identify the medical practice where he or she is employed, and ask to speak with the intended person.
- If the patient is not available, it is acceptable to leave a live or recorded message asking the patient to return the call. It is important, however, that the message does not contain any medical information and does not mention the purpose of the call. If the name of the practice indicates the nature of the call, do not disclose the name.
- When the patient is contacted, it is acceptable to discuss their medical information over the phone. Test results and other PHI must not be given to anyone other than the patient or a person designated as the patient's representative.

Procedure 4-1 Identifying Community Resources

PURPOSE:
To have a list of community resources readily available for referral to patients.

EQUIPMENT/SUPPLIES:
Computer and printer
Following is a list of information sources to consider when beginning to put together a Community Resource Reference:
- Local Public Health Department
- Internet
- Community service numbers in the local telephone directory
- State/federal agencies
- Visiting nurses
- Counselor/social workers at local hospitals
- Nursing home associations
- Local charities

PROCEDURE STEPS:
1. Determine the type of information to be in your database. RATIONALE: Only resources useful to your specific office should be maintained to save time and space.
2. Contact the sources listed previously and request any listings they may have. RATIONALE: This will save time.
3. Search the Internet using your favorite search engine. Enter under the city, state, and community resources. You may have to modify the subject of your search to obtain the desired resources. RATIONALE: This is an effective way to access information quickly.
4. Develop a database on your computer so you can search easily for the resource when needed by a patient and simply print it out. You may wish to have a notebook with the information printed and indexed, so other office staff can simply copy a page for a patient. Your data should include as many resources for assistance as you can find for each type of resource. RATIONALE: To have a listing of community resources readily available for office use.

Case Study 4-1

It is a typically active day at the offices of Drs. Lewis and King. Despite the three emergencies in the early afternoon and the full schedule of patients, everything is running smoothly with Dr. Lewis, and the entire staff is responding quickly but thoroughly to patient concerns.

At 4:00 PM, another emergency patient arrives; at the same time, Jim Marshal, an architect in a downtown firm, comes in early for a routine appointment and demands to be seen immediately. Jim, a regular patient, has a history of being difficult and impatient; being a bit arrogant, he tends to put his needs first. However, Dr. Lewis is occupied with another patient. It is critical to treat the patient with the emergency as soon as possible, and Jim is half an hour early.

Joe Guerrero, CMA, the office's administrative and clinical medical assistant, calmly asks Mr. Marshal to please wait until his scheduled appointment time. When he threatens to leave, Joe explains to Mr. Marshal that there are two patients ahead of him, but that the doctor will see him at his scheduled appointment time.

CASE STUDY REVIEW

1. What communication roadblocks did medical assistant Joe Guerrero avoid in reacting to Jim Marshal's demands to see the doctor?

2. With another student, role-play the scenario, with one student taking the role of patient and one student the role of the medical assistant. Identify roadblocks to communication imposed by the patient. How is the medical assistant using the five Cs of communication to deal with the situation?

3. Do you think the medical assistant reacted appropriately? What else could he have done? What should he *not* do in this situation?

Case Study 4-2

You have learned in this chapter that communication has not been successful until the cycle is complete. Consider the following scenario:

An 82-year-old woman with moderate dementia and a hearing impairment is brought to the surgeon's office for a follow-up appointment after hip replacement surgery. The woman's daughter accompanies her. The goal of the appointment is to make certain the hip is healing nicely and to discuss precautions before the patient returns to her assisted-living apartment. Almost immediately, the conversation is directed toward the daughter because it is so much easier to explain to her what should be done.

CASE STUDY REVIEW

1. What might the staff do to help the patient understand the following?
   - Use the walker consistently.
   - Shoes must be leather tennis shoe type or uniform style; consider Velcro closure as opposed to laces that have to be tied.
   - Do not wear pantyhose.
   - You will not be able to walk your dog on a leash.

2. Should the patient be left out of the conversation? Should the daughter be included?

3. In cases such as these, is something other than verbal communication indicated?

SUMMARY

Throughout this text you are reminded of the importance of effective communication techniques. Good communication takes practice. Use the techniques identified in this chapter with your family and with your peers. Watch for roadblocks, be aware of defense mechanisms, and remember the five Cs of communication.

STUDY FOR SUCCESS

To reinforce your knowledge and skills of information presented in this chapter:

- ❏ Review the Key Terms
- ❏ Practice the Procedure
- ❏ Consider the Case Studies and discuss your conclusions
- ❏ Answer the Review Questions
  - ❏ Multiple Choice
  - ❏ Critical Thinking
- ❏ Navigate the Internet by completing the Web Activities
- ❏ Practice the StudyWARE activities on the textbook CD
- ❏ Apply your knowledge in the Student Workbook activities
- ❏ Complete the Web Tutor sections
- ❏ View and discuss the DVD situations

REVIEW QUESTIONS

Multiple Choice

1. Culture influences which of the following?
   a. biases and prejudices
   b. ethnic heritage, age, and sex
   c. educational and life experiences and value systems
   d. b and c only

2. In the cycle of communication, encoding means:
   a. deciphering a message
   b. creating the message to be sent
   c. sending the message
   d. receiving the message

3. Body language:
   a. is used to express feelings and emotions
   b. is not as important as verbal communication
   c. only makes up 7% of the message
   d. is only used in Eastern cultures

4. A comfortable social space is defined as:
   a. touching to 6 inches
   b. 1½ feet to 4 feet
   c. 12 to 15 feet
   d. 4 to 12 feet

5. A reassuring cliché is:
   a. a way of calming down a patient
   b. a means of rationalizing a decision
   c. a roadblock to communication
   d. always useful in daily communications

6. Redirecting a socially unacceptable impulse into one that is socially acceptable is an example of which of these defense mechanisms?
   a. sublimation
   b. rationalization
   c. projection
   d. displacement

7. When using an open-ended question with a patient, we expect:
   a. a yes or no answer
   b. him or her to tell us the truth
   c. a response that permits the patient to elaborate
   d. only the right answers

8. Buffer words:
   a. help us get through the day
   b. are meant to soothe a patient's feelings
   c. are expendable words used in answering a telephone call
   d. are important in face-to-face communication

Critical Thinking

1. A 15-year-old girl awaiting a sports physical examination says that she is overweight and has pimples. How will you respond therapeutically?

2. Bill, who is 28 years old, comes for his annual checkup. When reviewing his social data sheet, you discover he is now living in an apartment and has a

new phone number. He mumbles to you that his wife left him and won't let him see the kids. How will you respond therapeutically?

3. You try to be gentle and gracious with Edith. She is fragile and difficult to please. While positioning her for a radiograph, she sneers and says, "You are about the roughest person who ever cared for me." How will you respond therapeutically, and how will you control your body language?

4. When you report to Herb that his cholesterol is quite high and that the doctor wants to discuss medication and diet, he responds, "That is impossible; you must have made some mistake." Which defense mechanism is Herb using? How will you respond therapeutically?

5. How might the unequal relationship between physician and client/patient impact therapeutic communication?

WEB ACTIVITIES

Select three cultures of particular interest to you personally and search the World Wide Web for information regarding these cultures and communication traditions. How might this new information be applied to the physician whose clientele is primarily made up of these cultures? How might this new knowledge benefit a medical assistant employed in this type of setting?

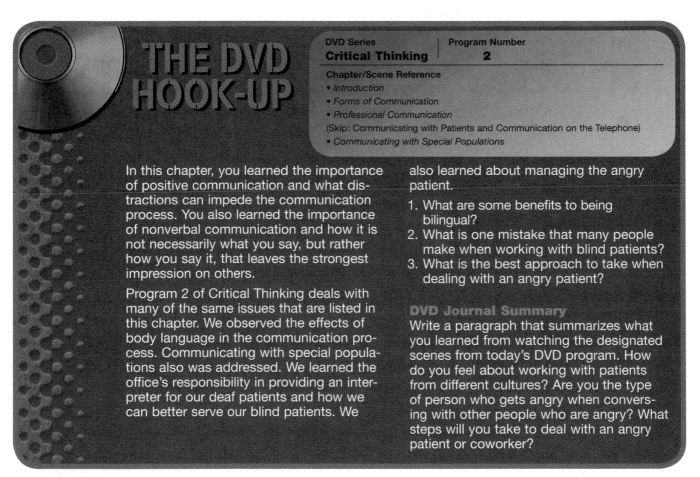

THE DVD HOOK-UP

DVD Series **Critical Thinking**	Program Number **2**

Chapter/Scene Reference
- *Introduction*
- *Forms of Communication*
- *Professional Communication*
(Skip: Communicating with Patients and Communication on the Telephone)
- *Communicating with Special Populations*

In this chapter, you learned the importance of positive communication and what distractions can impede the communication process. You also learned the importance of nonverbal communication and how it is not necessarily what you say, but rather how you say it, that leaves the strongest impression on others.

Program 2 of Critical Thinking deals with many of the same issues that are listed in this chapter. We observed the effects of body language in the communication process. Communicating with special populations also was addressed. We learned the office's responsibility in providing an interpreter for our deaf patients and how we can better serve our blind patients. We

also learned about managing the angry patient.

1. What are some benefits to being bilingual?
2. What is one mistake that many people make when working with blind patients?
3. What is the best approach to take when dealing with an angry patient?

DVD Journal Summary
Write a paragraph that summarizes what you learned from watching the designated scenes from today's DVD program. How do you feel about working with patients from different cultures? Are you the type of person who gets angry when conversing with other people who are angry? What steps will you take to deal with an angry patient or coworker?

REFERENCES/BIBLIOGRAPHY

Blair, G. M. (January 23, 2000). *Conversation as communication.* Retrieved from http://www.ee.ed.ac.uk/~gerard/Management/art7.html

Luckmann, J. (2000). *Transcultural communication in health care.* Clifton Park, NY: Thomson Delmar Learning.

National Center for Cultural Competence, Georgetown University Center for Child and Human Development, Georgetown University Medical Center. (Spring/Summer 2004). Bridging the cultural divide in health care settings: The essential role of cultural broker programs. Washington, DC: Author.

Taber's cyclopedic medical dictionary. (19th ed.). (2004). Philadelphia: F. A. Davis.

Tamparo, C. D., & Lindh, W. Q. (2000). *Therapeutic communications for health professions.* Albany, NY: Delmar.

Webster's new twentieth century dictionary. (2nd ed.). (1983). New York: New World Dictionaries/Simon and Schuster.

Wilkes, M., & Crosswait, C. B. (1995). *Professional development: The dynamics of success.* San Diego: Harcourt Brace Jovanovich.

CHAPTER 5

Coping Skills for the Medical Assistant

OUTLINE

What Is Stress?
  Adaptation to Stress
Management of Stress
What Is Burnout?
  Stages of Burnout
  Burnout in the Workplace

What to Do If You Are Burned
  Out
Prevention and Recovery from
  Burnout
Goal Setting as a Stress
Reliever

OBJECTIVES

The student should strive to meet the following performance objectives and demonstrate an understanding of the facts and principles presented in this chapter through written and oral communication.

1. Define the key terms as presented in the glossary.
2. Differentiate between stress and stressors.
3. Describe Hans Selye's General Adaptation Syndrome theory.
4. Identify several approaches to managing stress in the ambulatory care setting.
5. Identify three characteristics associated with burnout in the workplace.
6. Describe the four stages of burnout.
7. List a minimum of five ways to reduce the risk for burnout.
8. Differentiate between long-range and short-range goals.

KEY TERMS

Burnout
Goal
Inner-Directed People
Long-Range Goals
Outer-Directed People
Parasympathetic Nervous
  System
Self-Actualization
Short-Range Goals
Stress
Stressors
Sympathetic Nervous
  System

**FEATURED
COMPETENCIES**

ABHES—ENTRY-LEVEL

COMPETENCIES

Professionalism

- Be a "team player"
- Adapt to change
- Conduct work within scope
  of education, training,
  and ability

SCENARIO

At the office of Drs. Lewis and King, there are four full-time medical assistants who collaborate to make the office run smoothly, both administratively and clinically. One day a month, though, office manager Marilyn Johnson, CMA, is out of town, leaving Ellen Armstrong, CMA, the administrative medical assistant, in charge of a busy reception area and an ever-ringing telephone.

On these days, Ellen is particularly careful to organize her work so that things run as they should. She organizes some work the night before, she sets priorities so that she is confident that the critical work will get done, and she tries to maintain her calm by taking a short break every couple of hours to review new needs that have come up during the day. Although Ellen cannot anticipate every emergency, she does try to influence the situation rather than let events control her.

INTRODUCTION

Even in the most well-managed ambulatory care setting, medical assistants and other health providers are likely to feel the effects of stress from time to time. They may be overworked on certain days, they may face difficult patient situations, and they may find that the administrative and paperwork load is getting ahead of them.

This chapter helps today's busy, multifaceted medical assistant pinpoint the symptoms of stress and provides ideas for coping with stress as it occurs. The better equipped the medical assistant is to confront and solve the sources of stress, the less likely stressors will become so overwhelming as to lead to burnout on the job. Goal setting, recognizing one's limitations and potentials, setting priorities, and keeping a balanced perspective can work together to reduce stress and enable the medical assistant to take pleasure in working with patients and colleagues.

WHAT IS STRESS?

The body's response to mental and physical change is termed **stress.** Adaptive behavior patterns we assume in response to real physical threats or emotional effects result in either eustress, positive feelings; or distress, negative feelings. Moving to a new city or receiving a promotion usually are perceived as positive events, whereas going through a divorce or losing a job are conversely negative events; however, each of these events can result in inducing stress in the body. These events are called **stressors.**

According to Hans Selye, who first conceived the theory of nonspecific reaction as stress, the body does not differentiate positively and negatively induced stress. It is only the level of the stress and its duration that affect the body. Some stress is beneficial and adds anticipation and a feeling of "being alive," for example, when we experience a roller coaster ride or bungee jump off a cliff. The short-lived adrenaline rush brings the world into sharper focus and enhances our lives. Short-duration stress is beneficial and helps us focus on details, achieve difficult goals, and perform at our best. When we have a last-minute rush in the office or are hurrying to get an assignment finished for school, we are experiencing short-duration stress. Short-duration stress is experienced when the telephone rings, the examination rooms are full, and the physician is called to the hospital on an emergency. Immediately, the body's stress mode is activated and adrenaline is produced, enabling you to make quick judgements and decisions, to be organized and efficient, and to accomplish tasks within minimal time limits.

Longer duration stress, normally associated with negative events, can be harmful to the body, resulting in illness such as headaches, insomnia, allergies, cancer, acute indigestion, stomach ulcers, hypertension, blood clots, stroke, and immune system disorders. Psychologically, the body also is influenced by long-term stress. Onsets of depression and anxiety, as well as eating problems resulting in weight loss or gain, are associated with the body's psychological response to stress. Anorexia and bulimia are common eating disorders attributed to long-term stressful events. Long-duration stress can also affect our ability to think clearly, and objectivity may be impaired. Physical symptoms of these emotional effects may include cigarette smoking, obesity, lack of interest, and excessive sexual activity.

Adaptation to Stress

The body's response to stress goes back to early human development. That response was designed to help humans survive whatever they were experiencing that caused a fearful response. The **sympathetic nervous system** prepared the body for "fight or flight" to allow humans the best chance of survival. The brain inhibits short-term memory, promotes long-term memory, and releases hormones such as adrenaline into the bloodstream. The respiration rate becomes more rapid, blood flow increases, red and white blood cells are released by the spleen, the immune system is altered to allow immune-boosting bodies to be sent to the body. Blood vessels in the skin are contracted to minimize blood loss from wounds, blood vessels in the muscles dilate to increase circulation, and fluids are diverted from nonessential locations; the metabolism rate is diminished to permit all available energy to be focused on the event that triggered the fight-or-flight response.

All of these caveman responses to stress are with us today, even though they may no longer be needed in the twenty-first century. The symptoms of headache, stomach ache, diarrhea, cold clammy hands, heart palpitations, indigestion, and short-term memory loss that we experience are the result of our body's reaction to stressors that has been developed over millennia. Short term, these responses are not harmful, and the body's **parasympathetic nervous system** returns to normal after the stressor has been removed. Long term, these responses are harmful to the body. See Figure 5-1 for an illustration of the adaptive stages related to stress.

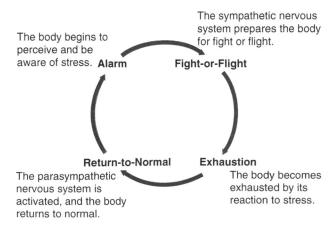

Figure 5-1 Hans Selye's General Adaptation Syndrome (GAS) theory proposes that four stages are involved in adapting to stress.

MANAGEMENT OF STRESS

Stress cannot be prevented; in fact, life would be dull without short-term stress. Anticipating the birth of a child, planning an upcoming wedding, or graduating from school are all stressful changes, albeit pleasant ones, that make life interesting. Long-term stressful situations are not desirable, but the situations leading to them can be managed if we understand the causes. Some causes of long-term stress are:

- *Powerlessness:* inability to control expectations, workload, and duties; feelings of frustration and panic because of schedules

- *Round peg in square hole:* not suited for the position you hold

- *Traumatic events on the job:* not emotionally prepared for trauma involved in the job

- *Environmental:* physical conditions such as noise, lighting, or temperature influence work

- *Management style:* your manager's style causes uproar or instability in work demands

- *Failure to satisfy needs:* job conditions do not permit achievement of Maslow's needs (see Chapter 4 for information related to Maslow's hierarchy of needs)

Requesting that you have a written job description can control powerlessness. You will then know the duties and responsibilities, and you will not experience sudden change when you least expect it. A job description will also help to avoid some of the instability resulting from a manager who is too sanguine or manages from one crisis to another. If you know what your job entails, you can anticipate the events and take action to prevent a crisis.

Planning and prioritization can help to avoid panic and reduce stress when faced with the inevitable situation of too much work and too little time. A job that looks

Critical Thinking—Practice in Time Management Analysis

List all of the tasks you do in a typical day. Beside each task write down how many minutes/hours you spend on each task. At the conclusion of the exercise, draw a histogram showing the percentage of each day spent on each task. This will quickly show where you spend most of your time. How could you save time? Develop a plan to reduce time spent in nonproductive, unessential activities.

impossible can be broken down into elements that are manageable. Prioritization of the smaller elements and proceeding without wasting time procrastinating usually results in getting the job finished in the allotted time or at least with a minimum amount of stress.

Managing your lifestyle also becomes part of stress management. Finding time to relax and divert your mind from the worries of the job is an effective tool in managing stress. Instead of working during lunch to solve a problem, taking a break away from the problem will reduce the stress to the point that you will actually increase your productivity. This is probably a good time to discuss worry. Worry is defined as undue concern for problems over which you have no control. Worry causes stress, yet it does nothing to resolve the problem causing your worry. Therefore, just remembering this definition and thinking about it every time you are inclined to worry will help you to stop worrying and actually will help you become more focused and better able to resolve the stressful event.

Mental attitude plays a role in tolerance to stress. Individuals who can focus on the positive can offset the depression often associated with stress. Identifying what is being accomplished versus focusing on what is not being accomplished or what does not meet your expectations is what is meant by focusing on the positive. Maintaining an active social network that allows you to discuss your problems is also quite helpful. The network should not include persons of negative personality who have common problems. This situation is likely to have as its outcome a "complain session."

Physical condition affects your body's tolerance to stress. Maintaining a regular sleep cycle, eating a proper diet, and getting regular exercise contribute to improving your body's tolerance to stressors (Figure 5-2). Stress can affect sleep and appetite, but intentionally not getting enough sleep or not eating a balanced diet makes you more susceptible to stress in the first place. Anything that "bugs" you contributes to stress. Some people believe that soft background music will reduce stress, but for a job requiring intense concentration, any distraction contributes to stress. Clothes or shoes that are uncomfortable can "bug" you and contribute to stress. The color of the walls in your office can contribute to stress. If the color "bugs" you, it will contribute to stress. Telephone interruptions can result in a stressful situation. All of these "minor" things that contribute to stress are manageable and should be considered as part of a plan to manage stress. See Table 5-1 for suggested techniques for reducing stress at work.

Maintaining a good interpersonal relationship with fellow employees or fellow students and faculty is important to achieving a satisfying work or school experience. Before a strong interpersonal relationship is established with others, a positive self-attitude is needed. The choices we make effect our positive attitude. Making positive decisions will affect our school and work environment, and hence the level and duration of stress experienced. Following are choices we all make in our lives:

- To be respectful of others

- To be a diligent worker

Critical Thinking—Checking Your Success-Oriented Attitude

Select three attitude attributes for which you are quite negative and develop a plan of action to make them more positive. Implement your plan; after two weeks, review whether your actions have impacted the stress level associated with that activity.

Negative Attributes	20%	40%	60%	80%	100%	Positive Attributes
Bored						Enthusiastic
Unhappy						Joyful
Never						Can do
Lethargic						Energetic
Cut corners						Honest
Out of control						Under control
Lack of confidence						Confident
Selfish						Selfless
Unyielding						Flexible
Loner						Part of a group
Know it all						Open to suggestion

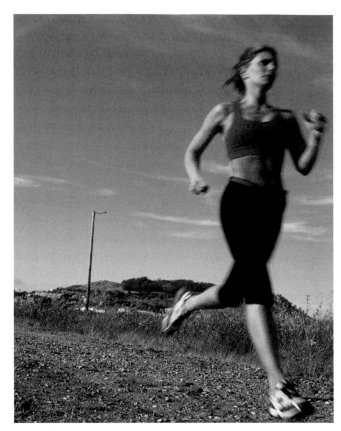

Figure 5-2 Regular exercise in some form improves the body's tolerance to stress.

- To be willing to learn
- To be honest
- To be willing to assume responsibility for actions
- To express appropriate humor
- To have an attitude of humility

TABLE 5-1 **TECHNIQUES FOR REDUCING STRESS AT WORK**
• Stretch or change positions.
• Slowly roll your head from side to side and forward and back.
• Slowly rotate your shoulders forward and backward several times.
• Turn away from the computer, or close your eyes for several seconds.
• Walk around and deliver charts or laboratory specimens, and so on.
• Stand or sit tall and take a few deep breaths.
• Meditate for 30 seconds.
• Know your limits and be aware of your body's needs.

- To be goal directed
- To understand Maslow's needs

By anticipating how an organization can cause stress, we can be prepared and minimize its effects. Following are common causes of stress in an organization:

- *Low salary:* Salary plays an important role in our needs. It leads to frustration if we believe it is too low, and this contributes to a negative attitude. Positive job conditions can overshadow low salary; however, if combined with other negative feelings, it is an overpowering cause of stress.

- *Little opportunity for career growth:* This reason results in frustration and leads to stress and burnout.

- *Overspecialization:* This problem results in the employee never seeing the overall picture and receiving little or no satisfaction from his or her work.

- *Workload:* Continual work level beyond your capability to complete it results in frustration, and ultimately burnout.

- *Job complexity versus skill level:* Expectation to perform beyond your skill level leads to long-term stress.

- *Responsibility delineation:* Lack of delineation of responsibility leads to continual questioning of whom is responsible for what job, and ultimately to frustration.

Critical Thinking—Self-Evaluation

- List several situations in your life that are stressful. Select the *one* that is most stressful.
- List as many things as possible about the situation that make it stressful to you.
- How would you change each of the things you have listed to make them less stressful?
- List the things you "could do" to effect the changes you listed.
- Rank the items in your "could do" list in terms of achievability.
- Select one or two of the items that are achievable and discuss them with a classmate. Now attempt to put them into practice for a week. Report back to your classmate on how effective these items were in reducing stress in your life.

- *Organization size:* Some individuals can get lost in a large organization.

- *Discrimination:* This illegal activity leads to bad feelings and frustration.

- *Poor time management skills:* The inability to prioritize and manage time effectively can lead to work overload.

- *Technological changes:* Change, even good changes, can cause stress.

- *Not being in control of your situation:* Lacking control leads to frustration.

WHAT IS BURNOUT?

Burnout is the result of stress and frustration, principally brought about by unrealistic expectations. Fatigue and exhaustion resulting from trying to meet unrealistic expectations compound it. Because burnout is so damaging, it needs to be discussed as a unique topic.

Stages of Burnout

Burnout has four stages:

- *Honeymoon:* love your job and have unrealistic expectation placed on you either by your manager or by yourself if you are a perfectionist; take work home and look for all the work you can get, cannot say "no" to accepting additional work

- *Reality:* begin to have doubts you can meet expectations; feel frustrated with your progress, work harder to meet expectations; begin to feel pulled in many directions; may not have a role model to follow, and established guidelines may not be defined

- *Dissatisfaction:* loss of enthusiasm; try to escape frustrations by binges of one sort or another, drinking, partying, shopping, or excessive eating or sex; fatigue and exhaustion develop.

- *Sad state:* depression, work seems pointless, lethargic with little energy, consider quitting, and look on yourself as a failure; represents full-blown burnout.

All of these stages are part of the process leading to burnout. The honeymoon stage might seem desirable, and it is pleasant, however, the seeds of the illness are present in the unrealistic expectations and the workaholic attitude of the employee. Unless these causes are eliminated, the progression to full burnout is assured.

Burnout in the Workplace

Burnout happens to people who previously were enthusiastic and bursting with energy and new ideas when first hired on the job or beginning a new experience. When individuals with a high need to achieve do not reach their goals, they are apt to feel angry and frustrated. Failing to recognize these signs as symptoms of burnout, they may throw themselves even more fully into work-related goals. Unless there is some type of revitalization outside of the workplace, burnout occurs.

Three characteristics associated with burnout in the workplace include:

- *Role Conflict:* When employees have conflicting responsibilities, they feel pulled in many directions. The perfectionist tries to do everything equally well without setting priorities. Fatigue and exhaustion associated with burnout begin to set in after time.

- *Role Ambiguity:* The employee does not know what is expected and how to accomplish it because there may not be a role model to follow or ask, or established guidelines to follow.

- *Role Overload:* If the employee cannot say no and continues to accept more responsibility than they can handle, burnout is sure to set in.

What to Do If You Are Burned Out

When you recognize the signs and symptoms of burnout, it is time to do some self-analysis by asking yourself some hard questions. Recall and analyze when you began feeling so tired and unable to relax and enjoy your work. Have you always been a perfectionist? Have you always had a higher need than most of your peers to do a job well? Are you irritable toward coworkers or patients? At what point did you lose your sense of humor? Do you always see work as a chore? Are you so intensely striving to achieve your goals that if you do not succeed you consider yourself a failure? Are you physically and emotionally exhausted?

The next step is to make some changes.

- Make a list of negative words or phrases that you most often use. Now replace the negatives with more neutral words or phrases.

- Create some job diversity for yourself. Drive to work via a different route; enter the building through a different door; change your work routine slightly; change your start time.

- Become creative. Redecorate your area.

Critical Thinking

Negative attitudes combined with low pay are a formula for burnout. Why?

- Establish some long- and short-term realistic goals and write them down.

- Take care of yourself; change your eating habits; exercise more; get more sleep.

- Renew friendships; go to lunch with coworkers; laugh with them.

- Implement time management techniques.

- Delegate responsibility to others who are capable.

Prevention and Recovery from Burnout

All of the techniques used for stress management are applicable for prevention and recovery from burnout. Following are the basic steps that need to be taken by a person who experiences burnout:

- Get some rest and relaxation away from the job for as long as is practical.

- Develop outside interests and an active social life.

- Set realistic goals for your life and your job.

- Negotiate a job description with your manager that has achievable expectations.

- Do not take work home.

- Develop time management techniques.

- Take steps to achieve regular sleep habits, nutritious diet, and physical exercise.

- Concentrate on thinking positively regarding job success.

GOAL SETTING AS A STRESS RELIEVER

Do you direct your life, or do you allow others to influence and make decisions for you? **Outer-directed people** let events, other people, or environmental factors dictate their behavior. By contrast, **inner-directed people** decide for themselves what they want to do with their lives. Laurence Peter, author of *The Peter Principle*, states,

"If you don't know where you are going, you will end up somewhere else" (Wilkes & Crosswait, 1995).

Discoveries prove that goal-oriented employees are more effective and assertive than colleagues with no goals or future objectives. Recognizing the value of goal planning, many employers arrange planning sessions or seminars to encourage goal setting as a practical application for coping with stress and burnout and to develop career objectives. If your employer does not offer these outlets, seek your own seminars for goal setting. Such an activity not only "centers" you in your current employment, but helps you clearly picture your future plans and hopes.

What is a **goal?** According to *Merriam-Webster's Collegiate Dictionary*, a goal is "the result or achievement toward which effort is directed." To reach a desired goal, a person must implement planning together with a sincere desire to work hard. Skill in goal setting allows the medical assistant to clarify what must be accomplished and to develop a strategic plan to successfully achieve the goal.

A goal must be specific, challenging, realistic, attainable, and measurable. Specific goals are focused and have precise boundaries. A goal that is challenging creates enthusiasm and interest in achievement. Realistic goals are practical or beneficial for the present and for future **self-actualization.** An attainable goal refers to the fact that the goal is possible to fulfill. Measurable goals achieve some form of progress or success. By reflecting on the process, one is encouraged to establish additional goals.

Long-range goals are achievements that may take three to five years to accomplish. Long-range goals give direction and definition to our lives and serve to keep us "on track" so to speak. Much discipline, perseverance, determination, and hard work will be expended in accomplishing long-range goals. Some adjustment and readjustment to your goals may be necessary, however. The rewards of goal achievement include satisfaction, pride, a sense of accomplishment, and a job well done.

Short-range goals take apart long-range goals and reassemble the required activities into smaller, more manageable time segments. The time segments may be daily, weekly, monthly, quarterly, or yearly periods.

As a graduate and new employee, one of your long-range goals might be to become the office manager in the ambulatory care setting in which you are currently employed. You may wish to attain this goal within the next three to five years; by breaking it into three longer range goals and a series of short-range goals, you will be able to measure progress and feel a sense of accomplishment. Examples of long- and short-range goals might include:

Long-range goal 1:

To become proficient in all back-office clinical skills during the first year of employment.

Short-range goals necessary to achieve this:

- Practice accuracy and proficiency when performing tasks and skills.

- Practice efficiency by planning ahead for the equipment and supplies needed for each task performed.

- Evaluate your progress on a regular basis, and identify areas that need improvement.

Long-range goal 2:

To add front-office administrative tasks and skills to your routine during the second year of employment.

Short-range goals necessary to achieve this:

- Practice accuracy and proficiency when performing all front-office tasks and skills.

- Practice efficiency by planning ahead for the equipment and supplies needed for each task performed.

- Evaluate your progress on a regular basis, and identify areas that need improvement.

Long-range goal 3:

To begin to focus on office management during the third year of employment.

Short-range goals necessary to achieve this:

- Develop a procedure manual for all back- and front-office tasks and skills.

- Enroll in office management classes.

- Focus on team-building skills.

By the fourth year, you will be ready to move into the office manager position.

Long- and short-range goals work together to help make changes in our lives. Goals keep life interesting and give us something for which to strive. We can all reach goals successfully with some planning, hard work, discipline, and dedication.

Case Study 5-1

Ellen Armstrong, CMA, is an administrative medical assistant with Drs. Lewis and King. This is her first job. She is just two years out of school, and she is trying to learn everything she can to achieve her long-range goal of becoming office manager at this or some other ambulatory care setting.

Ellen has a great deal in her favor, for she is good with patients, both face-to-face and over the telephone. She is not daunted by the complexity of administrative work her job requires. Ellen knows she has a great deal yet to learn and, although she is a bit intimidated by her, Ellen looks to Marilyn Johnson, CMA, the office manager, for guidance and advice.

CASE STUDY REVIEW

1. How would you advise Ellen to go about achieving her long-term goal of office manager?

2. What are some of the short-term goals Ellen should set? Why are short-term goals important to her success?

3. Besides learning on the job, what else can Ellen do to achieve her goal?

Case Study 5-2

Ellen Armstrong, CMA, has been employed for five years as an administrative medical assistant with Drs. Lewis and King. Ellen is a perfectionist and has pushed herself to achieve many of her short- and long-term goals. The office staff has become aware that Ellen does not have a sense of humor lately. She seems frustrated and irritable, and is becoming critical of herself and others. Ellen has felt physically and emotionally exhausted, yet she continues to focus on her high standard of job performance; however, work is becoming a chore. At the end of the day, if everything has not been completed to her satisfaction, she feels like a failure.

CASE STUDY REVIEW

1. Do you feel Ellen is stressed or experiencing burnout? On what do you base your conclusions?
2. What might Ellen do to differentiate these two conditions?
3. What changes might Ellen implement to resolve this problem?

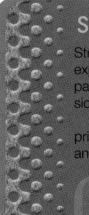

SUMMARY

Stress is very much a part of the medical profession. Each individual working in a medical career experiences consecutive days of demanding, emotionally and physically draining interactions with patients and staff members. This highly technical and ever-changing career requires its professionals to maintain a high level of skill and training and to be familiar with the newest technology.

Goal setting is one approach to reducing stress and burnout and promoting a sense of pride in the workplace, self-actualization, and possible employment promotion. Both long-range and short-range goal planning work together to help make changes in our lives.

STUDY FOR SUCCESS

To reinforce your knowledge and skills of information presented in this chapter:

- ❑ Review the Key Terms
- ❑ Consider the Case Studies and discuss your conclusions
- ❑ Answer the Review Questions
  - ❑ Multiple Choice
  - ❑ Critical Thinking
- ❑ Navigate the Internet by completing the Web Activities
- ❑ Practice the StudyWARE activities on the textbook CD
- ❑ Apply your knowledge in the Student Workbook activities
- ❑ Complete the Web Tutor sections

REVIEW QUESTIONS

Multiple Choice

1. Which answer is *not* true about stress?
   a. It does not occur suddenly.
   b. It has physical and emotional effects on the body.
   c. It may be positive or negative on its effects on the body.
   d. It is the body's response to change.
2. Hans Selye's General Adaptation Syndrome theory proposes that adaptation to stress occurs in how many stages?
   a. 2 stages
   b. 3 stages
   c. 4 stages
   d. 5 stages
3. Which is *not* a stage in the General Adaptation Syndrome?
   a. fight-or-flight
   b. exhaustion
   c. burnout
   d. alarm
4. Signs and symptoms of burnout include all of the following *except:*
   a. emotional and physical exhaustion
   b. hair-trigger display of emotion
   c. feelings of accomplishment and pride in work
   d. irritability and impatience
5. Long-range goals are easy to achieve if:
   a. they are not too challenging
   b. they are divided into a series of short-range goals
   c. they don't involve too much hard work
   d. you never change or adjust them

Critical Thinking

1. You have just graduated from a two-year medical assisting program and have been hired by a pediatric practice as a receptionist. The practice is busy with many telephone calls daily and many new patients who need charts created and information entered into the database. While in school you learned that you enjoyed the laboratory and clinical work much more than the front-office procedures. How do you think this position will impact your short- and long-term stress?
2. Identify two long-range goals you personally would like to attain within the next five years. How will you achieve these goals?
3. After you have been on the job for five years, you begin to recognize signs of burnout. How will you manage these symptoms?

WEB ACTIVITIES

Search the World Wide Web for additional information on burnout in the workplace. Compile your information into a report for your instructor. Be sure to include a bibliography identifying your Web sources.

REFERENCES/BIBLIOGRAPHY

Keir, L., Wise, B. A., & Krebs, C. (2003). *Medical assisting: Administrative and clinical competencies* (5th ed.). Clifton Park, NY: Thomson Delmar Learning.

Merriam-Webster's collegiate dictionary (10th ed.). (1994). Springfield, MA: Merriam-Webster.

Stress. (September 2001). Retrieved from http://www.reutershealth.com/wellconnected/doc31.html. Accessed April 5, 2005.

Stress management. (2000). Retrieved from http://www.ivf.com/stress.html. Accessed April 5, 2005.

Tamparo, C. D., & Lindh, W. Q. (2000). *Therapeutic communications for allied health professions.* Albany, NY: Delmar.

What you need to know about stress management. (2004). Retrieved from http://stress.about.com/cs/workplacestress/a/?once=true&. Accessed May 16, 2005.

Wilkes, M., & Crosswait, C. B. (1995). *Professional development: The dynamics of success.* San Diego: Harcourt Brace Jovanovich.

CHAPTER 6

The Therapeutic Approach to the Patient with a Life-Threatening Illness

KEY TERMS

Durable Power of Attorney
   for Health Care
Living Will
Physician's Directive
Psychomotor Retardation

OBJECTIVES

The student should strive to meet the following performance objectives and demonstrate an understanding of the facts and principles presented in this chapter through written and oral communication.

1. Define the key terms as presented in the glossary.
2. Describe possible patient perspectives when facing a life-threatening illness.
3. Define "life-threatening" illness.
4. Discuss cultural manifestations of life-threatening illness.
5. Identify the strongest cultural influence in the life of a patient.
6. List at least four choices to be made when facing a life-threatening illness.
7. Briefly describe the use of living wills and physician directives.

(continues)

FEATURED COMPETENCIES

CAAHEP—ENTRY-LEVEL COMPETENCIES

Professional Communications

- Recognize and respond to verbal communications
- Recognize and respond to nonverbal communications

Patient Instructions

- Identify community resources

ABHES—ENTRY-LEVEL COMPETENCIES

Professionalism

- Exhibit initiative
- Adapt to change
- Be courteous and diplomatic

Communication

- Be attentive, listen and learn
- Be impartial and show empathy when dealing with patients
- Adapt what is said to the recipient's level of comprehension
- Serve as a liaison among physician and others
- Recognize and respond to verbal and nonverbal communication

Legal Concepts

- Use appropriate guidelines when releasing records or information

Competency Components

- Seek patient's written authorization for release of any medical information

Psychology

- Recognize cultural influences on behavior
- Help patients adjust to illness

Instruction

- Instruct patients with special needs

OBJECTIVES (continued)

8. Discuss the range of psychological suffering that accompanies life-threatening illnesses.
9. Discuss additional concerns/fears when the life-threatening illness is AIDS, cancer, or end-stage renal disease.
10. Recall a number of challenges faced by the medical assistant when caring for people with life-threatening illnesses.

SCENARIO

You have seen the medical reports and agonize with your physician who must tell Suzanne Markis, a long-time patient, when she comes in today that she has inoperable pancreatic cancer. When she arrives, you treat her as you normally would, making certain she suspects nothing from you. When she emerges from the physician's room, you make certain to meet her, take her arm, and ask if you can call someone for her. You do not present her with a bill or make another appointment at this time. You recognize that anything you say probably will not be remembered, so you focus entirely on this patient and her immediate needs. In a day or two, as instructed by your physician–employer, you will make a phone call to set up an appointment for Suzanne and anyone she might want present at her visit with the physician so any questions can be answered.

You remind yourself to have Suzanne sign the necessary paperwork defining any designees she might identify to receive her medical information.

INTRODUCTION

Everything you learned in Chapter 4 regarding therapeutic communications is heightened and considered more difficult when the patient has a life-threatening illness. If you were told today that your life would probably be shortened because of a serious illness, your perspective would likely change. What was important yesterday may mean little or nothing now. Something that meant nothing to you yesterday suddenly takes on great importance to you now. It is essential for the medical assistant to remember this difference in perspective and what is likely to be important to patients with a life-threatening illness.

It also must be remembered that no two individuals respond to a life-threatening illness in the same way. Some respond with denial and act as if the information had never been shared with them. Others alter their lives radically and drastically change their priorities. Still others quietly continue their lives changing little outwardly but recognize that their choices may now be limited (Figure 6-1).

LIFE-THREATENING ILLNESS

A life-threatening illness is not easily defined. Some will use the word *terminal*; others refuse to use that word because they believe it removes any hope from the situation. Also, what is life-threatening for one individual may not be for another. For our purposes, life-threatening is used to imply a life that in all probability will be shortened because of a serious or debilitating illness or disease. It may be defined as death that is imminent; it may be defined in terms of a serious illness that one will battle for many years but will ultimately shorten his or her life.

Cultural Perspective on Life-Threatening Illness

 Strong cultural manifestations will be seen in the treatment of a life-threatening illness and for anyone facing death. Culture is defined as how we live our lives, how we think, how we speak, and how we behave. Cultures can be accepting, denying, or even defying of death. Death can be considered either as the end of existence or as a transition to another state of being or consciousness. Death can be considered as profane or sacred. In some cultures, a life-threatening illness may be viewed or referred to as a "slow-motion" death because of degenerative diseases that often exhaust the resources and emotions of patients and their families.

Some cultures prefer that the life-threatening illness not be shared with the patient in the beginning, but with the family who helps to prepare the patient for the inevitable. A few cultures generally do not seek care for an illness until it is quite advanced; this practice can make pain management and treatment more difficult or impossible in some cases. Some cultures surround the person who is ill with great attention, never leaving the person alone. Other cultures view the illness as something that must be removed from the body, perhaps even believing

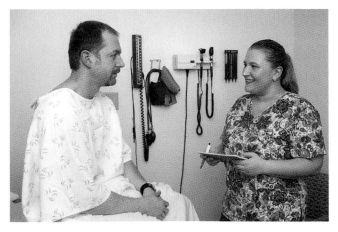

Figure 6-1 Establishing a caring and trusting relationship can help the patient come to terms with a life-threatening illness.

Spotlight on Certification

RMA Content Outline
- Patient relations
- Other personal relations
- Patient resource materials

CMA Content Outline
- Basic principles (Psychology)
- Hereditary, cultural, and environmental influences on behavior
- Adapting communication to individual's ability to understand
- Professional communication and behavior
- Patient advocate

CMAS Content Outline
- Professionalism

that the individual has been given this illness because of some past sin or transgression.

Pain is viewed in the same manner. Some cultures believe it is to be endured quietly without complaint; others believe there is to be no pain, and family members will go to great lengths to have health care providers relieve the pain. When questioning a patient about the pain level, it must be within a cultural perspective. For example, cultures with an Asian influence are more likely to describe pain in general terms related to the imbalance of the body than in terms of "piercing, intermittent, or throbbing" or on a scale of 1 to 10.

It must also be remembered that the strongest influence in managing any life-threatening illness in the life of the patient is *not* the health care team; it is the family and those closest to the patient. Therefore, great care must be taken to determine and understand the patient's cultural perspective as much as possible, and the patient must be given great respect. Often, the cultural influence may contradict the standard of care preferred by the health care provider. It is better to understand the culture and work within it than to deny it and continually work against the patient's belief system and influence of family.

CHOICES IN LIFE-THREATENING ILLNESS

Many choices are available to a patient with a life-threatening illness, but many decisions are to be made, also. The urgency of the decisions will depend, in part, on possible life expectancy. Sometimes these decisions may seem contrary to recommended medical intervention.

Patients have the right to choose or to refuse treatment in most cases. Some rush into a treatment protocol only to discover later that their choices have brought them pain, disability, and expense far beyond what originally was assumed. Although it is the health care professional's goal to heal, if healing is not likely or possible, patients ought not to be "urged" into treatment protocols that are likely to be contrary to their personal wishes for the sake of treatment only.

Although health care professionals seem less comfortable with death than they are with saving life, there are some issues appropriate to discuss with patients especially when facing life-threatening illness. Those issues include the following:

1. Alternative methods of treatment should be discussed, as well as the outcome if no treatment is sought. At some point, many patients will want to know *all* the treatment protocols that are feasible. This is a logical time to discuss any alternative therapies or integrative medicine that have shown success. Explanations should be made in language that the patient can understand. Illustrations and diagrams can be beneficial. Referrals might be made to integrative medicine practitioners, and patients are to be encouraged to discuss any chosen alternative therapies with their primary care physician. Patients may also ask what happens if no treatment is chosen. This question can be difficult for health care providers who are anxious to provide some form of treatment for patients, but patients may have a number of reasons not to seek treatment. Sometimes treatment alternatives the patient may consider are not within the realm of recognized medical acceptability, but it is better to have that discussion than to ignore the possibility. Remember the earlier statement indicating that family members and friends bring more influence to bear than does the health care professional.

2. Discussion of pain management and treatment is essential. The major fears patients have in facing life-threatening illness are pain and loss of independence. A frank discussion of pain control and how that can be accomplished can alleviate a fair amount of concern. Physicians should be ready to discuss loss of independence related to any life-threatening illness, or make a referral to someone who can be helpful. Patients have concerns such as wanting to know how long before the disease takes its toll, how long can they drive, what kind of care or assistance will be necessary, can they remain in their own home, and how long before they must have someone make decisions for them.

3. A **durable power of attorney for health care** allows an individual to make decisions related to health care when the patient is no longer able to do so. In the best of circumstances, this document will carry out the decisions the patient has already made in a **living will** or **physician's directive** regarding terminal conditions and whether to prolong life. Advances in medicine allow patient's lives to be sustained even when they are unlikely to recover from a persistent and vegetative state. The living will and the durable power of attorney for health care allow patients to make decisions before becoming incapacitated or whether life-prolonging medical or surgical procedures are to be continued, withheld, or withdrawn, as well as if or when artificial feeding and fluids are to be used or withheld. The living will and the durable power of attorney for health care documents are legal in all 50 states. Although states may vary somewhat

in the wording of these documents, they provide the same overall benefit to patients. (See Chapter 7 for more information.) The federal government passed the Patient Self-Determination Act in 1990 giving all patients receiving care in institutions receiving payments from Medicare and Medicaid written information about their right to accept or refuse medical or surgical treatment. The act also requires that patients be given information about their options to create living wills and to appoint someone to act on their behalf in making health care decisions (durable power of attorney for health care). Any documents of this nature that the patient has should be copied in the medical chart that goes with the patient when admitted to the hospital. At any time the patient makes a change in such a document, the old document is to be replaced with the new one.

4. Finances are to be considered. What will insurance cover (if there is insurance)? Who makes the decisions in a managed care environment? What family resources can or will be used? Finances are no one's favorite subject, especially physicians. However, such a discussion is important. Often, patients fear not being able to meet their financial obligations and leaving large debts to surviving family members almost as much as the life-threatening illness itself. As a medical assistant, you can help patients understand the parameters of their health insurance and any restrictions there might be on particular illnesses or treatments. Can medical insurance be canceled if employment pays a portion of the health insurance and the patient is no longer able to work? If there is a life insurance policy, help patients determine if any portion of the policy can be used for end-of-life expenses. Any services you can provide to the patient or family members in relieving the financial stress can bring great relief to everyone involved.

5. Emotional needs of the patient and family members are important. Emotional support is vital when dealing with a life-threatening illness. Health care professionals will want to determine where that support comes from for the patient. Should a support group be suggested for the patient and family members? For some patients and families, an individual giving spiritual guidance is seen as a member of the family and a member of the health care team. For others, no spiritual influence is recognized or sought.

It is not the responsibility of the health care professionals treating the individual with life-threatening illness to provide all these services, but a health care professional who raises these issues for patients and families to deal with is more closely in tune with a patient's power in the illness.

THE RANGE OF PSYCHOLOGICAL SUFFERING

The range of suffering associated with a life-threatening illness is extensive. Patients feel extreme distress. Anxiety and depression are common. At the time of diagnosis, patients' responses may include denial, numbness, and inability to face the facts. Sadness, hopelessness, helplessness, and withdrawal often are exhibited.

The range of psychological suffering leads to physical symptoms, such as tension, tachycardia, agitation, insomnia, anorexia, and panic attacks. The physician may be so intent on treating the physical ramifications of the illness that the psychological suffering is mostly ignored.

Relationships of individuals with a life-threatening illness often change. Close friends may feel uncomfortable with someone who is dying. Some fear touching or caressing the dying and become aloof and distant. However, new friendships can often be made as well, if patients meet others with the same or similar life-threatening issues and help maintain each other's self-esteem. Relationships are important because they provide support and encouragement beyond any other source. Patients experience a loss of self-esteem when they are ill, are in pain, and have a body that is failing them. When self-image is lost, patients feel useless, see themselves as burdens, and have difficulty accepting help from anyone. The psychological effect of this "loss of self" can even hasten death.

It is often helpful to encourage patients to set goals for themselves. These can be small goals such as walking around the block, eating all their dinner, and connecting with a friend. The goals may also be much larger, such as staying alive until a son graduates from college, or putting all financial matters in order for surviving family members. Personal goals give the patient something other than their illness to plan for and work toward.

Careful listening to patients and seeking clues for what *may not* be said is essential for the medical assistant and support staff caring for patients. Putting yourself in their shoes and asking what would be helpful is often beneficial. Be ready with a list of community resources that may benefit patients at this time.

It is not the intention of this chapter to specifically identify the many life-threatening illnesses and their particular needs. However, three threatening illnesses are identified in the following sections with some specific information.

THE THERAPEUTIC RESPONSE TO THE PATIENT WITH HIV/AIDS

Patients testing positive for human immunodeficiency virus (HIV) and those with acquired immune deficiency syndrome (AIDS) feel great stress from the infection, the disease, and the fear of other life-threatening illnesses. Persons with HIV infection may have only a short time before the onset of AIDS; others may have a much longer period. AIDS is a disease that can have many periods of fairly good health and many periods of serious near-death illnesses. Recent developments in the treatment of HIV infection and AIDS help patients to live longer, but their lives are greatly compromised because of their suppressed immune system.

In some cases, guilt develops about past behavior and lifestyles, or the possibility of having transmitted the disease to others. Members of the gay community or individuals addicted to intravenous drugs who are at high risk for the disease may also be estranged from their family's support system. Individuals with HIV infection may feel added strain if this is the first knowledge their families have of any high-risk behaviors they have that are associated with the transmission of the disease. When the disease is contracted by individuals who feel they are protected or safe from the disease, anger is paramount. HIV has affected mostly individuals who are relatively young. Thus, they are not as likely to have substantial financial resources or permanent housing. Treating HIV is expensive, and many patients have little or no insurance coverage.

Patients with HIV may experience central nervous system involvement. Forgetfulness and poor concentra-

Critical Thinking

What can be done to help individuals with HIV to cope with their emotional roller coaster?

tion may be followed by **psychomotor retardation,** or the slowing of physical and mental responses, decreased alertness, apathy, withdrawal, and diminished interest in work. Some patients later experience confusion and progressive impairment of intellectual function or dementia. When HIV-infected patients contract other opportunistic diseases, those symptoms are experienced as well.

THE THERAPEUTIC RESPONSE TO THE PATIENT WITH CANCER

The first reaction patients with cancer usually have is the fear of loss of life. Patients think, "Cancer equals death. Am I going to die?" After that, issues begin to differ for each person. Some may choose no treatment and allow life to take its course. Most, however, will wonder about what treatment to choose, how to make that choice, and how effective will it be. Many patients are empowered by taking a major role in the decision making related to their cancer. Research can be helpful in studying the many options that may be available in treatment. The fact is that many patients diagnosed with cancer will die, whereas others diagnosed will live many years after diagnosis and treatment.

The three most likely treatments for cancer are surgery, radiation, and chemotherapy. Often, treatment is a combination of the three. Patients can experience serious side effects from both radiation and chemotherapy. Alternative practitioners have shown that meditation or acupuncture can help relieve the side effects for some patients. Loss of hair, nausea, vomiting, and pain are quite disconcerting to patients trying to cope. The American

Critical Thinking

Many individuals in the end stages of both AIDS and cancer have lost their image of themselves. Their bodies have been diminished; they may have lost a great deal of weight from the disease or gained much weight from medications taken. They may have no hair. They may have lost their ability to speak or to control bodily functions. What can you do or say to help them feel like a human being?

Cancer Society (http://www.cancer.org) has a number of resources for patients.

The most common signs and symptoms of advanced cancer are weakness, loss of appetite and weight, pain, nausea, constipation, sleepiness or confusion, and shortness of breath. Make certain your patients understand your physician's willingness to relieve and treat these symptoms. Even when there is "nothing more to do" related to the cancer, there is still "much to do" to maintain comfort and to give patients the chance to do the things that are meaningful to them and their families.

THE THERAPEUTIC RESPONSE TO THE PATIENT WITH END-STAGE RENAL DISEASE

Loss of kidney (renal) function leads to serious illness known as end-stage renal disease (ESRD). When the kidneys fail completely, patients cannot live for long unless they receive dialysis or a kidney transplant. A successful kidney transplant relieves the person of kidney failure. However, there are not enough transplants for every person who needs one, and not all transplants are appropriate or successful. Dialysis is the name of the process of artificially replacing the main functions of the kidneys—filtering blood to remove wastes. Choosing dialysis as a treatment plan can sustain life for years and is covered by Medicare, but it does have complications that burden patients and their caregivers.

Depending on age, a patient's general health, and other circumstances, some patients will opt not to have dialysis and to let death come from kidney failure. The by-products of the body's chemistry accumulate in renal failure and cause an array of symptoms. Mild confusion and disorientation are common. Upsetting hallucinations or agitation can occur. Certain minerals concentrated in the blood can cause muscle twitching, tremors, and shakes. Some patients experience mild or severe itching. Appetite decreases early, and there can be rapid, shallow breathing. Many patients with kidney failure pass little or no urine. Fluid overload results in edema, or swelling of the body, particularly of the legs and abdomen. Patients with some urine output may live for months even after stopping dialysis. People with no urine output are likely to die within a week or two. Patients will lose energy and become sleepy and lethargic. Typically, patients slip into a deeper sleep and gradually lose consciousness. Kidney failure has a reputation for being a gentle death.

Life-threatening illnesses are family illnesses. There are primary (the person suffering from the illness) and secondary (family and friends) patients. Stress on a spouse or partner is enormous as they think about taking over the other person's role and as they try to deal with their own feelings. Patients and their families and friends cannot avoid feeling angry. The situation is tragic and, in some instances, might have been avoided (for example, a long-time smoker dying of lung cancer). There needs to be time to grieve. Depression is common among patients with life-threatening illness and warning signs should be reported to the physician. Remember that how patients live their last days is just as important as the numbers on the laboratory reports.

The Stages of Grief

There are a number of different philosophies on grief and the stages patients are apt to experience when they know their lives are about to end, but none is so widely known as that of Dr. Elisabeth Kubler-Ross, who was one of the first to conduct research and determine possible stages of grief. Those stages are:

Denial—"This *cannot* be happening to me."

Anger—"Why is this happening to me?"

Bargaining—"Okay, but only if I can just watch my last child graduate from college."

Depression—"I feel sad, blue, and prefer not to be around anyone."

Acceptance—"If this must be, then I am ready."

Dr. Kubler-Ross reminds health care professionals that not all patients go through all five stages; some patients go through all five stages many, many times, and still others get stuck in one stage, usually the denial stage. Grief and dying is personal. No two patients will follow the same pattern. The stages are identified so that you can be more aware of what is happening in the process to both the patients and their loved ones. Clashes are likely among family members and patients when they are in different stages.

THE CHALLENGE FOR THE MEDICAL ASSISTANT

As a medical assistant, you face the challenge of caring for people with a life-threatening illness; you must comfort those who face great suffering and death. You will become a source of information for patients and their support members. You must be particularly sensitive

Critical Thinking

What steps would you personally take to make certain you do not burnout from caring for patients with a life-threatening illness?

and respectful toward individuals who may be viewed as social pariahs. You will have to examine your own beliefs, lifestyle, and biases. You must be comfortable treating all patients, no matter what the illness is or how it was contracted.

As well as assisting your physician–employer in providing the best possible medical care, many nonmedical forms of assistance may be required by patients suffering from a life-threatening illness. You may need to make referrals to community-based agencies or service groups. Health departments, social workers, trained hospice volunteers, and AIDS volunteers may also be helpful to you, your patients, and their families.

The best therapeutic response to the patient with a life-threatening illness will build on the person's own culture and coping abilities, capitalize on strengths, maintain hope, and show continued human care and concern. Patients may want up-to-date information on their disease, its causes, modes of transmission, treatments available, and sources of care and social support. Be prepared to recommend support groups where patients can discuss their feelings and express their concerns. Treat patients with concern and compassion and assure them everything will be done to provide continuity of care and relief from distress. Patients may be encouraged to call on clergy for spiritual support.

Case Study 6-1

The extended family of Wong Lee is concerned about his illness and his care. Chronic obstructive pulmonary disease (COPD) has ravaged his body. He is on oxygen all the time now. He wants to remain at home to die; his family wants that, too. The family has been with him and has been involved in his care plan all along. Yet you are still uncertain of how much information to give to members of his expanded family when they call.

CASE STUDY REVIEW

1. Are the questions the extended family members raise intended to harm or help Mr. Lee?
2. Is there a durable power of attorney for health care in place?
3. Which, if any, of the family's desires are related to the culture?
4. What can you and your physician–employer suggest to be of help to everyone involved?

Case Study 6-2

Inner City Health Care, a multidoctor urgent care center in a large city, has a large roster of patients, some of whom have AIDS. Although clinical medical assistant Bruce Goldman tries not to be, sometimes he is nervous about assisting with patients who are gay. When Bill Swartz is seen by the physician for a change in a mole on his calf, Bruce does his best to interact in a professional manner even though Bill is gay. After this patient exchange, Bruce Goldman decides it is time to deal with his prejudices against gay and lesbians, as well as his fear of AIDS and all patients with AIDS.

CASE STUDY REVIEW

1. Although Bruce Goldman may not admit it, he is fearful of AIDS. What should he know about HIV transmission that may reduce his fears?
2. In the future, Bruce would like to be more open and supportive when he is dealing with an HIV-infected patient. What are some of the things he can do to help patients?
3. What are some things Bruce can do to reduce wariness regarding patients who are gay?

SUMMARY

Medical assistants must be aware that when caring for patients with a life-threatening illness, having even the slightest fear of death can undermine the ability to respond professionally, with empathy and support. If you feel yourself losing the ability to be helpful, it is time to briefly step aside. This does not mean withdrawal from your position or refusal to care for your patients. It means that you do whatever is necessary so that your perspective is not lost. It may mean taking a day off from work to "fill up your psyche" and to give yourself a rest. If the ambulatory care setting has an abundance of patients with life-threatening illnesses, it may require that you spend some time in a support group of your own so that you are better able to cope. Never be afraid to feel sad or weep with your patients. It is better to sense their pain and, at times, feel the pain with them, than it is to be so clinically objective you miss their true needs.

STUDY FOR SUCCESS

To reinforce your knowledge and skills of information in this chapter:

- ❑ Review the Key Terms
- ❑ Consider the Case Studies and discuss your conclusions
- ❑ Answer the Review Questions
  - ❑ Multiple Choice
  - ❑ Critical Thinking
- ❑ Navigate the Internet and complete the Web Activities

- ❑ Practice the StudyWARE activities on the textbook CD
- ❑ Apply your knowledge in the Student Workbook activities
- ❑ Complete the Web Tutor sections
- ❑ View and discuss the DVD situations

REVIEW QUESTIONS

Multiple Choice

1. When a practice treats patients with HIV/AIDS, cancer, or ESRD, it is important for medical assistants to:
   a. warn other patients about the dangers of transmission
   b. segregate these patient reception areas from other patient areas
   c. be supportive and free of prejudice
   d. deny any information to patients regarding the seriousness of the illness

2. The Patient Self-Determination Act:
   a. allows a patient to have a choice of physicians
   b. ensures a patient's right to accept or refuse treatment
   c. gives patients the right to formulate advance directives
   d. all of the above
   e. only b and c

3. The strongest influence on a patient with a life-threatening illness is:
   a. the physician
   b. the hospital
   c. the family
   d. the patient

4. Life-threatening illness may be defined as:
   a. a life shortened because of serious illness or disease
   b. death that is imminent
   c. serious illness to battle for many years but may shorten life
   d. all of the above

5. Culture may be defined in part as:
   a. how we choose a friend
   b. how we think and live our lives
   c. how we select a medication
   d. all of the above

6. Therapeutic communication with a patient with a life-threatening illness:
   a. is no different than communicating with any patient
   b. is heightened and considered more difficult
   c. is left to nonmedical support staff
   d. comes naturally and requires no special skill
7. Cultural influence may in part determine:
   a. when/how to involve family members
   b. whether spiritual support is sought
   c. how the illness and its pain is managed
   d. all of the above
8. Durable power of attorney for health care:
   a. enables someone other than the patient to make only health care decisions
   b. enables someone other than the patient to make any decisions for the patient
   c. makes certain that patients' financial responsibilities are met
   d. makes certain an attorney's wishes are followed
9. The confusion, disorientation, and mental deficiency seen in some patients with life-threatening illness:
   a. may make communication difficult or impossible
   b. is a good reason for a durable power of attorney for health care
   c. is made easier if patients expressed earlier their desires in a physician's directive
   d. all of the above
10. Effective pain management may depend on:
    a. patient's medical insurance
    b. family wishes and patient's needs
    c. professional nursing criteria
    d. all of the above

Critical Thinking

1. Research other sections in this text that discuss end-of-life legal documents. Describe additional information you find.
2. Discuss with a friend what cultural influences might affect each of you if you were facing a life-threatening illness. What choices would each of you make?
3. List common psychological reactions people might have from learning they have a life-threatening illness.
4. List the advantages/disadvantages of the physician directives available.
5. Discuss with a nurse or a nursing student in your school how nurses deal with the psychological suffering in patients with a life-threatening illness.
6. Discuss with a classmate your concerns in dealing with patients with a life-threatening illness. Would you choose to work where you seldom lost a patient to a life-threatening illness? If so, what are your reasons?
7. Research the agencies available in your community that can provide support for people and family members facing life-threatening illness.
8. At Inner City Health Care, Dr. Ray Reynolds is known for his compassion and great warmth toward people. On difficult days at the center, this attitude holds him in good stead. Sometimes, he tends to take on the more challenging cases: patients with life-threatening diseases, often young people with AIDS who should be in the prime of their lives. Clinical medical assistant Wanda Slawson always tries to learn from Dr. Reynolds' example. Although she is quieter and not as outgoing as Dr. Reynolds, Wanda hopes to be both courteous and comforting to patients, especially those who are anxious. She makes it a point to help patients discover a new way to cope with debilitating diseases. What resources might she use?
9. Teri Montague, RMA, is the office manager for a pediatric oncologist. In the past several months there seem to have been more patient deaths than usual. She notices that the entire staff seems "low and a little depressed." She discusses this concern with her physician–employer, Dr. Anita Glenn. The decision is made to close the office for a 2-hour lunch on Wednesday. The lunch will be catered, and a very good friend of Dr. Glenn will be invited to join everyone. Dr. Penny Hein has a PhD in psychosocial nursing and years of experience in grief counseling. Teri and Dr. Glenn believe she can give everyone some helpful information. Is this a good plan? Why or why not?

THE DVD HOOK-UP

DVD Series	Program Number
Critical Thinking	**2**

Chapter/Scene Reference
• *Communicating with Patients*

This chapter introduces you to the concept of using a therapeutic approach when working with patients.

In the designated DVD clip, we observed Mrs. Smith become quite anxious about her abnormal mammogram results. We also observed how Gwen, the medical assistant, addressed Mrs. Smith's concerns.

1. Do you feel that Gwen demonstrated a therapeutic approach toward Mrs. Smith's concern over her abnormal mammogram results?
2. List some gestures that Gwen used that illustrated her concern and compassion toward the patient.
3. Did Gwen overstep her boundaries as a medical assistant when she discussed the mammogram results with Mrs. Smith, or do you think that Gwen was trying to help the patient understand what the physician had already explained?

DVD Journal Summary
Write a paragraph that summarizes what you learned from watching the designated scene from today's DVD program. Did you empathize with Mrs. Smith regarding her anxiety over her abnormal mammogram? What will you do when you are faced with similar challenges in the industry? Do you think that you could ever work in an oncology practice? Why or why not?

WEB ACTIVITIES

1. Using your favorite search engine, key in American Cancer Society and look for statistics for the current year. Pay particular attention to the area reporting how long patients survive after diagnosis. What are the major changes in the last two years?
2. Many sites will come on your screen when you search for end-stage renal disease (ESRD). Seek out the site that identifies the six warning signs of kidney and urinary tract diseases. Identify the functions of the kidneys and what happens in ESRD. How many people in the U.S. population have ESRD?
3. Using search words "HIV Today" will take you to an AEGIS site that includes the latest press releases and statistics on AIDS. Browse around a bit. In what countries of the world is AIDS the greatest threat? Did you find a fact sheet providing a list of opportunistic infections related to AIDS? Print copies of a resource or two that might help patients.
4. Using the World Wide Web can be challenging, especially if you find more that 270,000 sites to browse. That is what you will find if you key in "Helping the Dying." Choose a couple of the topics that are especially helpful to you or might help other students studying this chapter. Write a brief paragraph on each.

REFERENCES/BIBLIOGRAPHY

Lewis, M., & Tamparo, C. (2002). *Medical law, ethics, and bioethics for ambulatory care*. Philadelphia: F. A. Davis Company.

Purnell, L., & Paulanka, B. (1998). *Transcultural health care: A culturally competent approach*. Philadelphia: F. A. Davis Company.

Tamparo, C., & Lindh, W. (2000). *Therapeutic communications for health professionals*. Clifton Park, NY: Thomson Delmar Learning.

UNIT 3
Responsible Medical Practice

Legal Considerations

OUTLINE

OBJECTIVES

The student should strive to meet the following performance objectives and demonstrate an understanding of the facts and principles presented in this chapter through written and oral communication.

1. Define the key terms as presented in the glossary.
2. List and briefly describe the five sources of law.
3. Compare/contrast civil and criminal law.
4. Identify the three major areas of civil law that directly affect the medical profession.

(continues)

KEY TERMS

(continues)

FEATURED COMPETENCIES

CAAHEP—ENTRY-LEVEL COMPETENCIES

Patient Care
- Maintain medication and immunization records

Legal Concepts
- Identify and respond to issues of confidentiality
- Perform within legal and ethical boundaries
- Demonstrate knowledge of federal and state health care legislation and regulations

ABHES—ENTRY-LEVEL COMPETENCIES

Professionalism
- Maintain confidentiality at all times
- Be cognizant of ethical boundaries
- Conduct work within scope of education, training, and ability

Legal Concepts
- Use appropriate guidelines when releasing information
- Follow established policy in initiating or terminating medical treatment

(continues)

OBJECTIVES (continued)

5. Recall at least seven of the nine administrative law acts important to the medical profession.
6. Compare/contrast administering, prescribing, and dispensing of controlled substances.
7. Describe the measures to take for disposal of controlled substances.
8. Recall the three main goals of HIPAA.
9. Explain the differences between expressed and implied contracts.
10. Identify the three main reasons for the physician/patient contract to be terminated.
11. Define and give examples of torts.
12. List and describe the 4Ds of negligence.
13. Discuss what constitutes battery in the ambulatory care setting.
14. Describe the two forms of defamation of character and how it might occur.
15. Recall how medical assistants can help to maintain a patient's privacy.
16. Identify at least 10 practices to help in risk management.
17. Discuss informed consent and its importance.
18. Compare/contrast the types of minors.
19. Outline the necessary steps in civil litigation and how a medical assistant might be involved.
20. Discuss how and when subpoenas are used.
21. Recall the special considerations for patients related to issues of confidentiality, the statute of limitations, public duties, and AIDS.
22. Describe procedures to follow in reporting abuse.
23. Discuss Good Samaritan laws.
24. Identify various forms of physician's directives.
25. Recall maintenance of advanced directives in the ambulatory care setting.
26. Discuss HIPAA regulations for confidentiality in physician's directives.

SCENARIO

Gwen, the office manager in Dr. Gold's office, is reviewing legal concerns in a staff meeting. Even though each employee is well aware of privacy, confidentiality, and the many ways their actions are legally binding, Gwen has noticed occasional carelessness creeping into their busy activities. Employees are reminded of how far their voices may carry in a phone conversation with a patient, they review placement of patients' medical charts for Dr. Gold, and they discuss how to protect confidentiality in filing insurance claims.

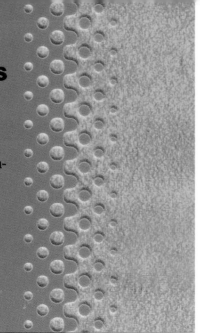
INTRODUCTION

The law as it relates to health care has grown increasingly complex in the last decade. The agendas of federal and state governments include an investigation of quality health care, a desire to control health care costs (whereas hoping to ensure equitable access to health care), and an interest in protecting the patient. A full discussion of health law requires several volumes; therefore, the aim of this chapter is awareness of the law and its implications and establishment of sound practices and procedures to both safeguard patient rights and protect the health care professional.

SOURCES OF LAW

 Law is a binding custom or ruling for conduct that is enforceable by an agency assigned that authority. The highest authority in the United States is the U.S. Constitution. Adopted in 1787, this document provides the framework for the U.S. government. The Constitution includes 27 amendments, 10 of which are known as the Bill of Rights. This authority is sometimes referred to as **constitutional law.** The U.S. Constitution calls for three branches of the federal government:

- Executive branch: the President, Vice President (elected by U.S. citizens), Cabinet officers, and various other departments of the federal government

- Legislative branch: members of the U.S. Senate, the House of Representatives (elected by U.S. citizens), and the staffs of individual legislators and legislative committees.

- Judicial branch: the courts, including the U.S. Supreme Court, Courts of Appeals for the nine judicial regions, and District Courts

Laws enacted at the federal level are called acts or laws. An example is Title XIX of Public Law established in 1967 to provide health care for the **medically indigent.** This program is known as Medicaid.

Statutory Law

Constitutions in the 50 states identify the rights and responsibilities of their citizens and identify how their state is organized. States have a governor as the head and state legislatures (both elected by the state's citizens), as well as their own court systems with a number of levels. The body of laws made by states is known as **statutory law.** All powers that are not conferred specifically on the federal government are retained by the state, yet states vary widely in their interpretation of that power. State law cannot override the power of any laws defined in the U.S. Constitution or its amendments.

Common Law

Common law is not so easily defined, but is essential to understanding law in the United States. Common law was developed by judges in England and France over many centuries and was brought to the United States with the early settlers. Common law is often called judge-made law. The law consists of rulings made by judges who base their decisions on a combination of a number of factors: (1) individual decisions of a court, (2) interpretation of the U.S. Constitution or a particular state constitution, and (3) statutory law. These decisions become known as **precedents** and often lay down the foundation for subsequent legal rulings.

Criminal Law

Criminal law addresses wrongs committed against the welfare and safety of society as a whole. Criminal law affects relationships between individuals and between individuals and the government. Another term that might be used to describe a criminal act is **malfeasance.** Malfeasance is conduct that is illegal or contrary to an official's obligation. Criminal offenses generally are classified into the basic categories of a **felony** or a **misdemeanor** that are specifically defined in statutes.

Felonies are more serious crimes and include murder, larceny or thefts of large amounts of money, assault, and rape. Punishment for a felony is more serious than for a misdemeanor. A convicted felon cannot vote, hold public office, or own any weapons. Felonies often are divided into groups such as first degree (most serious), second degree, and third degree. Sentences are generally for longer than one year and are served in a penitentiary. Misdemeanors are considered lesser offenses and vary from state to state. Punishment may include probation or a time of service to the community, a fine, or a jail sentence in a city or county facility. Misdemeanors also can be divided into groups or classifications, such as A, B, or C class misdemeanors, denoting the seriousness of the crime (Class A is the most serious).

For a person to be found guilty of a crime, a judge or jury must prove the evidence against the individual "beyond a reasonable doubt." In a criminal case, charges are brought against an individual by the state with the intent of preventing any further harm to society. For example, a physician practicing medicine without a proper license may be subject to criminal action by the courts for endangering a patient's life.

Civil Law

Civil law affects relationships between individuals, corporations, government bodies, and other organizations. Terms that may be used in civil law are **misfeasance,** referring to a lawful act that is improperly or unlawfully executed, and **nonfeasance,** referring to the failure to perform an act, official duty, or legal requirement. The punishment for a civil wrong is usually monetary in nature. When a charge is brought against a **defendant** in a civil case, the goal is to reimburse the **plaintiff** or the

person bringing charges with a monetary amount for suffering, pain, and any loss of wages. Another goal might be to make certain the defendant is prevented from engaging in similar behavior again. In civil law, cases need to show that a "preponderance of the evidence" is more than likely true against the defendant. The most common forms of civil law that directly affect the medical profession are **administrative law, contract law,** and **tort law.**

ADMINISTRATIVE LAW

Administrative law establishes agencies that are given power to specialize and enact regulations that have the force of law. The Internal Revenue Service is an example of an administrative agency that enacts tax laws and regulations. Health care professionals are bound by federal administrative law through the Medicare and Medicaid program rules administered by the Social Security Administration.

There are a number of other regulations in administrative law governing physicians and their employees. It is important that medical assistants be informed of legislation and any federal or state regulations that are critical to patients and the medical profession. Membership and attendance at meetings of professional organizations supporting the medical professions is a good way to remain current in health care issues. Identified here with a brief description are additional administrative acts, some of which also are referred to in other chapters in this textbook.

Title VII of the Civil Rights Act

Title VII of the Civil Rights Act of 1964 protects employees from sexual harassment. The office of Equal Employment Opportunities Commission (EEOC) guidelines make the employer strictly liable for the acts of supervisory employees, as well as for some acts of harassment by coworkers and clients. A written policy on sexual harassment detailing inappropriate behavior and stating specific steps to be taken to correct an inappropriate situation should be established. The policy should include: (1) a statement that harassment is not tolerated, (2) a statement that an employee who feels harassed needs to bring the matter to the immediate attention of a person designated in the policy, (3) a statement about the confidentiality of any incidents and specific disciplinary action against the harasser, and (4) the procedure to follow when harassment occurs.

Federal Age Discrimination Act

The Federal Age Discrimination Act of 1967 states that an employer with 15 or more employees must not discriminate in matters of employment related to age, sex, race, creed, marital status, national origin, color, or disabilities. Some states are more restrictive in their law and identify employers with eight or more employees. Valid reasons to decline applicants include: (1) health issues that may interfere with the safe and efficient performance of the job, (2) unavailability for the work schedule of the particular job, (3) insufficient training or experience to perform the duties of the particular job, and (4) someone else is better qualified.

Uniform Anatomical Gift Act

The Uniform Anatomical Gift Act of 1968 allows persons 18 years or older and of sound mind to make a gift of all or any part of their body (1) to any hospital, surgeon, or physician; (2) to any accredited medical or dental school, college, or university; (3) to any organ bank or storage facility; and (4) to any specified individual for education, research, advancement of medical/dental science, therapy, or transplantation. The gift may be noted in a will or by signing, in the presence of two witnesses, a donor's card. Some states allow these statements on the driver's license.

Regulation Z of the Consumer Protection Act

Regulation Z of the Consumer Protection Act of 1967, referred to as the Truth in Lending Act, requires that an agreement by physicians and their clients for payment of medical bills in more than four installments must be in writing and must provide information on any finance charge. This act is enforced by the Federal Trade Commission. These guidelines are often seen in prearrangements for surgery or prenatal care and delivery in fee-for-service plans, because patients may not be able to pay the entire fee in one payment.

Occupational Safety and Health Act

 The Occupational Safety and Health Act (OSHA) of 1967 is a division of the U.S. Department of Labor. Its mission is to ensure that a workplace is safe and has a healthy environment. Penalties can be quite high for repeated and willful violations assessed by OSHA. These guidelines make certain that all employees know what chemicals they are handling, know how to reduce any health risks from hazardous chemicals that are labeled 1 to 4 for severity, and have Material Safety Data Sheets (MSDSs) listing every ingredient in the product. Other sections of this law protecting medical assistants and patients are detailed in additional chapters. They include Clinical Lab Improvement Amendments of 1988 (CLIA), Blood-

borne Pathogens Standard of July 1992, and the Needle Stick Prevention Amendment of 2001.

Controlled Substances Act

The Controlled Substances Act of 1970 became effective in 1971. The act is administered by the Drug Enforcement Administration (DEA) under the auspices of the U.S. Department of Justice. The Controlled Substances Act lists controlled drugs in five schedules (I, II, III, IV, and V) according to their potential for abuse and dependence, with Schedule I having the greatest abuse potential and no accepted medical use in the United States. This act and the U.S. Code of Federal Regulations regulate individuals who administer, prescribe, or dispense any drug listed in the five schedules. Every physician who **administers, prescribes,** or **dispenses** any controlled substance must be registered with the DEA. The DEA supplies a form for registration and mandates that renewal occurs every three years.

A physician who only prescribes Schedule II, III, IV, and V controlled substances in the lawful course of professional practice is not required to keep separate records of those transactions. Physicians who regularly administer controlled substances in Schedules II, III, IV, and V or who dispense controlled substances are required to keep records of each transaction.

An inventory must be taken every two years of all stocks of the substances on hand. The inventory must include: (1) a list of the name, address, and DEA registration number of the physician; (2) the date and time of the inventory; and (3) the signatures of the individuals taking the inventory. This inventory must be kept at the location identified on the registration certificate for at least two years. All Schedule II drug records must be maintained separate from all other controlled substance records. These records must be made available for inspection and copying by duly authorized officials of the DEA. Some states are even more restrictive than the federal requirements.

Any necessary disposal of controlled substances, usually occurring when they become outdated or when a physician's practice is closed, requires specific action. The physician's DEA number and registration certificate should be returned to the DEA. Specific guidelines for destruction of the controlled substances will need to be

Critical Thinking

Identify the type of doctors or medical specialties most likely to prescribe and dispense controlled substances.

obtained from the nearest divisional office for the DEA. Using the Internet, search using the words "Controlled Substances Act of 1970" for a listing of sites providing more information. You will find a listing of drugs in each of the five schedules that change from time to time as new drugs come on the market and are classified.

Americans with Disabilities Act

The Americans with Disabilities Act (ADA) of 1990 prohibits discrimination of individuals who have physical or mental disabilities from accessing public services and accommodations, employment, and telecommunications. A disability implies that a physical or mental impairment substantially limits one or more of an individual's major life activities. ADA is identified in five titles. Title I, enforced by the EEOC, prohibits discrimination in employment (see Chapter 23 for further details). Essentially, Title I requires a potential employer to identify and prove that certain disabilities cannot be accommodated in performing the job requirements. Individuals who formerly abused drugs and alcohol and those who are undergoing rehabilitation also are covered by the ADA and cannot be denied employment because of their history of substance abuse.

Titles II, III, and IV mandate disabled individuals access to public services, public accommodations, and telecommunications. ADA protects persons with HIV infection or AIDS, making certain they cannot be refused treatment by health care professionals because of their health status. Generally speaking, health care professionals with HIV infection or AIDS cannot be kept from providing treatment either, unless that treatment could be found to be a significant risk to others. Title V covers a number of miscellaneous issues such as exclusions from the definition of "disability," retaliation, insurance, and other issues. The ADA law applies to businesses with at least 15 employees, but some states have more stringent laws.

Family and Medical Leave Act

The Family and Medical Leave Act (FLMA) of 1993 is important for large ambulatory care centers and hospitals. FLMA requires all public employers and any private employer of 50 or more employees to provide up to 12 weeks of job-protected, unpaid leave each year for the following reasons: (1) birth and care of the employee's child, or placement for adoption or foster care of a child; (2) care of an immediate family member who has a serious health condition; and (3) care of the employee's own serious health issue. Employees must have been employed for at least 12 months and have worked at least 1,250 hours in the 12 months preceding the beginning of the FMLA leave.

Health Insurance Portability and Accountability Act

The Health Insurance Portability and Accountability Act (HIPAA) of 1996 requires the Department of Health and Human Services to adopt national standards for electronic health care transactions. The law also requires the adoption of privacy and security standards to protect an individual's identifiable health information. The goal of HIPAA is also to assist in making health insurance more affordable and accessible to individuals by protecting health insurance coverage for workers and their families when they change or lose their jobs.

HIPAA law is identified in seven titles. They are summarized briefly as follows:

I. Health Insurance Access, Portability, and Renewal: Increases the portability of health insurance, allows continuance and transfer of insurance even with preexisting conditions, and prohibits discrimination based on health status.

II. Preventing Health Care Fraud and Abuse: Establishes a fraud and abuse system and spells out penalty if either event is documented; improves the Medicare program through establishing standards; establishes standards for electronic transmission of health information.

III. Tax-Related Provisions: Promotes the use of medical savings accounts (MSAs) used for medical expenses only. Deposits are tax-deductible for self-employed individuals who are able to draw on the accounts for medical expenses.

IV. Group Health Plan Requirements: Identifies how group health care plans must plan for portability, access, and transferability of health insurance for its members.

V. Revenue Offsets: Details how HIPAA changed the Internal Revenue Code to generate more revenue for HIPAA expenses.

VI. General Provisions: Explains how coordination with Medicare-type plans must be carried out to prevent duplication of coverage.

VII. Assuring Portability: Ensures employee coverage from one plan to another; written specifically for health insurance plans to ensure portability of coverage.

As of April 14, 2004, all covered health care entities were to have been in compliance of HIPAA's regulations. Each time a newly formed agency with regulations to practice appears, there is concern about how to comply and what costs will be involved. However, once the electronic codes and transactions for electronic filing of health insurance claims have been identified and put in place, the required security and privacy of all patient information is not as complex. If medical facilities and physician practices have been consistently diligent about protecting patient confidentiality, complying with HIPAA is not difficult. Many helpful Web sites are available simply by keying in HIPAA and having your favorite search engine identify sites. Look for a site that explains or summarizes this public law. You will see mention of HIPAA throughout this text as identified by the HIPAA icon as shown on the left.

CONTRACT LAW

The contractual nature of the doctor–patient relationship necessitates a discussion of contracts, which is an important part of a physician's practice. A contract is a binding agreement between two or more persons. A physician has a legal obligation, or duty, to care for a patient under the principles of contract law. The agreement must be between competent persons to do or not to do something lawful in exchange for a payment.

A contract exists when the patient arrives for treatment and the physician accepts the patient by providing treatment. An example of a valid contract occurs when a patient calls the office or clinic to make an appointment for an annual physical examination. Assuming both physician and patient are competent, and that the physician performs the lawful act of the physical examination and the patient pays a fee, all aspects of the contract exist.

There are two types of contracts: expressed and implied. An **expressed contract** can be written or verbal and will specifically describe what each party in the contract will do. A written contract requires that all necessary aspects of the agreement be in writing. An **implied contract** is indicated by actions rather than by words. The majority of physician–patient contracts are implied contracts. It is not required that the contract be written to be enforceable as long as all points of the contract exist. An implied contract can exist either by the circumstances of the situation or by the law. When a patient reports a sore throat and the physician does a throat culture to diagnose and treat the ailment, an implied contract exists by the circumstances. An implied contract by law exists when a patient goes into anaphylactic shock and the physician administers epinephrine to counteract shock symptoms. The law says that the physician did what the patient would have requested had there been an expressed contract.

For a contract to be valid and binding, the parties who enter into it must be competent; therefore, the mentally incompetent, the legally insane, individuals under heavy drug or alcohol influences, infants, and some minors cannot enter into a binding contract.

Medical assistants are considered **agents** of the physicians they serve, and as such must be cautious that their actions and words may become binding for their physi-

cians. For example, to say that the doctor can cure the patient may cause serious legal problems when, in fact, a cure may not be possible.

Termination of Contracts

A broken contract or breach of contract occurs when one of the parties does not meet contractual obligations. A physician is legally bound to treat a patient until:

- The patient discharges the physician
- The physician formally withdraws from patient care
- The patient no longer needs treatment and is formally discharged by the physician

Patient Discharges Physician. When the patient discharges the physician, the physician should send a letter to the patient to confirm and document the termination of the contract. The notice should be sent by certified mail with return receipt requested. Keep a copy of the letter in the patient's record (Figure 7-1).

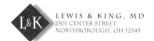

LEWIS & KING, MD
2501 CENTER STREET
NORTHBOROUGH, OH 12345

January 6, 20XX

CERTIFIED MAIL

Jim Marshal
76 Georgia Avenue
Millerton, TX 43912

Dear Mr. Marshal:

This will confirm our telephone conversation today in which you discharged me as your attending physician in your present illness. In my opinion your condition requires continued medical supervision by a physician. If you have not already done so, I suggest that you employ another physician without delay.

You may be assured that after receiving a written request from you, I will furnish the physician of your choice with information regarding the diagnosis and treatment which you have received from me.

Very truly yours,

Winston Lewis

Winston Lewis, MD
WL:ea

Figure 7-1 Letter confirms physician's discharge by the patient.

Inner City Health Care
222 S. First Avenue
Carlton, MI 11666

May 9, 20XX

CERTIFIED MAIL

Lenny Taylor
260 Second Street
Carlton, MI 11666

Dear Mr. Taylor:

You will recall that we discussed our physician-patient relationship in my office on May 6, 20XX.

Your son, George Taylor, and Bruce Goldman, my medical assistant were also present. As you know, the primary difficulty has been your failure to cooperate with the medical plan for your care.

While it is unfortunate that our relationship has reached this stage, I will no longer be able to serve as your physician. I will be available to you on an emergency basis only until June 10, 20XX. Meanwhile, you should immediately call or write the Medical Society, 123 Omega Drive, Carlton, MI 11666, Tel. 123-456-7899 and obtain a list of gerontologists. Any delay could jeopardize your health, so please act quickly.

Your physical (and/or mental) problems include: hypertensive heart disease, decreased kidney function, and arteriosclerosis. You could have additional medical problems that may also require professional care. Once you have found a new physician have him or her call my office. I will be happy to discuss your case with the physician assuming your care, and will transfer a written summary of your case to them upon the receipt of a written request from you to do so.

Thank you for your anticipated cooperation and courtesy.

Very truly yours,

James Whitney

James Whitney, MD
JW:kr

Figure 7-2 Letter reiterates "for the record" the physician's decision to withdraw from the case discussed during a previous meeting with patient.

Physician Formally Withdraws from the Case.

To avoid any charges of abandonment, the physician should formally withdraw from the case when, for example, the patient becomes **noncompliant** or the physician feels the patient can no longer be served. Again, notice should be sent to the patient by certified mail with return receipt

Inner City Health Care
222 S. First Avenue
Carlton, MI 11666

December 5, 20XX

CERTIFIED MAIL

Rhoda Au
41 Academy Road
Carlton, MI 11666

Dear Ms. Au:

I find it necessary to inform you that I am withdrawing further professional medical service to you because of your persistent refusal to follow my medical advice and treatment.

Since your condition requires medical attention, I suggest that you place yourself under the care of another physician without delay. If you so desire, I shall be available to attend you for a reasonable time after you have received this letter, but in no event later than January 7, 20XX. This should give you sufficient time to select a physician from the many competent practitioners in this area.

You may be assured that, upon receiving your written request, I will make available to the physician of your choice your case history and information regarding the diagnosis and treatment which you have received from me.

Very truly yours,

Mark Woo

Mark Woo, MD
MW:kr

Figure 7-3 Letter notifies patient of physician's withdrawal as attending physician.

requested and a copy of the notice should be filed in the patient's record (Figures 7-2 and 7-3).

The Patient No Longer Needs Treatment.

Unless a formal discharge or withdrawal has occurred, a physician is obligated to care for a patient until the patient's condition no longer requires treatment.

TORT LAW

A **tort** is a wrongful act, other than a breach of contract, resulting in injury to one person by another.

Medical Practice Acts

Each state has medical practice acts that regulate the practice of medicine with the intent of protecting its citizens from harm. These statutes govern licensure, standards of care, professional liability and negligence, confidentiality, and torts. Medical assistants sometimes are asked to maintain their employer's records of continuing education for license renewal and to process the renewal at the proper time. In some states, the renewal may be done on-line if the license is active and in good standing.

States also may regulate personnel who are employed in the ambulatory care setting. Generally, medical assistants perform their duties and responsibilities under the direct supervision of the physician or doctor, and therefore are governed by Medical Practice Acts or the Board of Medical Examiners. Medical assistants employed and supervised by independent nurse practitioners are governed by the Nurse Practice Act and the Board of Nursing. Also, some states require that medical assistants be licensed or certified to perform any invasive procedures. Other states require additional training in radiology for the medical assistant to be able to take radiographs. Furthermore, some states are so strict in their regulations that medical assistants mostly perform clerical functions and noninvasive clinical duties.

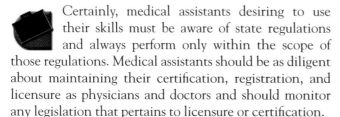 Certainly, medical assistants desiring to use their skills must be aware of state regulations and always perform only within the scope of those regulations. Medical assistants should be as diligent about maintaining their certification, registration, and licensure as physicians and doctors and should monitor any legislation that pertains to licensure or certification.

Standard of Care

To better understand torts, we must consider the standard of care and the four Ds of negligence. Physicians, medical assistants, and all health care providers have the responsibility and duty to perform within their scope of training and to always do what any reasonable and prudent health care professional in the same specialty or general field of practice would do. That is what is expected of every physician when a contact is made by a patient. Failure to do what any reasonable and prudent health care professional would do in the same set of circumstances can be seen as a breach of the standard of care.

Negligence is defined as the failure to exercise the standard of care that a reasonable person would exercise in similar circumstances. Negligence occurs when someone experiences injury because of another's failure to live up to a required duty of care. This is a primary cause of malpractice suits. **Malpractice** is professional negligence.

Four Ds of Negligence. The four elements of negligence, sometimes called the 4 Ds, are:

1. Duty: duty of care
2. Derelict: breach of the duty of care
3. Direct cause: a legally recognizable injury occurs as a result of the breach of duty of care
4. Damage: wrongful activity must have caused the injury or harm that occurred

If an individual has knowledge, skill, or intelligence superior to that of a layperson, that individual's conduct must be consistent with that status. Medical assistants are held to a high standard of care by virtue of their skills, knowledge, and intelligence. As professionals, medical assistants are required to have a standard minimum level of special knowledge and ability. This is what is known as duty of care.

The Medical Assistant's Role in Negligence. Medical assistants may commit a tort that may result in **litigation.** If it can be proven that the injury resulted from the medical assistant (or other health care professional) not meeting the standard of care governing their respective professions, then litigation is a possibility. If, however, the medical assistant (or other health care professional) commits a wrongful act but the patient experiences no injury or harm, then no tort exists. If, for example, the medical assistant changes a wound dressing, breaks sterile technique, and the patient suffers a severely infected wound, the medical assistant has committed a tort and can be held liable, and legal action can be taken. In contrast, if the medical assistant changes a wound dressing, breaks sterile technique, and the patient's wound does not become infected, no harm has occurred, and a tort does not exist. If a medical assistant fails to report to the physician an abnormal result on a blood test that causes the physician to fail to make an early diagnosis of a disease, the assistant's omission of an act has caused a breach in the standard of care.

There are two major classifications of torts: intentional and negligent. Intentional torts are deliberate acts of violation of another's rights. Negligent torts are not deliberate and are the result of omission and commission of an act. Malpractice is the unintentional tort of professional negligence; that is, a professional either failed to act in a reasonable and prudent manner and caused harm to the patient or did what a reasonable and prudent person would not have done and caused harm to a patient.

There are two Latin terms that can be used to describe aspects of negligence. These are known as **doctrines.** *Res ipsa loquitur,* or "the thing speaks for itself," is the term used in cases that involve situations such as a nick made in the bladder when the surgeon is performing a hysterectomy. The negligence is obvious. The other doctrine, *respondeat superior,* "let the master answer," expresses that physicians are responsible for their employees' actions. If a medical assistant violates the standard of care, therein lies the basis for a suit of medical malpractice. For example, the medical assistant used the incorrect solution to clean the patient's wound and the patient sustained injuries to the wound. The physician–employer can be sued under the doctrine of *respondeat superior* because the physician–employer is responsible for the acts of employees committed in the scope of their employment. The medical assistant also can be sued because individuals are responsible for their own actions.

Risk Management

 Some common areas of negligence may result in torts when adherence to the standard of care has not been carried out; practicing good **risk management** makes the medical assistant and the physician–employer less vulnerable to litigation.

Following are some ways to avoid incidents that may lead to litigation:

* Perform only within the scope of your training and education.

* Comply with all state and federal regulations and statutes.

* Keep the office or clinic safe and equipment in readiness.

* Never leave a patient unattended; if you must leave, pass the responsibility for the patient's care on to another individual.

* Keep all patient information confidential.

* Follow all policies and procedures established for the office or clinic.

* Document fully only facts; formally document withdrawing from a case and discharging clients.

* Log telephone calls and return calls to clients within a reasonable time frame.

* Follow up on missed or canceled appointments.

* Never guarantee a cure or diagnosis, and never advise treatment without a physician's order.

* Secure informed consent as necessary.

* Do not criticize other practitioners.

* Explain any appointment delays.

* Be particularly watchful with patients who have special needs, such as the elderly, pediatric patients, and those with physical and emotional disabilities.

* Report any error that may have occurred to your physician–employer.

Critical Thinking

Identify the suggestions in the previous column that are most likely not performed if the staff in the ambulatory care setting find themselves overworked, overwhelmed, and behind. What might be done to prevent carelessness brought on by such circumstances?

Some specific examples of common torts that can occur in the office or clinic are battery, defamation of character, and invasion of privacy.

Battery. The basis of the tort of battery is unprivileged touching of one person by another. A patient must consent to being touched. When a procedure is to be performed on a patient, the patient must give consent in full knowledge of all the facts. It does not matter whether the procedure that constitutes the battery improves the patient's health. Patients have the right to withdraw consent at any time.

One example of battery is when a medical assistant insists on giving the patient an injection the physician ordered for the patient even though the patient refuses the injection. Another example can be seen when a physician performs additional surgery beyond the original procedure (the surgeon performed a hysterectomy, for which consent was given, but is liable for battery for removing an abdominal nevus from the patient's abdomen without consent). It does not matter that the physician does not charge for the additional procedure. It also does not matter if the patient would have given consent if asked in advance.

Defamation of Character. The tort of defamation of character consists of injury to another person's reputation, name, or character through spoken or written words for which damages can be recovered. Two kinds of defamation are **libel** and **slander.** Libel is false and malicious writing about another, such as in published materials, pictures, and media. An example can be seen when the medical assistant writes in the patient's record, "Mr. O'Keefe's wife and her negative attitude appear to be the cause of his ulcer." A copy of Mr. O'Keefe's records were later sent to a new physician who reviewed the record and reads the remarks quoted by the medical assistant.

Slander is false and malicious spoken words. Slander can be seen in the following comment directed by a patient toward the physician, "Dr. Woo is incompetent. He should have his license revoked." The statement is overheard by the office receptionist and other patients waiting in the reception area.

For a tort of defamation of character (either libel or slander) to exist, a third party must see or hear the words and understand their meaning.

Invasion of Privacy. Invasion of privacy is another kind of tort. It includes unauthorized publicity of patient information, medical records being released without the patient's knowledge and permission, and patients receiving unwanted publicity and exposure to public view. For example, if a minor unmarried girl has been examined for possible pregnancy, and the medical assistant telephones the girl's home and inadvertently gives the laboratory results to someone other than the patient, her privacy has been invaded. A second situation exists when persons other than those providing care and performing examinations and procedures (essential or nonessential personnel) are allowed to be present without the patient's consent. Yet another example of the patient's right to privacy being violated is when the patient is asked to walk from the examination room across the hall to a treatment room while wearing only a patient gown in full view of other patients and personnel.

Medical assistants and other health care professionals should:

* Close a door, pull a curtain, or provide a screen when looking at, handling, or examining the patient

* Expose only body parts necessary for treatment (drape the patient, exposing only the part that is being treated)

* Discuss patients with no one except those individuals involved in the patient's care, and then discuss only those aspects of care that relate to the needs of the patient

It is not an invasion of privacy to disclose information required by a court order **(subpoena)** or by statute to protect the public health and welfare, as in the reporting of violent crime.

INFORMED CONSENT

Documentation of **informed consent** becomes an important part of the patient care process. Every patient has a right to know and understand any procedure to be performed. The patient is to be told in language easily understood:

1. The nature of any procedure and how it is to be performed
2. Any possible risks involved, as well as expected outcomes of the procedure
3. Any other methods of treatment and those risks
4. Risks if no treatment is given

It is the responsibility of the health care provider to make certain the patient understands. If an interpreter is necessary, the physician must procure one.

Often, consent forms will be signed if there is to be a surgical or invasive procedure performed (Figure 7-4). The medical assistant may be asked to witness the patient's signature and may be expected to follow through on any of the physician's instructions or explanations, but is not expected to explain the procedure to the patient. The signed consent form is kept in the medical chart, and a copy also is given to the patient.

Implied Consent

Two circumstances related to consent are worth mentioning at this point. **Implied consent** occurs when there is a life-threatening emergency, or the patient is unconscious or unable to respond. The physician, by law, is allowed to give treatment without a signed consent. Implied consent also occurs in more subtle ways. The patient who rolls up a shirtsleeve for the medical assistant to take a blood pressure reading is implying consent to the procedure by the action taken.

Consent and Legal Incompetence

Consent for treatment is not valid if the patient is legally incompetent to give consent. Legal **incompetence** means that a patient is found by a court to be insane, inadequate, or to not be an adult. In such instances, consent must be obtained from a parent, a legal guardian, or the court on behalf of the patient. Consent for treatment may be given only by the natural parent or legal guardian as determined by the court for a **minor** child. A minor is a person who has not reached the age of majority (18–21 years old), depending on the laws of each state. Generally, a minor is considered unable to give effective consent for medical treatment; therefore, without proper consent from parents or guardians, medical professionals can be held liable for battery if medical treatment is given. Exceptions to this rule are in cases of emergency and for mature and **emancipated minors.** Emancipated minors are younger than 18 years who are free of parental care and are financially responsible, married, become parents, or join the Armed Forces. **Mature minors** are persons, usually younger than 18 years, who are able to understand and appreciate the nature and consequences of treatment despite their young age. Nearly every state allows minors to give consent for treatment for pregnancy, drug or alcohol addiction, and sexually transmitted disease. Some states have passed legislation that name minors as statutory adults at 14 years old for the purpose of receiving medical care. In these states, minors may consent and

CONSENT TO
OPERATION, ADMINISTRATION OF ANESTHETICS AND
RENDERING OF OTHER MEDICAL SERVICES

1. I hereby authorize and direct Dr. _____, my physician, and

   whomever he/she designates as his/her assistants (associates and/or resident physicians), to perform upon

   (state name of patient or myself)_____

   The following procedures: _____

   _____

   _____

   If any unforeseen condition arises in the course of this operation for the physician's judgment to perform procedures in addition to or different from those now contemplated, I further request and authorize him/her to do whatever he/she deems advisable and necessary in these circumstances. Such additional services may include, but are not limited to, the administration and maintenance of anesthesia and the performance of services involving pathology and radiology.

2. The following information has been explained to me to the degree that I wish to have it discussed:
   - The nature and character of the proposed treatment or procedure;
   - The anticipated results;
   - Possible recognized alternative methods of treatment, including non-treatment;
   - Recognized serious possible risks, complications, and anticipated benefits involved in proposed and alternative treatments, including non-treatment.

   My questions have been answered to my satisfaction. I acknowledge that no guarantee, warrantee, or assurance has been made as to the results or cure that may be obtained.

3. Federal Regulations (21 CFR Part 821) require manufacturers to track certain medical devices, and assist the U.S. Food and Drug Administration (FDA) with notification to individuals in the event that a certain medical device presents serious health risks. I authorize and agree to the release of my contact information to the manufacturer: _____ for this tracking purpose only. I understand that the manufacturer may notify me, if necessary, of important safety information about my medical device, and may release my information to the FDA if ordered to do so. I understand that this consent is valid for the life of the medical device.

Any sections below that do not apply to the proposed treatment may be crossed out. The patient must initial any section crossed out.

4. I consent to the administration of blood and blood products if deemed medically necessary. I understand that all blood and blood products involve the risk of allergic reaction, fever, hives, and in rare circumstances infectious diseases such as hepatitis and HIV/AIDS. I understand that precautions are taken by the blood bank in screening donors and in matching blood for transfusion to minimize those risks.

5. I hereby consent to the disposal or use for research purposes any tissues, parts, or products of conception, which may be removed.

6. I authorize and agree to the presence of observers during my surgical procedure. These observers may include persons other than the medical staff that are considered appropriate by my health care provider during my care and treatment. The purpose of these individuals observing would be for instruction and medical study.

I certify that I have read this form and understand its contents.

PATIENT NAME & ID #	Signature of Patient or Legally Responsible Party
	Relationship to patient, if not signed by patient
	Signature of Witness
	Printed Name of Witness
	Date_____Time_____a.m. / p.m.

MRD: HOSP1
DISTRIBUTION: 1-**WHITE** – CHART   2-**CANARY** – PATIENT COPY

Figure 7-4   Model formal consent for treatment form.

Critical Thinking

Identify problems that may occur in the ambulatory care setting when a minor seeks treatment for drug or alcohol addiction or a sexually transmitted disease, or is determined to be pregnant. What is the role of the medical assistant?

be protected by confidentiality and privacy even though their parents or legal guardians may still be financially responsible for their medical bills.

Questions of ability to give consent related to minors and emancipated minors often must be determined on a case-by-case basis because state statutes vary. Placing a telephone call to the state attorney general's office can help clarify issues, questions, and concerns that involve consent and treatment of minors.

CIVIL LITIGATION PROCESS

Despite all the best efforts of health care professionals and their employees, litigation can occur. Litigation is the process of taking a lawsuit or a criminal case through the courts. It is helpful to understand the steps taken for civil litigation to occur. The greatest amount of any litigation seen in the ambulatory care setting occurs when relationships between individuals break down for one reason or another. When this happens, the party, or plaintiff, bringing the action, usually a patient, seeks an attorney who agrees to bring the complaint to the courts. The physician, or defendant, is summoned to court. This summons or subpoena notifies the physician of the plaintiff's suit and allows the defendant to file an answer with the court.

Subpoenas

A portion of a medical record or the entire medical record may be subpoenaed or the physician and health care provider (*subpoena duces tecum*) may be subpoenaed to testify in court, or both may be subpoenaed. The subpoena is an order from the court naming the specific date, time, and reason to appear. The staff in the ambulatory care setting usually will have ample time to make certain the record is current and complete before its inclusion in court. Out of courtesy, the physician will notify patients whose records have been subpoenaed. If, for any reason, the patient does not want the record released, the physician must call for legal advice on how to respond to the subpoena.

Certain records, because of their sensitive nature, may require more than a subpoena to be released. These include records related to sexually transmitted diseases, including AIDS and HIV testing; mental health records; substance abuse records; and sexual assault records. For the courts to have access to these records, a court order is required in some states.

 HIPAA law requires clinics to identify in written policies and procedures what information they will release regarding patients. Before patient information is released, the following must be identified: (1) the purpose or need for the information, (2) the nature or extent of the information to be released, (3) the date of the authorization, and (4) the signature(s) of the person(s) authorized to give consent. Release only what the subpoena or court order specifically requests rather than releasing the entire medical record. Many practitioners keep a patient's consent information in a specific section of the medical record for quick referral and to demonstrate HIPAA compliance.

The care taken with subpoenas and court orders for certain information is to assure patients of confidentiality. The information in the medical record, including the information a patient shared with the physician and medical assistant, is private.

No patient information can be given to another (another physician, patient's attorney, insurance company, federal or state agency) without the expressed written consent of the patient. Care must be exercised at all times to ensure that the patient's right to confidentiality is not breached. For example, information given to unauthorized personnel associated with the physician's or clinic's practice in regard to the patient's condition or financial status regarding payment of bills violates the patient's right to confidentiality. Likewise, when discussing issues over the telephone that can be overheard, such as the patient's account being turned over to a collection agency, the patient's right to confidentiality has been violated.

There are certain disclosures of information about a patient's conditions and suspected illnesses that are required by law. Legally required disclosures are necessary when the public needs to know certain information for its safety and welfare. The disclosures supersede the patient's right to privacy and confidentiality. See "Public Duties" in this chapter.

Discovery

A time of **discovery** follows the subpoenas. This is the time in which both parties are allowed access to all the information and evidence related to the case. Rules of discovery vary from state to state, but may include the following:

1. An **interrogatory** is a written set of questions that can come from either the plaintiff or the defendant

that must be answered, under oath, and within a specific time period.

2. A **deposition** is oral testimony taken with a court reporter present in a location agreed on by both parties. Both attorneys are usually present when depositions are taken.

Medical assistants may be asked to respond to an interrogatory or may be deposed by the plaintiff's attorney. The defendant's attorney will provide specific instructions in both situations. Because both are done under oath, honesty is an absolute. The medical assistant may be asked to refer to certain documents, recall specific information, or identify documentation in a medical record.

Expert Witnesses. Physicians and members of their staff may be called to testify in court to the standard of care. In such a case, they are usually considered **expert witnesses.** An expert witness is one who has enough knowledge and experience in a field to be able to testify to what is the reasonable and expected standard of care. Expert witnesses are expected to tell what they know to be fact and are best counseled to use lay terms rather than complicated medical language. The goal is for jurors and judges to understand the nature of any medical information shared. Visual aids, charts, and computer simulations often are used to illustrate or clarify testimony given by expert witnesses.

Pretrial Conference

A pretrial conference is generally held close to the trial date to decide if there is just cause for the suit, to make certain that both parties are ready, and to determine if there might be an out-of-court settlement. If a trial seems imminent, **alternative dispute resolution (ADR)** may be suggested. **Mediation** allows a neutral facilitator to help the two parties settle their differences and come to an acceptable solution. If no settlement is reached, the case can still look to the court for satisfaction. **Arbitration** allows the neutral party to settle the dispute. This arbitration can be binding or nonbinding. In binding arbitration, both parties agree at the outset to accept the neutral party's decision as final. In nonbinding arbitration, the case can look to the court for settlement. ADR saves money, time, and adverse publicity that can come from a trial.

Trial

A trial can be held before a judge or a judge and a jury. When the trial begins, opening statements outlining the details of the case are made by both sides. The plaintiff's attorney calls witnesses to produce evidence first. This is known as direct examination. In cross examination,

the defendant's attorney questions the witness. When the plaintiff's case is finished, the defendant presents the case in the same manner. When all the information has been presented, the case is turned over for judgment.

If the plaintiff's case is successful, the judge or jury may award a specific amount of money or damages. The judge will instruct a jury regarding the kinds of damages that can be considered in that state. A number of states have placed limits on monetary awards in malpractice cases. If the defendant's case is successful, the case is dismissed. After a court decision, the party that has lost the case can begin an appeal process. The appeal requests an opinion from higher courts that reviews cases usually on the basis of a faulty legal process or action.

Figure 7-5 outlines the civil case process.

Statute of Limitations

No discussion of negligence, malpractice, or medical records is complete without a brief statement regarding the statute of limitations that will, in part, determine how long medical records are kept. Generally, all records should be retained until after the statute has run, usually three to six years. Statutes of limitations most commonly begin at the time a negligent act was committed, when the act was discovered, or when the care of the patient and the patient–physician relationship ended. It is easy to understand why many physicians choose to keep their records indefinitely.

State and federal statutes set maximum time periods during which certain actions can be brought or rights enforced; there is a time limit for individuals to initiate legal action. The statute of limitations varies from one jurisdiction to another and a lawsuit may not be brought after the statute of limitations has run. For example, in the Commonwealth of Massachusetts, the statute of limitations for an act of medical malpractice committed on an adult is three years. If harm to a patient resulted from a medical assistant administering the wrong dose of medication to a patient in Massachusetts, a lawsuit must be brought within three years from the time the medication error was made, with the three years commencing at the time the negligent act was committed.

PUBLIC DUTIES

Reportable Diseases/Injuries

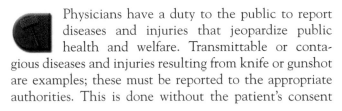

Physicians have a duty to the public to report diseases and injuries that jeopardize public health and welfare. Transmittable or contagious diseases and injuries resulting from knife or gunshot are examples; these must be reported to the appropriate authorities. This is done without the patient's consent

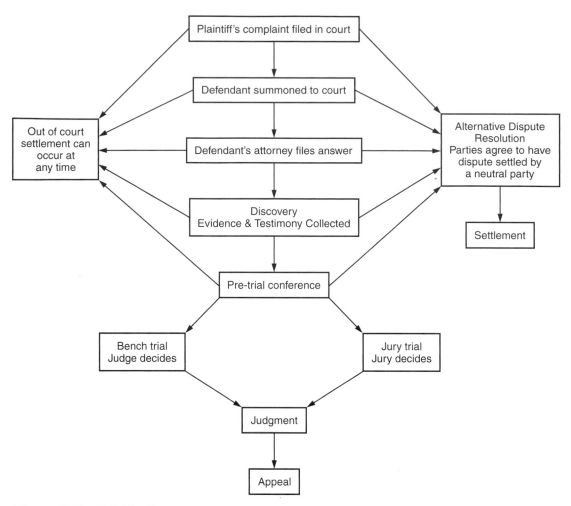

Figure 7-5 Civil litigation process.

because it is required by law. When reporting, it is important to do so properly and according to the laws of the state in which one is employed. Knowledge of which illnesses, injuries, and conditions to report, to whom to report, and the appropriate forms to submit is essential. Copies of all information must be kept for the office or clinic.

Medline Plus, a Web site sponsored by the U.S. National Library of Medicine and the National Institutes of Health, has an excellent site connected to the Medline Encyclopedia identifying guidelines for reportable diseases. Local, state, and national agencies such as the Centers for Disease Control and Prevention require such diseases to be reported when diagnosed by doctors or laboratories. States may vary in the diseases that require reporting, but their lists are likely to include the basic list provided on-line at http://www.nlm.nih.gov. Some diseases require written reports. Others require reporting by telephone; they include rubeola (measles) and pertussis (whooping cough). Still others ask only for the number of cases to be reported. Such reporting is beneficial to

society and all health care managers in tracking and preventing illness. The list changes from time to time as new diseases occur and are diagnosed.

Other generally required facts to report include births, deaths, childhood immunizations, rape, and abuse toward a child, elder, or domestic partner.

Some states have laws specific to the release of information relative to mental or psychological treatment, human immunodeficiency virus testing, acquired immune deficiency syndrome diagnosis and treatment, sexually transmitted diseases, and chemical substance abuse.

Local or state health departments can provide lists of diseases and injuries to report and will also provide the appropriate forms.

Abuse

Child abuse, domestic violence, and elder abuse are becoming more common in our society. As a result, patients experiencing such abuse may be seen in the ambulatory care setting. In all cases of abuse, medical records hold valuable information if a court procedure ensues. Careful documentation is critical. State laws are fairly specific in mandates to report child abuse, but laws related to elder abuse and domestic violence are not as detailed. In any case, the rights of victims must be protected.

Child Abuse. The law mandates, or requires, that physicians and health care professionals, teachers, social workers, and certain others who suspect child abuse report the incident to the proper authorities. Confidentiality in the physician–patient relationship does not exist when children are abused. If a person has a reason to suspect abuse and reports the abuse to the police, and in the case of child abuse to the child protective agency, this individual is protected against liability as a result of making the report. Failure to report could result in criminal or civil penalties. Usually, the Child Protective Unit of the State Department of Social Services is called to investigate suspected cases of child abuse. Some injuries that are commonly seen in child abuse are bruises, welts, burns, fractures, and head injuries. Evidence of neglect or intimidation also may be seen.

If a suspicion of abuse exists, the physician and health care professional should:

- Treat the child's injuries
- Send the child to the hospital for further treatment when necessary
- Inform parents of the diagnosis and that it will be reported to the police and social services agency
- Notify the child protective agency (keep phone number posted)
- Document all information
- Provide court testimony if requested

Elder Abuse. Elder abuse may consist of neglect, physical abuse, punishment, physical restraint, or abandonment. Examples are seen when elders are overmedicated or undermedicated, physically restrained, intimidated by shouting or profanity, sexually abused, neglected or abandoned, or in any other way have their rights and dignity violated. The person reporting the abuse is generally a health care professional, and the reporting agency is most likely one of a social service or welfare nature.

Domestic Violence. Incidents of spousal abuse have escalated since the 1970s. The battered women's syndrome is a significant problem. The violence of it is a criminal act, and failure to report it may be considered a misdemeanor in some states. Victims of domestic violence should be treated as soon as possible after the assault so as to preserve evidence for legal purposes. In the United States, domestic violence is a crime. Domestic violence, however, is considered acceptable behavior in many cultures, even in the United States. Some cultures believe the woman is chattel, or property, of her spouse, that she has no rights or authority, and that she must submit to her husband's, brother's, or father's demands. A woman who manages to come to the ambulatory care setting with signs of domestic violence is courageous. She probably is extremely frightened also, because she knows that reporting the violence puts her at increased risk for continued violence, and even death in some instances. Make certain there are community resources readily available for these women, even if they choose to stay in the abusive situation. In many cases, the abused patient's options are so few that leaving is more frightening than staying in the abusive relationship. Do not pass judgment on these women; they desperately need your understanding and your compassion. Your understanding and compassion is perhaps the only door through which they might feel comfortable enough to enter to leave the abusive relationship.

Good Samaritan Laws

 Most states have laws regarding the rendering of first aid by health care professionals at the scene of an accident or sudden injury. Good Samaritan laws, although not always clearly written, encourage physicians and health care professionals to provide medical care within the scope of their training without fear of being sued for negligence. In an emergency situation, medical assistants cannot be held liable should an injury result from some form of first aid rendered or from first aid they omitted to render as long as they acted in a reasonable way within the scope of their knowledge. Medical assistants and other health care professionals with skills in cardiopulmonary resuscitation (CPR) who are present when CPR is needed must perform the procedure on the victim or otherwise could be declared negligent. Emergencies that arise in the ambulatory care setting generally are not covered by Good Samaritan laws.

PHYSICIAN'S DIRECTIVES

 Medical assistants in the ambulatory care setting will be asked to attach physician's directives or living wills to patients' charts (Figure 7-6). These directives are legal documents in which patients indicate their wishes in the case of a life-threatening

Washington
Health Care Directive

Directive made this_____day of _____, _____.
           (date)   *(month)*   *(year)*

I,_____,
                                      (name)

having the capacity to make health care decisions, willfully and voluntarily make known my desire that my dying shall not be artificially prolonged under the circumstances set forth below, and do hereby declare that:

(a) If at any time I should be diagnosed in writing to be in a terminal condition by the attending physician, or in a permanent unconscious condition by two physicians, and where the application of life-sustaining treatment would serve only to artificially prolong the process of my dying, I direct that such treatment be withheld or withdrawn, and that I be permitted to die naturally. I understand by using this form that a terminal condition means an incurable and irreversible condition caused by injury, disease, or illness that would within reasonable medical judgment cause death within a reasonable period in accordance with accepted medical standards, and where the application of life-sustaining treatment would serve only to prolong the process of dying. I further understand in using this form that a permanent unconscious condition means an incurable and irreversible condition in which I am medically assessed within reasonable medical judgment as having no reasonable probability of recovery from an irreversible coma or a persistent vegetative state.

(b) In the absence of my ability to give directions regarding the use of such life-sustaining treatment, it is my intention that this directive shall be honored by my family and physician(s) as the final expression of my legal right to refuse medical or surgical treatment and I accept the consequences of such refusal. If another person is appointed to make these decisions for me, whether through a durable power of attorney or otherwise, I request that the person be guided by this directive and any other clear expressions of my desires.

(c) If I am diagnosed to be in a terminal condition or in a permanent unconscious condition (check one):

❑ I DO want to have artificially provided nutrition and hydration.

❑ I DO NOT want to have artificially provided nutrition and hydration.

(d) If I have been diagnosed as pregnant and that diagnosis is known to my physician, this directive shall have no force or effect during the course of my pregnancy.

(e) I understand the full import of this directive and I am emotionally and mentally capable to make the health care decisions contained in this directive.

(f) I understand that before I sign this directive, I can add to or delete from or otherwise change the wording of this directive and that I may add to or delete from this directive at any time and that any changes shall be consistent with Washington State law or federal constitutional law to be legally valid.

(g) It is my wish that every part of this directive be fully implemented. If for any reason any part is held invalid, it is my wish that the remainder of my directive be implemented.

(h) I make the folllowing additional instructions regarding my care:

Signed:_____

City, County, and State of Residence:_____

_____

The declarer has been personally known to me and I believe him or her to be capable of making health care decisions.

Witness:_____

Witness:_____

Figure 7-6   Health Care Directive (Washington State sample). Compassion & Choices Federation makes legally recognized documents available for interested persons. (Reprinted by permission of Compassion & Choices Federation, 6312 SW Capitol Hwy., #415, Portland, OR 97239.)

illness or serious injury. Such documents should always accompany the patients to the hospital for any treatment or care. They may be updated from time to time, and the patient can ask to rescind such a document at any time. Medical assistants must remember that these documents reflect the choices of their patients and are to be respected as such.

Living Wills

Living wills are necessary because advances in medicine allow medical professionals to sustain life even if the individual will not recover from a persistent vegetative state. Persons who prefer not to remain in that state can use the living will to make decisions about life support and direct others to implement their wishes in that regard. The living will allows individuals to indicate to family and health care professionals whether life-prolonging medical or surgical procedures are to be continued, withheld, or withdrawn, and if artificial feeding and fluids are to be used or withheld. The living will allows individuals to make this decision before incapacitation.

To be valid, the proper and particular form, different in each state, must be used, and it must be lawfully executed. States vary in the number of witnesses required and whether a Notary Public is required for those signatures. The form goes into effect when provided to a patient's health care provider *and* when the patient is no longer capable of making health care decisions. Examples of incapacity may include permanent unconsciousness, life-threatening illness in the latter stages, or inability to communicate. The U.S. Legal Forms Web site (http://USlegalforms.com) has samples of living wills for all 50 states and the District of Columbia under the heading "Living Will Forms."

Durable Power of Attorney for Health Care

Another document seen in the ambulatory care setting is the **durable power of attorney for health care** or Designation of Health Care Surrogate (Figure 7-7). This document allows a patient to name another person as the official spokesperson for the patient should the patient be unable to make health care decisions. The documents may allow another person to manage finances and personal matters (durable power of attorney) or just to make medical decisions.

Every state has different versions of the physician's directive. The American Bar Association has a section on their Web site (www.abanet.org) on "Law for Older Americans" and "Health Care Advance Directives" that is useful in answering many questions. Also, the Web site for the Compassion in Dying Federation (http://www.compassionindying.org; located in Portland, OR) is quite helpful. Individuals wishing to have their choices known should they suffer from severe dementia may execute a document similar to the sample in Figure 7-8. The "Alzheimer's Provision" may be included in the Living Will document as well.

In 1991, the federal government passed the **Patient Self-Determination Act (PSDA),** which applies to all health care institutions receiving payments from Medicare and Medicaid. PSDA requires that all adults receiving health care from these institutions be given the opportunity to provide information about their wishes in an advanced directive.

Copies of advance directives are to be provided to patients' physicians so they can be transferred to a hospital or nursing facility as necessary. Any named agent should have a copy, and family members also may have a copy.

Patient Education

Because of increased awareness of confidentiality as a result of HIPAA, medical assistants can be helpful by suggesting that any family member(s) who might be involved and need to know about the patient's care be indicated in the patient's chart with a signed release from the patient. There have been examples recently of adult children of elder adults who were either not informed when their ailing parent was taken to emergency services in another state, or were unable to get any information about their parent from a hospital or physician even though a durable power of attorney for health care was in place. If that directive does not go with the patient, no information can be given. For that reason, it is suggested that patients may want to keep a wallet card containing a notice of the advance directive, any appointed agent named, and any family member(s) who is allowed information.

Washington Durable Power
of Attorney for Health Care

I understand that my wishes as expressed in my living will may not cover all possible aspects of my care if I become incapacitated. Consequently, there may be a need for someone to accept or refuse medical intervention on my behalf, in consultation with my physician. Therefore,

I, _____ ,
as principal, designate and appoint the person(s) listed below as my attorney-in-fact for health care decisions.

First Choice: Name: _____

                               Address: _____

                               City/State/Zip Code: _____

                                                    _____

                               Telephone Number: _____

If the above person is unable, unavailable, or unwilling to serve, I designate:

Second Choice: Name: _____

                               Address: _____

                               City/State/Zip Code: _____

                                                    _____

                               Telephone Number: _____

1.   This Power of Attorney shall take effect upon my incapacity to make my own health care decisions, as determined by my treating physician and one other physician, and shall continue as long as the incapacity lasts or until I revoke it, whichever happens first.

2.   The powers of my attorney-in-fact under this Power of Attorney are limited to making decisions about my health care on my behalf. These powers shall include the power to order the withholding or withdrawal of life-sustaining treatment if my attorney-in-fact believes, in his or her own judgment, that is what I would want if I could make the decision myself. The existence of this Durable Power of Attorney for Health Care shall have no effect upon the validity of any other Power of Attorney for other purposes that I have executed or may execute in the future.

3.   In the event that a proceeding is initiated to appoint a guardian of my person under RCW 11.88, I nominate the person designated as my first choice (on page 1) to serve as my guardian. My second choice (on page 1) will serve as my guardian if the first person is unable or unwilling.

4.   I make the following additional instructions regarding my care:

By signing this document, I indicate that I understand the purpose and effect of this Durable Power of Attorney for Health Care.

Dated this _____ day of _____ , 20 _____ .
                    (date)   *(month)*   *(year)*

Signed: _____

The person named as principal in this document is personally known to me. I believe that he/she is of sound mind, and that he/she signed this document freely and voluntarily.

Witness: _____

Witness: _____

Figure 7-7   Durable Power of Attorney for Health Care (Washington State sample). (Reprinted by permission of Compassion & Choices Federation, 6312 SW Capitol Hwy., #415, Portland, OR 97239.)

The "Alzheimer's Provision"

Most advance directives become operative only when a person is unable to make health care decisions and is either "permanently unconscious" or "terminally ill." There is usually no provision that applies to the situation in which a person suffers from severe dementia but is neither unconscious nor dying.

The following language can be added to any Living Will. There it will serve to advise physicians and family of the wishes of a patient with Alzheimer's disease or other forms of dementia.

> **If I am unconscious and it is very unlikely that I will ever become conscious again, I would like my wishes regarding specific life-sustaining treatments, as indicated on the attached document entitled "My Particular Wishes," to be followed.**
>
> **If I remain conscious but have a progressive illness that will be fatal and the illness is in an advanced stage, and I am consistently and permanently unable to communicate, swallow food and water safely, care for myself and recognize my family and other people, and it is very unlikely that my condition will substantially improve, I would like my wishes regarding specific life-sustaining treatments, as indicated on the attached document entitled "My Particular Wishes," to be followed.**
>
> **If I am unable to feed myself while in this condition, I do/do not (circle one) want to be fed.**

I hereby incorporate this provision into my durable power of attorney for health care, living will, and any other previously executed advance directive for health care decisions.

_____   _____
Signature   Date

Figure 7-8   Compassion & Choices "Alzheimer's Provision" applies to the situation when a person has severe dementia but is neither unconscious nor dying. (Reprinted by permission of Compassion & Choices Federation, 6312 SW Capitol Hwy., #415, Portland, OR 97239.)

Case Study 7-1

Three weeks ago, Dr. King treated a new patient, Boris Bolski, for lower back pain, which the patient believed was the result of consistent heavy lifting at his job. Medical assistant Joe Guerrero assisted Dr. King during the examination and, today, both Joe and Dr. King were served with subpoenas by Mr. Bolski's attorney. Mr. Bolski is alleging that unsafe conditions at his workplace caused severe strain on his back, and he is suing his employer for damages. Dr. King and Joe Guerrero were called as expert witnesses to a civil hearing; Joe, especially, is a bit nervous about this, because he has never been on the witness stand in court and is not sure what is expected of him.

CASE STUDY REVIEW

1. How will Mr. Bolski's medical record help Joe answer questions at the hearing?
2. What information should Joe gather to be prepared to testify?
3. As an expert witness, what is Joe expected to communicate to the judge in this case?

Case Study 7-2

Wanda Hanson is working on a part-time basis in Hudson, Florida as an administrative medical assistant on the phone desk in the Emergency Department at Hudson Community Hospital when a frantic long-distance call is received. The caller is Larry Nelson from Cheyenne, Wyoming. He received a call from the nursing home where his 95-year-old mother was living informing him that she was taken by ambulance to your hospital. Larry wants to know if Muriel Nelson has arrived and what her condition is. You are aware of a patient's right to privacy, confidentiality, and the new HIPAA regulations. You observed Mrs. Nelson arrive at the emergency department quite incoherent and confused.

CASE STUDY REVIEW

1. What can Wanda tell Mr. Nelson, especially after noting that no records were with the elderly Mrs. Nelson when she arrived at the hospital?

2. What information would Wanda need from Mr. Nelson before complying to his request?

3. How can Wanda put Mr. Nelson at ease? What can Wanda do to help?

SUMMARY

Changing societal values have contributed to an increase of lawsuits in medical practice. Patients are more aware than ever of their rights, especially those of confidentiality and the right to privacy, consent, and records ownership. They are likely to seek redress when they perceive their rights have been violated.

A healthy relationship between physicians and patients and between medical assistants and patients, as well as respect for the patient's rights, reduces the likelihood of a lawsuit.

Additional knowledge of the laws that regulate medical and business practices in your state is necessary to be in compliance. Sources of information regarding state and federal laws can be obtained from the state medical society, the physician's liability insurance company, the state medical assistant society, the state attorney general's office, the Internet, or the public library.

STUDY FOR SUCCESS

To reinforce your knowledge and skills of information presented in this chapter:
- ❑ Review the Key Terms
- ❑ Consider the Case Studies and discuss your conclusions
- ❑ Answer the Review Questions
  - ❑ Multiple Choice
  - ❑ Critical Thinking
- ❑ Navigate the Internet and complete the Web Activities
- ❑ Practice the StudyWARE activities on the textbook CD
- ❑ Apply your knowledge in the Student Workbook activities
- ❑ Complete the Web Tutor sections
- ❑ View and discuss the DVD situations

REVIEW QUESTIONS

Multiple Choice

1. The type of contract that most often exists between physician and patient is:
   a. expressed
   b. implied
   c. privileged
   d. civil
2. The administrative law act that prohibits discrimination, has five sections, and is enforced by the EEOC is called the:
   a. Controlled Substances Act
   b. Federal Age Discrimination Act
   c. Americans with Disabilities Act
   d. Health Insurance Portability and Accountability Act
3. Slander is defamation through:
   a. spoken statements that damage an individual's reputation
   b. written statements that damage a person's reputation
   c. written falsehoods about an individual
   d. a, b, and c
4. Occasionally, a physician will be sued for the negligence of an employee, even though the physician is not guilty of any negligent act. This is done on the basis of the doctrine of:
   a. *res ipsa loquitur*
   b. *respondeat superior*
   c. proximate cause
   d. contract law
5. The standard of care expected of a physician is held by the courts to mean:
   a. on a par with all other physicians engaged in the same medical specialty anywhere
   b. reasonable, attentive, diligent care comparable with other physicians of the same specialty in the same or similar community
   c. the best possible under the circumstances
   d. the same as the national norm
6. Physician's directives:
   a. allow patients to direct how their billing is to be handled
   b. are designed to encourage physicians to render first aid in an emergency
   c. direct physicians based on a patient's wishes in life-threatening circumstances
   d. are not considered legal documents
7. A subpoena:
   a. is a court order requesting data, an appearance in court, or both
   b. is sufficient to enforce a release of any type medical record or information
   c. may be ignored without consequences

   d. allows the person being served to select a specific date or time to appear
8. The 4 Ds of negligence are:
   a. duty, danger, damage, and disaster
   b. derelict, direct cause, damage, and danger
   c. danger, direct cause, damage, disaster
   d. duty, derelict, direct cause, damage
9. Emancipated minors:
   a. are considered adults and can consent to treatment
   b. live on their own and are self-supporting
   c. may be married or serve in the military
   d. all of the above
   e. only b and c
10. Torts:
   a. include battery, defamation of character, invasion of privacy
   b. are always intentional in nature
   c. do not require that harm has occurred
   d. do not include malpractice

Critical Thinking

1. Chris is a 6-year-old girl who Dr. King treated for a broken leg. Chris' parents fail to follow Dr. King's treatment plan for Chris. What, if any, action can Dr. King take? What is the legal term for this situation?
2. Marijuana is presently listed as a Schedule I controlled substance and is identified by the DEA as having "no accepted medical use in the United States." As of May, 2005, eleven states have passed legislation allowing patients to use marijuana to alleviate pain, nausea, and other symptoms without fear of prosecution. Discuss the issue of the state's power overriding the federal administrative law. Can you recall what other legal battle recently occurred between the federal and state jurisdictions that involved the U.S. Attorney General in physician-assisted suicide? How was that issue resolved?
3. Jaime arrived in the clinic having sustained a serious laceration at his construction site. Dr. Woo ordered Demerol R 100 mg. 1.m - stat, which Wanda, the medical assistant, administers. Dr. Woo determines surgery is required. Should a consent form be prepared? If so, by whom, and what should be included?
4. Do you have a living will or a physician's directive? Why or why not? Identify to a family member or a loved one what your wishes might be if you were seriously injured in an accident and were still in what appears to be an irreversible coma after 10 months.
5. Discuss the medical assistant's obligations in regard to public duties.
6. What is the Good Samaritan law? What must a medical assistant and any other health care

professional remember when giving first aid at the scene of an accident?

7. Describe three types of abuse. Tell what your role as a medical assistant is when Juanita brings her 3-year-old son Henry to the clinic. Henry has bruises on his face and chest and appears quite frightened when you approach him. While you prepare Henry for the pediatrician's examination, Juanita's answers to your questions seem evasive.

WEB ACTIVITIES

1. Research the American Bar Association Web site (http://www.abanet.org). How often should an advance directive be renewed or reviewed, or is such renewal necessary? Is an advance directive valid when you cross state lines?

2. Using the Internet, determine if or when a medical clinic might be required to follow the federal guidelines of the Family and Medical Leave Act (FMLA). Identify reasons to follow the FMLA guidelines.

3. Using your favorite search engine, key in the words "Medical Malpractice Awards." A number of sites will appear. Has a national limit been set on malpractice awards? What makes this topic a political one? Identify those who favor malpractice award limits and also those who oppose these limits.

4. Research the World Wide Web for the statute of limitations related to claims injuries. What is the time span in your state?

THE DVD HOOK-UP

DVD Series	Program Number
Critical Thinking	**3**

Chapter/Scene Reference
- *Licensing and Scope of Practice*
- *Regulating Agencies OSHA, DEA, and CMS*

This chapter deals with legal considerations that must be adhered to when working in the medical industry. One of the most important legal responsibilities that you have as a medical assistant is to stay within the boundaries of your scope and training as a medical assistant.

In one of the scenes listed above, Barb, the office manager, reprimands Eileen for administering a Demerol injection. Eileen states that the doctor ordered her to give the injection, which is why she gave it. The office manager tells Eileen that medical assistants are not allowed to give controlled substances in that particular state. Eileen replies that she didn't know she could not give controlled substances, and that she gave controlled substances in the last office that she worked. Barb reminds Eileen that the information was posted in the office's procedures manual that she was suppose to have read at the time of orientation. Barb told Eileen that she had no other choice but to document this error in her personal record.

1. Why did Barb take such a hard approach with Eileen? What steps does Barb need to take in the future? What responsibility does the doctor have?
2. How could Eileen have avoided this awkward situation?
3. What will you do if a physician orders you to perform a procedure that medical assistants are not allowed to perform?

DVD Journal Summary
Write a paragraph that summarizes what you learned from watching the designated scenes from today's DVD program. What steps will you take to make certain that you know what medical assistants can and cannot do in the state in which you practice?

REFERENCES/BIBLIOGRAPHY

American Bar Association. Health Care Advance Directives. Retrieved from http://www.abanet.org. (Public Documents). Accessed April 4, 2005.

American Bar Association. Law for older Americans. Retrieved from http://www.abanet.org. Accessed April 4, 2005.

Balasa, D. A. (May/June 2004). Legal environment differs under independent nurse practitioners. *CMA TODAY*, Vol. 37, Issue 3, 24–25.

Compassion & Choices. The Alzheimer's Provision. Retrieved from http://compassionindying.org. Accessed May 23, 2005.

Compassion & Choices. Washington Durable Power of Attorney for Health Care. Retrieved from http://compassionindying.org. Accessed May 23, 2005.

Flight, M. (2004). *Law, liability and ethics for medical office professionals* (4th ed.). Clifton Park, NY: Thomson Delmar Learning.

Krager, D., & Krager, C. (2005). *HIPAA for medical office personnel*. Clifton Park, NY: Thomson Delmar Learning.

Lewis, M. A., & Tamparo, C. D. (2002). *Medical law, ethics, and bioethics for ambulatory care* (5th ed.). Philadelphia: F. A. Davis.

CHAPTER 8

Ethical Considerations

OUTLINE

KEY TERMS

Bioethics
Cryopreservation
Ethics
Genetic Engineering
Macroallocation
Microallocation
Surrogate

OBJECTIVES

The student should strive to meet the following performance objectives and demonstrate an understanding of the facts and principles presented in this chapter through written and oral communication.

1. Define the key terms as presented in the glossary.

2. Identify two reasons for Codes of Ethics.

3. Discuss the eight characteristics of principle-centered leadership.

4. Describe the five Ps of ethical power.

5. Recall the ethics check questions.

6. Relate the five principles of the AAMA code to patient care in the ambulatory care setting.

7. Discuss the ethical guidelines for doctors, giving at least four examples.

8. Restate the dilemmas encountered by the following bioethical issues: (a) allocation of scarce medical resources; (b) abortion and fetal tissue research; (c) genetic engineering/manipulation; (d) artificial insemination/surrogacy; (e) dying and death; (f) HIV and AIDS.

SCENARIO

On occasion, ethical dilemmas occur because patients are unsure of the role of the medical assistant. For example, the medical assistants of Inner City Health Care are truly multidisciplinary and have a range of administrative and clinical skills. However, patients sometimes think of them as nurses who have an entirely different set of skills. Although most of the medical assistants gently correct patients and make it a point to practice only within their area of expertise, occasionally newer members of the medical assistant staff may feel more "important" when patients regard them as nurses or physicians' assistants.

A few weeks ago, medical assistant Liz Corbin, who is in her early 20s, was taken aback when Walter Seals, the office manager, spoke up about Liz's tendency to let patients assume she was a nurse. Although Liz never deliberately intended to mislead patients, she never corrected them about their misconceptions. Walter pointed out that to present a good example of the medical assisting profession, Liz should gently but firmly help patients understand that she was a medical assistant with a specific range of skills that complemented, but did not substitute for, nursing skills.

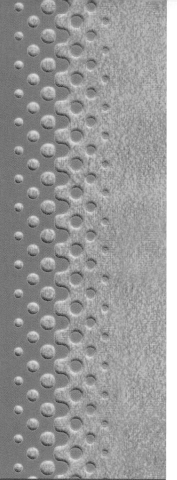
- Professional components
- Allied health professions
  and credentialing

Administrative Duties

- Schedule and monitor
  appointments
- Use physician fee schedule

Legal Concepts

- Determine needs for documentation and reporting
- Use appropriate guidelines
  when releasing records
  or information
- Maintain licenses and
  accreditation
- Monitor legislation related
  to current healthcare
  issues and practices

INTRODUCTION

It is impossible in today's world to function as a medical assistant without an awareness of the impact of ethics and bioethics on health care. Just as an understanding of the law and working within the law is vital information for the medical assistant, it is equally important to understand ethics and bioethics.

From Chapter 7, you have come to realize that there are many circumstances and situations that occur in health care that are guided and directed by state and federal laws. You, personally, are expected to be above reproach in all your actions in this regard. You must also work with your employer and other members of the health care team to assure that each member of the staff functions within the law—protecting both patients and providers.

Ethics plays a huge role in such an endeavor. To function ethically demands that you never function outside the law. Ethics, however, demands something more—ethics calls for honesty, trustworthiness, integrity, confidentiality, and fairness. To function ethically, you must know yourself well and understand weaknesses and any vulnerabilities that might prevent you from acting ethically.

The scenario described earlier is just one situation in which medical assistants may need to reflect on their actions and be sure that they are acting ethically and within the range of their skills. Medical assistants also need to recognize the warning signs that they, or some other staff member, may be

about to breach a code of ethics. Often, this kind of breach occurs when one has, or seeks to have, too much power; when one attempts to take on too much authority; and when one has too little knowledge and experience. When a breach seems about to occur, the individuals involved should be encouraged to step back and review their actions and the likely consequences of those actions.

ETHICS

Traditionally, **ethics** is defined in terms of what is considered right or wrong. Sometimes ethics is referred to as "morals." Professional organizations often identify their ethics in "codes," or a set of principles and guidelines. Physicians, through the American Medical Association (AMA), have established such a code of ethics called the Principles of Medical Ethics. This code can be reviewed by accessing the AMA Web site (http://www.ama-assn.org/ama/pub/category/2512.html). The Code of Medical Ethics Current Opinions with Annotations is published every two years; this document provides up-to-date information on a number of ethical dilemmas. Medical assistants have a code of ethics and a creed. The AAMA Mission Statement, AAMA Medical Assistant Code of Ethics, and AAMA Medical Assistant Creed appear on the AAMA Web site (http://www.aama-ntl.org). Clicking on the Mission Statement, Code, and Creed will identify these statements for you in an interesting fashion.

There are more than 50 differing codes of ethics for professional organizations, and most are related to medicine. There are seven ethical codes that relate to the entire world. These include such famous codes as the Declaration of Geneva, Declaration of Helsinki, and the International Code of Medical Ethics. A listing of these codes is found by searching the Internet for "world medical ethics codes." Another fascinating Web site identifies the characteristics of Traditional Chinese Medical Ethics when you use the Internet to search for "Chinese Medical Ethics." Chinese medical ethics emphasizes self-cultivation and personal ethics of practitioners rather than a strict organizational code of ethics.

Codes of ethics bring standards of moral and ethical behavior together in one place. They assist organizations and individuals in putting words to their expected behaviors and actions. There is a benefit to such codes when they become reminders to everyone regarding their conduct. Codes also can have a limiting affect, however. For instance, if an organization does not have a code of ethics, is that organization viewed as unethical? When one answers that question, there also comes the understanding that having a code of ethics does not necessarily create an ethical organization.

Medical assistants and medical professionals are asked to balance personal and professional areas of their lives in the middle of constant pressure and crises. At the same time, the quality of one's personal life is going to be shown in the quality of their service to others in their professional life. To be effective in the medical profession, there needs to be maturity in both the personal and the professional selves that creates the utmost of ethical conduct and professionalism.

Principle-Centered Leadership

Stephen R. Covey, author of *The 7 Habits of Highly Effective People* and *Principle-Centered Leadership,* has identified eight characteristics of principle-centered leaders. Leaders who know themselves and understand their principles more easily abide by a code of ethics. Consider the following questions as guides to how you might perform ethically in a medical setting.

Are you continually learning? Are you seeking training, taking classes, listening to others, learning from your peers? Are you curious? Do you realize that developing new knowledge and skills is a lifelong endeavor?

Are you service-oriented? Do you see your life as a mission rather than a career? Are you generally a nurturing individual who seeks service in the medical field? Can you see yourself working alongside a coworker and pulling together with that person toward a goal? Can you put yourself in the place of others?

Do you radiate positive energy? Are you cheerful, pleasant, optimistic, and positive? Is your spirit hopeful? If it is, you carry a positive energy field that allows you to neutralize or sidestep a negative energy source. Are you aware of your energy field and its impact on those around you? Do you see yourself as a peacemaker or one that can create harmony to undo negative energy?

Do you believe in other people? Can you keep from labeling, stereotyping, or prejudging other people? Can you believe in the unseen potential of others? Can you keep from overreacting to negative behaviors and criticism? Can you put aside any grudges?

The final three characteristics of principle-centered leaders identified in Covey's *7 Habits of Highly Effective People* are more personal but can help you maintain an understanding of yourself and how you might make ethical decisions in the medical field, and appear below.

Do you lead a balanced life? Do you keep up with current affairs and events? Do you know what is happening in the medical field and how that affects you? Do you have at least one confidant with whom you can be transparent? Are you physically active within your limits of age and health? Do you enjoy yourself? Do you have a good sense of humor? Are you open to communication?

Do you see life as an adventure? Are you able to rediscover persons each time you meet them? Are you interested in others? Do you listen well? Are you flexible and unflappable? Does your security come from within rather than from without?

Are you synergistic? Synergy is what happens when the whole of something is greater than the sum of its parts. Do you know your weaknesses? Can you complement your weaknesses with the strength of others on the team? Can you work hard to improve most situations? Are you trusting? Can you separate the person from the problem?

Do you exercise for self-renewal? In this element, Mr. Covey identifies four dimensions of the human personality that need exercise: physical, mental, emotional, and spiritual dimensions. How do you keep your body in shape? How do you keep your mind alert? Do patience, unconditional love, and accepting responsibility for your own actions keep you emotionally healthy? Do you have a way to meditate, pray, or "draw away" for a period to "fill up your spirit"?

These questions and your response to them can give you insight into your ability to function ethically and to be successful in the world of medicine.

Five Ps of Ethical Power

Kenneth Blanchard and Norman Vincent Peale, wrote a simple, but powerful little book called *The Power of Ethical Management.* In it they discuss the "Five Ps of Ethical Power." The five Ps are as follows:

Purpose: Understand your objective or your purpose. Your purpose may change from time to time, but it is something that requires you to behave in a way that makes you feel good about yourself.

Pride: Have pride in what you do. Feel good about yourself and your accomplishments. Nurture your self-esteem while remaining humble. Be proud to be a medical assistant.

Patience: It takes time to create an atmosphere where your objective can be obtained. Strive to believe that no matter what happens, everything is going to work out. Expect results from yourself and your work, but refrain from demanding it "now."

Persistence: To act in an ethical manner means to strive to act in that manner all the time, not just when you want to or it seems easy to do. Winston Churchill said, "Never! Never! Never! Never! Give Up!" That is what persistence is. If you make a mistake, admit it, correct it, learn from the mistake, and move on, but never give up.

Perspective: Keep your life and your purpose in perspective. Find time each day to maintain balance in your life (perhaps looking again at the eight characteristics of principle-centered individuals). Plan some quiet time, some fun time, but certainly some reflective time. The constant pressure and the crises will become overwhelming without keeping perspective.

Ethics Check Questions

Finally, those striving to act in an ethical manner can perform a little test each time they have a question about ethics. This, too, comes from Blanchard and Peale. The questions to ask are: (1) Is it legal? Is it against the law or any company policy? (2) Is it balanced? Is this the best possible approach for all concerned? Does it promote a win–win situation? (3) How will it make me feel about

myself? Will I feel good if my decision is published in a newspaper? Will my family and coworkers be proud of my decision?

Ethics are not easy. Performing ethically is hard work. Being ethical means determining who you are and how you will act. Laws are more clearly defined than ethics, but acting in an unethical manner can cause as much pain and difficulty as can acting illegally. The ideas of Covey, Blanchard, and Peale give guidance, thoughts to ponder, and perhaps goals to reach. Keep them in mind as you review the next section.

BIOETHICS

Bioethics brings the entire focus of ethics into the field of health care and into those ethical issues dealing with life. Never before in the history of medical care has bioethics been such a topic of concern. In the past, most bioethical decisions were made by physicians and esteemed members of the medical or legal profession. However, advancing technology giving patients and consumers numerous choices regarding their health care causes each one of us to take an active role in bioethics.

Medical assistants will encounter ethical and bioethical issues across the lifespan. In Figure 8-1, a few issues are identified for contemplation and discussion. Issues of bioethics common to every medical clinic are the allocation of scarce medical resources, abortion and fetal tissue research, genetic engineering or manipulation, and the many choices surrounding life, dying, and death.

For medical assistants to fully comprehend a discussion of ethics and bioethics, review of the Code of Ethics of AAMA (Figure 8-2) is beneficial.

KEYS TO THE AAMA CODE OF ETHICS

Medical assistants should consider the more salient points in the AAMA Code of Ethics and ask themselves the following questions:

A. *Render service with full respect for the dignity of humanity.*
  - Will I respect every patient even if I do not approve of his or her morals or choices in health care?
- Will I honor each patient's request for information and explain unfamiliar procedures?
- Will I give my full attention to acknowledging the needs of every patient?
- Will I be able to accept the indigent, the physically and mentally challenged, the infirm, the physically disfigured, and the persons I simply

A FEW ISSUES FOR CONTEMPLATION AND DISCUSSION

Infants

- In premature, deformed, or severely disabled infants, ethical issues include the decision to provide or withhold treatment. Health care professionals and parents are not always in agreement. Central to this issue, also, is the expense involved in certain treatments and deciding who pays the cost of treatment, because insurance usually does not.
- Vulnerability of infants can lead to issues of negligence, abuse, or rejection. Parents also are vulnerable because they may be unable to cope with the needs of the entire family.

Children

- Children who are ill-fed, housed, educated, and clothed exhibit great needs for preventive, curative, and rehabilitative health care. Obesity in children is becoming a serious issue.
- Minors with sexually transmitted diseases can seek treatment without the parents' knowledge. Treatment also must be offered without parental consent to pregnant, infected, or addicted minors.
- Child abuse presents an ethical dilemma, especially when a child confides physical, sexual, or emotional abuse to a health care worker but does not want the information divulged. Health care professionals, as mandated reporters, must report suspected child abuse. Will the child/patient view this as a violation of confidence or suffer dire consequences as a result of the reported abuse?

Adolescents

- Adolescents as young as 14 to 18 years of age may seek abortion without parental knowledge or consent. Is this a violation of parents' right to medical information regarding their children? Or should the adolescent, fearful of parental reaction, have the right to decide?
- The adolescent's growing autonomy, need for independence, changing values, and desire for peer acceptance lead to a number of ethical issues that may involve the health care environment. These include the adolescent's decision to be sexually active, to use birth control, to protect against sexually transmitted diseases, and to use drugs and alcohol.

Adults

- Many low-income women do not have sufficient access to prenatal care, which has proven to be a cost-saving medical measure that is critical to the health of both mother and infant.

- As employers seek to reduce the cost of health insurance benefit programs, many individuals and families are finding themselves shifted from one insurance program to another, leaving them with little or no continuity of care. Also, in some managed care programs, adults may receive medical services from a number of health care professionals with whom they have no opportunity to establish an ongoing physician-patient relationship.
- Even with a physician's directive or a living will, a dying patient's wishes may not be followed. Technological advances in medicine have created a situation where patients may not be able to exercise a choice in the death issue.

Senior Adults

- Dementia is a common problem that is physically and financially exhausting for the caregiver, who is usually a spouse or adult child. How do caregivers cope with their own needs and the needs of dependent adults? Often, the elderly may reject nursing home placement, and there may be limited funds for such long-term and specialized care.
- Elderly patients have the right to maintain dignity and privacy, but their dependency on others may deprive them of these basic rights.
- Physician-assisted suicide for terminally ill patients is a prominent issue in our society, especially when elderly patients sense a total loss of dignity.
- Oregon, the only state with voter-approved assisted dying legislation was threatened when the Attorney General John Ashcroft ruled physicians who used controlled substances to assist patients in dying would face federal prosecution. May 26, 2004 the Ninth Circuit Court of Appeals confirmed a lower court ruling that Oregon's law was valid and beyond the scope of Ashcroft's Department of Justice. Some believe the ruling is destined for the U.S. Supreme Court.

Figure 8-1 Ethical issues across the life span. (Compiled by Carol D. Tamparo, CMA, PhD, and Marilyn Pooler, RN, MEd.)

AAMA CODE OF ETHICS

The Code of Ethics of AAMA shall set forth principles of ethical and moral conduct as they relate to the medical profession and the particular practice of medical assisting.

Members of AAMA dedicated to the conscientious pursuit of their profession, and thus desiring to merit the high regard of the entire medical profession and the respect of the general public which they serve, do pledge themselves to strive always to:

A. render service with full respect for the dignity of humanity;
B. respect confidential information obtained through employment unless legally authorized or required by responsible performance of duty to divulge such information;
C. uphold the honor and high principles of the profession and accept its disciplines;
D. seek to continually improve the knowledge and skills of medical assistants for the benefit of patients and professional colleagues;
E. participate in additional service activities aimed toward improving the health and well-being of the community.

(A)

CREED

I believe in the principles and purposes of the Profession of Medical Assisting.
I endeavor to be more effective.
I aspire to render greater service.
I protect the confidence entrusted to me.
I am dedicated to the care and well-being of all people.
I am loyal to my employer.
I am true to the ethics of my profession.
I am strengthened by compassion, courage, and faith.

(B)

Figure 8-2 (A) American Association of Medical Assistants (AAMA) Code of Ethics. (B) AAMA Creed. (Copyright by the American Association of Medical Assistants, Inc. Revised October, 1996.)

do not like as equal and valid human beings with an equal right to service?

B. *Respect confidential information obtained through employment unless legally authorized or required by responsible performance of duty to divulge such information.*
- Will I refrain from needless comments to a colleague regarding a patient's problem?
- Will I refrain from discussing my day's encounters with patients with my family and friends?
- Will I always protect a patient's chart and everything in it from unnecessary observation?
- Will I keep patients' names and the circumstances that bring them to my place of employment confidential?

C. *Uphold the honor and high principles of the profession and accept its disciplines.*
- Am I proud of serving as a medical assistant?
- Will I always perform within the scope of my profession, never exceeding the responsibility entrusted to me?

- Will I encourage others to enter the profession and always speak honorably of medical assistants?

D. *Seek to continually improve the knowledge and skills of medical assistants for the benefit of patients and professional colleagues.*
- Will I always be willing to learn new skills, to update my skills, and seek improved methods for assisting the physician in the care of patients?
- Will I keep my credentials current and valid?
- Can I always remember that I am a member of a group of broad-based health care professionals, and that my goal is to complement rather than to compete with that team?

E. *Participate in additional service activities aimed toward improving the health and well-being of the community.*
- Will I be able to serve in the community where I reside and work to further quality health care?
- Will I promote preventive medicine?
- Will I practice good health care management for myself, being a model for others to follow?

ETHICAL GUIDELINES FOR DOCTORS

It is fairly common for each professional group of medical practitioners to have their own code of ethics. The AMA's Code of Medical Ethics and the "Current Opinions with Annotations of the Council on Ethical and Judicial Affairs" was mentioned earlier. The American Chiropractic Association has a Code of Ethics identified in six sections. Other practitioners may consider their mission and policies to be their code of ethics. Some have no specific written code of ethics, but rather call on their practitioners to refer to their culture as one based on ethics, mutual respect, and moral evaluation when ethical decisions are made. There are many similarities in these statements on ethics that are important for patients and medical employees.

Advertising

Physicians and professional people traditionally have not advertised; however, it is not illegal or unethical to do so if claims made are truthful and not misleading. Advertisements may include credentials of physicians and a description of the practice, kinds of services rendered, and how fees are determined. Managed care agencies may advertise their services and the names of participating physicians.

Confidentiality

 Physicians must not reveal confidential information about patients without their consent unless they are otherwise required to do so by law. Confidentiality must be protected so that patients will feel comfortable and safe in revealing information about themselves that may be important to their health care. The following list contains examples of the kinds of reports that allow or require health professionals to report a confidence.

- A patient threatens another person and there is reason to believe that the threat may be carried out.

- Certain injuries and illnesses *must* be reported. These include injuries such as knife and gunshot wounds, wounds that may be from suspected child abuse, communicable diseases, and sexually transmitted diseases.

- Information that may have been subpoenaed for testimony in a court of law.

When in doubt, it is always recommended that a physician have the patient's permission to reveal any confidential information.

 Extra caution must be taken to protect the confidentiality of any patient's data that are kept on a computer database. As few people as possible should have access to the computer data, and only authorized individuals should be permitted to add or alter data. Adequate security precautions must be used to protect information stored on a computer.

Medical Records

The medical chart and the information in it are the property of the physician and the patient. No information should be revealed without the patient's consent unless required by law. The record is confidential. Physicians should not refuse to provide a copy of the record to another physician treating the patient so long as proper authorization has been received from the patient. Also, physicians should provide a copy of the record or summary of its contents if a patient requests it. A record cannot be withheld because of an unpaid bill.

On a physician's retirement or death, or when a practice is sold, patients should be notified and given ample time to have their records transferred to another physician of their choice.

Professional Fees and Charges

Illegal or excessive fees should not be charged. Fees should be based on those customary to the locale and should reflect the difficulty of services and the quality of performance rendered. Fee splitting (a physician splits the fee with another physician for services rendered with or without the patient's knowledge) in any form is unethical. Physicians may charge for missed appointments (if patients have first been notified of the practice) and may charge for multiple or complex insurance forms. Physicians and their employees must be diligent to assure that only the services actually rendered are charged or indicated on the insurance claim. Only what is documented in the patient's chart is to be billed.

Increasingly, there are a number of physicians who now refuse any insurance payments and operate strictly on a cash only basis. Some others charge a yearly fee to care for a family, providing all services necessary at that flat fee. Physicians, upset by the rules and regulations of insurance, find this method of payment creates a simpler form of medical practice. Physicians and patients alike will be discussing the ethics of such a move for some time. Although physicians may choose whom they wish to serve, the cash only basis makes it difficult for low-income families and the poor.

Professional Rights and Responsibilities

As stated earlier, physicians may choose whom to serve, but may not refuse a patient on the basis of race, color, religion, national origin, or any other illegal discrimination. It is unethical for physicians to deny treatment to HIV-infected individuals on that basis alone if they are qualified to treat the patient's condition. Once a physician takes a case, the patient cannot be neglected or refused treatment unless official notice is given from the physician to withdraw from the case.

Patients have the right to know their diagnoses, the nature and purpose of their treatment, and to have enough information to be able to make an informed choice about their treatment protocol. Physicians should inform families of a patient's death and not delegate that responsibility to others.

Physicians should expose incompetent, corrupt, dishonest, and unethical conduct by other physicians to the disciplinary board. It is unethical for any physician to treat patients while under the influence of alcohol, controlled substances, or any other chemical that impairs the physician's ability.

Physicians who know they are HIV positive should refrain from any activity that would risk the transmission of the virus to others.

Any activity that might be regarded as a "conflict of interest" (for example, a physician holding stock in a pharmaceutical company and prescribing medications only from that company) should be avoided. Financial interests are not to influence physicians in prescribing medications, devices, or appliances.

Abuse

It is the responsibility of physicians and their employees to report all cases of suspected child abuse, to protect and care for the abused, and to treat the abuser (if known) as a victim also. This is not an easy task. Abuse is not easy to witness. Although there are specific laws regarding suspected child abuse, and in most states medical assistants are mandated to report abuse, the laws are vague or nonexistent for older adults or in domestic violence cases. However, whatever form the abuse takes, it is best to treat all forms of abuse in the same manner by providing a safe environment for those abused and seeking treatment for the abused and the abuser.

BIOETHICAL DILEMMAS

Guidelines for bioethical issues are even harder to define than are guidelines for ethics, because each of the bioethical issues calls on us to make decisions that directly affect a person's life. In some instances, the bioethical issue requires a choice about who lives and requires a definition of the quality of life. Such dilemmas are difficult, if not impossible, to approach from a neutral point of view even though medical assistants should strive not to impose their own moral values on patients or coworkers.

Allocation of Scarce Medical Resources

The issue faced daily by health care workers is the allocation of scarce medical resources. Even with the government's attempts at health care reform, medical resources still are not available to everyone. When the receptionist determines who receives the only available appointment in a day, when patients are turned away because they have no insurance or financial resources to pay for services, when Medicare/Medicaid patients are denied services because of low return from state and federal insurance programs, scarce medical resources are being denied.

Weightier decisions might include who gets the surgery, a kidney transplant, or the experimental bone marrow transplant. These allocations are being made and will continue to require decisions on the part of the health care team. As recent as the 2004 national meeting of the AMA, a proposal was made suggesting that physicians refuse treatment to lawyers and their family members or any patients who "threaten" a lawsuit if treatment is unsuccessful. The proposal did not pass, but it came from frustrated physicians trying to spotlight the access problems caused by professional liability cases. Rationing of health care may become more widespread as managed care operations try to achieve a balance between providing access to care while still curtailing costs.

Decisions made by Congress, health systems agencies, and insurance companies are termed **macroallocation** of scarce medical resources. Decisions made individually by physicians and members of the health care team at the local level are termed **microallocation** of scarce resources. No matter what the level, physicians and medical assistants will be involved.

Abortion and Fetal Tissue Research

It appears these issues associated with abortion and fetal tissue research will be with us for quite some time. Although the law is specific on abortion guidelines as set forth in *Roe v. Wade,* there is a continual challenge in the courts of its validity. Some states are more restrictive in how and if abortions might be performed in the second and third trimesters of pregnancy. However, the law stipulates that a woman has a right to an abortion in the first trimester without interference from regulations in any state.

A physician must decide whether to perform abortions within the legal parameters and under what circumstances. A physician cannot be forced to perform abortions, nor can any employee be forced to participate or assist the physician to perform an abortion. Employees not wishing to participate in abortions are advised to seek employment where they are not performed.

There are many unanswered ethical questions related to abortion that make it difficult for health care professionals. Should abortion be considered a form of birth control? If not, should birth control be readily available to all who seek it regardless of age? Should insurance pay for birth control? Is it ethical to deny a woman on welfare an abortion whereas providing one to a woman who either has money for the procedure or whose insurance pays for it? And, of course, the major unanswered question that must be determined by every physician is: When does life begin?

 The abortion issue raises another bioethical issue—fetal tissue research and transplantation. Fetal tissue research, as early as the 1950s, led to the development of polio and rubella vaccines. Today, fetal cells hold promise for medical research into a variety of diseases and medical conditions, including Alzheimer's disease, Huntington's disease, spinal cord injury, diabetes, and multiple sclerosis. There is some research to indicate that fetal retinal transplants may be a successful treatment for macular degeneration, which is the leading cause of old-age blindness in the United States. This issue is also political, as well as bioethical, and it changes with each major political shift in our government. Fetal tissue research gets caught up in the pro-life forces, also. About half of the states have laws regulating fetal research. Some ban the research using aborted fetuses. Federal law prohibits the sale of fetal tissue and requires all federally funded fetal tissue research projects to comply with state and local laws. Fetal tissue research is not to be used to encourage women to have abortions; rather, the tissue would be available only after a decision had already been made regarding abortion.

Genetic Engineering/Manipulation

So much is possible today in the area of **genetic engineering** and new discoveries increasingly are being seen. This biotechnology can be used in the diagnosis of disease, production of medicines, forensic documentation (DNA used in solving crimes), and for research. Some reasons to continue study in this area include to determine if anything can be done to prevent or cure some

4,000 recognized genetic disorders and major diseases that have large genetic components. Who among us would not want to be free of certain illnesses? But at what cost? How far do we go in genetic engineering? Would we prefer a society where everyone is healthy and beautiful? If it is determined that a fetus suffers from a serious defect, should abortion be encouraged? If we manipulate the genes before implantation, are we playing God? If fertilization takes place *in vitro,* is discarding defective embryos a reasonable and presumed choice?

Artificial Insemination/Surrogacy

For many individuals, artificial insemination is the only means by which they can conceive a child. Physicians are called on to perform artificial insemination for couples, single women, or lesbians who want a child. If artificial insemination is performed, it is recommended that the signed consent of each party involved be obtained. It is also recommended that physicians practicing AID (artificial insemination by donor), use many donors for semen, and that meticulous screening be performed before the insemination.

Surrogacy is another bioethical issue. Men have been used as **surrogates,** or substitutes, for decades with the practice of artificial insemination, but society seems to have a more difficult time accepting surrogate mothers who are artificially inseminated by a donor and carry the fetus to term for another parent. Gay men seek surrogates who are able to provide them a child who represents half their genetic makeup. How should the rights of each individual in the exchange be protected? For many of these issues, there is little protection or guidance under the law; therefore, physicians and their employees must make decisions on the basis of their own belief systems.

Artificial insemination and surrogacy were viewed as experimental and quite controversial just 20 years ago. Today, however, the procedures are widely practiced and available. Both artificial insemination and surrogacy are costly and can become legal tangles for all involved if careful steps are not taken.

Critical Thinking

When fertilization occurs outside the womb, additional embryos are stored and saved for future use. How long should they be stored? To whom do they belong? What happens if no one wants those embryos later? Should they be destroyed, given to some other hopeful parent, or used for research?

Dying and Death

Patients are making more choices regarding their own death. We all have the right to direct health care professionals regarding our death in the case of a life-threatening illness. Through a living will or a physician's directive, we can mandate that life support systems be removed. Review Chapter 7. Sometimes, patients make these decisions before physicians are ready to remove the life support. Other times, physicians can determine when a case is hopeless far quicker than the patient or the patient's family. What should be done then? When a physician is committed to sustaining life, it is difficult to make decisions to terminate life. Oregon, the only state to pass a physician-assisted suicide law has had great difficulties maintaining and putting the law into practice, partly because of a challenge by the United States Attorney General. Oregon voters have held firm, however, and so far the Attorney General has been unsuccessful in overturning the voters' wishes.

Choices available to patients who are dying always cause us to ask ourselves what is "quality of life"? Although the answer to that question is different for everyone, it is a question often in conflict with today's medical technology that can, in many instances, keep a patient alive much longer than the patient might prefer. The benefits of advanced technology will continue to be weighed against what many consider the right to die with dignity and a minimum of medical intervention.

HIV and AIDS

The general public's fear of AIDS has caused some serious bioethical issues. Patients who may suspect they have HIV or AIDS should be tested for the virus. Their confidentiality must be protected as much as possible because individuals with AIDS often face loss of employment, medical insurance, and even loss of family and friends. It is unethical to deny treatment to individuals because they test positive for HIV.

Although individuals with HIV/AIDS must be protected, so must the public. Therefore, if physicians suspect that an HIV-seropositive patient is infecting an unsuspecting individual, every attempt should be made to protect the individual at risk. Health professionals must first encourage the infected person to cease endangering any person. Second, if the patient refuses to notify the person at risk or wishes the physician to notify the person, the physician can contact authorities. Many states and cities have Partner Notification Programs that will anonymously notify the patient at risk, keeping the source confidential. The program informs them that it has been brought to their attention that they are a "person at risk" and provides them with free testing. Third, the physician can notify the person at risk.

Case Study 8-1

Harley Navarro is a new medical assistant in a busy internist's clinic. Harley is nervous and fairly intimidated by the other medical assistants who are female and have many years of experience. He is especially hesitant to ask for assistance or admit that he is having a problem. Twice today he was unable to get a good blood pressure reading on patients. One patient was very obese, and the other kept trying to carry on a conversation with him.

CASE STUDY REVIEW

1. If Harley's behavior does no harm to the patient, has he acted unethically? Illegally?

2. What might the office manager do if she senses Harley's lack of certainty?

3. Discuss the role of female and male medical assistants working together and how they might complement each other.

Case Study 8-2

Liz Corbin is a medical assistant in the fertility clinic of a large metropolitan medical clinic and hospital. Liz really likes her job and is delighted when parenthood is made possible for many of those seeking the clinic's advanced technology. The clinic also stores and maintains the unused frozen embryos that result from artificial insemination. She is a little alarmed when her physician–employer informs her that four of the embryos are to be destroyed. The physician has been unable to contact the owners (now parents of more than one child from artificial insemination) for directions, and space for storage is limited. The physician instructs Liz to destroy the embryos.

CASE STUDY REVIEW

1. Liz is rather hesitant to comply with her physician's orders, so she does a little research. She discovers that most fertility clinics ask couples using **cryopreservation** to decide early in the process how to handle their excess embryos. The choices are: (1) discard the embryos, (2) donate anonymously to other infertile couples, and (3) donate to scientific research. What might Liz do to influence the clinic's policy?
2. Can anything be done to ensure that couples do not abandon their embryos?
3. If embryos are given to other infertile couples, how is a decision made on who should have them?

SUMMARY

As medical technology continues to advance, a greater need for ethical guidelines will be necessary. Physicians and health care professionals at all levels must stay abreast of the issues and carefully consider all aspects before making any decision.

Medical assistants must, however, keep the following legal and ethical guidelines in mind: (1) always practice within the law; (2) preserve the patient's confidentiality; (3) maintain meticulous records; (4) obtain informed, written consent; (5) do not judge patients whose belief system differs from yours.

STUDY FOR SUCCESS

To reinforce your knowledge and skills of information in this chapter:
- ❏ Review the Key Terms
- ❏ Consider the Case Studies and discuss your conclusions
- ❏ Answer the Review Questions
  - ❏ Multiple Choice
  - ❏ Critical Thinking
- ❏ Navigate the Internet and complete the Web Activities
- ❏ Practice the StudyWARE activities on the textbook CD
- ❏ Apply your knowledge in the Student Workbook activities
- ❏ Complete the Web Tutor sections
- ❏ View and discuss the DVD situations

REVIEW QUESTIONS

Multiple Choice

1. Typically, ethics has been defined in terms of:
   a. what is right and wrong
   b. whether an action is legal
   c. the expedient thing to do
   d. professionalism in the workplace
2. Bioethics has to do with:
   a. biological reproduction
   b. the act of artificial insemination
   c. genetic engineering
   d. ethical issues that deal with life and health care
3. The AAMA Code of Ethics:
   a. is concerned with principles of ethical and moral conduct
   b. defines the duties the medical assistant can perform
   c. is intended for physicians only
   d. applies only to patient rights
4. When a physician or medical assistant suspects child abuse, they should:
   a. give the parent a warning
   b. report it to the proper authorities
   c. not impose their values on the parents
   d. give the child some hints on how to protect against abuse
5. When a patient has HIV:
   a. it is ethical for the physician not to provide treatment
   b. it is unethical for the physician not to provide treatment
   c. other patients should be warned of the possibility of infection
   d. all friends and family members of the patient should be notified
6. A copy of a medical record may be granted to:
   a. a physician the patient is being referred to
   b. a physician's attorney when subpoenaed or released by patient
   c. the patient
   d. all of the above
   e. only a and b
7. The eight characteristics of principle-centered leaders originates from the following author:
   a. James R. Jones
   b. Steven R. Covey
   c. Francis H. Ambrose
   d. Jason N. Diamond
8. The five Ps of ethical power are:
   a. Personality, performance, purpose, pride, patience
   b. Purpose, patience, perfection, personality, procrastination
   c. Patience, purpose, pride, persistence, perspective
   d. Purpose, pride, patience, perfection, perspective
9. Which of the following is true?
   a. A physician can choose whom to serve.
   b. A physician may charge for completing multiple and complex insurance claims.
   c. Physicians and their employees cannot be forced to perform abortions.
   d. All of the above
   e. None of the above
10. You are most likely to make ethical decisions correctly when:
    a. you have a clear picture of the situation
    b. you leave emotion out of the decision as much as possible
    c. you understand your weaknesses and vulnerabilities
    d. honesty and integrity are hallmarks of your entire life
    e. all of the above

Critical Thinking

1. In your own words, define ethics and bioethics.
2. A physician observes another physician put a patient at risk while under the influence of alcohol and does nothing about it. What would constitute ethical behavior?
3. A physician refuses to accept any more Medicaid patients for medical care. Is this the physician's right? Is it ethical? Why or why not?
4. A medical assistant whispers to the receptionist, "There goes the guy with AIDS." How should the receptionist view this behavior?
5. The services reported on the insurance claim are more complex than those actually rendered. Is this ethical or unethical? State your reasons.
6. The physician refuses to perform a legal abortion. Do you consider this an ethical issue? Why?
7. A physician performs artificial insemination for a lesbian couple; however, the medical assistant refuses to participate or assist the physician. What are the ramifications of the medical assistant's behavior? Do you believe the medical assistant has a right to refuse?
8. Referring to Figure 8-1, select an ethical issue with which you may have had some personal experience. Now, form a small group, with each student leading a discussion on a different issue.

WEB ACTIVITIES

1. Using the World Wide Web, print out the latest issue of the AMA Principles of Medical Ethics. Compare that with the AAMA Code of Ethics. Do you find this comparison helpful in more clearly understanding ethics, responsibility, and professionalism? Give your reasons.

2. Using the Web site given at the beginning of this chapter, select one additional code of ethics to compare with the AMA Principles and the AAMA Code. What are the similarities?

3. Using your favorite Internet search engine, key in two or three of the bioethical issues and do a small-scale review of items listed. From your research, identify at least three ethical/bioethical questions for your class to discuss.

THE DVD HOOK-UP

DVD Series **Critical Thinking**	Program Number **3**

Chapter/Scene Reference
• *Ethical Practice*

In this chapter, you learned about the importance of ethical behavior when working in the medical field. Ethics are not laws, but rather a set of morals or principles to which we adhere.

In the designated DVD clip, we observed Jen talking to Sarah about a patient that has diabetes. Jen feels that the patient has complications with her diabetes because she makes poor choices in her eating habits. Barb, the supervisor, overhears the conversation and talks to Jen and Sarah about the importance of being compassionate as health care providers. Even though this clip does not deal with some of the more noted ethical issues such as fetal tissue research or genetic engineering, judging the patient is a violation of ethical behavior and probably one of the more typical ethical issues that you will struggle with as a medical assistant.

1. As a medical assistant, you will make observations about your patients that can be helpful to the physician. What was inappropriate in the way Jen handled her observations?

2. Diseases such as emphysema, obesity, and diabetes can all be the result of unhealthy life styles. How will you as a medical assistant keep from judging a patient's actions or lifestyle that have resulted in illness?

DVD Journal Summary

Write a paragraph that summarizes what you learned from watching the designated scenes from today's DVD program. Ethical dilemmas may involve anyone in the medical office. For example, what would you do if you smelled alcohol on a coworker? What if you suspect the coworker is abusing alcohol? Are you obligated to say something? To whom? Why or why not?

REFERENCES/BIBLIOGRAPHY

American Medical Association. (2004–2005). Code of medical ethics. *Current opinions of the council on ethical and judicial affairs, 2004.* Chicago: American Medical Association.

Blanchard, K., & Peale, N. V. (1988). *The power of ethical management.* New York: William Morrow and Company, Inc.

Covey, S. R. (1991). *Principle-centered leadership.* New York: Simon & Schuster.

Flight, M. (2004). *Law, liability, and ethics for medical office personnel* (4th ed.). Clifton Park, NY: Thomson Delmar Learning.

Lewis, M. A., & Tamparo, C. D., (2002). *Medical law, ethics, and bioethics for ambulatory care* (5th ed.). Philadelphia: F. A. Davis.

CHAPTER 9

Emergency Procedures and First Aid

OUTLINE

OBJECTIVES

The student should strive to meet the following performance objectives and demonstrate an understanding of the facts and principles presented in this chapter through written and oral communication.

1. Define the key terms as presented in the glossary.
2. Learn to recognize, prepare for, and respond to emergencies in the ambulatory care setting.
3. Understand the legal and disease transmission considerations in emergency caregiving.
4. Perform the primary assessment in emergency situations.
5. Identify and care for different types of wounds.
6. Understand the basics of bandage application.
7. Discriminate among first-, second-, and third-degree burns.
8. Assess injuries to muscles, bones, and joints.

(continues)

KEY TERMS

Ambu Bag™
Anaphylaxis
Automated External
Defibrillator (AED)
Bandage
Cardiopulmonary
Resuscitation (CPR)
Cardioversion
Cauterized
Constriction Band
Crash Tray or Cart
Crepitation
Dressing
Emergency Medical
Services (EMS)
Explicit
First Aid
Fracture
Heimlich Maneuver
Hypothermia
Implicit
Lackluster
Normal Saline
Occlusion
Rescue Breathing
Risk Management
Shock
Splint
Sprain
Standard Precautions
Strain
Syncope
Systemic
Triage
Universal Emergency
Medical Identification
Symbol
Wound

CAHEEP—ENTRY-LEVEL COMPETENCIES

Patient Care

- Recognize and respond to emergencies
- Coordinate patient care information with other health care providers

Professionalism

- Demonstrate initiative and responsibility
- Work as a member of the health care team
- Prioritize and perform multiple tasks
- Treat all patients with compassion and empathy

Legal Concepts

- Comply with established risk management and safety procedures

ABHES—ENTRY-LEVEL COMPETENCIES

Professionalism

- Exhibit initiative
- Conduct work within scope of education, training and ability

Clinical Duties

- Recognize emergencies
- Perform first aid and CPR
- Prepare and administer medications as directed by physician

Legal Concepts

- Perform risk management procedures

OBJECTIVES (continued)

9. Describe heat- and cold-related illnesses.
10. Describe how poisons may enter the body.
11. Recall the eight types of shock.
12. Define a cerebral vascular accident.
13. Describe the signs and symptoms of a heart attack.
14. Demonstrate proficiency in Heimlich maneuver, rescue breathing, and cardiopulmonary resuscitation (CPR).

SCENARIO

Inner City Health Care, which is located in Carlton, Michigan, has its share of cold, snowy winters, and when the temperature drops near freezing, that snow sometimes turns to ice. Last night, as Clinical Medical Assistant Wanda Slawson, CMA, was leaving for the evening, she noticed a woman from an adjacent office slip and fall in the parking lot. Wanda immediately went over to the woman to lend assistance and saw that, in falling, the woman had cut the palm of her hand. Apparently, she had tried to break her fall with her hand only to sustain a wound that was now bleeding moderately. Fortunately, Wanda knew that one of the physicians was still in the office and she led the woman back to the building, reassuring her along the way. Once in the office, Wanda assisted Susan Rice, the physician, to examine the wound. After determining that sutures were not needed, Dr. Rice and Wanda cleansed the wound, applied a dry, sterile dressing, and covered it with an elastic bandage. The patient was instructed to call her physician first thing in the morning.

INTRODUCTION

Although the ambulatory care setting is primarily designed to see patients under nonemergency conditions, occasionally the physician will need to administer emergency care, and the medical assistant will be called on to assist the physician in this care. For the medical assistant who may need to triage or assess the patient's condition, the first and most critical step in responding to an emergency is developing the skill to recognize when emergency measures should be taken.

Whereas some emergencies can be treated in the office, others cannot, and the medical assistant must know when to call for outside help. If the emergency occurs in the ambulatory care setting, the physician usually provides immediate care. It is possible, however, that the medical assistant may be the first emergency caregiver should the physician be out of the office. The medical assistant also may be called on to provide care in an emergency outside of the office environment.

This chapter acquaints the medical assistant with types of emergency situations that may occur either inside or outside of the office. However, this chapter is merely an introduction to emergency topics and does not substitute for first aid and cardiopulmonary resuscitation (CPR) instruction taught either through the college curriculum or through the American Red Cross, the American Heart Association, the American Safety and Health Institute, or the National Safety Council. These hands-on classes are vital teaching tools, and all medical assistants should take them on a regular basis to continually update their skills.

RECOGNIZING AN EMERGENCY

An emergency is considered any instance in which an individual becomes suddenly ill and requires immediate attention. Most emergencies develop quickly and usually without warning. They can occur unexpectedly at any time to anyone. Some may be gradual, as seen with dehydration or slow blood loss, and become an emergency over time. Some common signs that an individual has an emergency include unusual noises, such as yelling, moaning, or crying. A person may appear to be behaving strangely when choking or if having difficulty breathing. To recognize when an emergency exists, it is important to have sharp senses of hearing, sight, and smell and be acutely sensitive to any unusual behaviors.

In the ambulatory care setting, medical assistants may encounter a range of emergency situations requiring first-aid techniques. **First aid** is designed to render immediate and temporary emergency care to persons injured or otherwise disabled before the arrival of a physician or transport to a hospital or other health care agency.

Spotlight on Certification

RMA Content Outline
- Body systems
- Disorders of the body
- First aid procedures

CMA Content Outline
- Performing telephone and in-person screening
- Preplanned action (Emergencies)
- Assessment and triage
- Establishing and maintaining an airway
- Identifying and responding (First Aid)
- Signs and symptoms
- Management (First Aid)

CMAS Content Outline
- Medical Office Emergencies

Emergency situations can be minor or severe and can include:

- Stroke
- Wounds
- Bleeding
- Burns
- Shock
- Fractures
- Poisoning
- Sudden illnesses such as fainting/falling
- Illnesses related to heat and cold
- Heart attack
- Choking and breathing crises

Some of these situations will be life-threatening; all will require immediate care. In either case, it is critical to remain calm, to follow the emergency policies and procedures established by the ambulatory care setting, and to be well-versed in first-aid and CPR techniques. The patient should not be further endangered.

Patient confidentiality must be maintained during an emergency situation, as it must at all times. Sometimes, when a situation is urgent and the patient is having trouble breathing, bleeding heavily, having a severe allergic reaction, or any other kind of emergency, in your eagerness to assist the patient, your voice when talking to other health care providers may be overheard by other patients. Be certain other patients cannot hear any conversations. Privacy must be maintained when faxing information to the emergency department. Also be cautious when speaking on the telephone. Do not give out information to a patient's family or to other practitioners without the patient's consent. Be cautious to keep the patient's anonymity protected.

Responding to an Emergency

Once it has been determined that an emergency exists, it is essential to act quickly. Before making any decisions about how to proceed, it is necessary to assess the nature of the situation. Does it include respiratory or circulatory failure, severe bleeding, burns, poisoning, or severe allergic reaction?

Sometimes, it is possible that more than one type of care must be administered. In this case, it is necessary to **triage** the situation, which is a method of prioritizing treatment. When an individual experiences more than one illness or injury, care must be given according to the severity of the situation. When two or more patients present with emergencies simultaneously, triage also determines which patient is treated first. The main principle of triage states that absence of heartbeat and breath and severe bleeding are immediate life threats. See Table 9-1 for the common ordering of triage situations.

To identify the nature of the emergency and respond effectively, it is critical that the patient be assessed. If the patient is conscious, ask for personal identification and identification of next of kin. Try to obtain information about symptoms being experienced to identify the problem. Always check for a **universal emergency medical identification symbol** (Figure 9-1) and accompanying identification card, which will describe any serious or life-threatening health problems that the patient has. Quickly observe the patient's general appearance, including skin color and size and dilation of pupils. Check pulse and blood pressure.

Primary Survey

If the patient is unresponsive, it is critical to assess the ABCs, which include:

- Airway
- Breathing
- Circulation

To assess whether the unresponsive patient is breathing and to determine if there is an open airway, place your face close to the patient's face and look, listen, and feel. Look at the patient's chest and notice whether the chest rises and falls with breathing. Listen for air entering and leaving the nose and mouth and feel for moving air.

If the individual is not breathing, first open the airway by either tilting the head and lifting the chin (Figure 9-2A); or by the jaw-thrust maneuver, which involves

TABLE 9-1	EXAMPLES OF TRIAGE SITUATIONS	
First Priority	**Next Priority**	**Least Priority**
Airway and breathing problems	Second-degree burns not on the neck and face	Fractures (simple)
Cardiac arrest	Major or multiple fractures	Minor injuries
Severe bleeding that is uncontrolled		Sprains, strains
Head injuries	Back injuries	
Poisoning	Severe eye injuries	
Open chest or abdominal wounds		
Shock		
Second- and third-degree burns		

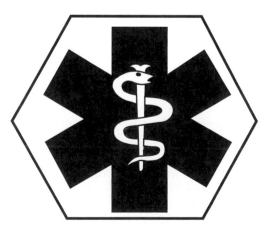

Figure 9-1 The universal emergency medical identification symbol.

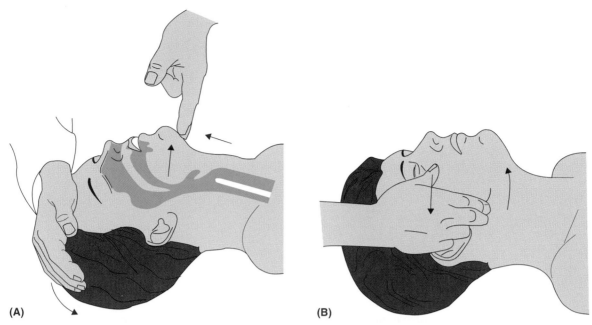

(A)   **(B)**

Figure 9-2 If the individual is not breathing, first open the airway (A) by tilting the head and lifting the chin, or (B) by the jaw-thrust maneuver, which involves placing both thumbs on the patient's cheekbones and placing the index and middle fingers on both sides of the lower jaw.

placing both thumbs on the patient's cheekbones and placing the index and middle fingers on both sides of the lower jaw (see Figure 9-2B). **CAUTION:** Do not attempt to tilt the head and lift the chin when the patient has a head, neck, or spinal cord injury.

If the patient still does not breathe after the airway has been opened, rescue breathing must be performed (discussed later in this chapter).

To assess circulation, check for the presence of a pulse at the carotid artery on the side of the neck below the ear. If no pulse is present, the patient may be in cardiac arrest and must be given CPR. Use of an **automated external defibrillator (AED)** may be necessary. CPR techniques are discussed in detail later in this chapter.

Patient Education

Alert patients to the importance of carrying the universal emergency medical identification symbol and its accompanying identification card if the patient suffers from severe heart disease, diabetes, or has other life-threatening illnesses or allergies.

Using the 911 or Emergency Medical Services System

The **Emergency Medical Services (EMS)** system is a local network of police, fire, and medical personnel who are trained to respond to emergency situations. Other community experts and volunteers also act as resources in an EMS system. In many communities, the network is activated by calling 911. Even when preliminary emergency care is provided by the ambulatory care physician, the patient may still need to be transported to a hospital for follow-up care. It is also possible that the physician may not be equipped to deliver the type of emergency care required, in which case, one person should call for EMS help while another stays with the patient until help arrives. Never leave a seriously ill or unconscious patient unattended.

While waiting for EMS to arrive, continuously check the patient for the following signs: (1) degree of responsiveness, (2) airway/breathing ability, (3) heartbeat (rate and rhythm), (4) bleeding, and (5) signs of shock. Monitor vital signs. Keep patient warm and lying down. If there are no head injuries, the legs can be elevated on pillows.

Good Samaritan Laws

 When delivering or assisting in delivering emergency care, the medical assistant may be concerned about professional liability. Most states have enacted Good Samaritan laws, which provide some degree of protection to the health care professional who offers first aid.

Most Good Samaritan laws provide some legal protection to those who provide emergency care to ill or injured persons. However, when medical assistants or any other individuals give care during an emergency, they must act as reasonable and prudent individuals and provide care only within the scope of their abilities. Remember that a primary principle of first aid is to prevent further injury.

Although Good Samaritan laws give some measure of protection against being sued for giving emergency aid, they generally protect *off-duty* health care professionals. Also, conditions of the law vary from state to state. As part of establishing emergency care guidelines, every ambulatory care setting should understand the **explicit** and **implicit** intent of the Good Samaritan law in its state. See Chapter 7 for more information on legal guidelines.

Blood, Body Fluids, and Disease Transmission

 When providing emergency care, medical assistants should always protect themselves and the patient from infectious disease transmission. Serious infectious diseases, such as hepatitis B (HBV), hepatitis C (HCV), and HIV can be transmitted through blood and body fluids.

By establishing and following strict guidelines, the risk for contracting or transmitting an infectious disease while providing emergency care is greatly reduced.

* Always wash hands thoroughly before (if possible) and after every procedure.

* Use protective clothing and other protective equipment (gloves, gown, mask, goggles) during the procedure.

* Avoid contact with blood and body fluids, if possible.

* Do not touch nose, mouth, or eyes with gloved hands.

* Carefully handle and safely dispose of soiled gloves and other objects.

Standard precautions were issued by the Centers for Disease Control and Prevention (CDC) in 1996 and combine many of the basic principles of universal precau-

tions with techniques known as body substance isolation. These augmented 1996 guidelines represent the standard in infection control and are intended to protect both patients and health care professionals.

PREPARING FOR AN EMERGENCY

Emergencies are unexpected but can and should be anticipated and prepared for in the ambulatory care setting. Being properly prepared assures that the office has the materials and resources needed to respond to emergencies.

An in-office handbook of policies and procedures should be developed and should be familiar to all staff members. Telephone numbers for the local emergency medical services (often this is 911) and the poison control center should be posted and kept in an established place so that there is no delay in calling for outside assistance. Materials and supplies should be maintained in proper inventory. All personnel should be trained in the basics of first aid and CPR, so that every staff member can respond to or assist the physician in providing care. Proper documentation should be completed after any emergency situation. The office environment itself should be a safe one and as accident-proof as possible. Wipe up spills to avoid falls on a slippery floor, keep corridors free of clutter, and keep medications out of sight. These basic **risk management** techniques will help medical personnel focus on giving emergency care and also will protect the facility from possible litigation.

The Medical Crash Tray or Cart

Every health care facility should have a **crash tray or cart,** with a carefully controlled inventory of supplies and equipment (Figure 9-3). These first-aid supplies should be kept in an accessible place, and the inventory should be routinely monitored to assure that all supplies are replaced and that all medications are up to date and have not reached their expiration dates.

A smaller practice may require only a portable tray for emergency and first-aid supplies; larger urgent care centers may respond more frequently to emergencies, and thus may need a cart that can hold a larger inventory and variety of supplies. Whether a tray or cart is used, supplies should be customized to the facility and the type of emergencies frequently encountered. Remember that only physicians can order medications or treatment.

Following is a brief list of some common supplies found on most trays and carts.

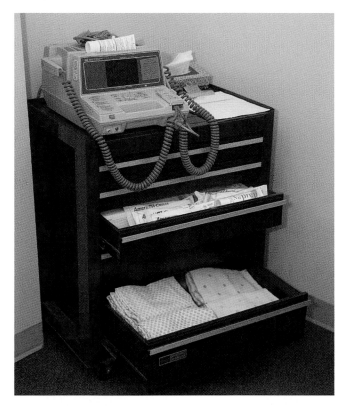

Figure 9-3 Medical crash cart with defibrillator.

General supplies:

- Adhesive and hypoallergenic tape

- Alcohol wipes

- Bandage scissors

- Bandage material

- Blood pressure cuff (standard, pediatric, large)

- **Constriction band**

- Defibrillator

- Dressing material

- Gloves

- Hot/cold packs

- Intravenous (IV) tubing

- Needles and syringes for injection

- Orange juice for diabetics (refrigerated)

- Penlight (with extra batteries)

- Personal protective equipment

- Stethoscope

Emergency medications	Uses
Activated charcoal	Poisonings
Aspirin	Fever, heart attack
Atropine	Slow heartbeat
Dextrose	Insulin reaction
Diazepam*	Antianxiety
Diphenhydramine	Antihistamine
Dopamine	Increases blood pressure
Epinephrine	Constricts blood vessels, increases blood pressure
Glucagon	Insulin reaction
Insulin	Hyperglycemia
Lidocaine	Local anesthetic, IV for cardiac arrhythmia
Nitroglycerin tablets, patches	Chest pain from angina pectoris
Phenobarbital*	Sedative
Verapamil	Hypertension, angina pectoris, irregular heartbeat, tachycardia
Xylocaine, Marcaine	Local anesthetics

*Controlled substance—must be kept in locked cabinet.

Respiratory supplies:

- Airways of all sizes for nasal and oral use

- **Ambu bag™**

- Bulb syringe for suction

- Oxygen mask

- Oxygen tank

This list represents just some of the supplies to be found on a well-stocked crash cart or tray. The type and list of supplies should always be overseen by facility physicians and tailored to the emergency demands of the practice. The medical assistant should be familiar with the equipment and medication on the crash cart or tray. Practice "drills" simulating various emergency situations are helpful for preparing staff members for actual emergencies.

COMMON EMERGENCIES

Included in this discussion of common emergencies are shock, wounds, burns, musculoskeletal injuries, heat- and cold-related illnesses, poisoning, sudden illness, cerebral vascular accident, and heart attack.

Shock

When a severe injury or illness occurs, shock is likely to develop. **Shock** is basically a condition in which the circulatory system is not providing enough blood to all parts of the body, causing the body's organs to fail to function properly.

Shock is always life threatening, and EMS should be activated. The body's attempt to compensate for a massive injury or illness, especially those involving the heart and lungs and severe bleeding, often lead to other problems. During shock, several things occur.

- The heart becomes unable to pump blood properly.
- Consequently, the body's cells, tissues, and organs do not get enough oxygen, which is carried by the blood.
- The body tries to compensate by sending blood to critical organs and reducing the flow of blood to arms, legs, and skin.

Signs and Symptoms of Shock. Learn to recognize the signs and symptoms of shock.

- Patient may be restless or feel irritable.
- Weakness, dizziness, thirst, or nausea may occur.
- Breathing may be shallow and rapid.
- Skin is cool, clammy, and pale.
- Pulse is weak and rapid.
- Blood pressure is low.
- Area around the lips, eyes, and fingernails may turn cyanotic (blue) from lack of oxygen.
- The patient may be confused or become suddenly unconscious, or both.
- Dilated pupils and **lackluster** eyes are obvious.

Types of Shock. There are eight major types of shock, including respiratory, neurogenic, cardiogenic, hemorrhagic, anaphylactic, metabolic, psychogenic, and septic. See Table 9-2 for a description of each.

Treatment for Shock. A person suffering from shock needs immediate medical attention. Call for outside emergency help first, then care for the patient until help arrives. **CAUTION:** Shock requires immediate medical help. Shock is progressive, and if not treated immediately, most types can be life threatening. Once shock reaches a certain point, it is irreversible.

To care for a patient in shock, follow these procedures:

- Lie the patient down. This minimizes pain and decreases stress on the body.
- Loosen clothing.
- Check for an open airway.

TABLE 9-2	EIGHT TYPES OF SHOCK WITH DESCRIPTIONS
Type of Shock	**Description**
Respiratory	Trauma to the respiratory tract (trachea, lungs) that causes a reduction of oxygen and carbon dioxide exchange. Body cells cannot receive enough oxygen.
Neurogenic	Injury or trauma to the nervous system (spinal cord, brain). Nerve impulse to blood vessels impaired. Blood vessels remain dilated and blood pressure decreases.
Cardiogenic	Myocardial infarction with damage to heart muscle; heart unable to pump effectively. Inadequate cardiac output. Body cells not receiving enough oxygen.
Hemorrhagic	Severe bleeding or loss of body fluid from trauma, burns, surgery, or dehydration from severe nausea and vomiting. Blood pressure decreases, thus blood flow is reduced to cells, tissues, and organs.
Anaphylactic	Results from reaction to substance to which patient is hypersensitive or allergic (allergen extracts, bee sting, medication, food). Outpouring of histamine results in dilation of blood vessels throughout the body, blood pressure decreases and blood flow is reduced to cells, tissue, and organs.
Metabolic	Body's homeostasis impaired; acid–base balance disturbed (diabetic coma or insulin shock); body fluids unbalanced.
Psychogenic	Shock caused by overwhelming emotional factors; i.e., fear, anger, grief. Sudden dilation of blood vessels results in fainting because of lack of blood supply to the brain. In most cases, not life-threatening unless it leads to physical trauma as a result of a fall.
Septic	An acute infection, usually **systemic,** that overwhelms the body (for example, toxic shock syndrome). Poisonous substances accumulate in bloodstream and blood pressure decreases, impairing blood flow to cells, tissues, and organs.

- Check breathing.
- Control any external bleeding.
- Help the patient maintain normal body temperature. A blanket over and under the patient can help avoid chilling. Do not overheat.
- Reassure the patient.
- Elevate the legs about 12 inches, unless you suspect head injury, spinal injuries, or broken bones involving the hips or legs.
- Do not give the patient anything to eat or drink.
- Ascertain that outside help has been called and stay with the patient until help arrives.
- Monitor vital signs.

Wounds

Typically, **wounds** are classified as open wounds or closed wounds. In the closed wound, there is no break in the skin; a bruise, contusion, and hematoma are common closed wounds. An open wound represents a break in the skin and can be classified as an abrasion, avulsion, incision, laceration, or puncture wound.

Closed Wounds. Most closed wounds do not present an emergency situation. If there is pain and swelling, the application of a cold compress can be effective. Protect the patient's skin by placing a cloth beneath the source of cold; apply the compress for 20 minutes, then remove for 20 minutes; continue for 24 hours. Then apply heat 20 minutes on and 20 minutes off for the next 24 hours. A common procedure for treating closed wounds is to RICE or MICE it.

RICE	MICE
• *Rest*	• Motion or Movement
• *Ice*	• Ice
• Compression	• Compression
• Elevation	• Elevation

Recently, some physicians, especially those who treat sport injuries, advocate motion or movement as a means of treating a closed wound injury. They also advise ice, compression (elastic bandage), and elevation (MICE). Check with the physician.

Some closed wounds, such as hematomas, can be dangerous and may cause internal bleeding. If the patient is in severe pain and was subject to an injury caused by high impact, call for help and keep the patient comfortable until the help arrives. Watch for symptoms of shock and monitor vital signs.

Open Wounds. Open wounds can be minor tears in the skin or more serious skin breaks, but all open wounds represent an opportunity for microorganisms to gain entry and cause an infection. Some major open wounds may involve heavy bleeding, which will need to be controlled, probably by suturing. A tetanus injection is indicated for an open wound if the patient has not had a booster in the last 7 to 10 years.

There are five common types of open wounds:

1. *Abrasions* are a superficial scraping of the epidermis. Because nerve endings are involved, they can be painful. However, they are not usually serious, unless they cover a large area of the body. Administer first aid by cleaning the area carefully with soap and water, apply an antiseptic ointment if prescribed by a physician, and cover with a dressing.
2. In an *avulsion*, the skin is torn off and bleeding is profuse. Avulsion wounds often occur at exposed parts: fingers, toes, ear. First, control bleeding (see Procedure 9-1) if necessary. Then clean the wound. If there is a skin flap, reposition it. Apply a dressing, then bandage as necessary. Note that pieces of the body may be torn away. If possible, save the body part, keep moist, and transport with the patient.
3. *Incisions* are wounds that result from a sharp object, such as a knife or piece of glass. Incisions may need sutures. The wound must be cleaned with soap and water and a dressing applied.
4. *Lacerations* tear the body tissue and can be difficult to clean; therefore, care must be taken to avoid infection. If there is not severe bleeding, which in itself is a cleansing mechanism, these wounds may need to be soaked in antiseptic soap and water to remove debris. If there is severe bleeding, it must be controlled immediately (see Procedure 9-1). Lacerations with severe bleeding usually need suturing.
5. *Punctures* pierce and penetrate the skin and may be deep wounds while appearing insignificant. Usually, external bleeding is minimal, but the patient should be assessed for internal bleeding. Because a puncture wound is deep, the risk for infection is great and the patient should be advised to watch for signals of infection, such as pain, swelling, redness, throbbing, and warmth.

Use of Tourniquets in Emergency Care. In the past, tourniquets were regularly used in the field to control hemorrhaging from an extremity when all other attempts to control bleeding were unsuccessful. However, because tourniquet application was meant to completely stop blood flow, many times this complete lack of blood flow resulted in the death of the arm or leg. Often, the affected extremity needed to be amputated.

To remedy this situation, a "constriction band" was substituted for the tourniquet and is now widely used. The constriction band is made of a material similar to that used in the tourniquet. When the band is applied to an extremity to control bleeding, it is applied tightly enough to stem the rapid loss of blood but loosely enough to allow a small amount of blood to continue to flow. A pulse should be felt distally to the constriction band. The use of the constriction band applied in this manner allows a blood supply to the remainder of the extremity unlike the tourniquet, which cuts off all blood flow.

Dressings and Bandages.
When a patient presents with an open wound, after the physician has treated the wound, it is critical to dress and bandage it properly to curtail infection. Covering of the wound is accomplished by a series of **dressings** and **bandages.**

Typically, dressings are sterile gauze pads placed directly on the wound; they often have nonstick, sterile surfaces, but they are absorbent and will soak up blood and protect the wound from microorganisms. They are often made of a gauze-type material.

Bandages, which are nonsterile, are placed over the dressing. They hold the dressing in place and are made to conform to the area to be covered. Sometimes, as in a Band-Aid®, the dressing and bandage are combined. Roller bandages, such as those made of elastic, can be placed over a dressing and used to help control bleeding or swelling.

Kling gauze, a type of gauze that stretches and clings as it is applied, and roller bandages, long strips of soft material wound on itself, are other types of bandage materials.

Bandages and their applications can take many shapes and forms, depending on the type of injury and the injury site. In all cases, a bandage must be secure, but not constricting. Avoid too tight or too loose a wrap.

- Spiral bandages are useful for injuries to the arms or legs (Figure 9-4).

- A figure-eight bandage will hold the dressing in place on a wound on the hand or wrist, knee, or ankle (Figure 9-5).

- Fingers, toes, arms, and legs can also be bandaged using a tubular gauze bandage (Figures 9-6, 9-7, and 9-8). Using a cylindrical applicator, a quantity of gauze is stretched over the wound site.

- Commercial arm slings are used to support injured or fractured arms (Figure 9-9). To apply, support the injured arm above and below the injury site while applying the sling.

Burns

Most burns are commonly caused by heat, chemicals, explosions, and electricity. Critical burns can be life threatening and require immediate medical care. Accord-

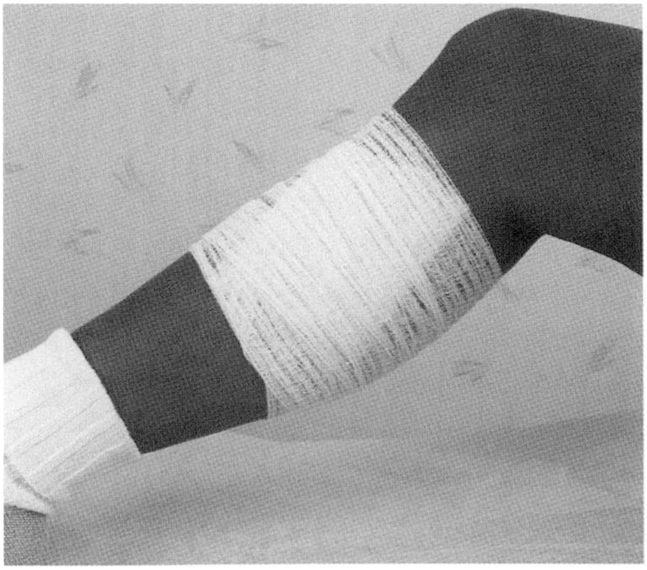

Figure 9-4 The spiral bandage is an option for arm and leg injuries.

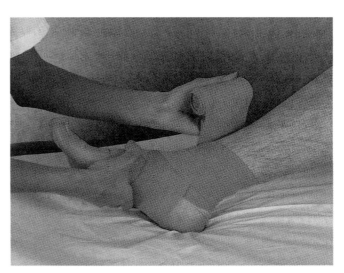

Figure 9-5 An elastic figure-eight bandage holds dressings in place or can be used for immobilization as with an ankle sprain.

ing to the American Red Cross, critical burns have the following characteristics:

- Involve breathing difficulty
- Cover more than one body part
- Involve the head, neck, hands, feet, or genitals
- Involve any burns to a child or older adult (other than minor burns)

To distinguish critical from minor burns, it is important to understand the degrees of burns and what they mean.

First-, Second-, and Third-Degree Burns.
First-degree burns are superficial burns that involve only the top layer of skin. The skin appears red, feels dry, is warm to the touch, and is painful. First-degree burns usually heal in a week or so with no permanent scarring.

In a second-degree burn, the skin is red and blisters are present. The healing process is slower, usually a month, and some scarring may occur. Second-degree burns affect the top layers of the skin, are very painful, and may take three to four weeks to heal. Some scarring may occur.

Third-degree burns are the most serious, affecting or destroying all layers of skin. It is not unusual for fat, muscles, bones, and nerves to be involved. These burns look charred or brown. There may be great pain or, if nerve endings are destroyed, the burn may be painless. Victims of third-degree burns must receive immediate medical attention both for the burn and for shock. Of serious con-

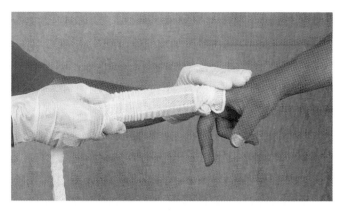

Figure 9-7 The gauze bandage is stretched over the appendage by pulling the applicator away from the base of the appendage. At the same time, the bandage should be held in place at the appendage base with the other hand.

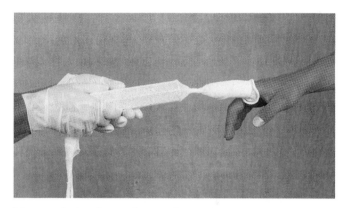

Figure 9-8 Once the applicator has been pulled off the finger, a layer of the bandage will remain on the appendage. To apply another layer, the applicator is again fitted over the finger and a new layer is applied in the same manner as before.

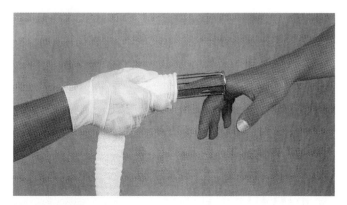

Figure 9-6 There are several types and sizes of tubular gauze applicators, including plastic, solid metal, and metal cage applicators; the metal cage is shown here. All applicators use a seamless elastic gauze bandage (also available in various sizes) that slides over the applicator. The applicator with the gauze then fits over the appendage to be wrapped.

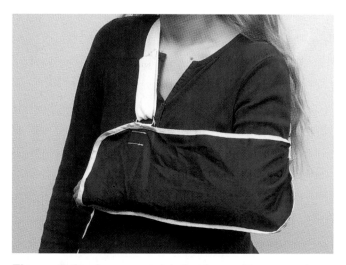

Figure 9-9 A commercial sling is used to support injured or fractured arms.

cern with a third-degree burn is the likelihood of infection and the amount of fluid loss. Scarring can result in loss of body function. Skin grafts may be necessary.

Figure 9-10 shows the relative penetration level of each degree of burn into the skin and underlying structures.

General Guidelines for Caring for Burns. Treatment for burns depends on the type of agent causing the burn. General treatment strategies for any degree of burn include the following:

- Cool the burn with large amounts of cool normal saline, or water if saline is unavailable.

- Cover the burn with a sterile dressing if one is available and burn is minor. Otherwise, cover the burn with a sheet or other smooth textured cloth for a burn over a large area of the body.

- Be sure the patient is protected from being either chilled or overheated.

However, it is important to follow these guidelines:

- Do not apply ice or ice water to a burn.

- Do not touch a burn, except with a sterile dressing.

- Do not clean a severe burn, break blisters, or use any kind of ointment.

- Do not remove pieces of clothing that may be sticking to the burn.

First Aid for Burns. First aid for burns is outlined in Table 9-3.

Types of Burns. Most burns are caused by heat; however, burns can also be caused by chemicals, electricity, and solar radiation.

Chemical Burns. Chemical burns can occur in the workplace or even in the home with "ordinary" household chemicals. To stop the burning process, you must remove the chemical from the skin. Have someone call an ambu-

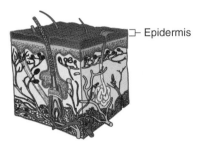
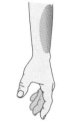

First-degree, superficial

Skin red, dry

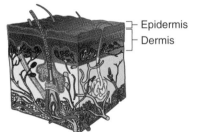
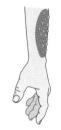

Second-degree, partial thickness

Blistered; skin moist, pink or red

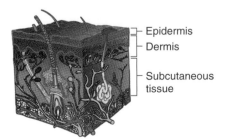
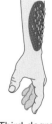

Third-degree, full thickness

Charring; skin black, brown, red

Figure 9-10 Classification of burn injuries.

Patient Education

Some burns can be prevented. Advise patients who insist on sunbathing to protect themselves against harmful rays by using a sunscreen and avoiding the sun between 10 AM and 2 PM.

Patient Education

Advise patients not to run should their clothing catch on fire. They should fall to the ground or wrap themselves in a blanket or rug and roll on the ground to extinguish the flames.

lance while you flush the skin or eyes with cool water. Remove any clothing contaminated by the chemicals unless they adhere to the skin. If clothing clings to the skin, it can be cut with scissors. Do not attempt to pull clothing away from a burned area.

Electrical Burns. Electrical burns can be caused by power lines, lightning, or faulty electrical equipment in the home or workplace. *It is important to remember never to go near a patient injured by electricity until you are sure the power has been shut off, because you*

TABLE 9-3 FIRST AID FOR BURNS

First-Degree Burn Response Guide

Questions	Responses	Action to Take	Rationale
Is skin reddened without blisters?	YES ⇨	Submerge in cool **normal saline** or ⇨ water 2–5 minutes.	Stops burning process.
NO ⇩			
Does area involve: • hands? • feet? • genitals? • face?	YES ⇨	Have patient come to office. ⇨	These are potential danger areas and require evaluation by the physician.
NO ⇩			
Is patient: • elderly? • very young?	YES ⇨	Have patient come to office. ⇨	These groups are susceptible to burn complications.
NO ⇩			
Consult physician.			Physician has final decision whether patient is seen.

Second-Degree Burn Response Guide

Questions	Responses	Action to Take	Rationale
Is skin reddened with blisters or splitting of the skin?	YES ⇨	Submerge in cool normal saline or ⇨ water 10–15 minutes if skin is intact. Use compresses if skin is broken. Do not break blisters. Do not use anesthetic creams or sprays.	Stops burning process. If blisters are broken, can allow infection in burn. Creams or spray may slow healing process and increase severity of a burn.
NO ⇩			
Does area involve: • hands? • feet? • genitals? • face?	YES ⇨	Have patient come to office or go to ⇨ the emergency department.	These are potentially dangerous areas and require medical attention.
NO ⇩			
Is the area involved larger than a child's hand?	YES ⇨	Have patient come to office or go to ⇨ the emergency department.	Burns of this size are susceptible to complications.
NO ⇩			
Is patient experiencing trouble breathing?	YES ⇨	Patient should go to emergency ⇨ department.	There may be swelling of the airways because of heat and noxious fumes.
NO ⇩			
Consult physician.			Physician has final decision whether patient is seen.

(continues)

TABLE 9-3 **FIRST AID FOR BURNS** (continued)

Third-Degree Burn Response Guide

Questions	Responses	Action to Take	Rationale
Is skin gray, black, or charred appearing? Can muscle, fat, or bone be seen in wound?	YES ⇨	Call EMS immediately. Do not ⇨ apply cold; do not remove burnt clothing from burn area.	Life-threatening emergency that requires prompt attention.
NO ⇩			
Is patient experiencing: • pallor • loss of consciousness? • shivering?	YES ⇨	Patient in shock: ⇨ • call EMS. • maintain airway. • maintain body temp. • elevate feet if appropriate. • monitor breathing. • may need oxygen and intravenous fluids while waiting for EMS to arrive.	Need to control shock caused by fluid loss.
NO ⇩			
Consult physician.			Physician has final decision whether patient is seen.

could be injured. If there is a downed line, call the power company and EMS.

A victim of an electricity burn may be suffering from two burns: one where the power entered the body, and one where it exited. Often, the burns themselves may be minor. Of more serious consequence are the possibilities of shock, breathing difficulties, and other injuries. CPR often is needed in this situation.

Solar Radiation. Most "sunburns," although not advisable or good for the skin, represent minor burns. If the patient has a severe burn, however, he or she should see a physician who will cover the burn area to reduce infection and protect the patient against chill.

Musculoskeletal Injuries

Most injuries to muscles, bones, and joints are not life threatening, but they are painful and, if not properly treated, can be disabling. Some injuries, such as those to the spinal cord, can be quite serious and can result in paralysis. These injuries are not typically seen in the ambulatory care setting.

Types of Injuries. A **sprain** is an injury to a joint, often an ankle, knee, or wrist, that involves a tearing of the ligaments. Some sprains are minor and heal quickly; others are more severe, include swelling, and may not heal properly if the patient continues to put stress on the sprained joint. Signs of a sprain are rapid swelling, discoloration at the site, and limited function. Many times it is difficult to

determine whether the patient has sustained a sprain or a fracture because the degree of pain may not be a true indicator of the patient's injury. As with most closed wounds, treating the injury with the RICE or MICE method is beneficial, and determined by the physician's choice.

A **strain** results from the overuse or stretching of a muscle or group of muscles, as with improper lifting or moving heavy objects. Applications of ice and heat (as described for treatment of sprains), as well as rest, are indicated for treatment of strains.

Dislocations are painful and involve the separation of a bone from its normal position. These usually occur from the kind of wrenching motion that might result from a fall, automobile accident, or sports injury.

Fractures involve a break in a bone and can be caused by a fall, by a blow, from bone disease, or from sports injuries. There are several types of fractures, but all are classified as either open or closed fractures. An open fracture involves an open wound and is characterized by a protruding bone. In a closed fracture, the skin is not broken. Signs and symptoms that occur with a fracture may include swelling, discoloration, pain, deformity, and immobility of the body part. It is not unusual for patients to tell you that they heard the bone break or that they sensed a grating feeling. **Crepitation** is the term that describes the grating sensation experienced or heard when bone fragments rub together. Fractures are further defined as follows:

- Incomplete or greenstick: fracture in which the bone has cracked, but the break is not all the way through; frequently seen in children

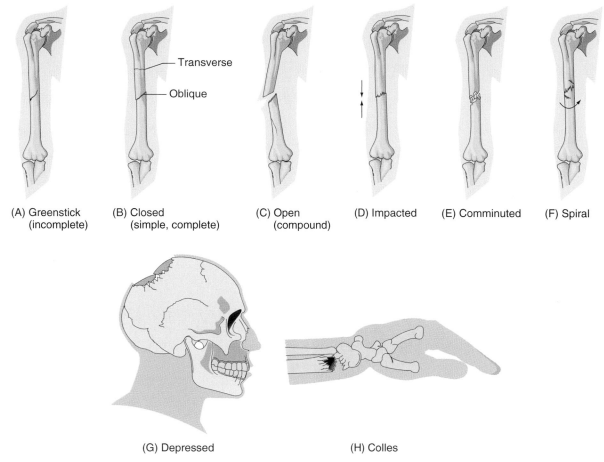

(A) Greenstick (incomplete)   (B) Closed (simple, complete)   (C) Open (compound)   (D) Impacted   (E) Comminuted   (F) Spiral

(G) Depressed   (H) Colles

Figure 9-11   Types of fractures.

- Simple: complete bone break in which there is no involvement with the skin surface

- Compound: fracture in which the bone protrudes though the skin surface, creating the possibility of infection

- Impacted: fracture in which the broken ends are jammed into each other

- Comminuted: more than one fracture line and several bone fragments are present

- Spiral: fracture that occurs with a severe twisting action, causing the break to wind around the bone

- Depressed: fracture that occurs with severe head injuries in which a broken piece of skull is driven inward

- Colles: fracture often caused by falling on an outstretched hand; involves the distal end of the radius and results in displacement, causing a bulge at the wrist

See Figure 9-11 for examples of these fractures.

Assessing Injuries to Muscles, Bones, and Joints. Sometimes it is difficult to determine the extent of an injury, especially in closed fractures. There are some assessment techniques to call on, however, to gauge the seriousness of an injury.

- Note the extent of bruising and swelling.

- Pain is a signal of injury.

- There may be noticeable deformity to the bone or joint.

- Use of the injured area is limited.

- Talk to the patient: What was the cause of the injury? What was the sound or sensation at the time of injury?

Caring for Muscle, Bone, and Joint Injuries. Most injuries to muscles, bones, and joints are treated in a similar way; some require rest, some motion, elevation of the injured part, immobilization, and the application of ice to the injury.

After calling for outside care (always check for life-threatening symptoms, such as breathing difficulties, bleeding, or head, neck, or back injuries), it is important to immobilize the injured area if the patient must be moved. EMS personnel use a variety of **splints** to immobilize bones and joints. See Procedure 9-2 for splinting an arm in the ambulatory care setting.

Heat- and Cold-Related Illnesses

The condition of patients who have been subject to extreme heat and cold can deteriorate rapidly, and either a heat- or cold-related illness can result in death. Individuals especially vulnerable to extreme exposures include the very young and very old, individuals who must work out of doors, and people who suffer from poor circulation.

Heat-Related Illnesses. Illnesses related to heat, in increasing degree of severity, include heat cramps, heat exhaustion, and heat stroke. Heat cramps, the least serious, involve cramping in the legs and abdomen caused by excessive body exposure or exercise in hot weather. Heat cramps should be considered a signal to stop, slow down, rest in a cool place, and drink plenty of water. Salt tablets should not be taken. The individual should lightly stretch the muscles. Heat cramps can progress to heat exhaustion or heat stroke, both of which are more serious conditions.

Heat exhaustion, often experienced by people who work or exercise in extreme heat, is a more serious reaction and is signaled by exhaustion, cold and clammy skin, profuse sweating, headache, and general weakness. The individual should come out of the heat immediately, apply cool, wet towels, and slowly drink cool water. The physician will advise the patient not to resume activity in the heat.

Heat stroke is the least common but the most dangerous of heat-related illnesses and requires immediate medical attention. Heat stroke is characterized by red, dry, hot skin; an abnormal, weak pulse; and breathing that is shallow and fast. In heat stroke, the body systems are extremely taxed. EMS should be alerted; until they arrive, stay with the patient, watch for breathing problems, and attempt to reduce body temperature by applying cool, wet towels or sheets.

Cold-Related Illnesses. Exposure to extreme cold for prolonged periods can lead to frostbite or hypothermia.

Frostbite, which typically affects the extremities such as fingers, toes, ears, and nose, involves the freezing of exposed body parts. Symptoms include skin that becomes off-color, is cold, or takes on a waxy appearance.

Severity can range from the superficial (frostnip) to more penetrating stages, which may require amputation.

Individuals with frostbite need immediate medical attention. To care for frostbitten extremities, warm the area of injury by wrapping clothing or blankets around the affected body part. Be careful in handling the frozen part. It is best to have the patient transported as soon as possible to emergency care. This type of facility is better able to properly rewarm the frozen part, preventing further tissue damage.

Hypothermia is a serious illness in which the body temperature decreases to a perilously low level. It can result in death if the individual does not receive care and if the progression of hypothermia is not reversed. Hypothermia occurs when a person falls through the ice or is exposed to cold temperatures, for example, after getting lost in the woods while hiking. Symptoms include shivering, cold skin, and confusion.

After checking for breathing problems and alerting EMS, care for the patient. Make the individual comfortable, provide a source of warmth, such as a blanket, and *gradually* warm the body. If clothing is wet or cold, remove and put on dry clothing. In extreme cases, it may be necessary to provide rescue breathing (discussed later in this chapter).

Poisoning

Poisons can enter the body in four ways:

- *Ingestion.* Ingested poisons enter the body by swallowing. Swallowed poisons may include medications, plant material, household chemicals, contaminated foods, and drugs.

- *Inhalation.* Poisons are inhaled into the body in poorly ventilated areas where cleaning fluids, paints and chemical cleaners, or carbon monoxide may be present.

- *Absorption.* Poisons absorbed through the skin include plant materials such as poison oak or ivy, lawn care products such as chemical pesticides, and other chemical powders or liquids.

- *Injection.* Drug abuse is the most common cause of injected poisons. The stingers of insects inject poisons into the body and can be extremely dangerous and can lead to anaphylactic shock in allergic individuals.

Whenever a patient calls regarding poisoning or there is a suspicion of poisoning, call the local poison control center or the local emergency number and ask for advice. Telephone numbers of the poison control center should be posted in a familiar and accessible place.

Patient Education

Remind patients who are parents of young children to remove any potential sources of poisoning from their homes or to keep them in locked cabinets. Also advise them to include the nearby poison control center in their list of emergency phone numbers. They should also keep activated charcoal on hand.

Patient Education

Advise all patients with known allergic reactions to be particularly careful when working or playing outdoors. Insects are not usually aggressive until their nests are approached; however, often these nests are not easy to detect, and an individual may approach one without being aware of its presence. Patients with allergies to insects should always wear shoes when outside, wear light-colored clothing, preferably with long sleeves and pant legs, look before taking a sip from a beverage when outdoors, and inspect lawn areas, shrubbery, and building walls periodically for evidence of stinging insect nests.

The treatment for poisoning will vary according to the source of the poisoning and must be tailored to the specific incident. The physician will have advised staff regarding specific poisoning antidotes. Generally, do not give the patient anything to eat or drink; try to determine what poison the patient was exposed to and, if ingested, how much was taken; if the patient vomits, save some of the vomitus for analysis.

If prescribed by a physician or recommended by the poison control center, medication used to treat poisoning is activated charcoal, which is used to absorb certain swallowed poisons.

Insect Stings. The medical assistant in the ambulatory care setting is likely to receive a number of calls every summer from patients who have been stung by insects, typically yellow jackets, hornets, honeybees, or wasps. In the nonallergic patient, the sting is likely to result in localized swelling and tenderness and slight redness. The physician will recommend that these localized symptoms be managed with a topical cream and oral antihistamines. Swelling can be significant and cause for serious concern if the sting occurred in a vulnerable area of the body such as the mouth or tongue. Swelling in these locations can be frightening and dangerous because it can impair breathing. An antihistamine, administered as soon as possible after the sting, may help to curtail symptoms somewhat. Treatment for insect stings in nonallergic individuals consists of removing the stinger by scraping it off with the edge of something rigid such as a credit card or your fingernail. Tweezers can cause more venom to be dispersed into the patient's body tissues, so this method should not be used. Wash the area with soap and water, apply a cold pack to the site, and watch for a possible severe reaction.

The individual who experiences an allergic reaction or hypersensitivity to a sting needs to be seen immediately, because in severe cases a sting may induce an anaphylactic reaction that can lead to death. If allergic, individuals who have been stung are likely to experience symptoms within a half hour of the incident. Symptoms are generalized throughout the body and may include hives, itching, and lightheadedness, and may progress to difficulty breathing, faintness, and eventual loss of consciousness.

For individuals with known allergic reactions, the physician will prescribe epinephrine, which patients should carry with them and self-inject should they not be able to get immediate emergency care. EPIPEN is a brand of epinephrine to self-inject. The patient should then seek immediate emergency treatment. For individuals who present at the ambulatory care setting with an apparent allergic reaction to a sting, the physician will prescribe epinephrine, an antihistamine, and corticosteroids if necessary. Attempt to allay patient apprehension and monitor vital signs while waiting for EMS personnel to arrive.

Sudden Illness

Sudden illness is, by definition, an unexpected occurrence. Although the cause of the illness may be inexplicable, it is important to respond sensibly and responsibly within the parameters of knowledge and resources.

Sudden illnesses include, but are not limited to, fainting, seizures, diabetic reaction, and hemorrhage.

Fainting. Also known as **syncope,** fainting involves a loss of consciousness, caused by an insufficient supply of blood to the brain. Loss of consciousness may simply be the result of a fainting episode, or it may indicate a more serious medical problem such as diabetic coma or shock. A fall during a fainting incident may result in bodily harm.

 If a patient in the office or clinic "feels faint," indicated by lightheadedness, weakness, nausea, or unsteadiness, have the individual lie down or sit down with head level with the knees. This may prevent a fainting episode.

If a patient faints, gradually lower the patient to a flat surface, loosen any tight clothing, check breathing and for any life-threatening emergencies, and apply cool compresses to forehead. Elevate the legs if there is no back or head injury. If vomiting occurs, place the patient on his or her side. Although fainting is typically not serious in itself, 911 or EMS may need to be called because the problem may be indicative of a more complex medical condition.

Seizures. Seizures or convulsions occur when normal brain functioning is disrupted, which can occur for a variety of reasons including fever, disease such as diabetes, infection, or injury to the brain. Epilepsy is a common cause of convulsions. Involuntary spasms or contractions of muscles characterize seizures.

To the onlooker, seizures look frightening and painful, which may lead inexperienced individuals to try to stop the seizure when they see it occurring in another individual. A patient experiencing a seizure should never be restrained; simply care for the victim of a seizure with compassion and medical understanding. The goal is to protect the patient from self-injury during the episode. Also, do not force anything between the patient's clenched teeth—individuals experiencing seizures cannot "swallow" their tongues.

 Most patients will recover from a seizure in a few minutes. During the seizure, protect the patient from injury, cushion the patient's head, and roll the patient to the side if any fluid is in the mouth. After the seizure subsides, calm and comfort the patient.

If a patient is known to regularly have seizures, and the patient's seizure subsides in a matter of minutes, EMS personnel usually do not need to be summoned. Repeated seizures during the same time frame, however, dictate a call to emergency services, as does any seizure if the patient is diabetic, pregnant, injured, or does not regain consciousness after the incident.

Diabetes. Diabetes is defined by the American Diabetes Society as the "inability of the body to properly convert sugar from food into energy."

Under normal functioning, the body produces a hormone called insulin, which transports sugars into body cells. In some cases, the body does not produce insulin at all or does not produce enough; this results in diabetes.

Diabetes occurs in two major types:

- Type I, or insulin-dependent diabetes

- Type II, or noninsulin-dependent diabetes, which usually occurs in adults; in type II, the body produces insulin in insufficient quantities

Complications from diabetes, which you may encounter in a medical office or clinic setting, include diabetic coma (acidosis) and insulin shock or reaction. The physician will prescribe either insulin or glucose before the patient is transported to the hospital. Both are serious emergencies that require immediate EMS assistance. See Table 9-4 for common causes and symptoms of diabetic coma or insulin shock.

Hemorrhage. The different sources of bleeding determine the seriousness of hemorrhage, or bleeding.

External Bleeding. External bleeding includes capillary, venous, and arterial bleeding. Capillary bleeding, often from cuts and scratches, usually clots without first-aid measures. Bleeding from a vein, which is characterized by dark red blood that flows steadily, needs to be controlled quickly (see Procedure 9-1) to avoid excessive blood loss. Bleeding from an artery produces bright red bleeding that spurts from the wound; this is the most serious type of bleeding and occurs when an artery is punctured or severed. Like venous bleeding, arterial bleeding requires immediate emergency care, because serious loss of blood and profound irreversible shock can quickly ensue.

Epistaxis, or nosebleed, may be the result of breathing dry air for a long period; result from injury or blowing the nose too hard; caused by high altitudes; caused by hypertension (high blood pressure); or result from overuse of medications such as aspirin and anticoagulants.

To control nosebleeds, seat the patient, elevate the patient's head, and pinch the nostrils for at least 10 min-

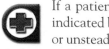

Patient Education

Advise the patient not to blow the nose for several hours after an epistaxis.

TABLE 9-4   CAUSES AND SYMPTOMS OF DIABETIC COMA AND INSULIN SHOCK

Diabetic Coma or Acidosis		Insulin Shock or Reaction	
Causes	Too little insulin, too much to eat, infections, fever, emotional stress	Causes	Too much insulin or oral hypoglycemic drug, too little to eat, an unusual amount of exercise
Symptoms	Skin: Dry and flushed	Symptoms	Skin: Moist and pale
	Behavior: Drowsy		Behavior: Often excited
	Mouth: Dry		Mouth: Drooling
	Thirst: Intense		Thirst: Absent
	Hunger: Absent		Hunger: Present
	Vomiting: Common		Vomiting: Usually absent
	Respiration: Exaggerated, air hungry		Respiration: Normal or shallow
	Breath: Fruity odor of acetone		Breath: Usually normal
	Pulse: Weak and rapid		Pulse: Full and pounding (gives patient feeling of heart pounding)
	Vision: Dim		
	Blood glucose greater than 200 mg/100 ml		Vision: Diplopia (double)
			Low blood glucose level (40–70 mg/100 ml or less)
First aid	Keep patient warm	First aid	If conscious, give patient sugar or any food containing sugar (fruit juice, candy, crackers)
	Obtain medical help immediately		Obtain medical help immediately

utes. Assist the patient to sit with head tilted forward so blood running down the back of the throat will not be swallowed. If bleeding cannot be controlled, the physician may request that you activate EMS. The patient's nostril may need to be **cauterized** or a gauze packing inserted.

Internal Bleeding. Internal bleeding may be minor or serious depending on the cause of the injury. A contusion, or bruise, will result in minor internal bleeding. A sharp blow may induce severe internal bleeding.

Because there is no visible blood flow, it is important to recognize other symptoms of internal bleeding. Symptoms are similar to those of shock and include a rapid and weak pulse, low blood pressure, shallow breathing, cold and clammy skin, dilated pupils, dizziness, faintness, thirst, restlessness, and a feeling of anxiety. There may be pain, tenderness, or swelling at the injury site. The abdomen may be boardlike.

If internal bleeding is suspected, ask another staff member to call EMS; until they arrive, stay with the patient and take measures to prevent shock. Monitor vital signs.

Cerebral Vascular Accident

The common term for a cerebral vascular accident (CVA) is stroke. A stroke is the result of a ruptured blood vessel in the brain; it can also be caused by the **occlusion** of a blood vessel or by a clot. Both these situations can result in blood spilling over brain cells and depriving them of oxygen, causing them to die. Symptoms of a stroke include numbness in face, arm, and leg on one side of the body; loss of vision; severe headache, mental confusion; slurred speech; nausea; vomiting; and difficulty in breathing and swallowing. Paralysis may be present. If a patient is suspected of having a stroke, call EMS, loosen tight clothing, lie the patient down, and keep him or her comfortable. Position the patient's head to facilitate the flow of secretion from the mouth to avoid choking and maintain an open airway. Do not give anything by mouth and monitor vital signs. Immediate emergency care is critical for all individuals experiencing strokes. If the stroke is caused by a clot that blocks blood flow, drugs may be able to protect the individual from permanent injury. Rapid transport to the hospital is important for treatment to be instituted as soon as possible. Treatment with the clot-dissolving drug must be given within a certain time frame after onset of symptoms for it to be effective.

Heart Attack

Heart attack, also known as myocardial infarction, is usually caused by blockage of one or more of the coronary arteries. Symptoms include tightness of the chest, pain radiating down one or both arms, or pain radiating into the left shoulder and jaw. Other signs include rapid and weak pulse, excessive perspiration, agitation, nausea, and cold and clammy skin. Heart attack symptoms in a woman may or may not be similar to those experienced by a man. Women may have symptoms such as abdominal discomfort, burning sensation in the chest, discomfort or pain in the lower chest or back, unexplained sudden fatigue, sweating, and breathlessness.

If you suspect the patient is experiencing a heart attack, contact EMS immediately, loosen tight clothing, and keep the patient comfortable. Prepare to give oxygen and other medications such as aspirin, as directed by the physician. Monitor vital signs. If the patient experiences an episode of cardiac fibrillation, **cardioversion** or defibrillation may be necessary with an automatic external defibrillator. Prepare to begin CPR if necessary.

PROCEDURES FOR BREATHING EMERGENCIES AND CARDIAC ARREST

Breathing or respiratory emergencies occur for a variety of reasons, including choking, shock, allergies, and other illnesses or injuries such as drowning and electrical shock. When an individual stops breathing, artificial or rescue breathing must be given quickly, for without a constant supply of oxygen, brain damage or death will occur.

When the breathing problem is accompanied by cardiac arrest, the rescue breathing must be accompanied by chest compressions. This is known as **cardiopulmonary resuscitation (CPR).** Cardiac emergencies may occur in the medical office because of the large number of patients who have heart disease.

 The procedures that follow will help you respond to breathing emergencies in your clinic or office until EMS arrives. The techniques vary for conscious and unconscious individuals, and for adults, children, and infants. These procedures are for review purposes only; it is essential that every medical assistant

attain provider-level CPR certification and take first-aid training courses as stated in the curriculum content of CAAHEP Standards and Guidelines. Frequent refresher courses and recertification in CPR are necessary.

Heimlich Maneuver (Abdominal Thrust)

A common cause of breathing difficulty results from choking. If an individual signals distress from choking, assist the patient in coughing up the object (Figures 9-12 and 9-13). If the patient cannot cough up the object, and the breathing airway is becoming completely blocked, act immediately. It is apparent that the airway is becoming blocked when the patient cannot cough or speak and the patient uses the universal sign for choking.

Have someone call an ambulance while you perform abdominal thrusts, known as the **Heimlich maneuver.** Patients can be taught to give themselves abdominal thrusts if they are alone and choking (Figure 9-14).

Procedures 9-3, 9-4, 9-5, 9-6, and 9-7 describe how to perform the Heimlich maneuver for adults, children,

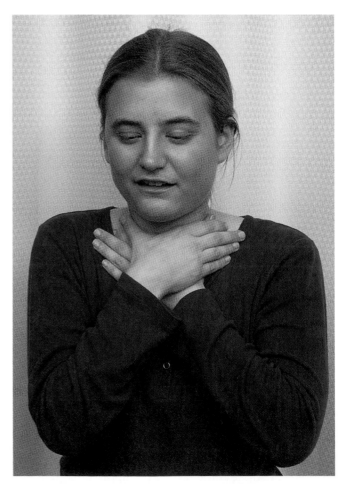

Figure 9-12 Universal sign for choking.

Patient Education

Teach patients to perform the abdominal thrust when they are alone and choking. To perform the Heimlich maneuver when alone, use the fist or thrust against a chair back or any other hard object of adequate height that reaches just below the navel. See Figure 9-14.

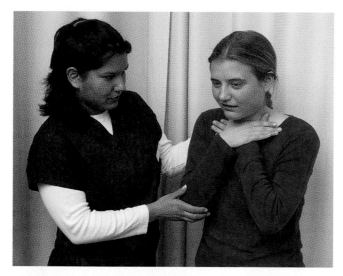

Figure 9-13 Assist the patient in coughing up an object by encouraging continuous coughing.

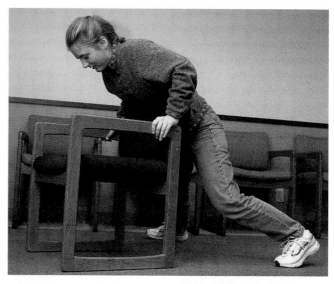

Figure 9-14 If alone, individuals can self-administer the Heimlich maneuver by using the back of a chair or similar hard object.

and infants. These reflect the American Red Cross latest updates, effective July 2000.

Rescue Breathing

Individuals in respiratory arrest require immediate emergency care. **Rescue breathing,** previously called mouth-to-mouth resuscitation, provides oxygen to the patient until emergency personnel arrive.

When performing rescue breathing procedures in the ambulatory care setting, it is recommended that resuscitation mouthpieces be used and that direct mouth-to-mouth (i.e., with no personal protective equipment) resuscitation never be used.

Procedures for rescue breathing differ for adults, children, and infants. See Procedures 9-8, 9-9, and 9-10.

Cardiopulmonary Resuscitation

The combination of rescue breathing and chest compressions is known as CPR. Alone, CPR cannot save an individual from cardiac arrest—it represents preliminary care until advanced medical help is available to the heart attack victim. See Procedures 9-11, 9-12, and 9-13.

When performing CPR, the rule is that you do not stop until

- another trained person can take over,

- EMS arrives and takes over care of the patient,

- you are physically exhausted and not able to continue, or

- the environment becomes unsafe for any reason.

Procedure 9-1 — Control of Bleeding

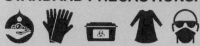

STANDARD PRECAUTIONS:

PURPOSE:
To control bleeding from an open wound.

EQUIPMENT/SUPPLIES:
Sterile dressings
Sterile gloves
Mask and eye protection
Gown
Biohazard waste container

PROCEDURE STEPS:
1. Wash hands.
2. Assemble equipment and supplies.
3. Apply eye and mask protection and gown if splashing is likely to occur.
4. Put on gloves.
5. Apply dressing and press firmly (Figure 9-15A).
6. If bleeding continues, elevate arm above heart level (Figure 9-15B).
7. If bleeding still continues, press adjacent artery against bone (Figure 9-15C). Notify the physician if bleeding cannot be controlled.

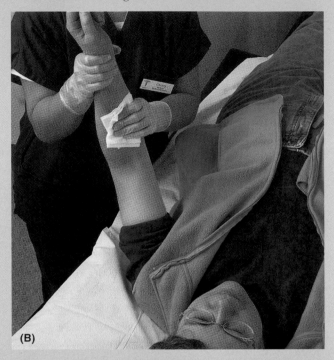

(B)

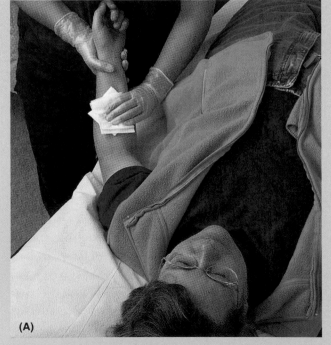

(A)

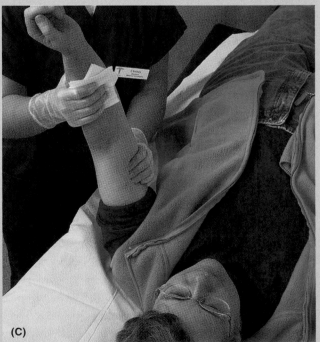

(C)

Figure 9-15 (A) Apply dressing and press firmly. (B) Elevate arm above heart level. (C) Press artery against bone.

(continues)

Procedure 9-1 (continued)

8. Apply pressure bandage over the dressing.
9. Dispose of waste in biohazard container.
10. Remove gloves, dispose of in biohazard container.
11. Wash hands.
12. Document procedure.

CAUTION: If wound is large and bleeding is not controlled, the patient may go into hemorrhagic shock. Be prepared to call EMS immediately.

DOCUMENTATION

4/4/20XX—10:00 AM Patient sustained small (1 cm) laceration on inside left forearm. Bleeding moderately. Pressure dressing applied to wound, left arm elevated above heart level. Bleeding continued. Pressure applied to brachial artery. Pressure bandage applied over dry sterile dressing. Bleeding seems to have subsided. BP 118/74, P 92. Dr. King notified. W. Slawson, CMA

Procedure 9-2 Applying an Arm Splint

STANDARD PRECAUTIONS:

PURPOSE:

To immobilize the area above and below the injured part of the arm to reduce pain and prevent further injury.

EQUIPMENT/SUPPLIES:

Thin piece of rigid board; cardboard can be used if necessary
Gauze roller bandage

PROCEDURE STEPS:

1. Place the padded splint under the injured area.
2. Hold the splint in place with gauze roller bandage. Pad gaps between arm and board (wrist) with gauze pads or other soft material.
3. After splinting, check circulation (note color and temperature of skin, color of nails, check pulse) to ascertain that the splint is not too tightly applied.
4. A sling can be applied to keep the arm elevated, which increases comfort and reduces swelling.
5. Wash hands.
6. Document the procedure.

DOCUMENTATION

4/4/20XX—2:00 PM Splint applied to right arm above and below injured area. Sling applied for comfort. Nail beds pink, hand warm, radial pulse easily palpated. Seen by Dr. Woo. J. Guerro, CMA

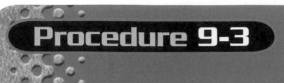

Procedure 9-3   Abdominal Thrusts for a Conscious Adult

STANDARD PRECAUTIONS:

PURPOSE:
To open up a blocked airway.

EQUIPMENT/SUPPLIES:
None needed

PROCEDURE STEPS:
1. Victim cannot cough, speak, or breathe.
2. Call 911.
3. Place the thumb side of your fist against the middle of the abdomen, just above the umbilicus and below the xiphoid process.
4. Grasp your fist with your other hand and give quick upward thrusts (Figure 9-16).
5. Repeat the procedure until the patient coughs up the object. If the person becomes unconscious,

perform abdominal thrusts for an unconscious individual (see Procedure 9-4).
6. Wash hands.
7. Document the procedure.

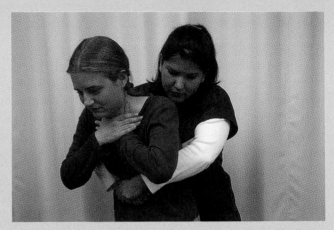

Figure 9-16   Grasp your fist with your other hand and give quick thrusts.

DOCUMENTATION

4/4/20XX—4:00 PM Patient was choking and coughing. Made the universal sign for choking with hands. Became unable to cough, speak, or breathe. Abdominal thrusts given several times. Patient coughed up a large piece of chicken. Breathing easily, color of skin good. BP 130/90, P 100. States she was very frightened but feels much better now. K. Hanson, CMA

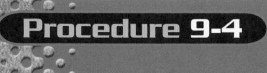

Procedure 9-4 Abdominal Thrusts for an Unconscious Adult or Child

STANDARD PRECAUTIONS:

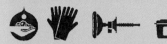

PURPOSE:
To open up a blocked airway in an unconscious victim.

EQUIPMENT/SUPPLIES:
Gloves
Resuscitation mouthpiece
Biohazard waste container

PROCEDURE STEPS:
1. Have someone call emergency services.
2. Put on gloves if available.
3. Lie person on back. Open victim's mouth and look for foreign object. Position resuscitation mouthpiece. Tilt back person's head (Figure 9-17A).

4. Give two breaths (Figure 9-17B).
5. If air will not go in, retilt head to try to give two breaths again. If air will not go in, give 15 abdominal thrusts.
6. Find hand position on breastbone 2 inches above xiphoid and compress 2 inches deep. (For child, give five abdominal thrusts, 1½ inches deep.)
7. Lift the jaw, look for object, and sweep it out of the mouth with finger, if seen (Figure 9-17C).
8. Tilt back the head, lift the chin, and give breaths again slowly. Continue giving breaths and thrusts, looking for object and sweeping it out if seen. Continue breathing until breaths go in. If the airway is cleared and victim does not begin to breathe on his or her own, prepare to perform CPR (see Procedure 9-11).
9. Check carotid pulse.
10. Dispose of waste in biohazard container.

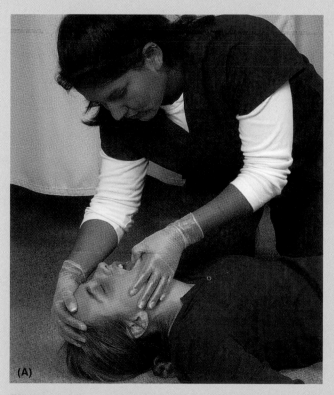

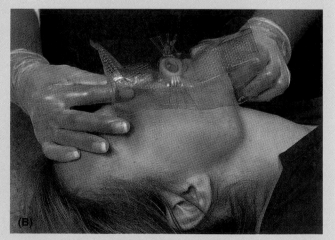

Figure 9-17 (A) Tilt back head. (B) Give breaths.

(continues)

Procedure 9-4 (continued)

11. Remove gloves, dispose of in biohazard container, and wash hands.
12. Monitor vital signs.
13. Document the procedure.

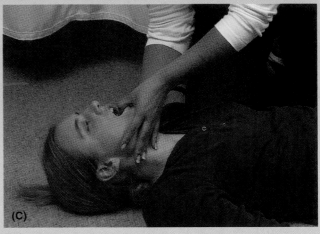

(C)

Figure 9-17 (C) Lift jaw and sweep out mouth.

DOCUMENTATION

4/5/20XX—9:00 AM While doing abdominal thrusts to a choking patient, the victim suddenly collapsed to the floor and lost consciousness. EMS notified by W. Slawson, CMA. No foreign object seen in mouth. Head tilted, breaths given, no air went into victim's body. Retilted head, gave two more breaths, and still no air could get through. Apparent foreign object in throat. Abdominal thrusts given, mouth swept, and large piece of apple found and removed. Breaths entered nose and throat easily, and patient regained consciousness and was breathing easily on own. BP 154/88, P 120, R 24. Color good. Advised to see her physician.

4/5/20XX—9:30 AM Blood Pressure recheck 144/82, P 102, R 20. K. Hanson, CMA

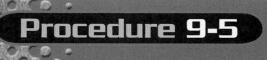 Abdominal Thrusts
for a Conscious Child

STANDARD PRECAUTIONS:

PURPOSE:
To open up a blocked airway.

EQUIPMENT/SUPPLIES:
None needed

PROCEDURE STEPS:

1. Place the thumb side of your fist against the middle of the child's abdomen, just above the umbilicus and below the xiphoid process (Figure 9-18A).

2. Grasp your fist with your other hand. Give quick upward thrusts (Figure 9-18B). Repeat the procedure until the object is expelled or until the patient loses consciousness (see Heimlich maneuver for unconscious child, Procedure 9-4).

3. Wash hands.

4. Document the procedure.

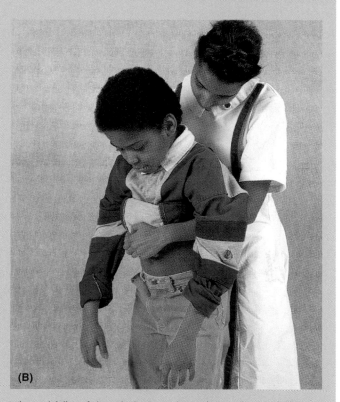

(A)

(B)

Figure 9-18 (A) Place the thumb side of your fist against the middle of the abdomen, just above the umbilicus and below the xiphoid process. (B) Grasp your fist with your other hand and give quick upward thrusts.

DOCUMENTATION

4/5/20XX—11:30 AM Child began choking while running with a hard candy in his mouth. Abdominal thrusts performed five to six times, and the candy was expelled onto the floor. Breathing easily. Color good. Dr. King notified. K. Hanson, CMA

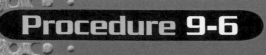

Procedure 9-6

Back Blows and Chest Thrusts for a Conscious Infant Who Is Choking

STANDARD PRECAUTIONS:

PURPOSE:
To open up a blocked airway and assist a conscious infant who is choking, and cannot cough, cry, or breathe.

EQUIPMENT/SUPPLIES:
None needed

PROCEDURE STEPS:
1. Call 911.
2. With the infant face down on your forearm, give five back blows between the infant's shoulder blades with the heel of your hand (Figure 9-19A).
3. Position the infant face up on your forearm.
4. Give five chest thrusts ½ to 1 inch deep, on about the center of the breastbone (Figure 9-19B).
5. Look in the infant's mouth for the object. Repeat the back blows and chest thrusts and look for object until the infant begins to breathe on own. If the infant becomes unconscious, use back blow and chest thrust techniques for unconscious infants (see Procedure 9-7).
6. Activate EMS if unconscious.
7. Wash hands.
8. Document the procedure.

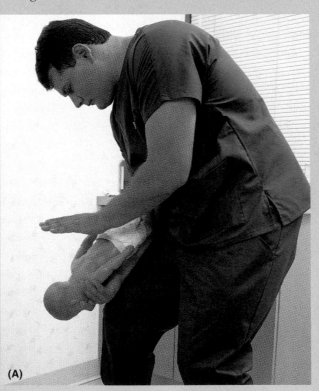
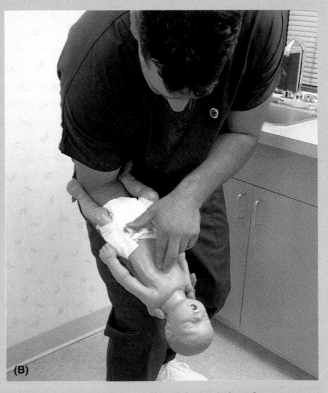

Figure 9-19 (A) With the infant face down on your forearm, give five back blows. (B) With the infant face up on your forearm, give five chest thrusts.

DOCUMENTATION

4/6/20XX—1:30 PM Baby appears to be choking. Back blows and chest thrusts given. Baby began to cry and forced object out of her mouth. Cried forcefully and color returned to pink. Checked by Dr. King. C. McInnis, CMA

Procedure 9-7 — Back Blows and Chest Thrusts for an Unconscious Infant

STANDARD PRECAUTIONS:

PURPOSE:
To open up a blocked airway.

EQUIPMENT/SUPPLIES:
Gloves
Resuscitation mouthpiece

PROCEDURE STEPS:
1. Have someone call emergency services.
2. Don gloves. Tap the infant gently to check for consciousness.
3. Gently tilt back the infant's head. Do not hyper-extend (Figure 9-20A).
4. Listen and watch for breathing.
5. Apply resuscitation mouthpiece. Give two breaths, covering infant's nose and mouth with your mouth (Figure 9-20B).
6. If air will not go in, retilt head, attempt to give breaths again.
7. If breaths still will not go in, give five chest compressions ½ to 1 inch deep.
8. Lift jaw and tongue and check for object. If you see the object, sweep it out (Figure 9-20C).
9. Tilt back head and give one breath again.

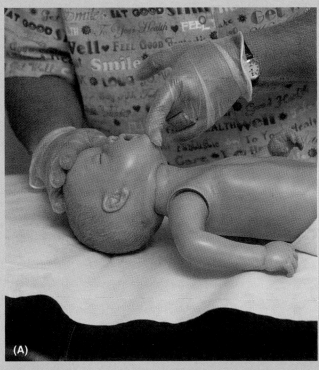

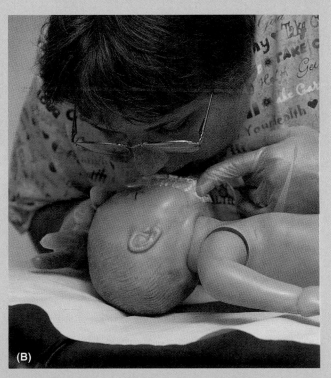

Figure 9-20 (A) Gently tilt back head. (B) Give two breaths, covering the infant's nose and mouth.

(continues)

Procedure 9-7 (continued)

10. Repeat breaths and five chest compressions, and check for object until breaths go in. If the infant does not begin to breathe on his or her own, prepare to perform CPR.
11. Remove gloves. Wash hands.
12. Document the procedure.

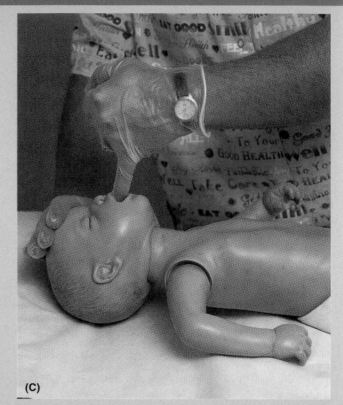

(C)

Figure 9-20 (C) Lift jaw and tongue. Check for object and, if seen, sweep out.

DOCUMENTATION

4/6/20XX—3:00 PM Mother stated that while her 1½-year-old was playing with a toy on the reception room floor, she noticed that the baby fell over, looked blue, wasn't breathing, and was limp. EMS activated. Dr. King notified. Baby unresponsive. Looked into baby's mouth, no object seen. Breaths given. Would not go in. Retilted head and two more breaths given. Still unable to get air into baby. Chest compressions given (½–1 inches deep). Breaths and compressions continued for about two minutes. Baby suddenly coughed up a small object. Crying and breathing on her own. Color pink, does not seem in distress. Seen and examined by Dr. King. W. Slawson, CMA

Procedure 9-8   Rescue Breathing for Adults

STANDARD PRECAUTIONS:

 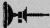

PURPOSE:
To respond to a breathing emergency.

EQUIPMENT/SUPPLIES:
Biohazard waste container
Resuscitation mouthpiece

PROCEDURE STEPS:
1. Have someone call emergency services.
2. Shout, "Are you all right?" "Are you all right?"
3. Look, listen, and feel for breathing.
4. No breathing . . .

5. Tilt back the head, lift the chin, position resuscitation mouthpiece, and pinch the nose closed (Figure 9-21A).
6. Give two short breaths. Breathe into patient until the chest gently rises. Turn your face to the side and listen and watch for air to return.
7. Check for pulse at the carotid artery (Figure 9-21B).
8. If pulse is present, but the person is not breathing, give one slow breath every five seconds. Do this for one minute.
9. Recheck pulse and breathing every minute.
10. Continue rescue breathing as long as pulse is present and the person is not breathing. Continue until breathing is restored or another person takes over.
11. Dispose of waste in biohazard container.
12. Wash hands.
13. Document the procedure.

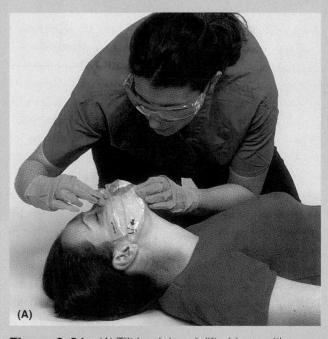

(A)

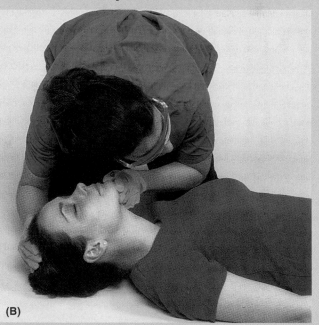

(B)

Figure 9-21   (A) Tilt back head, lift chin, position resuscitation mouthpiece, pinch nose closed, and give two short breaths. (B) Check for pulse at the carotid artery .

DOCUMENTATION

4/7/20XX—1:45 PM A few minutes after having blood drawn for laboratory work, Mrs. Edwards slumped to the floor. She was unresponsive. EMS activated. Dr. King notified. Airway opened, checked for breathing. No breathing. Gave breath. Checked carotid pulse. Pulse strong and regular. Still not breathing. Gave one breath every five seconds for one minute. Rechecked breathing and pulse. Patient breathing, shallow respirations. Dr. King examined patient.

4/7/20XX—2:00 PM BP 100/60, P 100, R 12. Color improved. A. Pemberton, CMA

Procedure 9-9 — Rescue Breathing for Children

STANDARD PRECAUTIONS:

PURPOSE:
To respond to a breathing emergency.

EQUIPMENT/SUPPLIES:
Gloves
Resuscitation mouthpiece

PROCEDURE STEPS:
1. Have someone call emergency services.
2. Don gloves.

3. Tilt back the head, lift the chin, position the resuscitation mouthpiece, pinch the nose closed, and give two short breaths (Figure 9-22A). If air does not go in, retilt head and breathe again.
4. Check for a pulse at the carotid artery (Figure 9-22B).
5. If pulse is present, but the child is not breathing, give one slow breath every three seconds. Do this for one minute.
6. Recheck pulse and breathing every minute.
7. Continue rescue breathing as long as pulse is present but the child is not breathing.
8. Remove gloves. Wash hands.
9. Document the procedure.

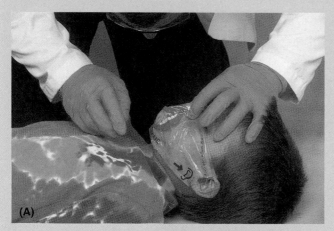
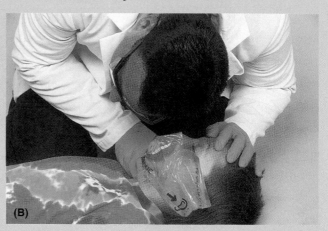

Figure 9-22 (A) Tilt back head, lift chin, position resuscitation mouthpiece, pinch nose closed, and give two short breaths. (B) Check for pulse at the carotid artery.

DOCUMENTATION

4/9/20XX—4:30 PM Seven-year-old JR was in the clinic today for his scheduled allergy desensitization injection. About 5–10 minutes after the injection, JR became weak, pale, and sweaty. He fell to the floor and was unresponsive. Rescue breathing began after activating EMS. Dr. Woo notified. After opening the airway, two slow breaths were given and after finding a carotid pulse, one breath was given every three seconds. JR began to breathe shallow breaths. Examined by Dr. Woo. EMS arrived, stabilized JR, and took him to the emergency department. C. McInnis, CMA

Procedure 9-10   Rescue Breathing for Infants

STANDARD PRECAUTIONS:

PURPOSE:
To respond to a breathing emergency.

EQUIPMENT/SUPPLIES:
Gloves
Resuscitation mouthpiece

PROCEDURE STEPS:
1. Have someone call emergency services.
2. Don gloves.
3. Tilt back the head (Figure 9-23A).

4. Position resuscitation mouthpiece. Seal your lips tightly around the infant's nose and mouth (Figure 9-23B).
5. Give two slow breaths. Breathe into the infant until the chest rises.
6. Check for a pulse at the brachial artery (Figure 9-23C).
7. If pulse is present, but infant is not breathing, give one slow breath every three seconds. Do this for one minute.
8. Recheck pulse and breathing every minute (Figure 9-23D).
9. Continue rescue breathing as long as pulse is present but the infant is not breathing.
10. Remove gloves. Wash hands.
11. Document the procedure.

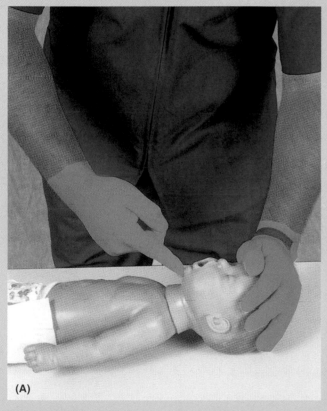

(A)

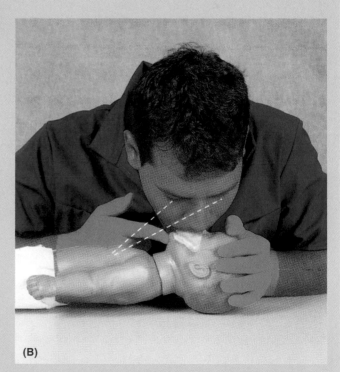

(B)

Figure 9-23 (A) Tilt back head. (B) Position resuscitation mouthpiece. Seal lips around nose and mouth and give two slow breaths.

(continues)

Procedure 9-10 (continued)

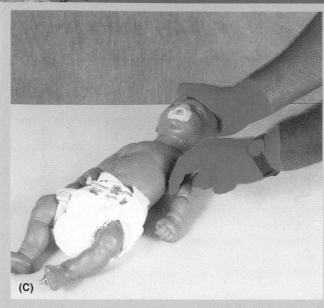
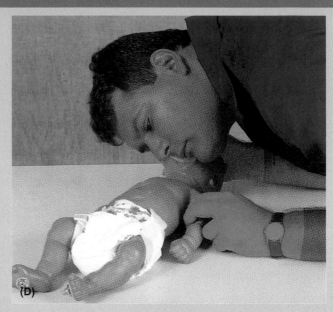

Figure 9-23 (C) Check for pulse at the brachial artery. (D) Recheck pulse and breathing every minute.

DOCUMENTATION

4/7/20XX—2:45 PM Six-month-old Samantha is seen by Dr. Woo in the pediatric clinic because she has "croup." T 102°F, P 124, R 32. While being examined by Dr. Woo, Samantha suddenly stops breathing. EMS activated. Rescue breathing begun. Two slow breaths given, pulse checked, and found pulse to be present. Breaths given every three seconds. Samantha began breathing after about three minutes of rescue breathing. Dr. Woo wants baby admitted to the hospital. Arrangements made with Gulf Shore Hospital. W. Slawson, CMA

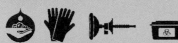
Procedure 9-11 CPR for Adults

STANDARD PRECAUTIONS:

PURPOSE:
To respond to a breathing and cardiac arrest emergency.

EQUIPMENT/SUPPLIES:
Biohazard waste container
Resuscitation mouthpiece
Gloves

PROCEDURE STEPS:
Ask, "Are you OK?" If no response:
1. Have someone call emergency services.
2. Put on gloves if available.
3. Tilt back head and lift chin.
4. Look, listen, and feel for breathing for 10–15 seconds. If the patient is not breathing, keep the airway open, pinch the nose, position the mouthpiece, seal your mouth over the device, and give two breaths through the mouthpiece into the patient's lungs.

5. Check the pulse at the carotid artery for 10 seconds. If the patient has a pulse, continue rescue breathing. If the patient does not have a pulse, start chest compressions.
6. After locating the area on the abdomen two inches above the xiphoid (Figure 9-24A), position your shoulders over your hands and compress the chest about 2 inches 15 times (Figure 9-24B).
7. Give two slow breaths, holding the nose (Figure 9-24C).
8. Do 3 more sets of 15 compressions and two breaths.
9. Check the pulse and breathing for about 10 seconds.

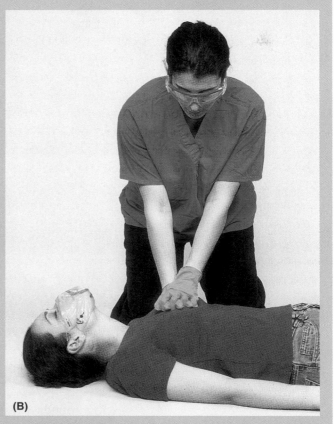

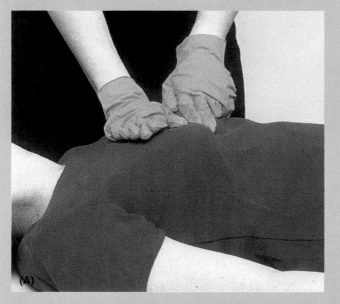

Figure 9-24 (A) Tilt back head and lift chin. Locate hand on the breastbone two inches above xiphoid process. (B) Position your shoulders over your hands and compress the chest 15 times.

(continues)

Procedure 9-11   (continued)

10. If there is no pulse or breathing, continue sets of 15 compressions and 2 breaths.
11. Use AED (Figure 9-25).
12. Dispose of waste in biohazard container.
13. Remove gloves, dispose of in biohazard container, and wash hands.
14. Document the procedure.

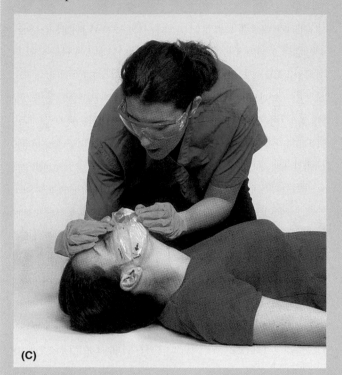

(C)

Figure 9-24 (C) Give two slow breaths, holding nose.

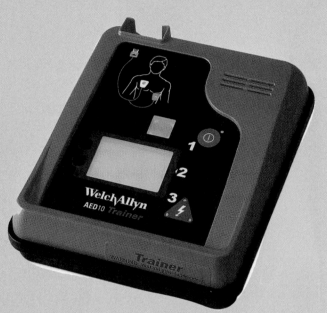

Figure 9-25 Automatic external defibrillator (AED). (Courtesy of Welch-Allyn.)

DOCUMENTATION

4/8/20XX—11:20 AM Fifty-four-year-old patient complaining of severe chest pain radiating down left arm and up into jaw. Nitroglycerin given sublingually. BP 100/70, P 116, R 28. Electrocardiography performed. Examined by Dr. Long. Suddenly patient stopped breathing. EMS activated. Two breaths given. Carotid pulse palpated and not present. CPR started. Fifteen chest compressions and two breaths given for four rounds. Pulse and breathing rechecked. Neither pulse nor breathing present. CPR continued. Oxygen given, automated electronic defibrillator (AED) used on patient. Patient's pulse returned. BP 90/60, P 100 (weak), R 8. Adrenalin given subcutaneously by Dr. Long. EMS arrived and stabilized patient for transport to emergency department. G. Burns, CMA

Procedure 9-12 CPR for Children

STANDARD PRECAUTIONS:

PURPOSE:
To respond to a cardiac arrest emergency in a child.

EQUIPMENT/SUPPLIES:
Gloves
Resuscitation mouthpiece

PROCEDURE STEPS:
1. Put on gloves.
2. Tap child to check consciousness level. Activate EMS.

3. Tilt head; look, listen, and feel for breathing. If there is no breathing, give two slow breaths. Check carotid artery for pulse.
4. Locate one hand on the breastbone and one hand on the forehead to maintain an open airway. Use heel of hand only above notch of xiphoid. Position your shoulders over the child's chest and compress the chest 1½ inches for five times (Figure 9-26A).
5. Position resuscitation mouthpiece. Give one slow breath, while pinching the nose (Figure 9-26B).
6. Repeat cycles of five compressions and one breath for about one minute.
7. Check the pulse and breathing for about 5 seconds (Figure 9-26C).

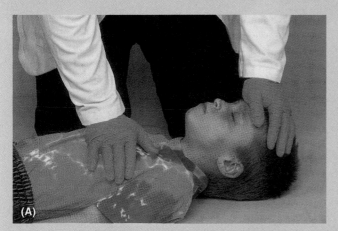

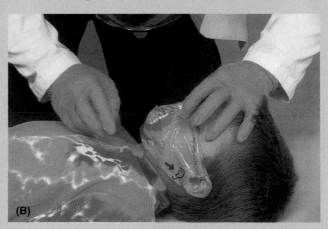

Figure 9-26 (A) Position your shoulders over the child's chest and compress the chest five times. (B) Give one slow breath, holding the nose.

(continues)

Procedure 9-12 (continued)

8. If there is no pulse, continue sets of five compressions and one breath.
9. Recheck the pulse and breathing every few minutes.
10. If child is 8 years or older and is 55 pounds, use AED.
11. Remove gloves. Wash hands.
12. Document the procedure.

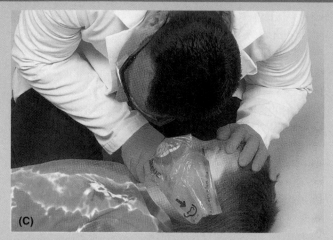

(C)

Figure 9-26 (C) Check pulse and breathing for 5 seconds.

DOCUMENTATION

4/8/20XX—3:20 PM Eight-year-old Sam was given allergy desensitization injection. Within four to five minutes, he collapsed. Checked for breathing, and it was absent. Two breaths given, carotid checked. Both absent. Dr. King notified and examined patient. EMS activated and CPR begun. Sets of one breath to five chest compressions continued for approximately three to four minutes. Patient began to move slightly. Shallow breathing and weak carotid pulse felt. BP 70/40, P 116 (weak), R 12 (shallow). Adrenaline, Benadryl, and oxygen given by Dr. Woo. Patient transported to emergency department after stabilization. C. McInnis, CMA

Procedure 9-13   CPR for Infants

STANDARD PRECAUTIONS:

PURPOSE:
To respond to a cardiac arrest emergency in an infant.

EQUIPMENT/SUPPLIES:
Gloves
Resuscitation mouthpiece

PROCEDURE STEPS:
1. Don gloves.
2. Gently tap the infant to determine consciousness level. Have someone activate EMS.
3. Tilt head. Look, listen, and feel for breathing. If there is no breathing, position resuscitation mouthpiece and give two slow breaths, covering mouth and nose. Check brachial artery for pulse for 5–10 seconds.
4. Find your finger position on the center of the sternum between the nipples.
5. Compress the infant's chest five times about ½–¼ inch.
6. Give one slow breath (Figure 9-27A).
7. Repeat cycles of five compressions and one breath for one minute.
8. Recheck brachial pulse and breathing for about 5–10 seconds (Figure 9-27B).
9. If there is no pulse, continue cycles of five compressions and one breath.
10. Recheck the pulse and breathing every few minutes.
11. Remove gloves. Wash hands.
12. Document the procedure.

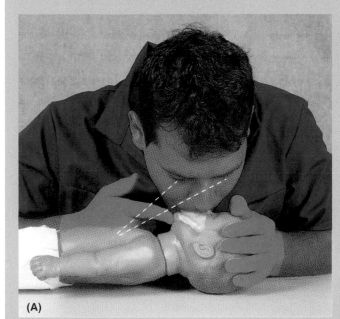

(A)

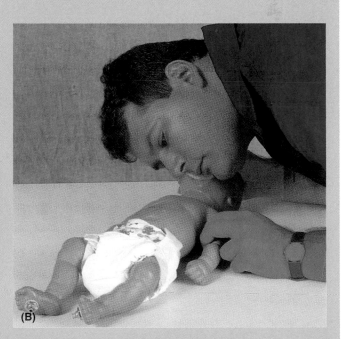

(B)

Figure 9-27 (A) Give one slow breath. (B) Recheck brachial pulse and breathing for 5–10 seconds.

DOCUMENTATION

4/8/20XX—4:30 PM Infant unresponsive. Mother states, "I think she was bitten by a spider." No breathing, no pulse. CPR began after activating EMS. Dr. Woo examined infant and directed CPR be resumed. One breath and five chest compressions given for about one minute. Rechecked patient in one minute. Still no pulse, no respirations. No blood pressure. Oxygen, adrenaline, and Benadryl administered by Dr. Woo. CPR continued. EMS arrived and stabilized infant with IVs and oxygen and transported infant and mother to emergency department. E. Nagle, CMA

Case Study 9-1

Annette Samuels, a regular patient at Inner City Health Care, is walking her dog one morning, stops to rest on a grassy knoll, and notices a wasp on her arm. She brushes it away, unthinkingly, and then realizes it has stung her. She receives two more stings and suddenly notices she is at a nest site. Annette is now a half-hour walk from home but is not really concerned because she has never had an allergic reaction to a wasp sting. However, a few minutes into her walk, her palms become itchy, her ears start to burn, and she feels light-headed. She is not having difficulty breathing. She is determined to get home and she does, at which point she notices she is covered with hives. She calls Inner City Health Care to ask: Should she come in?

CASE STUDY REVIEW

1. Wanda Slawson, CMA, is triaging calls the morning Annette is stung. What questions should she ask Annette?
2. Because Annette obviously is having a hypersensitive or an allergic reaction, she is advised to seek emergency care immediately. What first-aid measures might be taken?
3. What advice about precautions against getting stung again should Wanda give Annette?

Case Study 9-2

Abigail Johnson has arrived at Inner City Health Care for her scheduled appointment. As she checks in with Bruce Goldman, the medical assistant, she reports feeling nauseated, having some pressure in her chest, and being short of breath.

CASE STUDY REVIEW

1. What immediate actions should Bruce take to respond to Mrs. Johnson's complaints?
2. What equipment/supplies/medications should be ready and available for Dr. Lewis?
3. Because of the possibility of myocardial infarction, what action would Dr. Lewis direct Bruce to take after Mrs. Johnson has been stabilized?
4. What patient education can Bruce use in this situation?

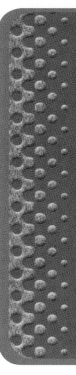

SUMMARY

Although many of the emergencies covered in this chapter may never be seen by the medical assistant in the ambulatory care setting, it is nonetheless important to develop a broad base of information about the various types of potential emergency situations. This knowledge gives the medical assistant the confidence and the preparation to manage the emergencies that do occur with speed, accuracy, and understanding until outside emergency help arrives. Staff will need to assess their response to emergencies on a continual basis. Was protocol followed? Were there difficulties in the delivery of care? Were staff and equipment prepared and ready to deal with these potentially life-threatening situations? Staff meetings should be held to discuss these and other questions that may have arisen and to allow staff the opportunity to talk about any fears or concerns they might have. It must be stressed that this chapter is at best an introduction to the topic of emergency procedures and first aid; it is essential medical assistants in all ambulatory care settings, whether large or small, enroll in a Red Cross, American Heart Association, American Safety and Health Institute, or National Heart Association first-aid and CPR program, attain provider level CPR, and take refresher courses to update skills.

STUDY FOR SUCCESS

To reinforce your knowledge and skills of information presented in this chapter:

- ❏ Review the Key Terms
- ❏ Practice any Procedures
- ❏ Consider the Case Studies and discuss your conclusions
- ❏ Answer the Review Questions
  - ❏ Multiple Choice
  - ❏ Critical Thinking
- ❏ Navigate the Internet and complete the Web Activities
- ❏ Practice the StudyWARE activities on the textbook CD
- ❏ Apply your knowledge in the Student Workbook activities
- ❏ Complete the Web Tutor sections
- ❏ View and discuss the DVD situations

REVIEW QUESTIONS

Multiple Choice

1. Good Samaritan laws:
   a. are designed to protect the public
   b. protect non–health care professionals
   c. require that all individuals providing assistance act within the scope of their knowledge and training
   d. protect health care professionals on the job
2. First-degree burns:
   a. are the most serious and penetrate all layers of skin
   b. affect only the top layer of skin
   c. often leave scar tissue
   d. usually take more than a month to heal
3. A fracture in which the bone protrudes through the skin is called:
   a. greenstick fracture
   b. compound fracture
   c. depressed fracture
   d. comminuted fracture

4. To control a nosebleed, it is important to:
   a. have the patient lie down
   b. tilt the patient's head back
   c. tilt the patient's head forward
   d. call 911 immediately
5. Another name for a heart attack is:
   a. cerebral vascular accident
   b. cardiac arrest
   c. angina pectoris
   d. myocardial infarction

Critical Thinking

1. Sixteen-year-old Cindy Roland, a patient newly diagnosed with seizures caused by epilepsy, came into the office for a follow-up appointment today. She approached the reception desk and said she can see flashing bright lights in both eyes and that she feels "weird." The receptionist alerted the

medical assistant, who immediately responded to the patient.

a. What actions should the medical assistant take?

b. Is there a significance to the flashing bright lights? Explain.

c. Address strategies the medical assistant can use to educate Cindy about her disease. Discuss at least five topics to include when teaching patients and others about epilepsy.

2. Mrs. Williams, a 75-year-old patient, came to the office today for a routine follow-up appointment for her diabetes. She suddenly collapsed onto the floor of the reception area.

a. What immediate steps did the medical assistant take to provide care for this patient in distress?

3. Define the purpose of a crash cart or tray and compile a list of the major supplies and medications it should contain.

4. Describe shock and tell how and why it is important to prevent a patient from going into shock.

5. Recall three types of bandages and give examples of their use.

6. Describe the difference between first-, second-, and third-degree burns.

7. Recall and describe the four ways that poisons may enter the body.

8. What is a hemorrhage? What kinds of bleeding may the medical assistant encounter? What are the symptoms of each?

9. Explain when and why Heimlich maneuver, rescue breathing, and CPR techniques are performed.

10. Explain steps to take if a patient has a laceration on the hand with moderate to heavy bleeding.

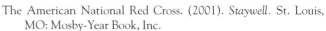

WEB ACTIVITIES

1. Search the Internet for sites and resources on the Emergency Medical Services (EMS) System. Are there any cities or towns within 100 miles of your place of residence that do not use the EMS System?

2. What sites can you recommend to patients and their families who are looking for first-aid information about diabetes and heart attack?

3. What organizations could you use to search for information that deals with first aid for convulsions?

4. Search the Internet for information regarding first aid for insect stings.

5. What sites are available for information about poisonings?

REFERENCES/BIBLIOGRAPHY

The American National Red Cross. (2001). *Staywell*. St. Louis, MO: Mosby-Year Book, Inc.

Taber's cyclopedic medical dictionary (21st ed.). (2003). Philadelphia: F. A. Davis.

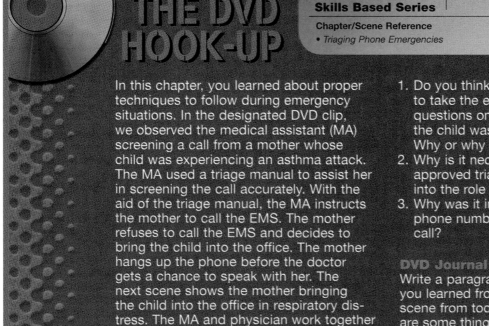

THE DVD HOOK-UP

DVD Series **Skills Based Series**	Program Number **8**

Chapter/Scene Reference
• *Triaging Phone Emergencies*

In this chapter, you learned about proper techniques to follow during emergency situations. In the designated DVD clip, we observed the medical assistant (MA) screening a call from a mother whose child was experiencing an asthma attack. The MA used a triage manual to assist her in screening the call accurately. With the aid of the triage manual, the MA instructs the mother to call the EMS. The mother refuses to call the EMS and decides to bring the child into the office. The mother hangs up the phone before the doctor gets a chance to speak with her. The next scene shows the mother bringing the child into the office in respiratory distress. The MA and physician work together as a team to get the patient's breathing stabilized.

1. Do you think that it was wise of the MA to take the extra time to ask screening questions once the mother stated that the child was having an asthma attack? Why or why not?

2. Why is it necessary for you to follow an approved triage manual if you are put into the role of screening patient calls?

3. Why was it important to get the patient's phone number at the beginning of the call?

DVD Journal Summary

Write a paragraph that summarizes what you learned from watching the designated scene from today's DVD program. What are some things you can do to help you know how to respond to emergencies before they happen?

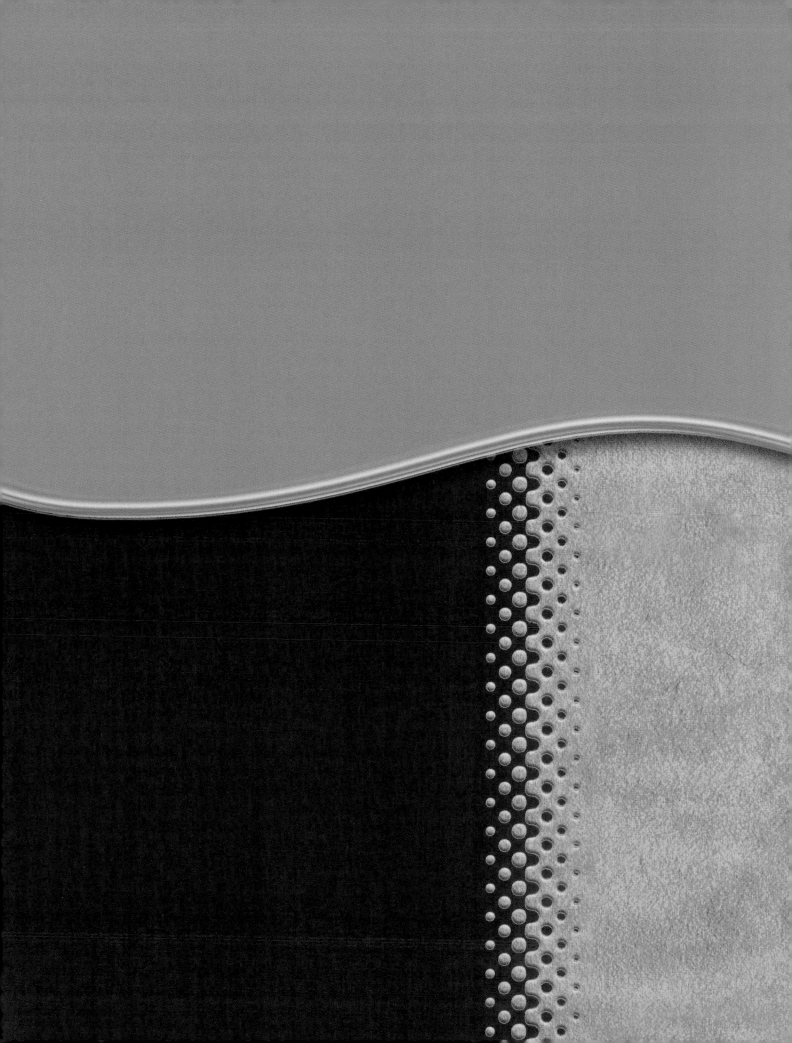

UNIT 4
Integrated Administrative Procedures

Creating the Facility Environment

KEY TERMS

Informatics

OBJECTIVES

The student should strive to meet the following performance objectives and demonstrate an understanding of the facts and principles presented in this chapter through written and oral communication.

1. Define the key terms as presented in the glossary.
2. Describe a comfortable and pleasing reception area.
3. Identify cultural aspects of the reception area.
4. Discuss the role of HIPAA in patient privacy.
5. Determine the number of patients a reception area should accommodate.
6. Describe the role of color in the office environment.
7. Recall essential elements of the Americans with Disabilities Act.
8. Discuss the importance of the physical office environment to the patient's care.
9. Identify the important personality characteristics the medical receptionist should possess.
10. Describe the procedure to use when an unexpected delay causes patients to wait for the physician.
11. List at least three tasks to perform on opening and closing the facility.
12. Identify two future characteristics of ambulatory health care.

SCENARIO

The design of any ambulatory setting often evolves as the needs of the office and patients change. In the office of Drs. Lewis and King, which is a two-doctor family practice, the environment has always been warm and welcoming, which is particularly important because the physicians see many children. However, the office was initially designed in the early 1980s, before the Americans with Disabilities Act (ADA) was passed by the U.S. Congress.

Once this act was passed in 1990, the office manager, Marilyn Johnson, CMA, was aware of the need to comply with its mandates. In addition, Drs. Lewis and King wanted to make all their patients, including those with disabilities, as comfortable as possible. Working with a local architect, Marilyn was able to incorporate changes into the practice's existing space: a ramp was added outside, doorways were widened to provide wheelchair access, and new Braille signage was installed outside for the visually impaired patients. Although the changes were not without expense, the staff of Drs. Lewis and King willingly complied with the ADA not only because it is law, but because it gave more access to more patients.

More recently, while making certain the clinic protocol was in compliance with the Health Insurance Portability and Accountability Act of 1996 (HIPAA), the clinic staff took another look at the facility to ensure it was favorable in light of protecting patient confidentiality. With only a simple modification of the reception counter, an open cubicle space was created at the side of the counter to use for greeting patients, discussing private information, and making return appointments.

INTRODUCTION

The environment of the medical office or clinic contributes almost as much to a patient's well-being as does the medical attention given by the physician and medical assistants. The physical environment can foster a feeling that embraces and welcomes patients or, conversely, can cause them to feel alienated and intimidated.

Interior designers and experts who specialize in medical space planning are advising all individuals involved in designing clinics, medical offices, and hospitals that patient comfort must be considered as important as the facility's functional utility and ease of maintenance. The ADA also must be taken into account when creating any medical office environment to make provisions to accommodate patients who are physically challenged.

 The creation of a health care facility involves many variables. Some are tangible elements, such as lighting, color choice, and furniture arrangement. Yet others are intangible and are expressed in a receptionist's greeting and attitude toward patients. Important components of patient satisfaction are a warm and caring staff, comfortable surroundings, and the ability of patients and visitors to find their way around the medical clinic without getting lost. Convenience of access and privacy is essential. The latter, although always important to patients, recently became a focus of HIPAA regulations that identify how a patient's privacy and confidentiality are to be protected. Together, these elements make an ambulatory setting the kind of environment where patients will feel comfortable and secure.

THE RECEPTION AREA

A reception area is just that—a place of reception; it should never be thought of as the waiting room. This is the area that can make the patient feel welcome, secure, and comfortable. Adequate and comfortable seating affords patients room to have their own space (Figure 10-1).

 Proper seating placement also respects cultural biases. For example, some people do not like to be touched by strangers. Middle Eastern and Latin cultures, by contrast, encourage closeness and touching, and individuals from these cultures may cluster themselves close together in the reception area. Cultural differences also will have an impact on the amount of space necessary for the reception area. Some ethnic populations are likely to bring several relatives with them to an appointment. This may be because of the need for emotional support, or the need for a language interpreter.

Space planners indicate that the reception area should accommodate at least one hour's patients per physician and a friend or relative who may accompany each

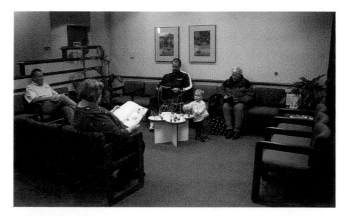

FIGURE 10-1 An inviting and pleasant reception area provides privacy and confidentiality for arriving patients and a comfortable setting while awaiting their appointments.

patient. Another quick rule of thumb to use is 2.5 seats in the reception area for each examination room. Clinics where physicians see patients without advance appointments will, of course, need a larger reception area.

If the clinic treats children as patients, or children are apt to accompany adult patients, a children's area is especially helpful and appreciated. A special table and chairs for children, interactive toys, and perhaps even a small television placed in a children's corner can be provided. This area needs to be away from doors that swing or hazards on which children might be injured. A children's area should always be in sight of the receptionist, who may be charged with keeping order, especially if a parent must be seen alone in an examination room.

Current magazines that are appropriate to the clinic clientele, plants, and other features such as a professionally maintained built-in aquarium will help set a welcome tone. A receptacle for litter or trash and a box of tissues can be helpful. Research has shown that patients and their families are more comfortable in surroundings that provide access to nature, natural sunlight, and the sound of moving water. Many clinics being built today include a courtyard or garden, perhaps with a relaxing waterfall, and skylights to provide natural sunlight.

Depending on the clientele of the ambulatory care setting, consider the following to help ease patients' time in the reception area or take their minds off current medical problems: a table and chairs with a "puzzle in progress," Internet access for busy employees, an entertainment center, or a juice bar. Although these items are not appropriate in every setting, they certainly can be in some. Refer to Case Study 10–2 at the end of this chapter.

The fabric and texture of draperies, upholstery, and carpet should be pleasing, comfortable, and easy to maintain. It is helpful if there is a place for patients to hang heavy coats or wet umbrellas.

Many physicians provide educational materials for patients in the reception area. For example, new parents always appreciate pamphlets related to raising children. It is also appropriate to have available in the reception area a patient information brochure that describes the services of the office, the function of medical staff members, measures to take in case of an emergency, and other issues that patients may need to consider. See Chapter 22 for more information on developing brochures for patient use.

OFFICE DESIGN AND ENVIRONMENT

Even when the office or clinic is housed in an older building not originally constructed as a medical facility, there is much that can be done to create an environment that enhances patient comfort. Remember to see things from the patient's point of view. If the facility is a labyrinth of corridors where patients can easily get turned around, make certain that directions are clear. Be sure that examination rooms are not made more frightening by an assortment of exposed medical equipment and strange-looking dials, hoses, and nozzles. Be alert to odors that are often distasteful to patients even if the odors are from necessary antiseptics. This can be accomplished with proper ventilation.

A reception window or desk should not make the patient feel closed off from the receptionist; it should provide privacy for the receptionist and total confidentiality for patients, whereas allowing a full view of the reception area. A poorly illuminated room may suggest poor housekeeping, dusty baseboards, soiled carpets, or faded draperies. Lighting can be soft and inviting while providing proper illumination. Natural light is best.

Some rooms in the facility, by their very nature, cause patients to feel intimidated. Consider the patient who is naked on an examination table except for a paper or cloth gown interacting with the physician who is fully clothed, wearing a white lab coat, and comfortably seated at a counter desk. Consider also the patient who is about to have a sigmoidoscopy and must be placed on a special examination table tilted into the knee-chest position. Both these situations place the patient at a disadvantage with the physician for discussion and negotiation. The goal in medical care should be to empower the patient with as much control as possible (Figure 10-2).

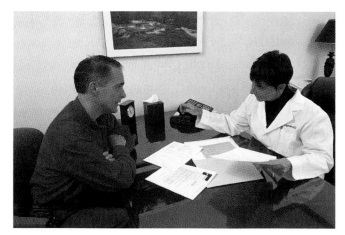

FIGURE 10-2 Patients should be afforded as much dignity and empowerment as possible. Many patients may feel more comfortable discussing conditions, procedures, or treatments in the physician's office rather than in the examination room.

Privacy is always important to patients. Provide space for them to hang their clothes and undergarments out of view. A mirror is especially helpful when dressing. Always ask if a patient needs help in disrobing, and always knock before entering a room. Remember, too, that privacy implies that the patient's conversation cannot be overheard in any other part of the facility.

Color can do much to establish an inviting environment. Greens and blues are good in areas that require quiet and extended concentration. Cool colors cause individuals to underestimate time and make heavier items seem lighter, objects smaller, and rooms larger. Warm colors with high illumination cause increased alertness and an outward orientation. The aged will have difficulty distinguishing pastels because of failing eyesight. (Access the Internet and visit the Lighthouse International Web site at http://www.lighthouse.org and go to information on "effective color contrast" for additional information on the effect of colors for those with vision difficulties.) Strongly contrasting patterns and extremely bright colors can be overwhelming and even intimidating or threatening in their effect.

Accessories and artwork can easily add a special touch to a facility. Whereas fresh flowers might be a nice touch, fresh flowers harbor microorganisms, and some patients may be allergic to them. There is the tendency to use living plants in the medical facility, but some silk plants and flowers also may be appropriate. It would be worth the investment to have a professional designer specializing in medical space planning look through the facility to make suggestions regarding color, artwork, and the general environment of the office.

Americans with Disabilities Act

Accessibility, or making facilities and equipment available to all users, is a major consideration when creating the health care environment. The ADA was passed by the U.S. Congress in 1990. The purpose of this act is to provide a clear and comprehensive national mandate to end discrimination against individuals with disabilities and to bring them into the economic and social mainstream of life. In addition to accessibility regulations identified in Titles II, III, and IV, this act also provides employment protection for persons with disabilities (Title I). ADA applies to businesses with 15 or more employees; however, some states may have stricter legislation. Even before ADA became legislation, most health care facilities attempted to make their premises barrier free and accessible to patients with special needs. Although many ambulatory care settings will have less than 15 employees, accessibility for all patients in all settings is important.

A professional designer can provide advice on how the facility must be accessible to people who are physically challenged. For example, all doors and hallways must accommodate a wheelchair. There must be a bathroom facility available for handicapped individuals. Signage in Braille accommodates patients with visual disabilities. Elevators must be provided if the facility is on more than one level. There must be at least one accessible entrance complying with ADA. It should be protected from the weather by a canopy or overhanging roof. Such entrances are to incorporate an accessible passenger loading zone. Ten percent of the total number of parking spaces at outpatient facilities must be accessible. (Visit the ADA home page at http://www.ada.gov for more information.) Be alert also to patients whose impairment is not obvious, for example, individuals with impaired hearing or vision and individuals whose infirmity (temporary or permanent) may prevent them from doing certain physical activities.

THE RECEPTIONIST'S ROLE

 The receptionist is the person on the health care team who must always keep a positive "We can help you" attitude, have a smile for each patient, and exude a genuine "I care about you" personality. This individual, who often is a medical assistant with other duties as well, must be able to perform telephone triage, retrieve records, greet patients, present a bill, make appointments, and log data into the computer all the while remembering that the patient's comfort is of primary concern. The receptionist must genuinely like people and not be upset when they are grumpy, irritable, or depressed and worried about an illness. The receptionist is the person who sets the social climate for the interchange between the patient and the physician and the rest of the staff (Figure 10-3).

 Some large clinics have a receptionist greet the patients on their arrival, and then direct them to a more private area where they are checked in, their insurance or payment plan is verified, and follow-up appointments are made. The telephones are in this more private area so conversations with callers cannot be overheard in the reception area.

Patients who are very ill, injured, or upset should not have to wait in the reception area, but rather should be shown to an examination room away from other patients. The receptionist or medical assistant may also have to monitor children who may be intent on disrupting patients. This is especially necessary if the parent seems unconcerned about keeping youngsters under control.

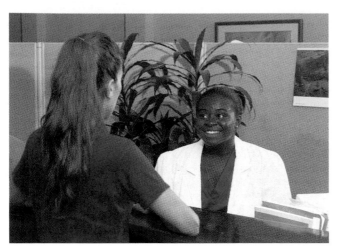

FIGURE 10-3 A friendly, warm greeting from the medical assistant who is serving as receptionist is reassuring to arriving patients.

Receptionists also are expected to maintain the tidiness of the reception area. Magazines can be straightened, litter picked up, and surface counters attended to. Counters, table surfaces, and toys in medical clinics are among those most infested with microbes; therefore, they should be sanitized daily, or sometimes twice a day, especially when arriving patients may have contagious diseases. Receptionists may be asked to place paper masks in the reception area and instruct patients when they make their appointments to pick up a paper mask on arrival at the front door.

If there are unexpected delays in the physician's schedule, hopefully never more than 20 minutes, be certain to notify patients of the delay tactfully and graciously and offer them the alternative of making other arrangements. Keep in mind that the patient's time is as valuable as the physician's.

OPENING THE FACILITY

When the facility is opened in the morning, everything should be in readiness. The receptionist or administrative medical assistant, who arrives at least 20 minutes before the first patient, will make a visual check of each room to be certain it is prepared and ready for the day.

Rooms should be of a comfortable temperature, well organized, pleasantly illuminated, and spotless. All necessary supplies and equipment should be checked for readiness. At all times, patient comfort and safety should be paramount. Patient charts for the day should be retrieved if not done so the prior evening. The receptionist will also check the answering service or machine for any telephone messages.

An effective way to check a room's readiness is to place yourself in the room as a patient. Ask yourself how you feel about being there, what mood the surroundings create for you, and whether you would feel welcome and comfortable as a patient.

CLOSING THE FACILITY

At the close of the day, each room should be checked to make certain all equipment is shut down and doors and windows are secured. Be sure that all materials of a sensitive nature are under lock and key. The preferred method of record storage is a lateral file cabinet with doors that can be closed and locked to insure patient confidentiality. Any drugs identified in the Controlled Substances Act list of narcotics and non-narcotics must be in a locked and secure cabinet and should also be checked when leaving the office. Petty cash kept on the premises must be locked in a safe container. It is best, also, to put each room and area in readiness for the next day.

 Local law enforcement officers can advise you on appropriate indoor and outdoor lighting, as well as any other security measures to make both during and after office hours.

Always contact the answering service to notify them that the office is closed and where and how the medical staff can be reached in an emergency.

THE FUTURE OF AMBULATORY CARE

In 2001, the Institute of Medicine (IOM; http://www.iom.edu), a private, nonprofit institution that provides health policy advice under a congressional charter granted to the National Academy of Sciences, has as one of its projects the "Identifying and Preventing Medical Errors." The project identifies medical errors as the eighth leading cause of death in the United States. Since 2001, steps have been made to improve that statistic. Medical **informatics** and avoiding handwritten physicians' orders solves some of the problems. Electronic medical records that make a patient's chart available at any location and provide access to information such as patient allergies, negative drug interactions, and physician referrals will decrease the likelihood of errors. Although electronic medical records have been implemented in many areas, this change may still be a few years in the future for some clinics.

At least one expert, Kirby Vosburgh, Associate Director of the Center for the Integration of Medicine and Innovative Technology in Boston, believes health care is moving into the home. Internet-enabled medicine allows patients and practitioners to communicate in cyberspace. This event has been referred to as "mouse" calls rather than "house" calls. Doctors can listen to a patient's heart or lungs and monitor blood pressure while verbally and visually communicating through specialized home telemedicine monitoring devices that include a blood pressure cuff and a telephonic stethoscope. This technique can be especially useful for consultations with physicians located in rural areas of the country. The American Medical Association (AMA) predicts that within 5 years, about 50% of physicians will treat patients through on-line methods. Electronic mail (e-mail) communication between patients and doctors is now commonplace

in many areas; however, patients are asked to give written permission for the transmission of e-mail information because privacy cannot always be guaranteed.

At the same time, medical providers work diligently to decrease the number of medical errors made, and advancing technology creates new patterns of health care. Also, patients are becoming astute consumers. These new consumers are better educated; they seek value and are comparison shoppers. They know that managed care has its limitations, and that doctors can be wrong. These patients believe they know their own bodies better than anyone, and that quality of life is important. They know, too, that cost containment and the complexities of the health care system leave them vulnerable to medical difficulties if they do not take responsibility for themselves and their medical care.

Today's patients are exposed to numerous Internet sites and magazine articles that provide medical information to them 24 hours a day, 7 days a week. These patients arrive at their appointments with the ability to discuss potential diagnoses and treatment plans. Hopefully, the health care team welcomes this new partnership, even if health care professionals have to assist patients in weeding out some of the invalid medical information available.

Case Study 10-1

Even though she appears collected on the outside, Abigail Johnson, who is about 75 years old, is quite nervous about having her annual physical. Clinical medical assistant Audrey Jones senses her patient's underlying tension and wants to do what she can to help Abigail relax. She knows that the patient has hypertension and may be feeling guilty about going off the strict diet that was designed to manage both her high blood pressure and her diabetes. At this moment, Audrey is helping Abigail get ready to see Dr. King, her physician. She does not want to intrude on her patient's privacy but does want her to relax a bit.

CASE STUDY REVIEW

1. What are some of the actions Audrey can take to ensure her patient's privacy?
2. In what ways can the physical environment itself become a calming influence for Abigail?
3. How will Audrey's sympathetic attitude affect her patient?

Case Study 10-2

The eighth-floor orthopedic surgery department in a large metropolitan city has an interesting approach to patient dynamics. Physicians and their assistants see patients for diagnosis and preparation for surgery. Patients likely are seen in this department three to five times before and after their procedures. The staff involves their patients to relieve any anxiety they might have.

Addison Burton approaches the reception desk; he is immediately greeted and asked to wait a moment until the receptionist clears a previous patient. There is a huge box filled with slightly used tennis shoes that patients and staff are collecting for needy children and the homeless. Addison remembers he has a couple of pairs at home he could bring. After checking in, he is directed to a counter where coffee, tea, and water are available, as well as the daily newspapers. Addison can take a seat in a chair, on a couch, at a window allowing him to put his feet and legs up, or at a table with chairs. The window seat gives a view of the city and a terrace garden four floors below. At the table there is an unusual puzzle being put together, and Addison takes a seat there. He is able to put four to five puzzle pieces together before being called for his appointment.

CASE STUDY REVIEW

1. When Jorja Anderson, CMA, calls Mr. Burton to the examination room, what might the conversation be? Would this conversation help to dispel anxiety? When the surgeon sees Mr. Burton for his hip problem, everyone has a good laugh—on the bottom of Addison's shoe is a puzzle piece.

2. What kind of mood has been established for this visit?

SUMMARY

Keep in mind that the environment in which patient care is given must promote health rather than aggravate illness and feed anxiety. The environment must be clean, fresh, cheerful, and nonthreatening with contemporary furnishings, appropriate colors, proper lighting, and soothing textures.

Even if patients are not consciously aware of the message they are getting from the office design and environment, they are subconsciously receiving it. The office environment reveals things that might subconsciously undermine a patient's confidence in the physician and the health care team.

STUDY FOR SUCCESS

To reinforce your knowledge and skills of information presented in this chapter:
- ❏ Review the Key Terms
- ❏ Consider the Case Studies and discuss your conclusions
- ❏ Answer the Review Questions
  - ❏ Multiple Choice
  - ❏ Critical Thinking
- ❏ Navigate the Internet and complete the Web Activities
- ❏ Practice the StudyWARE activities on the textbook CD
- ❏ Apply your knowledge in the Student Workbook activities
- ❏ Complete the Web Tutor sections

REVIEW QUESTIONS

Multiple Choice

1. Which of the following is appropriate for the reception area of an ambulatory care setting?
   a. heavily scented flowers
   b. medical journals with graphic colored pictures
   c. dim lighting
   d. live or silk plants
2. One of the goals in treating patients is:
   a. to give them as much control as possible
   b. to treat them as quickly as possible
   c. to disregard their desire for privacy
   d. to be sure they arrive on time for their appointment
3. One design element to avoid in a medical office is:
   a. a mirror for dressing
   b. the colors green and blue
   c. extremely bright, contrasting patterns
   d. accessories and artwork
4. The ADA is mostly concerned with:
   a. segregating individuals according to type of disability
   b. providing access and opportunity for physically challenged individuals
   c. only the work environment
   d. getting economic benefits for physically challenged people
5. In any medical office, the receptionist's key responsibility is to:
   a. not keep the physician waiting
   b. make sure all plants are watered
   c. greet patients in a friendly, warm manner
   d. be efficient, even if it means ignoring patient requests
6. Making a visual check of each examination room is a function of:
   a. weekly housekeeping and periodically through the day
   b. opening the office
   c. closing the office
   d. b and c
7. Space planners recommend the following for the reception area:
   a. three to four seats for each examination room
   b. seats to accommodate 1.5 hours of patients
   c. 2.5 seats for each examination room
   d. not bringing family members to appointments
8. ADA requires _____ of the total number of parking spaces in outpatient facilities be reserved for individuals with disabilities.
   a. 5%
   b. 10%
   c. 12%
   d. 7%
9. Telemedicine refers to doctors using the following for patient care:
   a. the Internet
   b. telemonitoring devices
   c. on-line services to treat patients
   d. all of the above
10. Children in the reception area:
   a. may need to be monitored by the receptionist
   b. must sit still and be quiet
   c. should have a play area for quiet activities
   d. a and c

Critical Thinking

1. What would an interior designer or space planner do to create a pleasant atmosphere for patients in a medical office? If there is an interior design program in your school, consult with their students on planning a medical office environment.
2. Describe the most pleasant office you have seen. What made it special? What were your first impressions?
3. Recall your physician's office. Is it accessible to all patients? If not, what would you do to make it accessible to all patients?
4. As the administrative medical assistant employed in a busy ambulatory setting, how will you keep your manner pleasant, warm, and genuinely friendly and caring even on days when you are having your own personal difficulties?
5. Discuss what you might do to monitor children aged 4 and 6 years while their parent is in the examination room.
6. If you believed the facility in which you are employed could benefit from the services of an interior designer either for minor adjustments or a major remodel, what suggestions would you make to your physician–employer to convince him or her of the benefits of such a suggestion?

WEB ACTIVITIES

1. Using your favorite search engine, key in "ADAAG" or "ADA Accessibility Guidelines for Buildings & Facilities." You will find a number of sites to research.
   a. Determine the correct placement for drinking fountains, wall mirrors, and sinks.
   b. What would you need to do to accommodate someone in a wheelchair in your own home? In your classroom?

2. The following Web site (the home page for Las Cruces, New Mexico) has an interesting section on medical offices and their ADA accessibility: http://www.las-cruces.org. Search for "ADA for Medical Offices."

a. What does this site suggest be done to conduct examinations for individuals in a wheelchair that require patients to lie prone or supine on an examination table?

b. What adjustments would be necessary to perform radiologic examinations?

c. How can medical assistants and other staff members assist in making persons with disabilities more comfortable in the situations described in this activity?

REFERENCES/BIBLIOGRAPHY

ADA *for medical offices.* (2004). Retrieved from http://www.las-cruces.org. Go to (1) "Departments," (2) "Human Resources," (3) "ADA Requirements for Business," (4) "Medical Offices." Accessed April 12, 2005.

Leibrock, C. (2000). *Design details for health.* New York: John Wiley & Sons.

Malkin, J. (2002). *Medical and dental space planning* (3rd ed.). New York: John Wiley & Sons.

Vosburgh, K. (2000, October). *The electronic outpatient/home environment—from house calls to mouse calls.* Lecture presented at the Beyond 2000: An international conference on architecture for health, Vancouver, British Columbia, Canada.

CHAPTER 11

Computers in the Ambulatory Care Setting

OUTLINE

OBJECTIVES

The student should strive to meet the following performance objectives and demonstrate an understanding of the facts and principles presented in this chapter through written and oral communication.

1. Define the key terms as presented in the glossary.
2. Describe the four fundamental elements of a computer system.
3. Identify the four main types of computers.
4. List four input devices and describe the function of each.
5. List three examples of data output devices.
6. Explain how storage devices might be used in ambulatory care settings.

(continues)

KEY TERMS

Algorithm
Antiglare Screen
Application Software
Backup
Benchmark
Booting
Central Processing Unit (CPU)
Compact Disk (CD)
Cyberspace
Data Storage Device
Data Storage Memory
Database Management System (DBMS)
Defragmentation
Digital Video/Versatile Disk (DVD)
Documentation
Driver
Ergonomics
Ethernet
Field
Firewall
Flash Drive
Floppy Drive
Footer
G-Hz Range
Gigabyte (GB)
Graphics Software
Hacking
Hard Drive
Hardware
Hard-Wired Network
Header
Information Retrieval System
Input Device
Internet
Jaz® Drive
License
Local Area Network (LAN)
Macro
Mainframe Computer
Megabyte
Memory
Merge Operation

(continues)

FEATURED COMPETENCIES

CAAHEP—ENTRY-LEVEL COMPETENCIES

Operational Functions

- Utilize computer software to maintain office systems

ABHES—ENTRY-LEVEL COMPETENCIES

Communication

- Application of electronic technology

Administrative duties

- Perform basic secretarial skills

- Apply computer concepts for office procedures

174

OBJECTIVES (continued)

7. Describe networking of computers and its purpose.

8. Differentiate between hard-wire and wireless networks.

9. Discuss the use of a flash drive and a tape drive and describe how each might be used in ambulatory care settings.

10. Identify three preventative measures to minimize computer viruses.

11. Discuss design considerations when computerizing a medical office.

12. Explain why ergonomics is important and recall at least five guidelines for setting up a computer workstation.

13. Explain the difference between system and application software.

14. Identify a minimum of four word processing features and describe how each might be used when creating documents in the ambulatory care setting.

15. Explain how database management concepts might be used in an ambulatory care setting.

16. Discuss patient confidentiality and guidelines for maintaining confidentiality while keeping in mind HIPAA requirements.

17. Discuss with a classmate the topic of professionalism as it relates to computers in the medical office.

SCENARIO

Inner City Health Care, an urgent care center in a large urban area, recently made the transition from a manual to a computerized system. It was a long overdue change, and it required a great deal of fact-finding and research before office manager Walter Seals could convince the center's physicians to purchase a network of computers for the five-physician center.

Once he persuaded his employers of the computers' potential value to the center, Walter, an administrative medical assistant, proceeded carefully. He spoke with other ambulatory care settings that were already computerized to establish benchmarks, or comparisons. He selected a computer vendor who was familiar with the software needs of a medical office. He made sure all staff would receive training in the use of the computers. Finally, he selected a two-week period when the office was routinely closed for summer vacation to have the computer system installed and operational.

INTRODUCTION

 *Computers have revolutionized our lives. You can order groceries, books, airline reservations, and theater tickets; make motel and car rental arrangements; register for college classes; and possibly find a romantic partner, all using the computer and what is called **cyberspace.** The medical office, hospitals, and even surgical procedures are increasingly dependent on the use of computers.*

Computers are no longer a luxury in the ambulatory care setting; they are an essential and sometimes mandatory part of doing business (e.g., filing Medicare statements for service). Today, the medical assistant must be computer literate, able to quickly learn how to use new programs, and knowledgeable of computer procedures that guard against loss or compromise of confidential medical records.

THE COMPUTER SYSTEM

Basic System

 All computer systems are composed of four fundamental elements (Figure 11-1):

1. *Input devices* that generate digital data used by the **central processing unit (CPU)** for processing
2. *CPU* that manipulates the data from the **input device,** that is, addition, subtraction, multiplication, and division
3. *Software* that instructs the CPU what operations to perform on the data from the input device and send the results to an **output device**
4. *Output devices* that display or store the results from the CPU

The details of each of these fundamental elements are highly technical and also involve support systems such as power supplies, time-keeping devices, **firewalls,** among others. The medical assistant will, under most circumstances, not need to develop his or her knowledge beyond understanding how to operate the elements, connect them together, ensure they are compatible with other elements in a system, and perform simple maintenance.

Types of Computer Systems

Although the medical assistant will be primarily using a microcomputer system, commonly called a **personal computer (PC),** it is helpful to understand some of the characteristics of the four major types of computer systems.

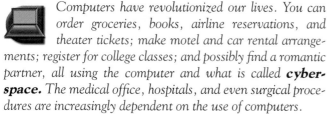

Supercomputers, the fastest and the most powerful computers, are used in medical research to combat cancer and to trace the genetic components for birth defects. They are the most expensive and complex of computers. Relatively few of these systems are up and running. Supercomputer technology is still under development but holds great promise for the advancement of sophisticated medical interventions.

Mainframe computers, the next largest in size and processing ability, are used for large volumes of repetitive calculations. With their high processing speeds, mainframes are invaluable for large governmental provider service programs such as Medicaid and Medicare.

Minicomputers, grouped between mainframes and microcomputers in terms of size, speed, and capacity, process data in health care facilities in a variety of ways, including patient account processing, insurance claim processing, and statistical analysis of research data. Minicomputers handle large amounts of processing and challenge the capabilities of older mainframe systems.

Microcomputers are the most widely used type of computer in today's health care facility. The smallest of the four types of computers, microcomputers range in size from easily transportable systems such as handheld **personal digital assistants (PDAs)** that physicians may use for hospital notes, laptop or notebook systems, to the more common desktop or personal computer (PC)

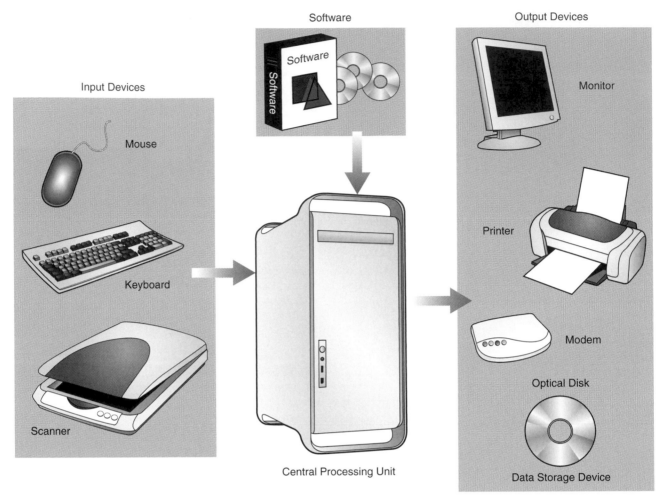

Figure 11-1 Components of a computer system.

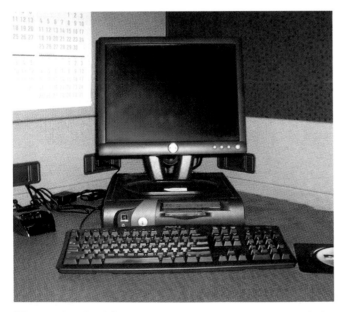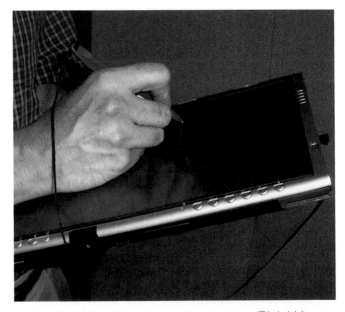

Figure 11-2 Microcomputers come in a variety of sizes and types. (Left) Desktop personal computer. (Right) Versatile laptop and handheld computer.

(Figure 11-2). See Chapter 16 for additional information related to PDA use.

The medical assistant will work with the computer on a daily basis in many different ways. Microcomputers may be used in a medical practice to schedule appointments, maintain patient accounts, and process insurance claims. Handheld micros may be used to input patient information during examination, with data downloaded to a minicomputer, server, or mainframe when it is convenient.

COMPONENTS OF A COMPUTER SYSTEM

A system is an assembly of parts that function together to perform a particular task. A computer system consists of hardware, software, and documentation of the installation.

Hardware

The components of a computer system that you can see, touch, or hear are referred to as **hardware.** Hardware consists of input devices, output devices, the CPU, as well as some firewalls and modems.

Data Input Devices. A data input device converts analog data such as keyboard keystrokes, motion, temperature, and mouse position into digital format understandable by the CPU, allowing it to manipulate the data in accordance with the software program. The most common examples of input devices are the keyboard and mouse. In addition to these common examples, touch screens, electronic tablets, scanners, pens, digital cameras, and many electronic clinical laboratory instruments are also input devices frequently encountered in medical settings. Input devices usually have their own software called a **driver,** which must be installed on the computer or provided by the **operating system (OS)** before they will function properly. Data storage devices frequently function as data input devices when raw data, which has been manipulated using the computer, is further processed using a different software program.

Central Processing Unit. The central processing unit (CPU) of a computer is the brain of the system. It carries out instructions defined by the program software on the data input and sends the result to the selected output device. The actual heart of the CPU is a silicon microchip approximately three inches square with sometimes hundreds of connections to other electronic components. The circuitry printed on the microchip contains logic **algorithms** for performing functions such as addition, subtraction, and multiplication. (Word processing example: The operator presses the letter *a* on the keyboard or data input device. The input device sends the numeric symbol for *a* to the CPU. The CPU then combines this input and whether the shift or caps key was pushed with data previously input when the word processing program was set up and sends the output to memory and to the monitor for you to view the letter *a*.)

Data Output Devices. The most common data output device is the monitor. The monitor, which looks like a television screen, allows the operator to see the output of the computer and make real-time correction to the input. The best example of this is in word processing of documents. Printers and fax machines are other examples of output devices used to produce hard-copy output. When hard copy is not required, digital data storage devices are used. As was the case with data input devices, data output devices require a driver, either loaded when the device is installed or provided by the OS.

A modem is a form of an input/output device, which alters the digital data from the computer in a manner that allows it to be transmitted over telephone lines or cable installations. A modem is required for dial-up Internet service and some cable services. Computer fax machines also require the use of a modem. Stand-alone fax machines have the modem feature built into them.

Data Storage Devices. Data storage devices are devices capable of permanently or temporarily storing digital data. Data storage device capacity is often referred to as **memory.** Together with computer speed, this area of the computer has seen the greatest improvement, with capability doubling every few years or less. Computers used by most of us today have no functional limitation for memory, with portable memory cartridges providing unlimited memory expansion.

Data storage devices consist of **read-only memory (ROM), random access memory (RAM),** and **data storage memory.** The computer manufacturer permanently writes data or instructions into the memory on ROM chips, which are installed directly onto the **motherboard.** They contain instructions for operations such as **booting** the computer when the power is turned on. RAM memory is also in the form of chips and is part of the motherboard. It provides the computer with registers in which to store in-process data. RAM memory is erased or "lost" when the computer is turned off or experiences a power failure. RAM memory is important to the user, in that a RAM capacity that is too small will cause the computer to run slow and sometimes will not run some software programs. Data storage memory is permanent and is not erased when the computer is turned off and can be either read-only or random access. Read-only data storage memory is used to store application programs for loading onto the computer. The following paragraphs describe several devices for providing data storage.

Hard drives are nonportable storage devices, usually installed directly into the computer cabinet that contains the CPU. A hard drive is a read-write device, and the memory is permanent unless the device experiences mechanical failure. Because of the failure potential of these devices, it is considered good practice to **backup** frequently the stored data by making a copy of files on a portable data storage device. The frequency for data backup is dependent on the rate at which data is entered into the system and on how long original records are maintained. Original records should never be destroyed until the stored data is backed up.

Floppy drives are portable memory storage devices where the storage media can be readily removed and transported. The most common floppies are 3.5 inches and hold about 1.4 **megabytes** of data, although minicomputers use larger drives that hold correspondingly more data. The use of floppy drives is being discontinued on many new machines because of newer technology.

Zip® drives and **Jaz® drives** are found on many computers. They are slightly thicker than a floppy drive but hold between 100 and 2,000 megabytes of data. They are portable and interchangeable from one computer to another.

Optical Drive. Two types of optical drives are used in computers: **compact disks (CDs)** and **digital video/versatile disks (DVDs),** which are sometimes referred to as digital versatile disks.

Compact Disk.
Computer data CDs are nearly identical to music CDs commonly used in home and automobile CD players. Whereas music CDs are read-only disks, those used in state-of-the-art computers have the capability for the computer not only to read a disk (CD-ROM), but to write on them (CD-R) and even erase data and rewrite new date (CD-RW). CDs store about 700 megabytes (MB) of data on a single disk. CD-ROMs are used as data input devices, usually for loading digital code for computer software programs.

Digital Video/Versatile Disk.
DVDs are identical with the DVD used to view home movies. They are similar to a CD, except that the format for writing the data to the DVD is different. Several formats for writing data are used at this time. DVDs store 4.7 **gigabytes (GBs)** or more of data. It is important that the storage media, the disk, and the drive are of the same format for the system to function.

Flash Drive. **Flash drive** is a solid-state memory device with no moving parts. It is usually connected to a computer using a **Universal System Bus (USB) port** or high-performance serial bus (IEEE1394). The device is small and can be carried on a key chain. It can store up to about 2 GB of data. It is used as a readily transportable data storage device when it is desirable to move data between computers that are not connected on a network.

Tape Drive. **Tape drives** are data storage devices capable of storing large amounts of data on replaceable reels of magnetic tape, much like a tape recorder but on a larger scale. Because they are much slower than many other storage devices, they are used when time is not usually too significant, such as in backing up a computer system. The storage media cost is significantly less with this type of storage device.

Servers are not true data storage devices. They usually contain or are connected to massive hard drives, but in many networked systems they become the storage devices for the user workstations. Servers may be located remote from workstations or even on the Internet. When servers are used, special protocols must be used to protect confidentiality of records. See the section on Patient Confidentiality in the Computerized Medical Office.

Drivers.
Drivers are computer programs that are designed to convert data output from one device into a format compatible with another device. They are required for most input and output devices and either are supplied with the device, must be downloaded from the **Internet,** or are contained in the OS software.

Networks.
Networking is the electronic connection of one or more computers, printers, software, and databases for the purpose of sharing information and resources. When properly networked, any computer on the network can share software, files, and peripheral devices contained or connected to other computers on the network. Conversely, certain sensitive files, such as financial and medical records can be limited in their accessibility. **Local area networks (LANs)** are the type most likely to be encountered in an ambulatory care setting, although a **wide area network (WAN)** could be encountered in a hospital-type clinic involving many computers and sites.

There are two types of networks: (1) **hard-wired networks** referred to as **Ethernet,** and (2) **wireless networks.** Hard-wired networks are capable of a much more rapid rate of data transmission than wireless networks, and the basic equipment is less expensive to purchase. Unless the office has been wired for a network, the cost of running cables can be expensive. Hard-wired systems are also more secure from **hacking** or other unauthorized access to data, because computers must be directly wired to the network to gain access. A note of caution is necessary: A system connected to the Internet provides an entry point for unauthorized access, necessitating incorporation of firewalls and virus protection systems, as well as requiring office personnel to use safeguards to ensure that they do not defeat system security protocols.

Wireless network equipment made by different manufacturers must be certified to **WiFi standards** of interoperability to ensure that different pieces of equipment are capable of exchanging data with each other. Even with WiFi-certified equipment there is no guarantee that the manufacturer's specifications for data transfer rates will be achieved because of outside radio interference in the surrounding area. A good rule of thumb is to assume that only half the specification rate will be achieved. If massive files will be transferred, such as downloading graphics from electronic imaging equipment, a wireless system may be too slow, resulting in maddening delays waiting for file download to be completed.

Power Outage, Electrical Surge, and Static Discharge Protection Devices

Protection devices must be an integral part of a medical office computer system. Computer systems should have an uninterruptible power supply, or battery backup, to prevent power outages from shutting down the system or destroying data. The power supply should also have a **surge protection** capability to prevent voltage surges on the utility line from damaging computer components. Static electricity can also be highly damaging to computers by transferring thousands of volts of electrical charge to components that are damaged by only a few hundred volts. This is the type of charge we all experience during dry weather when we get a shock from touching a grounded object and draw a spark. Nylon stockings, synthetic clothing, and walking on a synthetic fiber carpet all create static charges. To prevent damage from static discharges, grounding mats are required at all workstations.

Software

Software, frequently referred to as a computer program, can be thought of as a set of instructions that a computer follows to control computer hardware and to process data. System software and application software are both required by a computer to accomplish its tasks.

System software, frequently just called the operating system, tells the computer hardware what to do and when to do it. Most modern systems operate with a graphic interface that uses graphic symbols for input to the system and is much more user friendly than systems

requiring alphanumeric inputs. Microsoft Windows® and Macintosh® systems are probably the best known of the graphic interface operating systems.

Application software performs a specific data-processing function. Word processing, accounting, scheduling, and insurance coding are examples of application software functions.

Documentation

Computer system **documentation** consists of the manuals and documents that define how programs operate. Documentation tells how to execute specific functions and gives the specifications for specific hardware, such as the frequency of the internal clock, RAM, and hard drive available memory. Although it is more likely provided on an **optical disk** that contained the specific program documentation, it may also be in printed format.

Updates to program documentation are increasingly made available on the Web site of the company providing the program, together with **patches** for glitches discovered in the basic program. Third-party documents defining how to use application software are becoming increasingly popular and are frequently more user-friendly than documentation from the software supplier. All documentation, including **licenses,** recovery software, and program disks that come with the computer system, add-on hardware, and software should be maintained in a safe location for the life of the equipment and software, and then disposed of when the system or software is phased out of use.

Hardware and Software Compatibility

Hardware drivers and software of a computer system must be compatible. Many applications programs share files with the OS, and if there is a conflict with files having the same name, either the OS will not allow the applications program to load or it will not function properly. The

---

Critical Thinking

Your office has received legal notification requiring you to list all of the software used in your practice and to show proof that you have the necessary license granting use of the programs. You are successful in showing compliance, but your office procedures were disrupted for days in meeting this court mandate. Prepare an office protocol designed to ensure that all of your software is legal and that unauthorized persons have not installed illegal software on any office computers.

documentation for most applications programs define the versions of the operating system for which compatibility has been established and should always be checked before purchase of either a new applications program or a new version of the OS. Hardware driver requirements should also be checked for compatibility with the OS. The amount of RAM memory, CPU clock speed, and available drive storage space can affect whether a program will run satisfactorily.

Security Systems

 Security of a computer system must protect against two threats: (1) viruses and worms, and (2) unauthorized access to the computer.

 Virus Protection. Protection from viruses is important to prevent unauthorized transmission of confidential data; to prevent slowing, damage, or shutdown of the system; and to prevent loss of data. Viruses find their way onto a computer system through using uncontrolled software, downloading files from the Internet, and opening attachments to e-mail. There is no absolute means of preventing virus infections. However, the following preventative measures can minimize the problem:

- Install only authorized software on the computers.

- Do not open attachments received over the Internet that are not anticipated or are from an unknown person.

- Have the system equipped with an updated virus detection program and run the program on a scheduled basis.

- Keep OS and e-mail programs up to date with security patches.

 HIPAA requires the confirmation that all protected health information (PHI) data are accurate and have not been altered, lost, or destroyed in an unauthorized manner. Considerations include:
- Virus detection and elimination software must be installed.
- Inappropriate or unusual activity must be reported and investigated, and appropriate action(s) taken.
- Intrusion detection tools should be installed on all systems.

Unauthorized Access Prevention. It is necessary to prevent unauthorized access to computer files to protect patient confidentiality. Unauthorized access to the computer system from external sources may be minimized if not eliminated by using a firewall. Applying protocols that frequently require changing passwords minimize internal unauthorized access to computer data. Passwords also make access to data more difficult in the event of firewall penetration.

Firewalls come in two varieties: hardware and software. Both types function in a similar fashion; namely, they establish a list of acceptable sites based on a profile the device develops on the users of the system. It will then allow these sites access to your computer. All other sites are blocked. Some firewalls limit the type of files that can be transmitted. Other firewalls cloak specific network channels, making them invisible to hackers trying to gain access to your computer. Still others monitor the content of incoming packets of data.

System Backup. Viruses, equipment failure or damage, and hacker attacks make system backup mandatory. System backup devices are basically data storage devices that store the entire content of the nonportable computer memory so it can be recovered if a catastrophic system loss should occur. All office systems should use backup on a regularly scheduled basis. The frequency of the backup should be dependent on how much data the user can afford to lose. Magnetic tapes and optical drives are frequently used for this purpose. The backup is frequently done during hours when the system is not being used. Some of the system backup devices are automatic, requiring only that the tape or disk from the disk drive be changed in the morning and placed in safe storage. Current backup media should be stored in a secure off-site location.

COMPUTER MAINTENANCE BY CLINIC PERSONNEL

Maintenance of computer systems is generally limited to cleaning the monitor screens, replacing printer ink or toner cartridges, and refilling paper trays. However, two maintenance tasks that are within the capability of a computer-literate member of the health care team are file removal, disk **defragmentation,** and installation of security patches recommended by the supplier of the computer software.

The hard drive of a computer accumulates a host of old files ranging from old e-mails to obsolete programs and data files. If not removed, they use hard drive storage space and ultimately can slow the speed at which the computer stores and retrieves data. Simply right-clicking on the file with the mouse, and then selecting Delete from the menu can remove these old files. After removing files, you should also empty the recycle bin. Be careful with this step, however, because once the recycle bin has been emptied, the files can no longer be recovered without extraordinary means. A source for recovery efforts, including recovery of data from a crashed hard drive, is Drive Savers Data Recovery Inc. (http://www.drivesavers.com).

When files are deleted from the hard drive, blank spaces are left on the disk. For the computer to save new files it must sort through these blank spaces. The defragmentation process removes the blank spaces similar to the way you move all the books on a shelf to one side so new books can be added to the empty side. Defragmentation is easily done using a disk defragmenter that is included with the OS. Defragmentation takes a significant amount of time and should be performed when the office is closed.

The medical assistant may have as one of his or her responsibilities establishing a service agreement for maintenance of computers on a periodic basis, as well as any emergency repairs resulting from a major system failure. These agreements may also include personnel training and general technical support services. The medical assistant responsible for this contract should be sure that the vendor has signed the contracts required by the confidentiality protocols established by the medical office, and that all removable data storage media have been removed and secured before hardware is taken to the service company's facility.

DESIGN CONSIDERATIONS FOR A COMPUTERIZED MEDICAL OFFICE

The introduction of a computer system to perform many of the tasks that had been done with typewriters and manually can be a threatening experience for personnel who are not computer literate. If the change to a computerized system is well planned, with input sought from all affected personnel and with time allotted for training, the experience will be less stressful for all concerned. Involvement of all office personnel in the design of the system is extremely important because it creates a feeling of ownership and garners more willing support during the disruptive changeover period.

Software Selection

The first step in selection of software is to choose a knowledgeable and trustworthy vendor. The vendor should not only understand computers and software, but also the

Critical Thinking

Your office has obtained new medical management software. List as many options as you can think of for training office personnel to use the management software effectively. Identify the pros and cons for each option.

needs of the medical office. A reliable vendor should be able to assist you in anticipating and allowing for future needs as the medical practice grows and new diagnostic tools are introduced.

The next and most important step in developing a plan for computerization of a medical office is to determine what tasks will be computerized. This is done in conjunction with your vendor, by seeking input from your staff, and by talking with other people in medical offices similar to yours. Software available for each of the tasks should be identified and evaluated, preferably by actually using the programs on a trial basis. The best program for each task should be identified, and the hardware requirements for each program should be defined. Keep in mind that the program should be selected with operational commonality with all of the other software taken into consideration. Programs with similar menus and appearance on the monitor screen make training personnel much easier. Packaged programs that perform multiple tasks are commonly available. Microsoft® Office Suite is an example of a packaged program that includes word processing, spreadsheet, scheduling, e-mail, and database programs with commonality in menus and procedures. Similar programs tailored to the medical office are available. See Procedure 11-1 for installation steps.

Hardware Selection

Once the memory capacity (RAM, hard drive data storage capacity), CPU speed, and input and output device requirements have been identified for the software, the next step is to determine whether you are going to network. The type of network selected will be based on data transmission speed requirements and facilities considerations for running cables and the distance between computers and output devices. The hardware you select should meet or exceed the identified minimum requirements. If possible, get a computer system with substantially more memory than required by the software because inadequate memory or CPU speed may restrict the ability to use future software updates or improved programs. The CPU speed should be as fast as the technology permits at the time you make your purchase. The trend is toward using more memory and requiring greater CPU speed, especially if graphic programs will be used in your system. The more memory and CPU speed you can purchase, the longer your system will be viable without replacement of hardware. See Procedure 11-2 for installation steps.

Ergonomics

Although **ergonomics** in the medical office is an important consideration even without computerization, specific problems must be addressed when changing over to a computerized office environment. Safety issues and concerns specific to the computer, if addressed, can be minimized or avoided.

Eyestrain. Eyestrain can be a problem associated with the use of computers. The computer monitor should be positioned to prevent excessive glare entering from windows or reflecting from interior lighting. Attachment of an **antiglare screen** to the monitor further reduces eyestrain by reducing remaining residual glare. Computer operators should take a five-minute break each hour and focus on a distant object to prevent ocular accommodation and the headache and blurred vision associated with it. Using eye drops can minimize dry and itchy eyes. Figure 11-3 illustrates the proper positioning of the video display terminal (VDT) to prevent glare from artificial lights in a room and incoming light from windows.

Cumulative Trauma Disorder. The most widely known injury associated with individuals routinely using a computer is carpal tunnel syndrome. It is attributed to repetitive wrist motion. It can be prevented or the onset delayed by using a special keyboard that conforms to the natural position of the hands, or by using a conventional keyboard with wrist support as show in Figure 11-4.

Posture. Reports of back pain resulting from poor posture while using the computer are quite common. Carefully choosing and setting up computer equipment can minimize this type of injury. Computer operators should use a comfortable chair with lumbar support adjustment. A special chair with ergonomic features should be considered for individuals whose primary duty is keyboarding. Figure 11-5 shows the recommended computer operator position for proper posture to prevent back strain while operating a computer. The desktop should be 28 to 30 inches above the floor with an adjustable keyboard holder allowing adjustment for individual operator body size. A footrest may be helpful

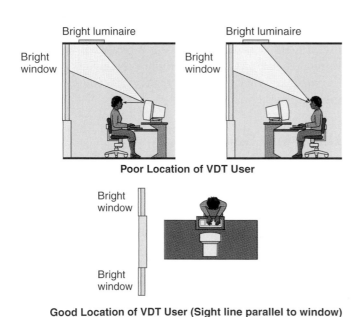

Figure 11-3 Proper positioning of the video display terminal/monitor (VDT) will prevent glare from incoming light from windows and artificial lights in the room.

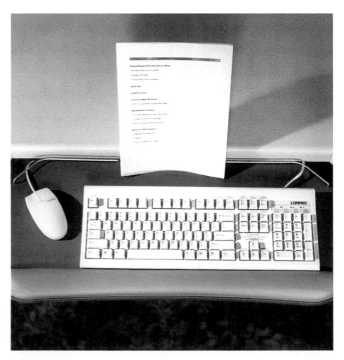

Figure 11-4 Keyboard with built-in wrist support. (Courtesy of Steelcase, Inc.)

in further minimizing posture problems (Figure 11-6). A document holder should be used to avoid excessive turning of the neck and looking downward (Figure 11-7). Operators who talk on the telephone while keyboarding or inputting data should use a headset telephone.

Scheduling the Changeover

The installation of a computer system is disruptive to office routine. Not only does it take time to install the hardware and load software, but it takes time to transfer files and data. Personnel may be intimidated by the computer and must be well trained to avoid being overly threatened. The installation of hardware should be scheduled during a down period such as a long holiday or vacation period. It is best to introduce the new system while continuing to use the old system. Start by transferring files and data, then when the staff is comfortable with the system and their computer skills, make the changeover. If your staff does not accept ownership for the system and is not trained and comfortable with it, disaster is almost guaranteed. The process cannot be rushed, and the short-term inefficiency must be accepted as a trade-off for the efficiency that will result from a computerized medical office.

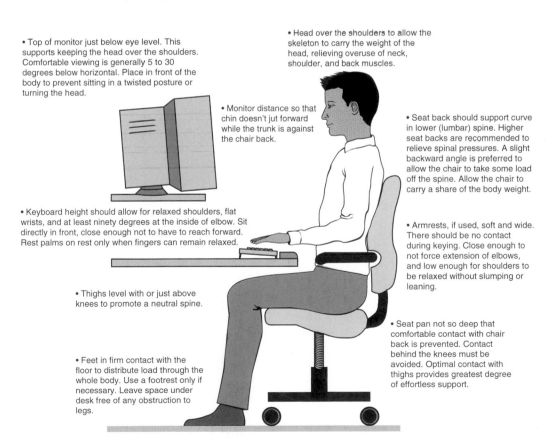

Sitting Diagram

This is the general diagram of the recommended sitting posture for computer users. Keep in mind that fixed postures contribute to the risk of cumulative trauma injury. Variety of posture is crucial, as is the habit of standing up often. The body needs movement. Nothing counts more than comfort, and this illustration is simply a tool to understand what is happening in your body at the computer. Keep these principles in mind as you develop a repertoire of comfortable postures to use throughout the workday, knowing that slumped and leaning postures demand more work from the body leading to early fatigue.

• Top of monitor just below eye level. This supports keeping the head over the shoulders. Comfortable viewing is generally 5 to 30 degrees below horizontal. Place in front of the body to prevent sitting in a twisted posture or turning the head.

• Head over the shoulders to allow the skeleton to carry the weight of the head, relieving overuse of neck, shoulder, and back muscles.

• Monitor distance so that chin doesn't jut forward while the trunk is against the chair back.

• Seat back should support curve in lower (lumbar) spine. Higher seat backs are recommended to relieve spinal pressures. A slight backward angle is preferred to allow the chair to take some load off the spine. Allow the chair to carry a share of the body weight.

• Keyboard height should allow for relaxed shoulders, flat wrists, and at least ninety degrees at the inside of elbow. Sit directly in front, close enough not to have to reach forward. Rest palms on rest only when fingers can remain relaxed.

• Armrests, if used, soft and wide. There should be no contact during keying. Close enough to not force extension of elbows, and low enough for shoulders to be relaxed without slumping or leaning.

• Thighs level with or just above knees to promote a neutral spine.

• Seat pan not so deep that comfortable contact with chair back is prevented. Contact behind the knees must be avoided. Optimal contact with thighs provides greatest degree of effortless support.

• Feet in firm contact with the floor to distribute load through the whole body. Use a footrest only if necessary. Leave space under desk free of any obstruction to legs.

Figure 11-5 Recommended computer operator position. (Courtesy of Gary Karp, Ergonomics Consultant, Onsight Technology Education Services, San Francisco, CA.)

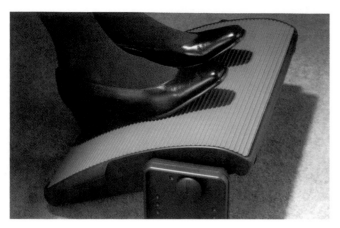

Figure 11-6 Using a footrest may help to avoid posture problems. (Courtesy of Steelcase, Inc.)

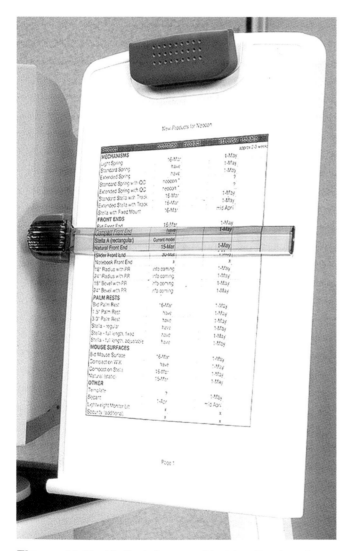

Figure 11-7 Vertical document holder. (Courtesy of Steelcase, Inc.)

COMMON SOFTWARE APPLICATIONS IN THE MEDICAL OFFICE

In a medical environment, application software can be used either for general or specialized purposes (Figure 11-8). When applications are needed to fulfill specific purposes, customized software might be used. Custom software can be purchased as a prewritten application designed for a specific industry, for example, The Medical Manager®, MedWare®, and Medisoft® software for the medical field (Figure 11-9). Although custom software can be expensive, it is valuable because it has many special features developed specifically for medical offices (Figure 11-10).

General-purpose software useful in the ambulatory care setting includes word processing, graphics, spreadsheet, database, and on-line communications programs.

Word Processing

Word processing is largely concerned with the production of textual material. Documents created using **word processing software** may include standard reports, medical transcription, memos, business letters, and articles.

Word processing software allows the medical assistant to produce a document that is needed quickly

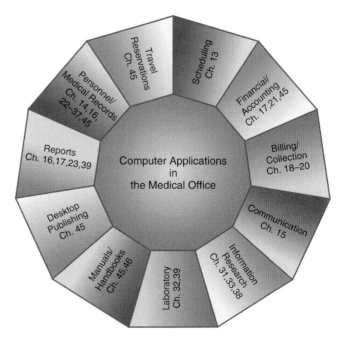

Figure 11-8 Examples of how computers may be used in the ambulatory care setting and correlation with chapter content.

and easily; the advantages of word processing versus typewriting are considerable, because corrections are easily made and material can be cut or copied and pasted from one file to another.

Common Word Processing Features. Common word processing features include:

- Block operations allow the user to highlight and move "blocks" of text to another position within the document. Text can be copied, appended, deleted, moved, and added to another document. It can be changed from lowercase to all caps, the font or typestyle can be altered, and it can be made italic or boldface.

- Page formatting can create a variety of looks for the printed page. Text can be right and left justified, centered, or aligned on the left with a ragged right. Other page format features include pagination, the placement of numbers on the page, **widow** and **orphan** control (where paragraphs end or begin on the page), and the use of **headers** and **footers** that mark each page of the document in some consistent way.

- Spell check is a feature of all word processing programs. Medical spell checkers can be added to most word processing programs and can be used to check medical terminology in word processed documents or transcribed medical reports. See also the transcription section in Chapter 16. Although spell checkers are useful tools, they are not a replacement for proofreading.

- **Macros** are keystrokes that have been saved separately so that the saved keystrokes may be inserted into any document. Macros are useful for increasing productivity when working with repetitive types of materials. For example, a letterhead used on every business letter could easily be saved in a macro format and used repeatedly.

- **Merge operations** are also time savers when working with repetitive material. Merges are often used on the individualized form letter. Ambulatory care settings may use merge operations in mailing patient education memos.

- **Sorting** refers to rearrangements of information. Sorts can be performed on alphanumeric (letters and numerals) or numeric (numerals) data. Frequently,

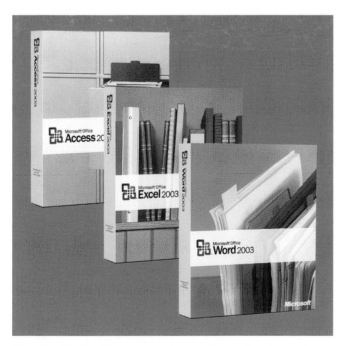

Figure 11-9 Examples of popular application software and documentation packages common to many medical offices.

FUNCTIONS OF MEDICAL MANAGEMENT SOFTWARE

- Provides immediate access to patient records, insurance information and eligibility, office notes, and reports
- Procedure entry routines capture information necessary for any type of claim or HMO report
- Electronic communications include ability to request, receive, and transfer information electronically. An example of this is electronic insurance claim filing
- Advanced billing features may include:
  - Capability for maintaining enrollment lists, automatically calculating co-pay amounts, and monitoring benefit limits for managed care
  - Capability for government reporting such as Worker's Compensation documents
  - Collection tracking system for patient bills and insurance claims
- Automates the scheduling of patient appointments, cancellations, and recalls
- Electronic medical records can store, organize, and present data on various aspects of a patient's medical history on demand
- Automated reporting allows practice to predefine reports and billing jobs to be printed automatically and even unattended

Figure 11-10 Some medical management software capabilities.

SIX OPERATIONS FUNDAMENTAL TO OPERATING SOFTWARE

1. File creation.
When alphanumeric or numeric data are entered, the information is stored in primary memory (RAM) and made available to the user for viewing on a monitor.

2. Formatting.
Formatting a file, depending on the software, usually refers to the arrangement of information so that its appearance is concise and easy to read. For word processing files, this process entails setting margins, line spacing, tab settings, and other variations. For a spreadsheet file, the process may involve choices about the size of the columns, the placement of headings over columns, and the placement of headings.

3. Editing.
Once a file has been created and formatted, modifications may be made to the original file. Spelling corrections can be made and formatting changes can be implemented. Sections of the document may be cut and pasted.

4. Saving.
If the file is to be retained permanently, it must be saved to a secondary storage medium. When working on any document, it is advisable to use the save command frequently; power interruptions and other events may cause the file to be deleted.

5. Printing.
A hard copy (printed page) is created when the file is complete and all changes have been made. Text viewed on the monitor is called a soft copy.

6. Retrieval.
Saved files may be retrieved from storage at any time. Accessing them is a process known as retrieval.

---

sorts are used to arrange labels for mailings by zip code.

- Importing and exporting data allow users to carry a text file into another applications program. Moving data from one program to another can be cumbersome, time consuming, and frustrating without the ability to import (bring in) and export (send out) easily and efficiently.

- Multicolumn output is the arrangement of text on a page in two or more columns for documents such as newsletters and patient education brochures. See Chapter 22 for techniques on developing patient information brochures.

- Desktop publishing refers to the ability to combine text and graphics into documents and produce them in a high-quality format, usually with the use of an inkjet or laser printer. Word processing packages vary greatly in their ability to provide all the options necessary for effective desktop publishing environments.

Graphics

Pictorial representations help to summarize and highlight important ideas and assist professionals in communicating material effectively. **Graphic software** is available to transform numeric data into graphs, pie charts, and other easy-to-read two- and three-dimensional formats (see Figure 11-11). It is also used to draw images and edit photographs for use in office newsletters or publications and to convert the output of imaging devices such as digital radiographs, computerized axial tomography scans, magnetic resonance imaging scans, and so on into graphic form on the computer monitor of the medical professional. New software currently is being developed to plot patient chart data and perform analysis on the data in near real time. In the future, graphics software applications will be increasingly used in the medical office, necessitating having computer systems with clock speeds in the high **G-Hz range** with massive data storage and data manipulation capability. It is probable that graphical data handling will be a new program area for medical assistants to support the advances in imaging technology. Just as the medical assistant places photographic X-rays into the patient's folder for the physician to have available before a visit with the patient, he or she will in the future pull up the data from imaging devices for reference by the physician.

Spreadsheets

Spreadsheet software crunches or calculates numbers. These programs act as electronic calculators, performing mathematical calculations and recalculations. These calculations occur so quickly and accurately that financial and other types of numeric data can be summarized and analyzed in ways that previously were difficult and time consuming. In fact, the introduction of spreadsheets began what we now know as the computer revolution.

Spreadsheets take the form of a worksheet, much like an accountant's columnar pad. The worksheet consists of empty rows and columns. Each row and each column is labeled, either numerically or alphabetically, to give entries a title. The intersection of row and column has a unique location, identified by the coordinates of the row and column, for example, D5 or AA7760. This intersection is called the cell location or cell address.

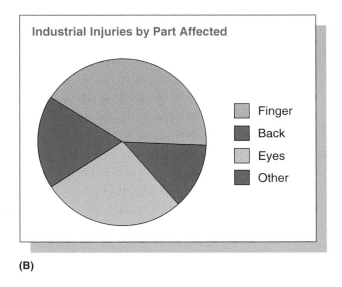

(B)

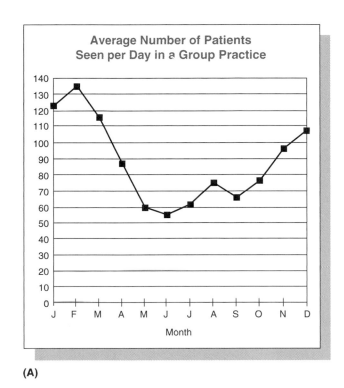

(A)

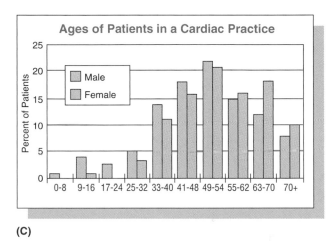

(C)

Figure 11-11 Graphs and charts are excellent for presenting information that can be interpreted at a glance: (A) line graph, (B) pie chart, (C) bar graph.

Common features found in most spreadsheet packages include the ability to format numbers. Values can be displayed in decimal format, in a currency format with a dollar sign, or as a percentage sign. Labels can be formatted to be left justified over a column of cells, right justified over a column of cells, or centered over the column.

Spreadsheets are useful for expense sheets, tax reporting, and other financial reporting. Medical billing packages are usually based on spreadsheet software.

Databases

Databases serve to organize large quantities of related data into manageable, useful forms. Database management software is used to manage employee information,

inventories, patient charts and records, possible drug interactions for patients, and so on.

Database Management Systems

Database management systems (DBMS), or databases, are built on the concept of data organization at its simplest component based on a **field** of data common to all other fields. A patient's clinic number may be the common base field. The patient's first name, middle initial, and surname would be related to the clinic number. Similarly, disease categories, prescribed drugs, and so forth would be other relational fields. Hence, the most common form of DBMS is called a relational database.

Structuring or Defining the Database. The first step in working with a database is the creation of the database structure itself.

Creating an imaginary patient database for a medical practice will be helpful for illustrative purposes. Consider a two-physician practice with 1,000 patients. The office maintains information on all its patients, including general identifying information, accounting information, and medical records.

A database is needed that will maintain the general identifying information. Minimally, the fields necessary for the database are:

- Patient name
- Patient address
- Work phone
- Home phone
- Patient insurance

Other fields might also be included, such as:

- Sex
- Social Security number
- Date of birth
- Occupation
- Place of employment

These headings provide the basic structure for the database.

The variables involved in health care databases are numerous and might include identification of the patient, identification of the insurance carrier or carriers, type of insurance, limits in plan benefits, diagnosis and procedure codes, and information concerning the primary care physician.

 With the influence of managed care, databases that identify patient insurance variables become increasingly important. These databases might include the identification numbers of insurance policies and the insurance carriers or managed care operations that provide coverage for the patient. In developing this database, it is important to consider the following questions:

- Is the patient insured?
- Is there more than one insurance policy?
- Who is the insurer? Does this insurance supplement governmental forms of insurance such as Medicare or Medicaid?

- Does the patient's insurance require co-payments or deductibles?
- What will be covered by which insurance policy?
- Does the patient assign (turn over) benefits directly to the provider?
- Is the patient covered through Workers' Compensation?

Once established, databases can provide invaluable information in little time. The key is to know what information you need readily available, and then structure a database to that objective.

Information Retrieval Systems. DBMS can be adapted to a variety of medical settings. In addition to DBMS's capability of processing patient data, databases are used within the health care environment as information retrieval systems. Through the Internet, it is possible to connect electronically with **information retrieval systems** to reference topics in health sciences literature. Most medical libraries and many hospitals have the capacity to use the MEDLARS (Medical Literature Analysis and Retrieval Systems) literature database. This database, through the National Library of Medicine, allows researchers to conduct literature reviews on any of their 20 on-line bibliographies.

Information systems that complete biomedical journal searches are also becoming available on a subscription service basis to individual purchasers for use on their microcomputers. One on-line service is Medline; it contains more than six million references on journal articles relevant to health care professionals.

Information retrieval systems are also available for patient use. Cancer treatment protocols, descriptions of treatment regimens, and prognosis information by diagnostic category are now available to individuals who wish to gather information on cancer diagnoses and treatment options. These information retrieval systems should not be used for complete medical care, but rather are a resource to patients who are frequently bewildered by treatment choices.

PATIENT CONFIDENTIALITY IN THE COMPUTERIZED MEDICAL OFFICE

 The computer and other electronic transmission media are powerful tools, but they are equally powerful in their potential to jeopardize patient confidentiality. A record or test result faxed to a loca-

HIPAA Security Checklist*

- Identify a person responsible for security
- Conduct risk assessment
- Implement security measures to address risks
- Implement a security audit and tracking system
- Implement a sanctions policy for violators

*Final rule Health Insurance Reform Security Standards

tion where the fax is not contained in a secured area can be read by anyone passing by. A fax also can be accidentally sent to the wrong phone, possibly the office fax of the patient, because this information is commonly in the patient record. Records sent over the Internet to an external location can be intercepted by a hacker and posted on the Web for all to see. These are just a few of the possible scenarios that can occur if protocols are not in place to ensure maintenance of confidentiality.

The starting point for a meaningful information security system is a comprehensive security policy that adheres to HIPAA policies and procedures and that is understood and supported by staff and employees. All staff, employees, and vendors having access to the computer system should be educated on the security policy and asked to sign a contract affirming that they will adhere to the policy before they are given access to confidential data. The signed contract affirms that they have received training and have been instructed in proper procedures to protect medical records. The signed contracts together with the protocols become a part of the facility's documentation showing compliance with HIPAA regulations.

The next essential step is to ensure that computer-literate personnel are employed to set up and structure databases. Protocols should be established defining who can access and modify databases, providing identification, dating, and authenticating mechanisms for those changes and additions. Procedures should be in place to ensure that people other than the intended recipient cannot accidentally read misdirected files, and that firewalls are in place or precautions are taken to prevent people from hacking into the system through Internet or **network interfaces.** Antivirus programs should be part of the system to prevent loss of the database or the unintentional dissemination of files.

Passwords incorporating employee personal identification numbers (PIN) or passwords that are specific

to individual employees are quite successful in controlling access to files and providing an authentication mechanism.

Output devices, such as printers and fax machines, should be located where unauthorized personnel cannot view them. Unauthorized persons should not be allowed to wander around the facility unescorted. Data storage media should be secured, and accountability records of persons accessing the media should be maintained.

Both the sender and the recipient can make sending files on the Internet secure by the use of encryption programs. Development of a firewall to allow outside computers to access your computer whereas restricting access to your databases is essentially impossible. The U.S. government, with unlimited facilities, has not been able to develop a foolproof system, thus other approaches are required for an office of limited resources. Probably the best approach is not to allow outside computers access to your database computers and to communicate to an outside network or Internet using a dedicated computer. Files to be transferred would be loaded into the dedicated computer using one of the portable data storage devices. This would also limit damage in the event a virus invaded your system.

The American Medical Association (AMA) supports the adoption of standards to protect individual confidential information. Figure 11-12 summarizes AMA Policy E5-07, "Confidentiality—Computers," issued before April 1977 and updated in 1994, 1998, and July 2002.

HIPAA STANDARDS FOR SAFEGUARDING PATIENT HEALTH INFORMATION

HIPAA standards for safeguarding PHI include:

- Preparation and implementation of written confidentiality protocols and procedures regarding PHI
- Staff training in implementation of all protocols
- Identification of authentication protocols for all personnel
- Access control of computer output, modification, or destruction of files
- Security of transmitted data
- Control of discarded records, storage media, and computer hardware

E-5.07 Confidentiality: Computers. The utmost effort and care must be taken to protect the confidentiality of all medical records, including computerized medical records.

The guidelines below are offered to assist physicians and computer service organizations in maintaining the confidentiality of information in medical records when that information is stored in computerized databases:

(1) Confidential medical information should be entered into the computer-based patient record only by authorized personnel. Additions to the record should be time and date stamped, and the person making the additions should be identified in the record.

(2) The patient and physician should be advised about the existence of computerized databases in which medical information concerning the patient is stored. Such information should be communicated to the physician and patient prior to the physician's release of the medical information to the entity or entities maintaining the computer databases. All individuals and organizations with some form of access to the computerized databases, and the level of access permitted, should be specifically identified in advance. Full disclosure of this information to the patient is necessary in obtaining informed consent to treatment. Patient data should be assigned a security level appropriate for the data's degree of sensitivity, which should be used to control who has access to the information.

(3) The physician and patient should be notified of the distribution of all reports reflecting identifiable patient data prior to distribution of the reports by the computer facility. There should be approval by the patient and notification of the physician prior to the release of patient-identifiable clinical and administrative data to individuals or organizations external to the medical care environment. Such information should not be released without the express permission of the patient.

(4) The dissemination of confidential medical data should be limited to only those individuals or agencies with a bona fide use for the data. Only the data necessary for the bona fide use should be released. Patient identifiers should be omitted when appropriate. Release of confidential medical information from the database should be confined to the specific purpose for which the information is requested and limited to the specific time frame requested. All such organizations or individuals should be advised that authorized release of data to them does not authorize their further release of the data to additional individuals or organizations, or subsequent use of the data for other purposes.

(5) Procedures for adding to or changing data on the computerized database should indicate individuals authorized to make changes, time periods in which changes take place, and those individuals who will be informed about changes in the data from the medical records.

(6) Procedures for purging the computerized database of archaic or inaccurate data should be established and the patient and physician should be notified before and after the data has been purged. There should be no commingling of a physician's computerized patient records with those of other computer service bureau clients. In addition, procedures should be developed to protect against inadvertent mixing of individual reports or segments thereof.

(7) The computerized medical database should be on-line to the computer terminal only when authorized computer programs requiring the medical data are being used. Individuals and organizations external to the clinical facility should not be provided on-line access to a computerized database containing identifiable data from medical records concerning patients. Access to the computerized database should be controlled through security measures such as passwords, encryption (encoding) of information, and scannable badges or other user identification.

(8) Backup systems and other mechanisms should be in place to prevent data loss and downtime as a result of hardware or software failure.

(9) Security:

A. Stringent security procedures should be in place to prevent unauthorized access to computer-based patient records. Personnel audit procedures should be developed to establish a record in the event of unauthorized disclosure of medical data. Terminated or former employees in the data processing environment should have no access to data from the medical records concerning patients.

B. Upon termination of computer services for a physician, those computer files maintained for the physician should be physically turned over to the physician. They may be destroyed (erased) only if it is established that the physician has another copy (in some form). In the event of file erasure, the computer service bureau should verify in writing to the physician that the erasure has taken place. Issued prior to April 1977; Updated June 1994.

Figure 11-12 Computer confidentiality guidelines. (Source: *Code of Medical Ethics Current Opinions with Annotations*, 1994 Edition, American Medical Association, Copyright © 1995–2004.)

PROFESSIONALISM IN THE COMPUTERIZED MEDICAL OFFICE

Areas of professionalism directly related to the computerized medical office may include:

- Working as a member of the health care team: This means that you become actively involved in the process of upgrading medical software and implementating policies and procedures related to computerization, and that you follow all protocols adopted by your employer.

- Adapt to change: The medical assistant must adapt to change. Computerization in the medical office will stretch the comfort limits of all personnel. New procedures will result in office inefficiency until everyone is familiar with the new system and it becomes second nature in its use.

- Work ethic: The medical assistant should refrain from using the office computer for personal use. This includes sending and receiving personal e-mail and searching the Internet. Passwords should never be shared, and unauthorized software should not be loaded onto the office computer. Protocols should be carefully followed in transmission of patient confidential information.

- Enhance skills through continuing education: Introduction of a computer system and periodic updates to program revisions will require continued education and training on the part of the medical assistant. A professional will approach these minor disruptions with a positive attitude.

Critical Thinking

The physician–employer has informed the office manager that he or she has observed employees visiting Web sites not connected with office requirements and is concerned about the practice becoming widespread. You have been asked to prepare a draft guideline for a policy on business and personal Internet use on office equipment during business hours. You have been further told that the policy should not be totally prohibitive, but it does need to address performing personal tasks during business hours and exercising propriety in the sites visited.

Prepare a draft policy proposal for computer use, and obtain written comments from several students regarding the policy guidelines. Prepare a final draft incorporating changes made to obtain consensus by the persons making comments and submit the original draft, the comments, and final draft to the instructor, together with your observations on the difficulty in achieving consensus on the policy.

Procedure 11-1   Software Installation

PURPOSE:
To add software programs to the computer system for later call-up and use. RATIONALE: To provide the computer with the necessary information to install the software.

PROCEDURE STEPS:
Software can be installed on Microsoft Windows® using an automatic "Installation Wizard" or by manual means.

Automatic Installation
- Close all open programs.
- Insert the CD supplied with the program into your CD drive. Shortly after the light on the drive shows activity, the Installation Wizard screen will appear. If more

than one disk is supplied (many programs have multiple disks because of the size of the program and files that must be stored to use the program), start with number 1 or the one marked "program." Usually, other disks will be marked disk 2, disk 3, or data.
- Follow the instructions given by your software documentation and the Installation Wizard screens that will appear. The wizard will usually ask for the following:
  1. the product registration number or serial number
  2. where you want the files to be stored on your hard drive (A default address is usually given and should be used unless your organization has a policy of storing programs in a specific drive or server. If that is the case, you probably have a system administrator for your computers and you should not be doing the installation.)

(continues)

Procedure 11-1 (continued)

3. whether you want the program icon on your desktop to aid in quickly starting the program (You should say YES to this question unless your desktop is quite cluttered. If you say NO, you will have to use the START button, then select PRO-GRAMS from the menu that appears, and then find the SOFTWARE NAME and click on it to start the program. If the program is frequently used, this becomes a nuisance.)

- At the completion of the installation, you may be asked to register the program if you are on-line, and then asked to restart your computer before the program will be operational. Just follow the instructions given by the wizard. It is a good idea to register the program so that you receive updates and announcements. If you are not on-line, you can register using ground mail.

Manual Installation
Sometimes the Installation Wizard will not recognize the program or the settings are not such that it will be automatic. In this case, you will need to perform the following steps:

- Close all open programs.

- Click START. Then select RUN from the menu. The CD should already be in the drive.
- A screen will appear that asks for the address and program name of the program you want to run for installation.
- The route will include the letter designation for the CD drive where the program disk is located. This is usually the D: drive, but it could differ depending on the configuration of your computer. The program documentation should specify the installation name. A common name is "setup." The route will look like the following when typed into the space: **D:\setup.** The answer is not case specific. If you do not know the drive designation, double-click on the My Computer icon on your desktop. The screen that appears will show the letter designation for the CD drive. If you have more than one drive, you may have to look carefully to identify which you have used.
- The setup program will result in some form of screen for installation. Follow the instructions and some of the advice given above for automatic installation.

Procedure 11-2 Hardware Installation

PURPOSE:
To add hardware programs to the computer system for later call-up and use. RATIONALE: To provide the computer with the necessary information to install the hardware.

PROCEDURE STEPS:
Microsoft Windows® normally identifies new hardware and asks you if you want to install it, or it simply starts and Installation Wizard. In some instances, the wizard will not recognize the new hardware, necessitating manual initiation of the wizard.

The wizard will request all or some of the following information:

- Close all open programs
- Manufacturer and Model Number of the hardware

- How it is connected to the computer (USB, Parallel, or IEEE 1394 cable)
- The driver supplied with the hardware or already registered with Microsoft (If not part of your operating system, you will need to install a CD into the drive for the computer to load into memory)

Follow the directions given by the wizard.
If the wizard does not appear, you will need to manually initiate the wizard to install the hardware. In this case, do the following:

- Close all open programs.
- Go to START, SETTINGS, CONTROL PANEL, and double-click ADD HARDWARE. The Add Hardware Wizard screen will start. Follow the instructions given on the screen. You may be asked to insert the CD with the driver supplied by the manufacturer.

Case Study 11-1

Once medical assistant Walter Seals received the go-ahead to order a computer system for Inner City Health Care, he immediately consulted a professional for advice on how to set up the workstations. As a health care professional, Walter firmly believes in preventive care, and he wants to ensure that staff members, especially those who might be using the computer extensively, do not develop some of the health problems associated with routine or prolonged computer use.

CASE STUDY REVIEW

1. Imagine that you are helping Walter design a typical computer workstation. Make a list of how the chair, monitor, and keyboard should be positioned. Sketch your diagram for a safe and effective workstation.

2. In addition to a proper workstation setup, what are other measures Walter should consider to ensure staff safety?

3. One of the center's medical assistants is reluctant to use the computer, not because of safety issues, but because she feels intimidated by the process. How should Walter help her overcome her timidity of the computer?

Case Study 11-2

Walter Seals, a CMA employed by Inner City Health Care, has been given approval to computerize the office. Walter is also concerned about confidentiality issues involved with a computerized medical office.

CASE STUDY REVIEW

1. Identify the areas where confidentiality is most likely to be jeopardized.
2. Suggest possible solutions to protect confidentiality in each of these areas.
3. Write a one-page summary, and submit it to your instructor.

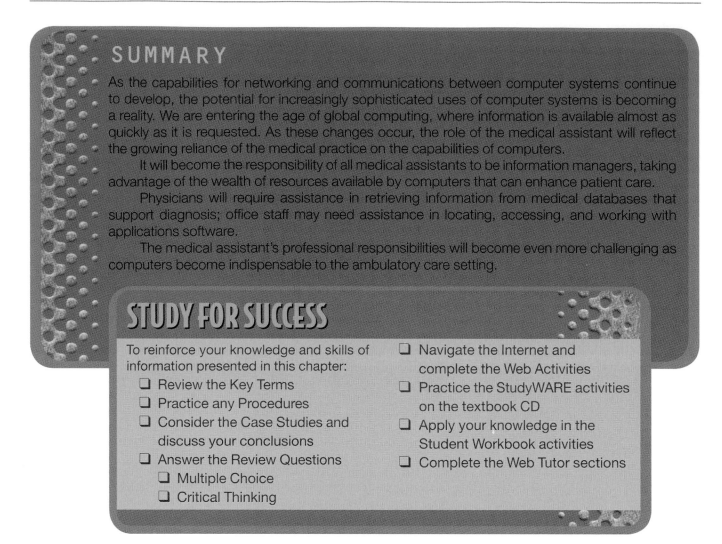

SUMMARY

As the capabilities for networking and communications between computer systems continue to develop, the potential for increasingly sophisticated uses of computer systems is becoming a reality. We are entering the age of global computing, where information is available almost as quickly as it is requested. As these changes occur, the role of the medical assistant will reflect the growing reliance of the medical practice on the capabilities of computers.

It will become the responsibility of all medical assistants to be information managers, taking advantage of the wealth of resources available by computers that can enhance patient care.

Physicians will require assistance in retrieving information from medical databases that support diagnosis; office staff may need assistance in locating, accessing, and working with applications software.

The medical assistant's professional responsibilities will become even more challenging as computers become indispensable to the ambulatory care setting.

STUDY FOR SUCCESS

To reinforce your knowledge and skills of information presented in this chapter:
- ❑ Review the Key Terms
- ❑ Practice any Procedures
- ❑ Consider the Case Studies and discuss your conclusions
- ❑ Answer the Review Questions
  - ❑ Multiple Choice
  - ❑ Critical Thinking

- ❑ Navigate the Internet and complete the Web Activities
- ❑ Practice the StudyWARE activities on the textbook CD
- ❑ Apply your knowledge in the Student Workbook activities
- ❑ Complete the Web Tutor sections

REVIEW QUESTIONS

Multiple Choice

1. Microcomputers:
   a. are the fastest and most powerful computers
   b. handle large amounts of processing and challenge the capabilities of old mainframe systems
   c. are widely used in today's health care facility
   d. are expensive and complex
2. The CPU:
   a. consists of electronic tablets with pointers, scanners, and touch screens
   b. is the brain of the computer system
   c. is often referred to as memory
   d. frequently is referred to as a computer program
3. Documentation:
   a. performs a specific data processing function
   b. is a set of instructions that a computer follows to control computer hardware and to process data

   c. frequently is called the operating system (OS)
   d. consists of the manuals and documents that define how programs operate
4. Data storage devices include:
   a. keystrokes, motion, temperature, and the mouse
   b. ROM, RAM, hard drives, and floppy drives
   c. hard copy, ROM, the mouse, and OS
   d. data input devices, hard copy, and OS
5. Networking includes:
   a. optical drives, compact disks, and digital video disks
   b. flash drives, tape drives, optical drives, and digital video disks
   c. LANs, WANs, and Ethernet
   d. CDs, DVDs, and LANs

6. When going from a manual to a computerized medical office, it is important to do all of the following *except*:
   a. know what the office needs in a computer system
   b. install the operation during a down period
   c. work with a trusted, knowledgeable vendor
   d. expect the computer system to be 100% operational immediately

7. Spreadsheets are used primarily in:
   a. document production
   b. financial analysis
   c. communications
   d. information retrieval

8. Formatting a document refers to:
   a. setting margins, tabs, and line spacing
   b. macros operations
   c. exporting features
   d. all of the above

9. Importing and exporting data:
   a. saves time when working with repetitive material
   b. allows users to carry a text file into another application program
   c. are keystrokes that have been saved separately so that the saved keystrokes may be inserted into any document
   d. allows the user to highlight and move blocks of text to another position within the document

10. Database management software may be used with which of the following?
    a. recording employee information
    b. managing inventory systems
    c. creating form letters
    d. all of the above

11. The beginning point for a meaningful information security system is a comprehensive security policy that:
    a. involves the use of LANs
    b. involves the use of WANs
    c. follows office policies and procedures
    d. adheres to HIPAA policies and procedures

Critical Thinking

1. Assume you work in an ambulatory care setting that operates on a manual system. Identify the functions you would have a computer perform in the office.

2. The same office is now going to make the transition to a computerized system. What steps would you take to make the transition as smooth as possible?

3. Discuss the study of ergonomics and identify steps to take to decrease or prevent computer-related injury.

4. Your physician has written authorization from a patient to fax laboratory test results to his or her home. You, the medical assistant, have just faxed the information and discovered that you sent it to the patient's office number instead of his or her home number. What legal implications does this create? What steps will you take to correct the error, and how will you document the incident?

5. Your physician–employer has asked you to research a particular medical topic on the computer. How do you proceed?

6. Discuss the importance of patient confidentiality in medical computing. What measures are you required to take to be HIPAA compliant? How are these documented?

WEB ACTIVITIES

Go to a software provider's Web site, such as www.microsoft.com, and list the name and purpose of each patch available for a selected application software program.

REFERENCES/BIBLIOGRAPHY

American Medical Association. (2004). *E-5.07 confidentiality: Computers.* Retrieved from http://www.ama-assn.org. Accessed April 7, 2005.

Humphrey, D. D. (2004). *Contemporary medical office procedures* (3rd ed.). Clifton Park, NY: Thomson Delmar Learning.

ingenix. (2003, December). *HIPAA Tool Kit.* Salt Lake City, UT: St. Anthony Publishing Medicode.

Karp, G. (1996). *Preventing computer injury.* Adapted from paper presented at the Association of American Medical Transcriptionists, Baltimore, MD.

Keir, L., Wise, B. A., & Krebs, C. (2003). *Medical administrative and clinical competencies* (5th ed.). Clifton Park, NY: Thomson Delmar Learning.

Krager, D., & Krager, C. (2005). *HIPAA for medical office personnel.* Clifton Park, NY: Thomson Delmar Learning.

Security Standards, Department of Health and Human Services. (Feb. 20, 2003). *Final rule health insurance reform.* The Federal Register: Retrieved from http://www.gpoaccess.gov/fr/index.html. Accessed April 8, 2005, pp. 8335–8381.

CHAPTER 12

Telecommunications

OUTLINE

KEY TERMS

OBJECTIVES

The student should strive to meet the following performance objectives and demonstrate an understanding of the facts and principles presented in this chapter through written and oral communication.

1. Define the key terms as presented in the glossary.
2. Describe useful rules for using proper telephone technique.
3. State at least five common telephone courtesies.
4. Discuss proper screening techniques.
5. Outline the proper procedure for answering incoming calls and transferring calls.

(continues)

Patient Care

- Perform telephone and in-person screening

Professional Communications

- Demonstrate telephone techniques

Legal Concepts

- Identify and respond to issues of confidentiality
- Perform within legal and ethical boundaries
- Document appropriately

Operational Functions

- Utilize computer software to maintain office systems

ABHES—ENTRY-LEVEL COMPETENCIES

Professionalism

- Project a positive attitude
- Maintain confidentiality at all times
- Be a "team player"
- Be cognizant of ethical boundaries
- Evidence a responsible attitude
- Be courteous and diplomatic
- Conduct work within scope of education, training, and ability

Communication

- Adapt what is said to the recipient's level of comprehension
- Use proper telephone techniques
- Application of electronic technology

(continues)

OBJECTIVES (continued)

6. Describe the information every message should contain.
7. Name at least three calls the medical assistant can take, and state the reasons why. Name three calls the medical assistant should refer to the physician, and state the reasons why.
8. Recall six questions that should be asked during telephone triage.
9. Elaborate on how calls from angry individuals should be handled in a professional manner, and give three steps to follow when this type of call is received.
10. Outline the proper procedure for placing outgoing calls.
11. Discuss the steps involved in preparing and recording a message on an answering device.
12. Discuss telephone documentation.
13. Identify ways to ensure patient confidentiality when using the telephone.
14. Discuss the impacts of HIPAA regulations on telecommunications.
15. Recall four examples of telephone technology, and describe their functions.
16. Discuss characteristics of professionalism related to telecommunications.

SCENARIO

At a busy two-doctor family physician's office, the telephone lines are rarely quiet. Yet, administrative medical assistant Ellen Armstrong has learned to maintain her composure when she is responsible for managing incoming calls. Ellen has in her favor a naturally warm telephone manner, but she has had to cultivate other traits so that she can represent the practice in a professional manner, help patients and other callers feel at ease, and efficiently screen or refer calls as necessary.

This is Ellen's first job since receiving her medical assisting credential, and initially she felt unable to properly screen calls. She was not sure when to refer callers to the physician; she did not know when she should record a message. With some advice from Marilyn, the office manager, Ellen devised a simple system to keep herself and her thoughts organized throughout a hectic day of telephone communications. Everyday before office hours, she gathers the materials she needs, including the appropriate message pad, a list of information needed to set a patient appointment, and any information she needs on prescription refills for patients and a copy of the office policy on referencing calls. With these few measures, Ellen feels organized and prepared, and thus able to focus her attention on interacting with the caller. To stay abreast of new telecommunication, Ellen attends conferences and seminars to learn how emerging technology can be used effectively in the medical office.

FEATURED COMPETENCIES (continued)

Administrative Duties

- Perform basic secretarial skills

Clinical Duties

- Perform telephone and in-person screening

Legal Concepts

- Document accurately
- Use appropriate guidelines when releasing records or information

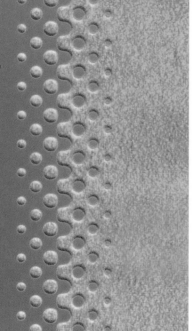

Spotlight on Certification

RMA Content Outline
- Medical secretarial–receptionist
- Oral communications

CMA Content Outline
- Adapting communication to an individual's ability to understand
- Professional communication and behavior
- Evaluating and understanding communication
- Receiving, organizing, prioritizing and transmitting information
- Telephone techniques
- Legislation
- Equipment operation
- Appropriate referrals
- Instructions for patients with special needs

CMAS Content Outline
- Office Communications

INTRODUCTION

As in many office settings, the telephone is the lifeline of the ambulatory care setting. By means of telecommunication, which can also include fax and e-mail transmissions, patient appointments are scheduled, referrals made, critical information related, and the practice personality conveyed.

Medical assistants, more multiskilled than ever, have a wealth of knowledge to bring to their telecommunications. Over the telephone, they will welcome new patients, reassure current patients, collaborate with other organizations on patient care, and calmly and efficiently deal with emergencies. They will need to draw on their vast resource of administrative and clinical knowledge; they will also need to cultivate a telephone personality that is warm and accessible while also being efficient and organized.

In this chapter, medical assistants will come to understand the principles basic to successful telecommunications, whether initiating or answering calls; will learn the extent and limits of their authority as medical assistants; will discover how to prepare themselves for making or receiving calls; and will be introduced to telephone systems and new technologies.

BASIC TELEPHONE TECHNIQUES

Telephone answering techniques are rapidly changing in all offices, even the smaller single-physician practices. The medical assistant responsible for answering the telephones previously was the first contact most people had with the practice, but today the first contact is usually with an automated phone system. Just as with a human answering the phone, first impressions are lasting. The program setup in the automatic phone system should be user friendly. It is not uncommon for a person unfamiliar

with a menu-driven telephone system to be unable to find the menu that applies, and it is extremely frustrating if they cannot find a way to connect with a human operator. An option to speak with a receptionist should always be offered. An automatic answering system should begin with a message instructing the caller what to do if the call is an emergency. In most locations, the caller is instructed to hang up and dial 911. After this should be a list of menus for such items as prescription refill, billing, scheduling an appointment, and so forth. If at all possible, the menu system should only be one level deep; for example, the billing selection should not lead to another menu for Medicare, HMO, or other finance categories.

Regardless of whether the automated system or a medical assistant makes first contact with the caller, at some point the medical assistant will usually speak with the caller. The impression the patient forms of the practice will depend on your telephone personality and how you answer incoming calls. To create a positive impression, try to answer the telephone by the end of the first ring if at all possible, and certainly within three rings. If your station has more than one incoming line, it may be necessary to interrupt a conversation to answer another call. Some guidelines to follow in this instance include:

- Excuse yourself to the first caller by saying, "Excuse me, another line is ringing. May I put you on hold for a moment?" This may be done only once, not repeatedly during the conversation.

- When, and not before, the first caller has given permission to be put on hold, answer the second call. Ascertain who is calling and determine that it is not an emergency if you are not using an automated system. Ask the second caller if you can put them on hold and return to the first call. Never try to quickly resolve the second call before returning to the first call.

- Return to the first caller and thank the person for holding.

- Explore the possibility of an automated message after three rings to put the calls into a waiting queue with a message that you are on another line and will answer the next call momentarily.

Telephone Personality

First impressions are usually conveyed through verbal and nonverbal communication. (Refer to Chapter 4 for a review of these communication modes.) In telephone communications, however, personality and attitudes are conveyed only through the tone in which words are spoken and the words themselves. Remember, callers are not an interruption of your work but the reason for your job. Even in a large practice, it is rare that someone just answers the telephone and has no other duties. No matter what other duties are pressing, the primary responsibility of every employee in a physician's office is patient care; everything else is secondary. Whoever answers incoming calls should be prepared to give the caller complete attention.

Use a voice that is pleasant and well **modulated** (one that varies in pitch and intensity) and conveys interest in the caller's needs. Hold the handpiece correctly, about 1 to 2 inches away from the mouth, and project your voice *at* the mouthpiece not *over* it. The use of headsets permits the mouthpiece to be positioned appropriately and frees the hands to locate and record information easily.

Volume, enunciation, pronunciation, and speed all have a profound effect on how you sound to the person on the other end of the line.

- Volume should be the same as when speaking conversationally.

- **Enunciation** implies speaking your words clearly and **articulating** carefully.

- **Pronunciation** involves saying the words correctly.

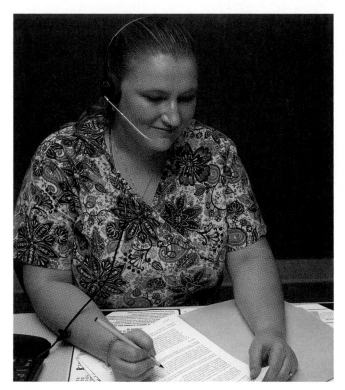

Figure 12-1   The headset type telephone frees the medical assistant's hands to document and record while maintaining an ergonomic position.

- Speed should be at a normal rate, neither too fast nor too slow.

Posture, the way the body is carried, also affects the voice. If slumped in a chair, the diaphragm (the muscle separating the abdominal and thoracic cavities) is compressed and breathing may be restricted. Using the headset speaker with the phone promotes good ergonomic position because it decreases neck and shoulder stress by allowing you to sit up straight (Figure 12-1). If you are less tired and tense, you can focus more easily on professional alertness, which comes across to the caller in the sound of your voice.

Being organized and prepared in advance for each telephone call enables the medical assistant to respond to each caller as if there is nothing else to do. By taking a breath before answering the telephone and putting on a smile, a pleasant vocal impression can be delivered to the caller.

Medical assistants who enjoy their work and want to be of assistance to patients communicate enthusiasm. Enthusiasm conveys interest to the caller and projects a sincere, caring attitude that can be "heard" over the telephone (Figure 12-2).

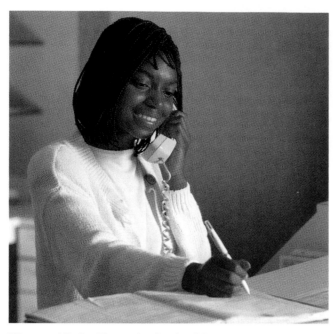

Figure 12-2 Tone of voice is able to put people at ease in a telephone conversation. People can hear an unpleasant mood, just as they can hear a warm smile.

 Though some callers will be upset, frightened, or even angry, the medical assistant must always be patient and in control. Some calls may be life-threatening emergencies; medical assistants need to remain calm to be of help to the caller, remembering their professional role as health care providers.

Medical assistants can concentrate on improving telephone communications by setting up a small tape recorder next to the telephone and setting it to record for one or two hours each day. At the end of the day, recorded calls will present an accurate representation of volume, articulation, and tone of voice. After using the tape as a self-improvement exercise, be sure to erase all messages to respect the confidentiality of callers.

Telephone Etiquette

Telephone **etiquette,** as with all good manners, simply involves treating others with consideration. Medical assistants have chosen a profession in which care and concern for others are paramount, so it is especially important to keep the patient's feelings in the forefront at all times.

TELEPHONE COURTESIES

- Always use callers' names and titles (e.g., Mrs. O'Keefe or Dr. King) during the course of a conversation when confidentiality is assured; this shows interest in them as individuals.
- Do not use technical terms if simpler ones will convey the information adequately. Using professional **jargon,** or terminology, is an easy trap to fall into because this terminology is used daily with coworkers. Jargon only confuses people outside the profession; the goal in communication is mutual understanding, not **obfuscation.**
- Do not use slang or nonstandard terms in a business setting. Slang terms may have entirely different meanings to individuals from another generation or cultural background. Use of slang is not professional and tends to indicate a poor vocabulary range or lack of education. However, patients may use slang in their communications. It is important not to be offended by slang terms; also, be certain that patients who use slang understand any common medical terminology you may use.
- The "hold" button on the telephone is probably the most misused piece of equipment in the practice; always use it sparingly. Never put a caller on hold until you know who is calling and why. Never place an urgent or emergency call on hold. Never put a caller on hold without asking for and receiving permission to do so. No call should be left unattended for more than 20 to 30 seconds. If it is necessary to keep callers waiting longer, go back to the caller and give the option of continuing to hold or receiving a call back in a few minutes.
- When it is necessary to get additional information and call back later, let the person know when to expect the call. If for some reason the information is not available when the time for the call back arrives, call anyway to let the person know when to expect another call.
- When taking a message for someone in the office, give the caller an idea of when to expect a return call. If the person will be out of the office for an extended period, see if someone else can help or if the caller would rather wait to hear from that specific individual. Never promise to have someone call back when you cannot control if or when this will happen.
- Pay attention to what the person is saying and *how* they sound. Do not interrupt or finish sentences for slow talkers. The caller may have difficulty putting some things into words, but give the person a chance to explain the problem or question. Listen with empathy for the caller. Also listen to what the tone of voice expresses.
- Never talk to someone in the office while on an open line. This is confusing to the caller, and confidential information could be inadvertently overheard.
- Do not attempt to work on other things while talking on the telephone.
- Never eat or chew gum when talking on the telephone. This impedes enunciation and is distracting to the caller.
- Say "good-bye" when closing the call, and allow the caller to hang up first.

Basic telephone courtesies should be kept in mind when answering any professional call.

ANSWERING INCOMING CALLS

Most calls received in an ambulatory care setting are from patients or prospective patients, though many also are from other physicians or medical facilities. The remainder will be from family members, salespeople, and miscellaneous others. Personal calls should not be permitted in the medical office because the busy lines are intended for business. Occasional personal emergency calls are appropriate.

Preparing to Take Calls

Before answering incoming calls or making outgoing calls, medical assistants should devise a simple system to keep organized throughout the hectic day of telephone communications. Collect pertinent materials, such as a message pad, information regarding office policies and scheduling of patients and prescription refills, internal and outside referral forms, listing of frequently used telephone numbers and extensions, and several sharpened pencils and working pens.

Answering Calls

When answering incoming calls, the name of the facility should be clearly identified, as well as the name of the person with whom the caller is speaking. The name of the office is important, because the caller wants to know the correct number has been reached. To avoid clipping off the office name, practice using **buffer words.** Buffer words are expendable words and may consist of introductory words, phrases, or statements. They allow a caller an opportunity to collect their thoughts and focus on what is being said.

Obtain the caller's full name and correct spelling, and ask if this is an emergency call. Determine how you can be of assistance, and complete the call efficiently by following all established office protocols. (Refer to Procedure 12-1.)

Screening Calls

One of the medical assistant's responsibilities is to screen incoming calls. The purpose of screening is twofold: (1) to be sure the caller talks to the person who will be most helpful (this is not necessarily the person asked for); and (2) to ensure the physician's time with calls is efficiently managed.

Many people who call an ambulatory care setting will ask to speak to the doctor. Patients calling for appointments or with billing problems or insurance questions will sometimes ask to speak to the primary physician, assuming he or she is the person in charge, and therefore should answer any question or solve any problem. In most practices, this is not the case. Medical assistants and other administrative employees are equipped to deal with front-office functions; usually, physicians are not involved in these procedures and sometimes may not be aware of administrative routines.

Proper Screening Techniques. Screening is usually a simple process of asking the caller's name and the reason for the call. There are situations, however, that will require tactful persistence to get the information needed to properly direct the caller. Sometimes callers hesitate to give information because the questions are of a confidential and possibly even embarrassing nature.

Occasionally, a caller flatly refuses to give any information or will just say, "I'm a friend." If it is a patient who refuses to give information after gentle prodding, respect the patient's privacy and take a message. If you do not know who the caller is and you are unable to get any information, take the message and give it to the physician. If the physician does not know the person, he or she can decide whether to return the call. In any event, do not argue with the caller. Be polite and professional at all times.

Transferring a Call

During the screening process, calls may mistakenly be directed to someone who is unable to assist the caller adequately. This call will need to be transferred to someone with more expertise in a particular area. Guidelines that ensure successful transfer of calls include:

- Get the caller's full name, telephone number, and any other situation-associated information before attempting to transfer the call.

- Determine who would be the best person to assist with this situation.

- Ask if you may place the caller on hold while you collect any pertinent data and make a call to confirm that the person best suited to assist is available.

- Return to the caller, thank him or her for holding, and give the name and extension of the person to whom you will be transferring the call.

- Follow your telephone system's procedure for transferring the call.

- Follow up to be sure the call transferred correctly.

See Procedure 12-2 for steps and rationale in transferring a call.

Taking a Message

When taking messages, it is advisable to use a standard telephone message pad with a carbonless copy that allows the office to maintain a record of all incoming calls (Figure 12-3). The information that should be recorded for *every* message includes:

1. Date and time call is received
2. Who the call is for
3. Caller's name and telephone number
4. When the caller can be reached
5. Nature and urgency of the call
6. Action to be taken (e.g., will call back, returned your call, please call back)
7. Message, if any
8. Your name or initials (in case there are questions)

Be sure to repeat the information back to the caller to verify that you have heard and copied it correctly. When taking a message, give callers an approximate time when they might expect to receive a call back if there is an established policy and all staff understand and follow that policy. ("Dr. King will be returning calls between 4:30 and 5:00." "Ellen is out of the office today, but I'll ask her to call you before 10 AM tomorrow.")

Always attach a message from a patient to the patient's chart before placing the message on the physi-

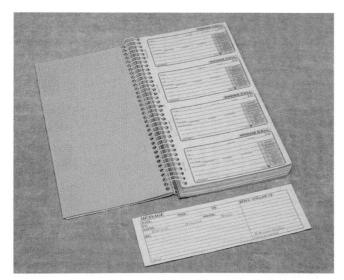

Figure 12-3 Message pads with a carbon allow the office to maintain a written record of all incoming calls.

cian's desk. The physician cannot discuss the patient's condition or answer questions without this information.

Procedure 12-3 identifies the steps and rationale in taking a telephone message.

Ending the Call

Ending the telephone call is as important as answering the call promptly. Bring the conversation to a courteous close and repeat any pertinent information back to the caller. ("Your appointment is scheduled for Friday, January 12, at 9 AM with Doctor King.") Pause just a moment to see if the caller has any additional questions. If not, say "Good-bye." Never use slang terms such as *bye-bye, see you later,* or *so long.* These terms do not reflect a positive professional image. You should always stay on the line until the caller hangs up. The caller might think of something else he or she wanted to ask or verify, and staying on the line gives the caller the opportunity to verbalize a thought rather than have to call back.

TYPES OF CALLS THE MEDICAL ASSISTANT CAN TAKE

Keep in mind that, no matter how experienced, the medical assistant has definite limitations of authority and knowledge. Most calls can be handled by the knowledgeable medical assistant, but there are situations that only the physician should manage simply because the physician ultimately is responsible for what happens in the practice. Examples of calls the medical assistant can take are as follows:

1. Established patients: When an established patient calls to set up an appointment, record the patient's name, daytime telephone number, and the reason for the appointment.
2. New patients: Require the same information as the established patient plus some additional information, including:

   - Address
   - Age/birth date
   - Employer
   - Insurance carrier or HMO
   - Insurance ID number of subscriber
   - Name of insured (self, spouse, or parent)
   - Name of referral source

   This information serves as a source for the establishment of the chart and may lead to a discussion regarding payment of fees. The information should be entered into the appointment book for both new and established patients.

3. Scheduling appointments: A major portion of telephone communications is spent scheduling patient appointments. See Chapter 13 for detailed information on patient scheduling and rescheduling.

4. Scheduling patient tests: Scheduling tests for patients can involve a great deal of coordination. Often appointment times need to be arranged among physicians, the patient, and the facility where a test may be conducted.

5. Billing questions: Billing questions can be involved and complex, and medical assistants should be prepared to answer questions by retrieving information on the patient's insurance and billing status.

6. Insurance information: Calls will come from patients about insurance, as well as from insurance carriers and HMOs with questions about patients or their treatment. If the call is from an insurance company or HMO, be sure there is a signed Release of Information in the patient's chart before giving information.

7. Requests for prescription refills: If a patient or family member is requesting that a prescription be refilled, medical assistants may take the call. However, they may not authorize a refill or tell the patient that a prescription will be refilled without the physician's approval. Most offices ask that the patient call their refill requests into the pharmacy; the pharmacy then calls or faxes the physician's office for approval. Messages taken on these calls should be attached to the patient's chart and given to the physician for review and for permission to refill. When the physician approves the refill, the pharmacy may be called with an approval. Some policies give authority to the CMA to refill standard medications with appropriate guidelines, for example, oral contraceptives, blood pressure medications, among others. Procedure 12-4 identifies the steps for calling a pharmacy to refill an authorized prescription.

8. Receiving routine progress reports: Frequently, physicians will ask patients to report on their progress. *If the patient is doing well,* it is acceptable for you to take that information on a message form to be given to the physician.

9. General information about the practice: People may call requesting information about hours, location, financial policies, or areas of practice.

10. Salespeople: The medical office should have policies regarding the scheduling of pharmaceutical and medical supply representatives.

TYPES OF CALLS REFERRED TO THE PHYSICIAN

Examples of calls that should be referred to the physician are as follows:

1. Requests for test results: Only the physician should give this information. A seemingly simple report may frighten or confuse the patient; at the very least it will probably generate questions that medical assistants are not qualified to answer. Many physicians allow medical assistants to report on satisfactory test results; always follow office policy.

2. Medical emergencies: There should be standard procedures for dealing with emergencies. The physician, when present, should be interrupted and notified of all emergency calls.

3. Medical questions: Medical assistants may not give medical advice without risking practicing without a license. Standing orders should correspond with written office policy.

4. Other physicians: When other physicians call, always ask if they need to speak to the physician immediately or if they would like a call back. Be sure to ask if the call is regarding a patient; if so, attach a message to the chart.

5. Patients who refuse information: If a patient will not provide information about a problem, take a message for the physician to call them back. Some patients are not comfortable discussing physical problems with anyone except the physician; they have a right to that privacy.

6. Complaints about medical treatment or care: In a medical office, all patient complaints should be viewed as potential malpractice suits. A patient with complaints about the office or the quality of care is best referred to the physician.

7. Poor progress reports: If a patient calls to report that a treatment regimen is not working, the information should be given to the physician immediately. Changes in the treatment or medication may need to be made, or the patient may need to be seen right away. This is a medical judgment that medical assistants are not qualified to make.

8. Requests for patient information from a third party: Unless there is a signed release, patient information may not be given to anyone. Any such requests (other than from the patient's insurance carrier or HMO) must be referred to the physician.

9. Requests for referrals (unless the physician has given the front office a list of specialists to use).

10. Requests for medication (other than standard refills).

SPECIAL CONSIDERATION CALLS

 Answering the telephone in an ambulatory care setting thrusts the medical assistant into contact with a variety of callers: those needing referrals to other facilities; emergency calls; callers who may be angry, older, or speak English as a second language. As a professional, your goal is to treat every individual with courtesy and respect and to respond to their queries appropriately or to transfer the caller to another team member who can assist.

Referral Calls to Other Facilities

If it is necessary to refer the caller to someone outside the office, such as to a laboratory or another physician, be sure to tell the caller:

- Why they should speak to someone else

- The telephone number to call (be sure to include the area code and extension)

- Who, specifically, to speak with at that number

- What information to have ready when they make the call

- When to call

- If you would like a call back after the other contact is made

Study the example of calls to other facilities.

Emergency/Urgent Calls

An emergency is a serious or life-threatening condition in which the patient requires immediate medical assistance that may or may not be delivered by the ambulatory care setting because of time constraints or because a hospital would be better equipped to handle the emergency. Tell the caller to hang up and call 911 immediately. It is appropriate to ask for a caller's name and telephone number so that you can dial 911 for the caller who is a child or seems confused or unable to dial for himself or herself. Keep the caller on the line and use another line to call 911. Then connect the two calls so the information exchange can take place. Be sure to have the patient's name and number in case they are disconnected. Sound judgment must always be used when making such decisions.

Triage is the act of evaluating the urgency of a medical situation and prioritizing treatment. Keep in mind that most patients when ill or injured, or if a family member is calling about a patient who is ill or injured, feel the situation requires immediate medical attention. Triage is one of the most important functions for the person answering the telephone. Triage requires skill and experience. An urgent condition is one that requires medical intervention that can be handled in a timely manner at an ambulatory care center.

To determine if a call is truly a medical emergency, keep a list of questions near the telephone to assist in evaluating the situation. Standard triage questions can determine the nature of an emergency. Not all questions are appropriate to every call; suitable questions depend

---

EXAMPLE: CALLS TO OTHER FACILITIES

Herb Fowler needs to have a glucose tolerance test done at the laboratory next door and make an appointment in your office for one week after the test is done.

Poor Technique

Medical Assistant: Mr. Fowler, you need to call Johnston Labs to arrange for those tests. We'll see you after the tests are done.

Correct Technique

Medical Assistant: Mr. Fowler, Dr. King has ordered a glucose tolerance test for you with Johnston Laboratory in Suite 516 of this building. Since you are working, we felt it would be better to have you call them yourself to make the appointment. If you have a paper and pencil, I'll give you the information you need.

The lab is open from 6:30 AM to 7 PM Monday through Friday. The phone number is (800) 555-1234 and you should ask for Susan at Extension 23; she makes the appointments. She will need your name, address, phone number, age, Social Security number, the name and address of your insurance company, and your insurance ID and Plan numbers.

After you make your appointment with Susan, please call me back so we can make an appointment for you here for one week later. Dr. King will have your test results by then and will want to go over them with you at that time.

Do you have any questions or do you need any of the information repeated? Fine, I'll speak to you after you talk to Susan and we'll set up your appointment with Dr. King.

on the nature of the situation. Triage questions to ask may include:

- What happened?
- Who is the patient? (Ask name and age.)
- Is the patient breathing?
- Is there bleeding? How much? From where?
- Is the patient conscious?
- What is the patient's temperature?
- If the patient ingested something:
  - What did the patient take?
  - How much?
  - Are there poison or overdose instructions on the bottle?

Triage does not only pertain to emergency calls. Triage techniques can also help determine when a patient with symptoms should be seen by asking the caller questions such as:

- How long have you had the symptoms?
- Is there any fever?
- Are you taking any medications?

This information helps determine whether an appointment should be scheduled immediately or if it can wait a few days.

 The practice should periodically review procedures for handling emergency/urgent calls. If an office situation involves a great deal of telephone triage, the staff should enroll in an advanced first-aid course. This will enable all participants to more accurately give instructions or to handle these calls if there is no physician in the office at that moment. In-service training provided by the physicians is a great tool to make telephone triage run smoothly. Remember, you should only render aid *within the areas of your training and expertise*. **Good Samaritan laws** do not cover paid employees, only uncompensated situations. All ambulatory settings should also post a list of numbers to be used in case of emergencies, such as the poison control telephone number. See Chapter 9 for more information on triage.

Angry Callers

Medical assistants will probably have occasion to speak with callers who are angry or upset. Though these calls may eventually need to be referred to the office manager

or the physician, medical assistants need techniques for managing problem calls.

 The first priority is to diffuse the situation. This cannot be accomplished if you become angry or upset. As a professional, it is important to remain calm and in control at all times. Like most skills, diffusing a difficult situation becomes easier with practice. See Procedure 12-4.

Older Adult Callers

There are several issues that may arise when dealing with older adult patients, such as impaired hearing, confusion, and an inability to understand procedures or technical information.

Do not assume that all older adults are senile or hard of hearing. This is a dangerous pitfall into which many people stumble.

If the individual has a hearing impairment, speak more slowly, more clearly, and a little louder than normal. Do not shout. If uncertain that the person has heard everything, ask if there are any questions, or ask the person to repeat information back to you.

If the person has difficulty understanding you, simplify the information, ask frequently if there are any questions, and try to explain in simple, concrete terms. At times, if it is difficult to communicate with an older adult patient, someone from the patient's family should be given certain information. Discuss this option with the office manager or physician first, and be sure signed documentation is on file.

English as a Second Language Callers

 In any ambulatory care setting, it is possible to have contact with many patients whose primary language is not English.

It is extremely helpful to have at least one person in the office who is bilingual, particularly in an area such as the Southwest where many people speak a language other than English. For the nonbilingual medical assistant, certain techniques may help when communicating with all but totally non-English speaking patients.

- A patient who does not *speak* **fluent** English may still *understand* as well as anyone. Do not assume that individuals with strong accents cannot understand you.
- Speak at a normal volume; raising the voice does not increase the other person's ability to comprehend.
- If the other person has difficulty understanding, speak more slowly. Avoid complicated words when simple ones will express the meaning just as well.

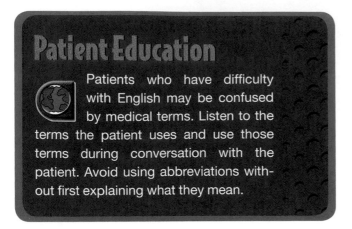

- Ask the person if clarification is needed. Be willing to review the information again.

- Be patient.

If these techniques are not successful, it is the responsibility of your physician–employer to provide an interpreter (who may or may not be a member of the patient's family) if necessary.

PLACING OUTGOING CALLS

When making calls for the medical office, whether to patients, health care facilities, or other physicians, know what information is needed and have it at hand before making the calls.

For example:

- If arranging for a patient to receive care at another facility, have the patient's chart and insurance information. Determine physician instructions as to the diagnosis and type of care (specific tests, radiographs, and so on) that need to be ordered.

- If calling insurance companies for claim follow-up, gather copies of all claim forms in question so you can answer specific questions regarding each claim.

- If scheduling meetings or outside appointments for office physicians, have their schedules in front of you.

Arrange to make outgoing calls from a telephone in a location that is free of distractions. If the calls concern patients (whether bills, insurance, or care), it is mandatory that the calls be made from a telephone where you cannot be overheard by other patients or people in the reception area.

Always choose a time when calls can be made without interruption. Arrange for someone else to cover incoming calls during this period and to take messages on any calls that you need to handle personally.

It is best to establish a routine for making various types of outgoing calls. Most offices call the next day's patients to confirm appointments near the end of each day. Collection and insurance calls, as well as pharmacy callbacks, are usually done either before the office is open for patients in the morning, during the period from noon to 2 PM when the office is closed for lunch, or after the last patient has been seen. Procedure 12-5 summarizes guidelines for placing outgoing calls.

PLACING LONG-DISTANCE CALLS

Placing Calls

Most long-distance calls medical assistants make are likely to be direct dialing calls; that is, calls placed without the help of an operator. To direct dial a local long-distance call, which is a call within the area code but out of the local calling area, dial 1 plus the telephone number; in some parts of the country, it is no longer necessary to dial 1 before the seven-digit telephone number.

For long-distance calls out of the area code, dial 1 plus area code plus telephone number. Nationwide area codes are usually listed in your telephone directory before alphabetical entries. When giving another party the medical office number, always include the area code. Many clinics issue scan numbers to staff allowing them to dial long-distance numbers directly. Without the scan number, employees are not authorized to make long-distance phone calls using clinic telephones. Be sure to use 800 or toll-free numbers whenever possible to minimize expense.

When it is necessary to make an operator-assisted call, dial 0 plus area code plus telephone number. Operator-assisted calls, many of which are automated, include collect calls, person-to-person calls, and occasionally credit card calls.

Time Zones

When making a long-distance call out of the area code, it is likely that a time zone change may occur (Figure 12-4). When scheduling the day's calls, it is important to

Critical Thinking

Your office is located in Seattle, WA, and you are calling Charleston, NC. What are some important considerations before placing the call?

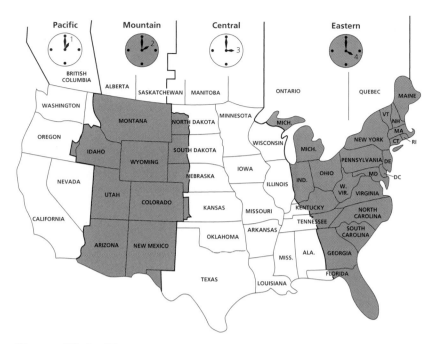

Figure 12-4   Time zone map.

keep in mind the location of the call and plan accordingly. Time zones include Pacific, Mountain, Central, and Eastern times and usually span a three-hour difference. If it is noon in New York, it is 11 AM in Illinois, 10 AM in Arizona, and 9 AM in Washington state.

Long-Distance Carriers

Many companies, some well-known, others new to the market, are competing for long-distance business. Judging the offers and services of long-distance companies can be a complex task, but a wise choice can save an ambulatory care setting hundreds of dollars a year or more in telephone charges. It is important to analyze the medical office long-distance requirements, and then make comparisons among several long-distance companies. Company representatives are usually more than willing to discuss their services in light of specific needs to help you comparison shop. The decision of which service to use will usually be made by the physicians and the office manager with feedback from all employees.

TELEPHONE DOCUMENTATION

Requests for medical information over the telephone should be discouraged. A physician or facility that needs the information to treat the patient usually places an emergency request. A call-back verification procedure should be implemented for this type of request. Request the caller's name and telephone number, and state that you will call back with the necessary information. Then call back to verify the identity of the caller and provide or fax the information. It is important to follow this procedure during routine telephone interchanges that take place between facilities/provider offices and laboratories seeking test results or consult findings.

All telephone requests for medical information should be documented either in a log reserved for that purpose or in the patient's medical record. This information is important in case of litigation to protect yourself and the medical practice. Documentation includes the following:

- Date of the request
- Name of the requestor
- The information requested
- Patient's name (and patient number)
- Name of the treating physician
- The information released
- To whom the call was referred (if applicable)

When a patient telephones the office to request prescription refills, is displeased with medical treatment, or expresses some form of a complaint, documentation of the call should always be recorded in the medical chart.

USING TELEPHONE DIRECTORIES

The medical assistant should have on hand in the office a variety of telephone directories and be skilled in their use. The telephone directory contains an organized, accurate, and complete listing of the name, address, zip code, and area code with telephone number for most individuals with telephone service. Often, the pages within the directory are color-coded; residences are listed on white pages, business numbers on blue pages, and advertisements on yellow pages. The front pages of many directories contain other useful information such as:

- Information that provides emergency and non-emergency numbers.

- The Internet guide makes it easy to get on-line.

- Information guide and consumer tips provide a variety of free facts and answers about the things you want to buy and the services you need.

- Community pages provide attractions, events, and the general-interest information unique to a particular area. Often, maps are provided on these pages.

- Phone service pages answer questions you may have regarding your phone service.

- Government pages contain information about county, state, tribal, and federal government office, as well as information regarding public schools and voter registration information.

- An index makes finding what you need easy.

Many metropolitan medical centers and hospitals produce another type of directory. These directories list important telephone numbers specific to that facility. Examples of information available within these directories include:

- Physician referral information

- Community education services

- Nurse counseling service/nurse line

- Main hospital/facility telephone number

- Automated operator

- TTY line for the hearing impaired

- Medical center departments

- Medical staff including department and photo of physicians and their names with credentials

Some of these publications list physicians no longer maintaining their active/associate privileges at the facility. Often, a map of the facility is included within the front or back pages. The large facilities also may produce supplements to maintain current information.

Many online telephone directory services are also helpful resources. Examples of these include but are not limited to the following:
http://www.yellowpages.com
http://www.dexonline.com
http://www.realpages.com
http://www.switchboard.com
http://www.smartpages.com
http://www.whitepages.com
http://www.anywho.com

LEGAL AND ETHICAL CONSIDERATIONS

 Two of the most important issues in the medical setting are patient confidentiality and right to privacy. Respecting the confidentiality of all patient information is a legal and ethical obligation. No information about patients is to be discussed outside the office, with family or friends, or with other patients. Violations of confidentiality leave you and your physician open to lawsuits. More importantly, they are violations of patient trust.

When calling patients, whether to discuss treatment or finances, do so with respect for the patient's privacy at all times. The front desk is certainly not the place to make collection calls when other patients are in the reception room. Either make calls from another location or choose a time when other patients cannot overhear you. Always be aware of the surroundings and who may be able to overhear conversations.

There are many situations when individuals will call the office to discuss a patient. Parents, spouses, grandparents, other relatives, significant others, employers, and friends often will have questions about a patient's condition or finances. Usually these people are asking questions out of genuine concern and a desire to help. The information they request may seem harmless, but discussing anything about a patient can turn into an ethical and legal issue. See text box examples on the following page regarding legal and ethical considerations.

To ensure patient confidentiality and practice sensible risk management, never discuss a patient with:

- The patient's spouse or family, without specific permission and a signed release

- The patient's employer

- Insurance carriers, HMOs, or attorneys without a signed release

- Credit bureau/collection agency (reporting a patient to a credit bureau or collection agency is a violation of confidentiality)

- Other patients

- People outside the office (friends, family, acquaintances)

When necessary for medical or administrative reasons, you can discuss a patient with:

- Members of the office staff as necessary to the patient's care

- The patient's insurance carrier or HMO, if you have a signed release

- The patient's attorney (usually in accident or Workers' Compensation cases), if you have a signed release

- The patient's parent or legal guardian, except concerning issues of birth control, abortion, HIV, or

sexually transmitted disease (check the laws in each state regarding minors' right to privacy)

- Another health care provider (physician, laboratory, or hospital) that is providing care to the patient under orders from the patient's physician

- Referring physician's office

HIPAA GUIDELINES FOR TELEPHONE COMMUNICATIONS

 The following guidelines should be followed when communicating information to patients by telephone:

- Determine whether the patient has requested confidential communications. Specific instructions should be provided to staff members on how to determine whether the patient has requested and been granted special conditions for keeping communications with the medical practice confidential.

- If the patient has not requested confidential communication, the patient should simply be called at the normal phone number contained in his or her records. If the patient has requested confidential communications and has provided an alternative telephone number, care should be taken to ensure that only the alternative number is called.

- The caller should identify himself or herself by name and say that he or she is an employee of the medical practice (use the complete official name of the practice).

- If the patient is not available, it is acceptable to leave a live or recorded message asking the patient to return the call. Leave the telephone number, and if the medical practice is returning a call made by the patient, it is acceptable to state this in the message that is left for the patient. However, it is important that the messages do not contain any medical information or mention the purpose of the call. Never leave messages containing test results.

EXAMPLES: LEGAL AND ETHICAL CONSIDERATIONS

Situation 1

A medical assistant called the home of a patient inquiring about the delinquent status of his account. The patient was not home, but his wife answered the phone. The medical assistant discussed the situation with the patient's wife, who wanted to know what the charges were for. On checking the file, it was discovered the patient had been tested for a sexually transmitted disease.

Situation 2

A patient's employer calls to find out "how Boris is doing and when he can come back to work. We really miss that guy!" The medical assistant, who just saw Boris in the reception area yesterday, responds without thinking, "Oh, he seems to be doing great, I'll bet you'll have him back in a few days." If he or she had checked the patient chart, he or she might have seen that Boris was filing a disability claim, as well as a negligence suit against the employer for unsafe working conditions. The medical assistant might also have seen that Boris is still in physical therapy and on pain medication, or that he may have permanent problems as a result of the accident.

HIPAA regulations specify that information is to be kept to the minimum necessary. It is all right to leave a voice mail message reminding patients of an appointment because the date, time, and name of the doctor do not disclose protected information to unauthorized individuals. This also holds true for postcard reminders.

- When the patient is contacted, it is acceptable to discuss his or her medical information over the telephone. It is critical, however, that test results and other protected health information (PHI) *not* be given to anyone other than the patient or a person designated as the patient's representative.

AMERICANS WITH DISABILITIES ACT

The ADA requires that communication procedures are available for persons with disabilities. Combined with HIPAA requirements, this presents a challenging situation in dealing with patients who are deaf or hearing impaired. The act requires that health care providers give effective communication alternatives using auxiliary aids and services that ensure that communication to people with hearing loss is equal to others without this disability. This includes both patients, as well as caregivers of patients, guardians, or spouses.

Alternative devices or services include interpreters for individuals with a language problem, assistive hearing devices, note takers for individuals who have difficulty writing, written materials, and so forth. The health care provider can choose the device as long as the result is effective communication. The deaf or hard of hearing patient should be consulted on which device he or she finds to be most effective. The cost of alternative devices or services cannot be billed to the patient. The expense must be charged against the overhead of the clinic or practice.

Telephone service for hearing-impaired patients is required by the ADA. Many hearing-impaired individuals use a TTY device, which transmits a keyed-in message to a relay operator provided by the telecommunications company. That person relays an oral message to the hearing person. The only requirement is that the person in the clinic uses the relay operator when initiating a call to the hearing-impaired patient. In some instances, the office may have to provide a TTY device for the hearing-impaired patients if they are required to make calls to your office.

TELEPHONE TECHNOLOGY

Though much of this chapter has been dedicated to the interpersonal nature of telephone communications, astute medical assistants will also investigate and become knowledgeable about the technology of telecommunications.

Ongoing advances in telecommunications have had a tremendous impact on how the staff of a medical office communicates both within the office and with patients, hospitals, and others outside the office. These advances include telephone systems with automated routing units; electronic transmissions (fax and e-mail); cellular telephones; and paging systems.

Automated Routing Units

Many hospitals and larger ambulatory care settings have **automated routing unit (ARU)** telephone systems to manage heavy telephone traffic. The system answers the call, and a recorded voice identifies departments or services the caller can access by pressing a specified number on the Touch-Tone telephone. If callers indicate they are having a medical emergency, the system can be programmed to immediately route calls to the medical assistant. This saves patients with immediate medical problems from waiting during busy telephone times.

Some automated telephone systems have electronic mailboxes so the caller can leave a message if the person they are calling is unavailable. In many ARU systems, selecting any of the numbered choices often gives the caller a second, third, or fourth menu of choices. If the caller does not select an option, the ARU will usually switch the call automatically to a live operator.

A disadvantage with ARU systems is that the recorded voice may be difficult to hear, especially for older adult or hearing-impaired patients. Many patients may not understand the recorded options. Offices with an ARU system should provide to all patients an information sheet

---

When contacting a patient via telephone, it is acceptable to discuss his or her medical information once it has been ascertained that you are talking with the patient. Verifying Social Security number, birth date, or patient ID number are means of identifying individuals. Test results and other PHI must not be given to anyone other than the patient. However, if a designated patient representative has been established, PHI may be shared with that individual.

Critical Thinking

Your office has just installed an automated telephone answering system. What steps might you take to aid your patients in understanding and using the system properly?

explaining their options when calling the office and how to get through to the office quickly in an emergency.

Answering Services and Machines

One responsibility of the office manager/medical assistant is to ensure that patient calls are answered after office hours, both on evenings and weekends. Whereas in smaller ambulatory care settings it may not be possible to have staff on telephone duty 24 hours a day, nonetheless calls must be answered and messages taken. **Answering services**—typically staffed by a live operator—and answering machines are two methods of taking calls after hours.

Many ambulatory care centers favor answering services because a live operator is reassuring to patients and other callers. These services also can provide flexibility in routing calls and locating the physician for emergencies. Typically, fees for answering services are by the month or by the number of calls.

Answering machines are convenient but perhaps less reassuring for the caller. The machine must be checked frequently for messages should an emergency occur. Sometimes, the message may leave a telephone number where the physician can be reached, but this system is likely to be cumbersome, for too many nonemergency calls may be directed to the physician. If an answering machine is used, the message often contains a number, other than the physician's, that callers can use for emergencies. That call is answered by a live operator who then screens and refers the call appropriately. See Procedure 12-6 for instructions on recording a message on an answering device.

Facsimile (Fax) Machines

Fax machines are becoming more and more common in the ambulatory care setting as they are used to send reports, referrals, insurance approvals, and informal correspondence. A **fax** is a **facsimile** transmission sent over telephone lines from one fax machine to another or from a modem to a fax machine. A fax document may contain data such as typed characters, photographs, or line art.

 Although fax machines are a great time-saver for the ambulatory care setting, confidentiality is a critical issue because fax machines are typically located in centralized areas where documents may be seen by unauthorized personnel. Before sending any document, be sure it will not violate confidentiality, have permission to transmit it by fax, and attach a cover sheet that stipulates the information is for the intended recipient only. Review fax machine information presented in Chapter 15.

Electronic Mail

 Electronic mail (e-mail) is the process of sending, receiving, storing, and forwarding messages in digital form over computer networks. E-mail saves time and money and eliminates having to leave a phone message and the risk for missing a return call, making it the method of choice for many interoffice communications. E-mail is a non–real-time method of communication—it permits us to leave a message at our convenience and allows the other person to read and respond at their convenience. E-mails can be sent to multiple people at the same time, something a traditional telephone call does not allow. Keep in mind, however, that there is a professional e-mail etiquette that must be adhered to. It is not acceptable to forward e-mail messages without the permission of the original author, and caution must be taken to avoid sending information that is not appropriate in a professional setting.

Clinical e-mail is becoming increasingly common as a means of communication between patients and their primary care physician. It is typically used for communication that is not considered urgent or in situations that may cause the communication to continue over a period of time. Scheduling appointments, sending reminder appointment notices, providing follow-up instructions, explaining general medical information, answering questions regarding billing procedures, and refilling prescriptions are current procedures handled by clinical e-mail.

When using clinical e-mail, it is important for the physician to remember that the same ethical responsibilities to patients must be adhered to as for other types of encounters. The same standard of professionalism must also be satisfied. Together with the convenience offered through e-mail communications come some risks. Fortunately, following specific guidelines for use of clinical e-mail can minimize risks to a level considered acceptable by many practices.

Basically, the following three risks or concerns must be addressed when using clinical e-mail:

* E-mail communication should be limited to current patients, meaning patients who have been examined for a specific condition within the last six months. Forwarding e-mail to the physician from persons with whom no patient–physician relationship has been established exposes the physician to potential disciplinary or legal actions and should not be practiced.

- E-mail communication should be limited to patients within the state in which the physician is licensed to practice. This also applies to patients who have moved to other jurisdictions. Patients who are traveling also cause some risk for disciplinary action, and the medical assistant should be sure the physician is aware of the patient's location status.

- Persons other than the intended recipient can read e-mail if the target computer does not have adequate password protection. Anyone can log on to an unprotected computer and read e-mail, resulting in unauthorized dissemination of medical records and violation of HIPAA regulations. (Review Chapters 11 and 15 for additional information regarding computer security and HIPAA regulations.)

Patients who meet criteria for e-mail correspondence established by the practice should be identified, and an informed consent form should be signed by each patient desiring this mode of communication. The form may be part of the form used for handling release of PHI. The form should provide instructions to the patient in the secure use of e-mail, the security risks involved, practice e-mail communication policy, the fee charged for e-mail correspondence if any, and a disclaimer absolving the practice in the event of patient noncompliance or technical failure in the system. The original signed form should be filed in the patient chart and a copy given to the patient for their records.

To limit legal or disciplinary exposure, the practice should include the following restrictions when establishing the e-mail criteria:

- Patients should reside within the state in which the physician is licensed to practice.

- Consultations should be limited to conditions or problems for which the patient has been examined within the last six months.

- New prescriptions should not be provided via e-mail.

- E-mail should never be used to discuss HIV test results or treatment, mental conditions, drug or alcohol treatment, or any addiction.

A procedure should be established to automatically respond to the patients' e-mail messages informing them they have been received. The patient should also be requested to respond to your messages acknowledging

Critical Thinking

What legal and ethical issues should be considered when using clinical e-mail? How might the medical facility protect its employees and the patient with regard to clinical e-mail use?

their receipt. An automatic receipt option is available under the tools menu of most e-mail software.

All e-mail correspondence should have an electronic signature and a reminder of security guidelines. This includes informing unauthorized recipients that the information is confidential and that they should notify the sender of the unauthorized release. In the event of unauthorized receipt, the patient should be notified immediately.

E-mail communications allows the patient to self-document or describe in their own words the nature of the situation, which is critical for the integrity of the medical record. A copy of all e-mail messages between patients and physicians should be retained in the patients' charts for future reference.

Instant Messaging

Instant messaging (IM) is becoming a popular method of communication in workplace settings. Instant messaging is similar to e-mail except it is a real-time medium, meaning communications are sent instantly back and forth from one IM user to another. Typically, IM clients such as MSN Messenger, AOL Instant Messenger, and ICQ have a list of the people with whom they communicate regularly. If the user is currently on-line, they will be listed as active and ready to receive messages. This is a great way to quickly and directly communicate with someone without having to use telephones. See Figure 12-5 for a screen capture of IM.

Most medical clinics, hospitals, and ancillary services have a campus or office network that provides access to e-mail, IM, and the Internet. Smaller offices may need to subscribe to an Internet Service Provider (ISP) to have e-mail access. The largest ISPs are America Online, MSN, and Earthlink.

Interactive Videoconferencing

Interactive videoconferencing consultation permits a physician at a remote location to practice telemedicine and avail themselves of the services of a specialist at a large medical center, university, or teaching hospital. Utilizing the Internet, computer, and real-time transmission of patient observations, the

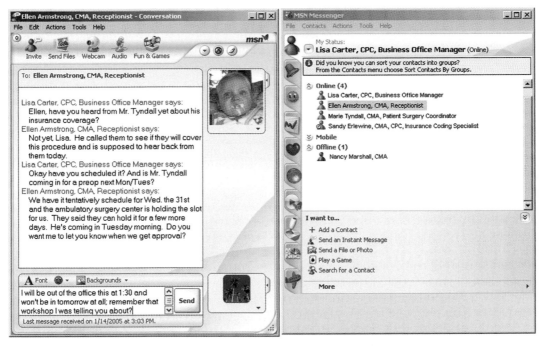

Figure 12-5 Instant Message screen capture.

specialist can examine the patient as if he or she were present in the specialist's examination room. Special stethoscopes, digitized radiographs and electrocardiograms, and digital videos are examples of equipment used to bring the specialist all the information required to make a diagnosis. A technician or a physician assistant is present with the patient and performs the tests and transmits observations viewed by the specialist in real time. The conference is frequently videotaped for future review by either the specialist or local provider.

 Care must be exercised when implementing interactive videoconferencing to ensure HIPAA compliance. The procedures outlined in Chapter 11 should be followed; in addition, the taped record of the conference must be protected and erased after reports have been written. The patient must also give written consent before interactive videoconferencing begins.

Cellular Service

Since the 1980s, **cellular telephones** have become increasingly popular and are now available and used in all populated areas of the country. Cellular communication offers convenient and flexible communication. The telephones themselves are available in many models and sizes and some can even fit in the palm of the hand. Many physicians have car and portable phones, allowing immediate verbal contact with their office or hospital staff.

 Cellular signals are not secure, which means that other people may be able to listen to the conversations with certain scanning radios. Therefore, staff and physicians should be careful not to use patients' full names or reveal any confidential information over the cellular phone.

Paging Systems

Another telecommunication option available is the use of **pagers** or beepers. Hospitals have used paging systems for many years both inside the hospital and for physicians on call. Several types of paging systems are available, and many physicians now use the same type of pagers available to individual consumers. Some paging system options include:

1. Voice alerts. The voice message is automatically heard by the person being paged. Not only does the person being paged hear the message, but anyone in the vicinity will hear it as well.
2. Beep alerts. The pager emits a beeping sound or silent vibration that notifies the person being paged to call a designated phone number to obtain the message.
3. Digital message display.
   a. Alphanumeric display: It displays the message on a digital screen. The message can include an entire typed message via a computer modem or

through an operator who will input the message and transmit it to the receiver. The receiver can scroll through the text message and save or delete messages as needed.

b. Numeric display: It displays the callback telephone number on small screen. The number displayed is selected by the person initiating the page.

Pagers are not always as convenient as cellular phones because about half allow only one-way communication. Two-way pagers are quickly gaining in popularity.

PROFESSIONALISM IN TELECOMMUNICATIONS

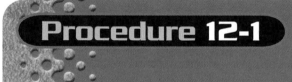

Professionalism in telecommunications is crucial in the medical office environment. The way in which the telephone is answered either conveys a message of sincerity to help or a message of interruption. Callers expect to have the phone answered in a professional manner and their concerns addressed promptly. Forwarding calls to someone else in the office who is more specialized in the callers' questions area and following up to see that the situation was resolved is evidence of a responsible attitude and of being a team player. One should always be courteous and diplomatic and work within the scope of one's education, training, ability, and legal boundaries.

Remember that personal telephone calls, other than emergency calls, should be avoided during working hours. When speaking with patients or other health care members, slang terms should not be used. Never eat or chew gum while answering the telephone. When completing a call, say "good-bye" and allow the caller to hang up before you do.

Additional attributes of professionalism include using appropriate guidelines when releasing information. Confidentiality issues must always be followed, as well as being aware of any ethical or legal responsibilities. Documentation is mandatory for follow-up care and for any legal implications. Continued education is important to stay on the leading edge of new technologies being implemented in the area of telecommunications.

Procedure 12-1 — Answering and Screening Incoming Calls

PURPOSE:
To answer telephone calls professionally, acquiring all necessary information from the caller, documenting it correctly, and properly acting on it.

EQUIPMENT/SUPPLIES:
Telephone
Appointment calendar
Message pad
Pen or pencil
Notepad

PROCEDURE STEPS:
1. Be prepared. Have materials such as a message pad, notepad, appointment calendar, sharpened pencils, and working pens nearby. RATIONALE: Being ready for calls conveys professionalism and lets the caller know you are prepared to assist.

2. Answer the telephone promptly. The phone should not ring more than three times before it is answered. RATIONALE: Callers may become annoyed and hang up if a call is not answered within a reasonable time.

3. Answer the call with the preferred office greeting, speaking directly into the mouthpiece. The mouthpiece should be 1 to 2 inches away from the mouth. For example, "Good morning. Doctors Lewis and King. Ellen speaking." RATIONALE: Take a breath before answering the phone, put a smile on your face, and use a pleasant tone of voice to convey a warm greet-

(continues)

Procedure 12-1 (continued)

ing. Holding the phone correctly and speaking directly into the mouthpiece aid the caller in hearing your message clearly.

4. Ask the name of the caller as quickly as possible, and determine if this is an emergency call. RATIONALE: Using the caller's name personalizes the call and acknowledges that you heard the name correctly. If this is an emergency call, follow emergency protocols.

5. Focus on the call. The caller may want to schedule an appointment, in which case you will need additional information to determine urgency and length of time required. RATIONALE: This gives the caller a sense that you are listening attentively, and information will be transmitted correctly.

6. Repeat information back to the caller. RATIONALE: This technique confirms facts are complete and accurate. The caller also has an opportunity to hear the message and confirm that it is accurate or may wish to modify the message meaning for clarity.

7. Follow written established triage protocols when screening telephone calls. RATIONALE: Assures that you are working within the scope of your training and that all pertinent information is collected.

8. When using a multiline telephone as shown in Figure 12-6, it is helpful to keep a notepad by the telephone. When you answer the phone and have the caller's name, jot down the name, which line the caller is on, and some quick notes about the content of the call. RATIONALE: Using this simple technique avoids problems if another line rings and you must put the first person on hold. No matter how many incoming lines there are, you will not forget who is on which line or what the call is about.

9. Ask if the caller has any other questions. RATIONALE: This saves you and the caller time. It is frustrating to have to place a second call because you forgot to ask something. It also ties up the telephone lines.

10. End the call courteously. Say "thank you" and "good-bye" (not "bye-bye"). RATIONALE: Saying good-bye conveys professionalism and leaves the caller with a positive image of the office.

11. Let the caller hang up before you disconnect. RATIONALE: Often callers think of questions just as they are ready to hang up. It is more time efficient to handle the question immediately rather than have the caller make another call.

12. Document information and record any future necessary actions. RATIONALE: This procedure is necessary for legal reasons. Remember, a deed not documented is a deed undone in a court of law.

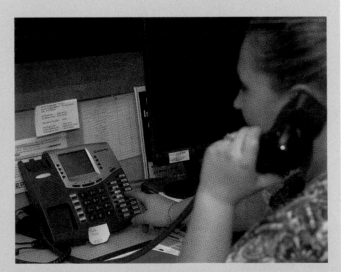

Figure 12-6 An example of a multiline telephone system.

Procedure 12-2 — Transferring a Call

PURPOSE:
To transfer a caller directly to the individual that can best solve the problem in an efficient and professional manner.

EQUIPMENT/SUPPLIES:
Telephone
Message pad
Black ink pen
Notepad
Interoffice telephone directory

PROCEDURE STEPS:
1. Answer the call following the steps outlined in Procedure 12-1. RATIONALE: Being ready for calls conveys professionalism. It confirms that the caller has reached the dialed number and to whom they are speaking.
2. Obtain the name and telephone number of the individual calling, and jot down notes regarding the situation/problem. RATIONALE: Provides you with appropriate information to forward to the transferee.
3. Determine the best person to assist this caller. RATIONALE: The situation/problem should be solved with only one transfer whenever possible.

This saves time in the long run and promotes positive public relations.
4. Ask the caller if you may put them on hold while you collect pertinent data, and then confirm that the best person suited to handle the problem is available. RATIONALE: Gives you an opportunity to collect any appropriate information and to determine if the correct person to assist the caller has been identified. They may direct you to someone else or may not be available.
5. Return to the caller and thank them for holding. RATIONALE: Expresses courtesy and promotes positive public relations.
6. Give the caller the name and extension of the person to whom you are transferring them. RATIONALE: If the transfer does not go through properly, the caller knows who to call directly.
7. Follow your telephone system's procedure for transferring the call. RATIONALE: Assures accurate transfer of calls.
8. Follow up to be sure the call transferred correctly. RATIONALE: Promotes positive public relations.

Procedure 12-3 — Taking a Telephone Message

PURPOSE:
To record an accurate telephone message and follow up as required.

EQUIPMENT/SUPPLIES:
Telephone
Message pad
Black ink pen
Notepad
Clock or watch

PROCEDURE STEPS:
1. Answer the telephone following the steps outlined in Procedure 12-1. RATIONALE: Being prepared and answering the phone promptly with the preferred office greeting prepares the medical assistant mentally to focus on the caller's needs. Using a pleasant tone of voice conveys a warm greeting.

(continues)

Procedure 12-3 (continued)

2. Using a message pad, take the telephone message, being sure to gather the following information:
   - Date and time call is received
   - Name of person calling, daytime and evening telephone number, including area code and extension when appropriate
   - Who the call is for
   - The reason for the call
   - The action to be taken
   - The name or initials of the person taking the call

   RATIONALE: Complete and accurate information is necessary to respond to the caller's requests efficiently.
3. Repeat the above information back to the caller. RATIONALE: To verify that the information was recorded accurately and to allow the caller to acknowledge that the message is correct.
4. If the call is from an established patient or concerns an established patient, pull the medical record/chart and attach the message to it before delivering the message to the intended individual. RATIONALE: Information about the patient is available should it be needed, and any required documentation can be made efficiently in the chart.
5. Maintain the old message book with all carbon copies intact. RATIONALE: Documents all telephone calls received by the office. This information could be useful in determining the need for additional telephone lines into the office.

Procedure 12-4 Handling Problem Calls

PURPOSE:
To handle calls in a positive and professional manner while providing necessary comfort, empathy, and information to the caller to resolve the problem.

EQUIPMENT/SUPPLIES:
Telephone
Message pad
Pen or pencil

PROCEDURE STEPS:
1. Answer the call as outlined in Procedure 12-1.
2. Remain calm and avoid becoming upset with an angry caller. Let the caller say what needs to be said without interruption (unless it is a medical emergency requiring immediate action). RATIONALE: This permits the caller to express concerns without having to repeat information or possibly forgetting something important.
3. Lower your voice both in pitch and volume. RATIONALE: This technique has a calming effect on an angry caller.
4. Listen to what the caller is upset about. Paraphrase information for verification that you have understood the problem. RATIONALE: This technique lets the caller know you are truly listening and have understood the problem.
5. Use the words "I understand" and show that you are interested in hearing the caller's concerns. RATIONALE: This does not necessarily mean you agree with the caller, but rather that you are willing to empathize and at least accept that, from a particular point of view, there is a reason to be upset.
6. Do not take the call personally. RATIONALE: It is the situation that made the caller angry; you have not done so.

(continues)

Procedure 12-4 (continued)

7. Offer assistance. RATIONALE: Ask what you can do to help, and then follow through.
8. Document the call accurately and properly. RATIONALE: Complete documentation promotes risk management and prevents lengthy litigation experiences.
9. When dealing with a frightened or hysterical caller, speak in a soothing voice; use a slower, lower tone than normal. RATIONALE: This often has a calming effect on the caller.
10. If the call is an emergency, begin triage procedures as needed. RATIONALE: Have a list of triage questions at hand to refer to or instruct the caller to dial 911. Be sure you have the name and telephone number for follow up.
11. Always have the caller repeat instructions. RATIONALE: People who are upset may not hear or comprehend much of what is said. Your instructions may deal with an emergency situation, thus it is important they are clearly understood.
12. Finalize and follow through on action to be taken, whether it is confirming emergency medical personnel are on the scene or scheduling an emergency appointment. RATIONALE: Ensure quality patient care.
13. Always report problem calls to the physician or office manager at once. RATIONALE: This will ensure appropriate action is taken, and it is important for risk management purposes.

Procedure 12-5 Placing Outgoing Calls

PURPOSE:
To place calls efficiently and effectively.

EQUIPMENT/SUPPLIES:
Notepad
Pen or pencil
All materials specifically applicable to the call

PROCEDURE STEPS:
1. Preplan the call by preparing all materials in front of you before making the call; for example, gather telephone number, chart, financial information, or appointment book. Also, have notes of questions you have or information you need to relay. RATIONALE: This technique uses time efficiently and conveys professionalism.
2. Make calls from a location and telephone that will not be disrupted with noise and distractions. RATIONALE: This type of location permits you to concentrate on the call without distractions or interruptions.
3. Try to schedule specific times of the day for calls, for example, early morning before patients arrive, midday, or after the last patient has been seen. Be aware of the time zone you are calling; you do not want to disturb people at inappropriate times. RATIONALE: Return calls to outside laboratories or consulting physicians may be done early in the morning before patients arrive and offices become busy with patient loads. Midday may be an appropriate time to call in prescription refills or reminders of appointments.
4. Use appropriate language and tone following proper telephone techniques. RATIONALE: Ensure that your message is conveyed clearly and understood accurately.

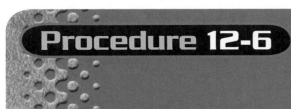

Recording a Telephone Message on an Answering Device or Voice Mail System

PURPOSE:
To provide clear and precise instructions to the caller when medical staff is not available to answer the call immediately. The words should be spoken clearly in a pleasant and well modulated tone.

EQUIPMENT/SUPPLIES:
Telephone and recording device
Prepared written message to record
Individual with pleasant tone of voice

PROCEDURE STEPS

1. Write out the message to be recorded including the following information:
   - Name of the facility
   - What to do in case of an emergency
   - Details of what information to leave in their message:
     Caller's name and complete telephone number
     Purpose for the call
     Action to be taken (return call, schedule appointment, and so forth)
     RATIONALE: To ensure accurate and clear directions are recorded.
2. Check for completeness and accuracy, and read the message aloud to determine its length.

RATIONALE: Collection of necessary information is required to process the message and return a call efficiently. If the message is too long, callers may become frustrated or confused as to what they are to do.

3. Record the message before or after working hours, or during a time when distractions and noise levels are at a minimum. RATIONALE: You will be able to concentrate on reading the message clearly, distinctly, and at a rate easily comprehended by the caller. Background noise will be kept to a minimum.
4. Play the message back while following your printed script to be sure that it was recorded accurately and includes all necessary information. RATIONALE: Assures a clear and concise message that is of good quality and is easily understood by callers.
5. Set the message device to the recorded message when you are not available to answer the telephone in a timely manner. RATIONALE: Avoids missing telephone messages when you are unavailable to answer the phone.

Case Study 12-1

Audrey Jones, the young clinical medical assistant for Drs. Lewis and King, was on telephone duty on a busy Thursday afternoon. This was only the third or fourth time Audrey was responsible for answering incoming calls, but her energy and quick judgment saw her through some difficult situations when all the lines were ringing at the same time. Audrey just received a call; a young man is calling about his mother, a patient of Dr. Lewis, who is having trouble breathing.

CASE STUDY REVIEW

1. What are the critical questions Audrey should ask the young man to triage the situation?
2. How will Audrey's training and background in Red Cross first aid help her assess the situation?
3. If Audrey needs to give medical information over the telephone, what limits should she respect?

Case Study 12-2

Wanda Slawson, Clinical Medical Assistant at Inner City Health Care, receives a telephone call from Claussen-Mason Laboratories requesting medical information about patient Juanita Hansen. Wanda is told by laboratory personnel that the information is needed to perform the tests scheduled by Dr. King. Wanda is not familiar with this request and asks if she can check the chart and return a call to the laboratory (callback verification procedure).

CASE STUDY REVIEW

1. What information will Wanda need from Claussen-Mason Laboratories?
2. What is the purpose of the callback verification procedure?
3. After the verification has been established, what should Wanda do?

DOCUMENTATION

In the log reserved for telephone documentation, the following entry could be made based on Case Study 12-2.

07/16/XX Claussen-Mason Laboratories requested previous laboratory findings from Qwik Lab in Nashville, Tennessee, for Juanita Hansen, patient number 306-30-7840. Juanita is a patient of Dr. King. The information was released to Janet Bailey, employee of Claussen-Mason Laboratories as directed by Dr. King. W. Slawson, CMA.

SUMMARY

Proper telephone techniques require the medical assistant to have excellent communication and listening skills. The ability to convey warmth and reassurance is vital to patient relationships. Efficiency and organization are also key elements in effectively managing the variety of telephone calls answered and placed in the ambulatory care setting. Medical assistants responsible for incoming and outgoing calls need to be able to perform telephone triage, screen calls, take messages, and refer calls professionally and efficiently.

Medical assistants also need to be aware of telecommunication technology to choose and productively manage the office's telecommunication systems. An understanding of technology can result in savings of both time and money for the efficient ambulatory care setting.

STUDY FOR SUCCESS

To reinforce your knowledge and skills of information presented in this chapter:

❑ Review the Key Terms
❑ Practice the Procedures
❑ Consider the Case Studies and discuss your conclusions
❑ Answer the Review Questions
   ❑ Multiple Choice
   ❑ Critical Thinking
❑ Navigate the Internet by completing the Web Activities
❑ Practice the StudyWARE activities on the textbook CD
❑ Apply your knowledge in the Student Workbook activities
❑ Complete the Web Tutor sections
❑ View and discuss the DVD situations

REVIEW QUESTIONS

Multiple Choice

1. Positive first impressions are conveyed over the telephone by:
   a. using the hold button sparingly
   b. being authoritative with the caller
   c. not permitting the caller too much leeway to speak
   d. working while talking on the telephone
2. Basic telephone techniques involve:
   a. volume, enunciation, pronunciation, and control of speed
   b. being assertive with the caller
   c. not spending too much time talking
   d. referring all calls to the physician
3. Buffer words:
   a. are necessary for clarity
   b. confuse the caller
   c. are used to avoid clipping off the office name
   d. are not considered introductory words, phrases, or statements
4. Guidelines that ensure successful transfer of calls include all of the following *except:*

   a. determine who would be the best person to assist
   b. follow your telephone system's procedure for transferring the call
   c. follow up to be sure the call transferred correctly
   d. getting the caller's name and telephone number is not necessary
5. Medical assistants should refer calls to the physician when:
   a. an appointment needs to be scheduled
   b. a patient has a billing question
   c. a salesperson is planning a call
   d. a patient requests test results
6. Triage:
   a. is the act of evaluating the urgency of a medical situation and prioritizing treatment
   b. is expressing oneself clearly and distinctly
   c. uses expendable words while answering the telephone
   d. is the ability to be objectively aware of and have insight into others' feelings, emotions, and behaviors

7. In handling a problem call, the medical assistant should:
   a. take it personally
   b. listen calmly to the upset person
   c. become upset to identify with the patient
   d. ask emotionally charged questions to calm down the patient
8. The callback verification procedure:
   a. should never be documented
   b. should always be documented
   c. should sometimes be documented
   d. is not appropriate in the ambulatory office setting
9. ARU telephone systems:
   a. transmit over telephone lines via modem
   b. involve transmissions sent from one fax machine to another
   c. use a recorded voice that identifies departments or services the caller can access by pressing a specified number
   d. process messages in digital form through telephone lines
10. Pagers or beepers are:
    a. useful for calling back patients
    b. older technology
    c. capable only of one-way transmission
    d. now replaced by fax machines

Critical Thinking

1. Telephone triage is important for all calls. Discuss or role-play with a classmate how to use triage effectively when answering the telephone in a medical office and practice this skill.
2. Answering the telephone professionally is critical in the health care profession. Meet with several class-mates who each have written a scenario appropriate for an ambulatory care setting phone call. Now take turns being the caller and the medical assistant answering the office phone. Follow the steps outlined in Procedure 12-1 to cultivate your skills.
3. You are the medical assistant assigned to answering the telephone today. You receive a call from an angry patient. He wants to know why his bill is so high when he was only in the office with the doctor for five minutes. What will happen if you become angry in retaliation? How should you handle this call in a professional manner?
4. Hearing-impaired patients and patients who speak English as a second language often become frustrated during telephone calls. How can you help improve communication and be more effective when dealing with these types of patients?
5. How would you go about writing a policy concerning the use of clinical e-mail in your office? What legal and ethical considerations must you consider? What information might be addressed in a disclaimer related to e-mail use?

WEB ACTIVITIES

Using the World Wide Web, search for current information relative to legal and ethical considerations when using telecommunications in the ambulatory care setting. Compile your information into a one-page report, and list your URL addresses for your instructor.

THE DVD HOOK-UP

DVD Series	Program Number
Critical Thinking	**2**

Chapter/Scene Reference
• *Communication on the Telephone*

In this chapter, you learned about the medical assistant's responsibilities when handling phone calls. Working the phones in a medical office is hard work. The medical assistant must become familiar with the telephone system, as well as office protocol for handling various types of phone calls. Patience is extremely important when working the telephones.

The designated DVD clips presented two separate scenarios. In the first scenario, we observed the medical assistant talking to Pat Morgan regarding an order for a possible prescription. The medical assistant checked to see if the physician left any orders in the chart for the patient's refill prescription. When the medical assistant saw that there was no order, she wrote down the patient's message and current symptoms so that she could share the information with the doctor. Before ending the phone call, the medical assistant told the patient that if the doctor approved the prescription, she would call it directly to the pharmacy, and that if there were any problems she would call her back; otherwise, she could pick the prescription up at the pharmacy after 3:00 PM.

1. Do you think that it was wise for the medical assistant to tell the patient that she would only call her back if the physician did not approve the prescription? Why or why not?
2. Did the medical assistant use a therapeutic approach when she spoke to the patient?

DVD Journal Summary
Write a paragraph that summarizes what you learned from watching the designated scenes from today's DVD program. In the last scene, the medical assistant tries to assist an older adult patient who is having problems with the telephone menu. How do you feel about telephone menus and older adult patients? Would you ever give out your extension to an older adult patient who was struggling with the phone menu? Why or why not?

REFERENCES/BIBLIOGRAPHY

Humphrey, D. D. (2004). *Contemporary medical office procedures* (3rd ed.). Clifton Park, NY: Thomson Delmar Learning.

ingenix. (2003, December). HIPAA Tool Kit. Salt Lake City, UT: St. Anthony's Publishing/Medicode.

Keir, L., Wise, B. A., & Krebs, C. (2003). *Medical assisting administrative and clinical competencies* (5th ed.). Clifton Park, NY: Thomson Delmar Learning.

Krager, D., & Krager, C. (2005). *HIPAA for medical office personnel.* Clifton Park, NY: Thomson Delmar Learning.

CHAPTER 13

Patient Scheduling

OUTLINE

KEY TERMS

Encryption Technology
Matrix
Modified Wave Scheduling
Stream Scheduling
Triage
Wave Scheduling

OBJECTIVES

The student should strive to meet the following performance objectives and demonstrate an understanding of the facts and principles presented in this chapter through written and oral communication.

1. Define the key terms as presented in the glossary.
2. Review six major scheduling systems.
3. Describe the six guidelines in scheduling appointments.
4. Explain the importance of triage in scheduling patient appointments.
5. Review proper cancellation procedures and explain the legal necessity of documenting cancellations.
6. Recall three types of reminder systems.
7. Choose an appropriate appointment scheduling tool and describe its advantages.

(continues)

FEATURED COMPETENCIES

CAAHEP—ENTRY-LEVEL COMPETENCIES

Perform Clerical Functions

- Schedule and manage appointments
- Schedule inpatient and out-patient admissions and procedures

Patient Care

- Perform telephone and in-person screening

Legal Concepts

- Identify and respond to issues of confidentiality
- Demonstrate knowledge of federal and state health care legislation and regulations

Patient Instructions

- Explain general office policies

Operational Functions

- Utilize computer software to maintain office systems

ABHES—ENTRY-LEVEL COMPETENCIES

Professionalism

- Project a positive attitude
- Maintain confidentiality at all times
- Be cognizant of ethical boundaries
- Adapt to change
- Be courteous and diplomatic

Communication

- Be impartial and show empathy when dealing with patients
- Interview effectively
- Application of electronic technology

(continues)

OBJECTIVES (continued)

8. Establish a matrix for a new year and a new practice.
9. Check in patients using a daily appointment sheet.
10. Schedule outpatient procedures and inpatient admissions.

SCENARIO

At Inner City Health Care, medical assistant Walter Seals is responsible for efficient patient flow. Because Inner City is an urgent care center, patients are seen as walk-in appointments, on a first-come, first-served basis unless there is an emergency situation. Inner City also operates specialty care clinics, and these clinics require scheduled appointments. Walter has found that the clustering system is most efficient for these specialized care clinics, with certain days dedicated to certain procedures.

Because of the high volume of patients and the need to coordinate multiple physician schedules, Walter's job is not an easy one. However, Inner City is computerized, so paperwork is easy to generate as appointments are made, canceled, or rescheduled. And although Walter manages a smooth patient flow, he makes it a point to remain flexible to accommodate patient needs and keep stress to a minimum.

FEATURED COMPETENCIES (continued)

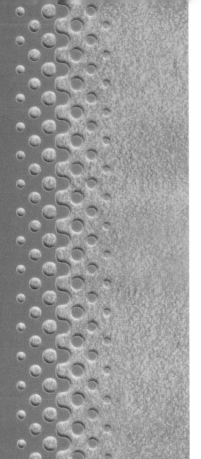

Administrative Duties

- Schedule and monitor appointments
- Apply computer concepts for office procedures
- Manage physician's professional schedule

Legal Concepts

- Determine needs for documentation and reporting
- Document accurately
- Monitor legislation related to current healthcare issues and practices

Instruction

- Orient patients to office policies and procedures

Spotlight on Certification

RMA Content Outline
- Reception
- Scheduling

CMA Content Outline
- Telephone techniques
- Equipment operation
- Computer applications
- Utilizing appointment schedules/types
- Appointment guidelines
- Appointment protocol
- Integrating meetings and travel with office schedule

CMAS Content Outline
- Medical Office Clerical Assisting
- Appointment Management and Scheduling

INTRODUCTION

Patient scheduling has undergone many changes. There was a time when the concern of the medical office staff was whether patients had a telephone. The concern now is whether the patient has a computer and is willing to use the computer for online appointment scheduling.

Patient scheduling is an integral part of the daily workload for medical assistants, whether in large family practices, urgent care centers, or single-physician offices. Scheduling becomes more complicated if doctors are practicing in more than one clinic and traveling between them. Scheduling patients can be stressful, especially when the telephone rings constantly and the medical assistant is unable to provide patients a convenient appointment.

Although patient appointment scheduling may seem like a routine function, a smooth patient flow often determines the success of a day in the ambulatory care setting. A variety of administrative skills are used in the performance of this vital office function. By effectively scheduling patients to fit a particular practice, it is possible to make profitable use of physician and staff time.

In addition, efficient patient flow is satisfying to the patient. A common patient complaint is the time spent waiting in the reception area or the examination room. Most patients appreciate an office that recognizes the value of patients' time. Accordingly, these patients do not hesitate to advertise their

experience *(good or bad) to friends and families—a fact of great significance to any medical setting.*

 In addition to the required administrative skills, medical assistants involved in scheduling patients must put into practice their best interpersonal and communication skills. Scheduling an appointment may be the first contact patients have with the medical office. They remember and value the treatment they receive from the time of first contact. The personality of the ambulatory care setting is always reflected in the treatment and respect accorded to patients.

Whether scheduling is done online, through a sophisticated computerized system, or in the paper appointment book (becoming rare these days), practitioners and their staff must remember the importance of that first impression and hopefully make it completely satisfying for patients.

TAILORING THE SCHEDULING SYSTEM

The schedule of each medical facility will determine the best method for scheduling appointments. A surgeon's office will have a much different flow of patients than a pediatrician's office. The key is to customize the system to best accommodate the practice. Primary goals in determining this should include:

- A smooth flow of patients with a minimal amount of waiting time

- Flexibility to accommodate acutely ill, STAT (or emergency) appointments, work-ins, cancellations, and no-shows

SCHEDULING STYLES

There are a number of methods for patient scheduling. The best method for a practice is the one that effects good patient flow and proper utilization of staff and physical facilities. Keep in mind that even the best computerized system will fail if the scheduling style does not comfortably fit the predetermined and necessary patient flow.

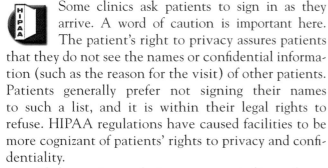 Some clinics ask patients to sign in as they arrive. A word of caution is important here. The patient's right to privacy assures patients that they do not see the names or confidential information (such as the reason for the visit) of other patients. Patients generally prefer not signing their names to such a list, and it is within their legal rights to refuse. HIPAA regulations have caused facilities to be more cognizant of patients' rights to privacy and confidentiality.

If the setting and circumstances indicate that a sign-in sheet for patients is the most efficient means of checking in patients, forms can be purchased that meet privacy and confidentiality expectations of patients.

Figure 13-1 illustrates a carbonized pack with perforations that allows a patient to sign in giving the necessary information. The receptionist then removes just the one strip at the perforation. The information remains on the bottom form only. The next patient to sign in does not see the information of the previous patient. These forms are available in shingled format as well.

A better policy may be to have the office staff create a list of names as patients arrive to check in. It is assumed, however, that the arrival of patients in person in a medical facility may mean that other patients recognize them and may know their names.

Open Hours

In open hours scheduling, patients are seen throughout a particular time frame; for example, 9:00 AM to 11:00 AM or 1:00 PM to 3:00 PM. Patients are seen on a first-come, first-served basis. Many clinics frequently choose this method because they are able, by their nature, to maintain a steady flow of patients. Open hours scheduling is likely a place where a sign-in sheet is helpful, because patients are seen on a first-come, first served basis. It is important to remember that a sign-in sheet can never replace a warm, welcoming greeting from the receptionist to set the tone for care given that day.

Double Booking

With the double-booking method, two or more patients are given a particular appointment time. This method is limited to a practice that can attend to more than one patient at a time. For instance, Maria Jover and Jim Marshal are both given a 9:30 AM appointment. Ms. Jover requires a complete checkup including lab tests, vitals, and so on. Mr. Marshal is being seen for suture removal. While the physician's staff conducts the lab tests on Ms. Jover, the physician can be treating Mr. Marshal. Obviously, this method requires a precise accounting for time and rooms and adequate staff. A good rule to remember is that if patients are consistently having to wait for staff to attend to them, double booking is not a wise choice of method.

Clustering

The clustering method applies the concept used in production line work, namely that performing only one step or process allows for efficient processing. In the ambulatory care setting, patients with similar problems are booked consecutively. Obstetricians and pediatricians commonly choose this method. A block of time, either hours or days of the week, is set aside for particular types of cases. For instance, an obstetrician might see only patients in their third trimester of pregnancy on Mondays and Fridays and gynecology patients on Tuesdays and Thursdays. A pediatrician's office might be organized for immunizations on Tuesday mornings and well-baby checkups on Monday and Friday afternoons.

Wave Scheduling

Wave scheduling is another method that can be used effectively in medical facilities that have several procedure rooms and adequate personnel to staff them. Using the wave scheduling system, patients are scheduled only in the first half hour of each hour. For example, three patients may be given the time of 11 AM. Generally, the first one to arrive is seen first. If they all arrive on time, the one who is most ill is usually seen first, and

NO.	Please Print Name Sign-in on next available #	Appt. Time	Time Seen	Appointment with	Note if first visit, new phone, address or insurance change

Patient Sign-In　　　　Date: _____

Please sign in and notify us if:
you are a new patient, your insurance, telephone number or address have changed.

NO.	Please Print Name Sign-in on next available #	Appt. Time	Time Seen	Appointment with	Note if first visit, new phone, address or insurance change
24	24				
25	25				
26	26				
27	27				
28	28				
29	29				
30	30				
31	31				
32	32				
33	33				
34	34				
35	35				
36	36				
37	37				
38	38				
39	39				
40	40				
41	41				
42	42				
43	43				
44	44				
45	45				
46	46				

Figure 13-1 Patient sign-in sheet that protects privacy of each patient while giving necessary information to office staff. (Courtesy of Bibbero Systems, Inc., Petaluma, CA; (800) 242-2376; www.bibbero.com.)

there will be a waiting time for the other two patients. Depending on the practice, some office receptionists will be instructed to schedule three patients at the top of the hour, and another two or three patients at the bottom of the hour (i.e., 11:30 AM). Patients who do not understand this system of scheduling may become irritated if they discover that another patient has the same appointed time with the same physician. This method takes into account that there will be no-shows and late arrivals. It can also

accommodate work-in appointments. However, it does require personnel who are able to triage patient problems precisely when establishing the appointments.

Modified Wave Scheduling

Modified wave scheduling is a variation of the wave method where patients are scheduled in "waves." In this method, two or three patients are scheduled at the beginning of each hour, followed by single appointments every 10 to 20 minutes the rest of the hour.

A variation of this method assesses major and minor problems. Major time-consuming problems are seen at the beginning of the hour (e.g., new patients). Minor problems are seen from 20 minutes past the hour to half past the hour (e.g., follow-ups, bandage changes, and other minor procedures), and walk-ins (e.g., a child with a 103°F temperature) are accommodated at the end of the hour. Again, good triaging will determine the success of this method.

With both the clustering and wave methods, empty or unscheduled periods can be used for dictation or the processing of paperwork.

Stream Scheduling

Stream scheduling is perhaps the best known and most widely used scheduling system. When this system works as it should, there is a steady stream of patients at set appointment times throughout the workday; for example, 30-minute appointment at 9:00 AM; 15-minute appointment at 9:30 AM; 15-minute appointment at 9:45 AM. Each patient is assigned a specific time. This can best be accomplished by establishing time guidelines for particular types of appointments, such as 45 minutes for consultations, 15 minutes for immunizations, and 30 minutes for a hearing test.

Practice-Based Scheduling

As discussed earlier in this chapter, some ambulatory care settings find it necessary to develop a system unique to their patient load. In these customized systems (practice-based), the practice determines the schedule. An orthopedist might schedule cast removals on Mondays and Fridays using double booking and stream scheduling for new patients, with each patient having a 45-minute appointment. A group of vascular surgeons might use both a double-booking and a modified wave system. They might double book patients for short rechecks and quick procedures, whereas using the modified wave for patients with preoperative and postoperative checks and long specialty procedures.

There are many variations of scheduling styles. An Oregon massage therapist who operates a private practice as a sole proprietor with no receptionist has found that an online welcome screen and appointment book is the best way for her patients to schedule a massage. Her online system also creates appointment reminder e-mail messages. This massage therapist and her patients are pleased. They believe that the self-service scheduling gives their therapist more time to take care of their needs.

ANALYZING PATIENT FLOW

When setting up a new practice or reviewing the current scheduling practice, a simple analysis can maximize an office's scheduling practices. This entails looking at appointment times, patient arrival times, the actual time a patient is seen, and the time a visit is completed. A simple grid chart can be produced for a given period; for example, one to two weeks (Figure 13-2). In addition, chart the number of no-shows and cancellations.

This analysis should provide a clear picture of patient flow and whether office personnel are being used efficiently. The data will assist in estimating how many patients to schedule and realistic time frames for particular problems or procedures. If the physician is scheduling return patients every 15 minutes yet the analysis shows these visits average 24 minutes, the scheduling method needs adjustment. This may mean either allowing 25 minutes for follow-up visits or building in slack time, or unscheduled time, where no appointments are made.

Develop a simple list of commonly scheduled visits with time estimates for each. This procedural sheet will be particularly useful when training new employees or when temporary help is used for scheduling (Figure 13-3).

Waiting Time

One of the most frequently voiced frustrations with physicians' offices is excessive waiting time. Obviously, emergencies and other unexpected interruptions cannot be anticipated. However, there are certain measures one can take when attempting to keep the schedule on target. If

PATIENT FLOW ANALYSIS

February 2, 20XX — Dr. King

Patient Name	Length of Appt.	Appt. Time	Time Seen	Time Out
Martin Gordon	15	10:20	10:22	10:45
Jason Jover	45	11:20	11:20	12:30
Nora Fowler	30	1:00	1:25	1:45
Jim Marshal	15	1:30	1:50	2:10
Herb Fowler	60	2:45	2:15	3:25

Figure 13-2 Patient flow analysis helps a practice determine realistic time frames for appointments.

> ## TYPICAL SCHEDULING TIMES FOR INTERNAL MEDICINE PRACTICE
>
> New patients . . . . 30 minutes
> Patients for consultation . . . . 45 minutes
> Patients requiring complete
>   physical examinations . . . . 45 minutes
> All other patients (minor illnesses,
>   routine checkups, etc.) . . . . 15 minutes

Figure 13-3 Most practices will have a list of typical visits with time estimates.

patients are kept waiting, it is a good strategy to explain the reason for the delay and give patients an estimate of how long the delay will be. *Never* ignore the delay hoping patients will not notice; this, in fact, seems to increase perceived waiting time. Find ways to make patients comfortable while they wait; for example, provide an appropriate choice of reading materials (or in the case of children, activities). Refer to Case Study 10-2. If a delay can be anticipated, for example, the physician was called away for a baby delivery or surgery, attempt to contact patients before they leave home to reschedule the appointments.

If the delay is likely to be a half hour or longer, provide patients with options, for example:

1. Offer patients the opportunity to run an errand, having them return at a specified time.
2. Offer to reschedule appointments for another day, or later that day, or to see another physician in the practice.

In any case, remember that good customer relations dictate your willingness to acknowledge the inconvenience to the patients and attempt to provide an acceptable solution. Remember also that some patients simply will not appreciate any efforts to apologize for a delay, in which case you must continue to act professionally toward them.

LEGAL ISSUES

 Information provided in any patient scheduling system may be used for legal purposes. A case of malpractice or questions regarding the physician's availability may require a copy of the daily schedule. It might become necessary to identify how many times a particular patient was a no-show or cancelled an appointment, never calling to reschedule. The appointment schedule could verify that a patient was seen and treated on a particular day, thus affirming the information in the patient's record.

All computerized systems provide a permanent record of patients seen, and any alterations to that schedule are saved on the hard drive or disk and are shown when a printout is produced. If an appointment book is still used, the staff will have to make certain there is a permanent record or daily appointment sheet that indicates cancellations, work-ins, urgent care needs, and no-shows. Any changes to the daily appointment sheet are to be made in pen; therefore, there will be no question regarding accuracy.

Remember that anyone looking into a practice will be looking at the record of documentation. Taking the time to accurately and consistently document all aspects of patient care makes a statement about the physicians in the practice and their staff and reflects positively on the presumed quality of patient care.

INTERPERSONAL SKILLS

Scheduling appointments requires interpersonal skills. Medical assistants convey a great deal to patients through attitude and actions. A hurried or disinterested manner communicates that the patient is not a priority. Because patients are often distraught or anxious when making appointments, it is extremely important to reduce rather than increase anxiety. Also, the medical assistant scheduling appointments may be the first contact a patient has with the office; patients do not easily forget rude or insensitive staff. A hurried, disinterested manner toward patients is just as often the basis for legal action than is a negligent act.

If any form of online scheduling is used, be certain that it is user friendly, has a rapid response time of no more than 24 hours, and provides patients an option if the online scheduling proves unsatisfactory for any reason. Make certain that staff are ready for online scheduling and that those responsible for assignments and backups are carefully prepared. It is important that the patients not be made to feel inadequate if they prefer not to use online scheduling or if they have difficulties making the transition.

The patient should always be made to feel worthy of attention. If scheduling a patient in the office and the phone rings, answer the call but excuse yourself first. Ask the caller to please hold for a moment. If you are on the telephone scheduling a patient and another patient walks in, acknowledge with a nod or signal that you will be right there—never let the person feel ignored. Today, patients have a variety of options for health care and tend to be much more consumer conscious of the treatment they receive.

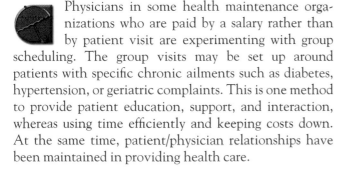

Critical Thinking

With another person in your class, identify two or three public encounters where you feel ignored or rushed as a customer. How does it make you feel? What suggestions would you make to the business to change that feeling?

GUIDELINES FOR SCHEDULING APPOINTMENTS

Whether completed by manual methods or computer technology, the process of scheduling appointments for patients and other visitors to the ambulatory care setting involves a number of variables, including (1) the urgency of the need for an appointment; (2) whether the appointment has a referral from another physician; (3) recording methods for new and established patients; (4) implementation of check-in, cancellation, and rescheduling policies; (5) use of reminder systems; and (6) accommodating visits from medical supply and pharmaceutical company representatives.

 Physicians in some health maintenance organizations who are paid by a salary rather than by patient visit are experimenting with group scheduling. The group visits may be set up around patients with specific chronic ailments such as diabetes, hypertension, or geriatric complaints. This is one method to provide patient education, support, and interaction, whereas using time efficiently and keeping costs down. At the same time, patient/physician relationships have been maintained in providing health care.

Triage Calls

Urgent calls will need to be **triaged,** or assessed, before they can be scheduled. In other words, the office personnel making the appointment will need to determine the actual urgency of that call and determine how the patient can best be scheduled. This requires a combination of both communication skills and medical knowledge.

Appropriate questions need to be asked to determine the actual urgency. Is the patient in immediate need of medical assistance? Is there any bleeding? Are there chest pains? The medical assistant needs to determine if this is a life-threatening matter, or if the problem is urgent in the patient's eyes but not a medical emergency.

While triaging, also obtain information that will assist in determining the urgent nature of the call. How long have the symptoms/complaint been present? If there is bleeding or discharge, where is the origin? How profuse is it? If it is pain, how intense is it? Is it localized? Precise information will assist the physician in determining the critical or noncritical nature of the call.

 In triaging the patient's urgency of care, be tactful in questioning and avoid making the patient feel that the need is insignificant. If questioning indicates this is a medical emergency, follow office policy for having the patient seen (whether it be an emergency appointment or referral to the emergency department). If referral to the emergency department or a call to 911 is necessary, make the call for the patient, being certain you have the correct address and telephone number available. Such a referral minimizes disruption to patients being seen in the ambulatory care setting. If it is determined that the best method in handling this emergency is to see the patient in the office, let scheduled patients know of the emergency and offer them the opportunity of rescheduling or waiting until the emergency has been resolved. A built-in slack time of 30 minutes in the morning and 30 minutes in the afternoon can provide some flexibility in last-minute emergency scheduling. If it is determined that the situation is not an emergency, work the patient into the schedule as the situation warrants and time allows, and make certain the patient is comfortable with the scheduled time. Be sure to leave the patient with the understanding that you have done your best to address the situation. See Chapters 9 and 12 for more information on triage.

Referral Appointments

 One of the primary sources for a physician's practice base is referrals from other physicians. This is especially true in a managed care climate, where patients usually must have a referral from their primary care physician and where physicians are part of an HMO network. It is important that these appointments be given special consideration and that referred patients be given an appointment as soon as possible.

Adequate information needs to be obtained to determine the urgency of scheduling. If the referring physician or office staff calls directly, the situation can be triaged at that time. However, if the referred patient calls, it is best to obtain necessary records and information from the referring physician's office to determine the urgency and appropriateness of an appointment. This can be done by obtaining general information from the patient, and then scheduling an appointment after the physician's office is contacted for complete information regarding the patient's condition. Be polite and assure the patient of an appointment as soon as the referring physician's office is contacted.

Recording Information

Patients can be sensitive to the amount of information they are required to provide to make an initial appointment. Keep the information as simple as possible and obtain only essential information. It should be tailored to fit the practice; for example, an obstetrician and a pediatrician will have different questions for the first-time patient.

Generally, these basic items should be obtained from a new patient, that is, someone being seen for the first time in the office:

1. The patient's full legal name (with the correct spelling)
2. A daytime telephone number
3. The chief complaint or reason for the visit
4. The referring physician, if relevant

In privacy, repeat this information back to the patient to assure accuracy.

 Offices with computerized scheduling and billing will require a few additional items, such as:

1. Date of birth
2. Type of insurance
3. Insurance number

The critical determination is whether the information is essential to the first contact or whether it could be obtained at the time of the visit.

An established patient, someone who has already been seen in the office, should require only the following information:

1. Full legal name
2. Chief complaint or reason for the visit
3. A daytime telephone number

When the information is recorded, print it legibly and accurately in a manual system, and check for accuracy in the same manner when using a computer system for scheduling. Record the appointment as soon as it is made—never rely on memory.

When scheduling an appointment time, ask the patient what day and time would be most convenient for them, and then make the appointment for the first available time stated. If possible, provide the patient with a choice of possible appointment times. Finally, confirm that the patient clearly understands the date and time of the appointment; be sure to repeat the date and time to ensure that both of you have recorded the same information. If the patient is making the appointment in person, provide them with an appointment reminder.

Scheduling an appointment for the office's available times for a parent who works outside the home, serves in a carpool, and is a coach for the gymnastics or swim team can require a great deal of patience. If the patient requests a particular appointment and this is not possible, courteously offer an explanation.

Many ambulatory care settings, especially those specializing in family practice and pediatrics, are providing alternative hours for scheduling appointments. Having evening appointments at least one day a week or Saturday morning appointments can be helpful for individuals whose work schedule does not permit weekday appointments.

Appointment Matrix

The appointment **matrix** must be established before patients can be scheduled. The matrix provides a current and accurate record of appointment times available for scheduling patient visits. Clinic hours are noted with times blocked off when the facility is closed. Doctor's schedules, vacations, holidays, hospital rounds, and any responsibilities that make doctors unavailable for appointments are recorded. The matrix of the scheduling plan might include slots for patients who need to see only staff members for their appointment; therefore, times when they are unavailable are impor-

---

DAILY APPOINTMENT WORKSHEET

Thursday, August 21

Time			
8:00	Hospital Rounds		
9:15	Chris O'Keefe	30 minutes	Immunizations
9:30	Jim Marshal	15 minutes	Blood pressure check
10:00	Martin Gordon	60 minutes	PE/lab work
11:00	Nora Fowler	30 minutes	URI
11:30	Lunch break		
12:30	Dentist Appointment, Dr. Schleuter		
2:00	Maria Jover	30 minutes	Suspicious rash
2:45	Meet with drug rep regarding new beta-blocker agents		
4:00	Joseph Ortiz	30 minutes	Choking problems

Figure 13-4 Daily appointment worksheet.

tant to the matrix. Any evening or weekend appointment slots available also are noted. See Figure 13-4 and Procedure 13-3.

 Typically, when using a computer system for scheduling, the program will search through a database of appointments, find an open appointment, and allocate an appointment time according to your instructions. These instructions can include finding an open appointment with a specific time length, on a specific day, or within a specified time frame. Once the appointment time is confirmed with the patient, patient data are keyed in, and the appointment is automatically scheduled.

Patient Check-In

Records of patient appointments serve a legal purpose. Establishing a procedure for checking in appointments simplifies tracking of the arrival of patients. (See Procedure 13-1.) This is particularly true in multiphysician settings or offices where a number of staff are attending to patients before, or instead of, seeing the physician.

 Even when the facility uses the open hours method of scheduling, it is a better policy for the office staff to create a patient list or to check the patients off of a list (Figure 13-5). When a patient checks

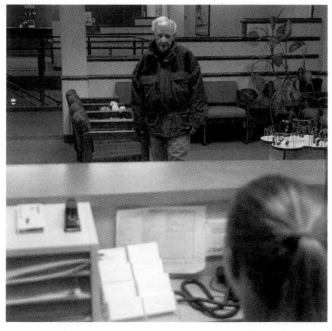

Figure 13-5 The medical assistant/receptionist should be able to see patients as they enter the office. Patients will be checked in by the medical assistant who will keep the patient check-in list current.

in, a red √ or other appropriate mark should be used in the appointment book or sheet.

Patient Cancellation and Appointment Changes

A permanent record of no-shows should be designated on the appointment sheet with a red **X**, or some other distinctive mark. Cancellations should be marked through on the appointment sheet with a single red line (Figure 13-6). Some facilities place a notation next to the patient's name. Computer scheduling will provide an area to indicate no-shows and cancellations also. No-shows and cancellations should always be noted in the patient's individual chart. Again, it is imperative that the physician's care of the patient be thoroughly documented. Should a patient develop complications and claim the physician was unavailable, the daily appointment sheet and chart should document the patient's failure to show.

Occasionally, a patient will not show up for an appointment because they simply forgot, or sometimes they might show up on the wrong day or at the wrong time. That can happen simply by human error or miscommunication. However, if one patient begins a pattern of getting the dates and times mixed up or forgets the appointment entirely, the physician should be made aware of the possibility that this patient might be affected by memory loss or general confusion. Sometimes, a pattern of missed and mixed-up appointments is your first sign that the patient may be experiencing memory loss and mental confusion.

 Many offices have established firm policies for multiple no-shows and cancellations. The general rule is that after three no-shows or cancellations in a row, the physician will review the records. For the physician to adequately treat a patient, the patient's cooperation is necessary. A no-show pattern may indicate that the patient is not truly committed to assisting in treatment. If a patient routinely cancels or does not show, the physician may write a letter terminating services and explaining why the physician is discontinuing care. This should be sent by certified mail, return receipt requested, to ensure that the patient received the notice. See Chapter 7 for more information on termination of services. Procedure 13-2 outlines the proper cancellation procedures.

 Although software programs differ, cancellations are typically performed by deleting the patient's name from the time slot; if the appointment is to be rescheduled, the name is then keyed in to the appropriate time, usually the first time open for other appointments.

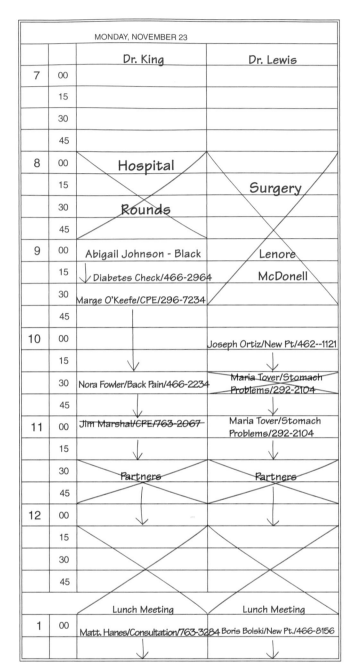

Figure 13-6 Multiphysicians' office where physicians' commitments and no-shows are marked with a red *X* and cancellations are marked with a single red line. Computer systems will have slightly different tracking systems, but all no-shows and cancellations also should be marked in the patient's record.

When canceling appointments by computer, be certain that the program maintains a list of canceled appointments including patient name, date, and time. This documentation is necessary for legal purposes; also record canceled appointments in the patients' charts.

Reminder Systems

Studies show that the national average of missed appointments is more than 10%. Reminding patients of their scheduled appointments results in a greater rate of fulfilled appointments. Give patients appointment card reminders when appointments are made at the medical facility. Those cards may easily be tucked in a wallet and forgotten, however. Many offices notify patients the day before the appointment with a reminder of their choice for the communication—telephone, pager, or e-mail.

 However, remember that this is confidential information and should never be left on such a recording device without the patient's express permission to do so. (When initially seeing the patient, obtain a number where a personal message could be left.) Finally, reminders can be mailed. This would be most appropriate for patients who come on a regular basis (e.g., once every six months).

Scheduling Representatives

Every medical office needs to schedule time with representatives of pharmaceutical and medical supply companies. These representatives provide a valuable service to physicians, and with clear guidelines regarding when and how often representatives can visit, a working partnership can develop. Most physicians set aside a specific time during the week to meet with these representatives; generally, a time allotment of 15 to 20 minutes is sufficient for these appointments. Some representatives try to establish a standard appointment once a month. If this is a representative your physician desires to see on a regular basis, that policy can be helpful to both the physician and the representative. However, this practice might not allow adequate time for other representatives; therefore, it is often discouraged.

SCHEDULING SOFTWARE AND MATERIALS

No matter what materials and which methods are used, the proper tools will enable patient scheduling to be a smoothly functioning, easily documented process. Materials needed for scheduling should be customized to the ambulatory care setting. For instance, a smaller practice may prefer a manual method involving appointment books; a large urgent care-type setting will use a computer program for patient scheduling.

Appointment Schedule

An appropriate appointment schedule system is essential to any medical practice in the ambulatory care setting. Each office has unique needs in its physical facility and for its staff. The physical arrangement of the scheduler, including the various combinations of time allotments, must be determined. Some have major headings for hours with minor spaces for 15-minute intervals, others have 10-minute intervals, and still others only hour intervals. An appointment sheet is necessary for both legal risk management and quality management purposes. Copies of the daily appointment sheet are made available to the doctors, medical assistants, and any other staff members. Using the daily appointment sheet, it is easy to check in patients as they arrive and indicate no-shows and cancellations. Indicating the check-in and checkout times can be useful for quality management purposes. More importantly, the daily appointment sheet assists the physician and staff and enables them to see the total scheme of the day's patient flow.

If a physician works between two clinics or a hospital and office, it is helpful to have this appointment schedule transferred to a handheld computer device for immediate referral. If a handheld computer is not used by the physician, reduce the dimensions of the appointment schedule sheet to pocket-size for the physician's easy access. Generally, if the physician makes hospital visits before coming to the office in the morning, this schedule is printed the previous evening before closing.

These daily appointment sheets can also be used to include other physician commitments such as meetings and visits from pharmaceutical representatives. Such a complete record of time assures that no patient appointments will be booked when, in fact, the physician is not available.

Computer Software and Hardware

Even the smallest of medical facilities today will find benefit from the use of computers. There are numerous software programs for the ambulatory care setting requiring only basic computer hardware that can save time for physicians and their staff members. Other programs are more sophisticated and may require on-site technical support.

Some scheduling software programs will schedule resources, equipment, examination rooms, and specialty staff, as well as patients and physicians. Some will show copayments due, authorization expiration dates, and insurance expiration dates. They can select the next available appointment, search for appointments by patient, copy and paste appointments, and specify minimum time increments between appointments. The staff can view multiple schedules daily, weekly, monthly, or even yearly. Reminder notes can be created for both physicians and patients.

Computerized scheduling systems that are a component of a completely computerized medical facility, including medical records, are able to indicate no-shows and cancellations in the system and the patient's chart at the same time. Facilities that are partially computerized will still want to indicate patients who do not keep their appointments on the daily worksheet and in the patients' medical records.

Online systems can handle prescription refill requests, patient–physician e-mail messages, and laboratory results. Some will allow patients to update insurance data and complete registration forms. All of the online systems are done within the physician's Web site, which includes security measures and sophisticated **encryption technology.** Therefore, security is less of a concern.

Electronic scheduling will continue to develop and become increasingly popular. Employers in ambulatory care settings who make certain patients understand computerized scheduling, have put time and effort into determining the best program for their use, and have trained their staff well, will not be disappointed with the outcome. Whatever system is chosen, keep in mind that the patient's time, the staff's time, and the physician's time are extremely valuable. The goal is to manage that time as efficiently as possible.

INPATIENT AND OUTPATIENT ADMISSIONS AND PROCEDURES

Often, patients are scheduled for either outpatient or inpatient hospital admissions or for special procedures performed in another facility. These appointments are most likely made while the patient is present in the ambulatory care center and has just been seen by the physician. It will be especially helpful if the patient has an appointment book identifying current responsibilities. Have a calendar handy for visualization of the days discussed.

Outpatient procedures may include endoscopy examinations and specialized radiologic examinations such as mammography, bone scans, and ultrasounds.

Computerized tomography (CT) scans and magnetic resonance imaging (MRI) procedures will also require specialized admissions. If a patient prefers to make his or her own arrangements for a procedure, indicate that the following information is necessary:

- Name, address, and telephone number of patient

- Name of physician ordering the procedure

- Name of patient's insurance, ID number, and Social Security number

Follow up in a day or two to make certain the required procedure has been scheduled.

Generally, a real service is done for the patients and staff when the medical assistant schedules the procedure. With the patient present, place a telephone call to the facility where procedures are to be performed. Identify yourself, your physician, and the clinic from where you are calling. Identify any urgency to the request and ask for the next available appointment. As dates and times are discussed, your patient is able to give an immediate response. Consider travel time for your patient and whether there is apt to be any uncomfortable examination procedures that might make travel difficult. Be certain to advise the patient if someone is needed to provide transportation home after the procedure. Often, there is a paperwork follow-up that indicates the nature of the illness and the reason for the specialty examination. Your doctor will tell you if a phone response to the examination is required, or if it is acceptable to wait for the written test results.

Once a date has been established, make certain the patient knows the correct date and time, as well as how to get to the place where the examination is to be per-formed. Inform the patient how and when he or she will receive test results.

Scheduling inpatient admissions to the hospital is similar. However, the majority of the time, the physician will want the patient in the hospital as quickly as possible. Call the preferred or designated hospital. Expect to provide pertinent patient and insurance information required by the hospital. Assist the patient in determining whether it is permissible to return home for some personal belongings and make home arrangements or admission is immediate. Some large facilities with surgical physicians are likely to have a surgery scheduler to make all these arrangements. In primary care, the medical assistant will be doing this kind of scheduling.

When a surgery is being scheduled, the medical assistant must sometimes coordinate several entities. Arrangement must be coordinated with an assistant in the surgeon's office, with the hospital or outpatient surgery center where the surgery will be performed, occasionally scheduling specialty equipment and personnel to be available, as well as with the patient's schedule. If any one of these entities is not available at the time requested, the process needs to begin again and can become quite convoluted. If the scheduling of the surgery is especially complex, the medical assistant should consider obtaining the patient's scheduling preferences and limitations and letting the patient go home to be contacted later when all the parts are in place.

Be sensitive to the patient's needs at this time. Rarely is scheduling a specialty examination or a hospital admission a convenience. More likely it is a great inconvenience to the patient, even when necessary. Anything you can do to make that scheduling more accommodating or pleasant for the patient will help in creating a beneficial atmosphere for all involved.

Procedure 13-1 — Checking In Patients and Explaining Office Policies

PURPOSE:
To ensure the patient is given prompt and proper care; to meet legal safeguards for documentation.

EQUIPMENT/SUPPLIES:
Patient chart
Black ink pen
Required forms
Check-in list or appointment book
Office policies brochure or flyer

PROCEDURE STEPS:
1. The previous evening or before opening the ambulatory care setting, prepare a list of patients to be seen and assemble the charts. RATIONALE: Provides a patient list to use as a guide through the day's schedule; charts are ready before patient arrival. If the task is left to the last minute, it may not get done.

(continues)

Procedure 13-1 (continued)

2. Check charts to see that everything is up to date. RATIONALE: Assures that physicians and their staff have all the necessary data before seeing a patient.
3. When patients arrive, acknowledge their presence. If you cannot assist them immediately, gesture toward a chair; thank them for waiting as soon as you are available. RATIONALE: Patients feel welcomed, their time is valued, and their presence is noted.
4. Check the patient in, reviewing vital information such as address, telephone number, insurance, and reason for visit. *Be certain to protect the patient's privacy by reviewing this information where doing so cannot be overheard by others.* RATIONALE: Assures that you have the latest personal information regarding your patient; provides patients with the privacy and confidentiality to which they are entitled.
5. Use a pen to check the patient's name off of the

daily worksheet if one is used for the permanent record. Place a check or the appropriate symbol in the computer space to indicate the patient's arrival. RATIONALE: Assures that there is a permanent record of the patient's arrival in the facility for an appointment. *Provides documentation for later referral if necessary.*
6. Give the patient an office policy brochure and let them know they can ask for clarification if they need to. Explain any specialized information in the brochure. Politely ask the patient to be seated and indicate the appropriate wait time, if any. RATIONALE: Provides direction to the patient and indicates how long a wait might be.
7. Following office policy, place the chart where it can be picked up to route the patient to the appropriate location for the visit. RATIONALE: The patient's chart is in readiness when the clinical medical assistant, laboratory personnel, or the physician is ready for the patient.

Procedure 13-2 Cancellation Procedures

PURPOSE:
To protect the physician from legal complications; to free up care time for other patients; to assure quality patient care.

EQUIPMENT/SUPPLIES:
Appointment sheet
Red ink pen
Patient chart

PROCEDURE STEPS:
Develop a system so it is evident to staff making appointments that, because of cancellations, time is now open to schedule other appointments.

1. Indicate on the appointment sheet all appointments that were changed, canceled, or no-shows by:
   - *Changes:* Note changes in the appointment sheet margin and directly in the patient's chart; indicate new appointment time. RATIONALE: Notifies all staff of a schedule

change; *documents same information in patient's chart.*
   - *Cancellations:* Note on both the appointment sheet and the patient's chart. Draw a single red line through canceled appointments. Date and initial cancellation in the patient chart. RATIONALE: Notifies staff of a schedule change; *documents cancellation in patient's chart, thus identifying a change in the patient's plans.* A cancellation may initiate a follow-up call from a staff member to determine the reason for the cancellation.
   - *No-shows:* Note on both the appointment sheet and the patient's chart. Date and initial notations in the chart. No-shows can be indicated with a red *X* on the appointment sheet. RATIONALE: Notifies the staff of a schedule change; *documents the no-show in the patient's chart.* Provides a reminder to a staff member to follow up on the reason for the no-show.

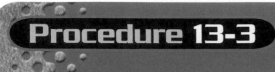

Procedure 13-3 Establishing the Appointment Matrix

PURPOSE:
To have a current and accurate record of appointment times available for scheduling patient visits.

EQUIPMENT/SUPPLIES:
Appointment scheduler
Physician's schedule
Staff schedule
Office calendar

PROCEDURE STEPS:
1. Block off times in the appointment scheduler when patients are not to be scheduled by marking a large **X** through these time slots. This establishes the matrix. Ideally, the whole year can be mapped out to avoid scheduling patients when the physician has other commitments or when the office is closed. RATIONALE: Identifies visually when patients cannot be scheduled for an appointment.
2. Indicate all vacations, holidays, and other office closures as soon as they are known. It may be helpful to indicate absences that might affect patient scheduling; for example, the vascular laboratory technician is gone April 20–23, so no Doppler procedures will be scheduled. RATIONALE: Informs all staff members of absences

from the facility and indicates when these members are not available to see patients.

3. Note all physician meetings, hospital rounds, appointments, conferences, vacations, and other prescheduled physician commitments. If the physician has routine items, such as a Medical Society meeting that is always held on the first Thursday of the month at 7:00 PM or daily hospital rounds at 8:00 AM, write these in. RATIONALE: Informs all staff members of prescheduled commitments when a physician is unavailable to see patients.
4. If the office has a scheduling system for certain examinations or procedures (e.g., all cast removals are done in the morning before 10:30 AM), these can be color-coded with highlighters. This way it is easily and quickly evident where particular types of appointments are available to be scheduled. RATIONALE: Allows all staff members to see at a glance where certain examinations or procedures can be scheduled. The color-coded highlighting helps prevent errors in establishing such specific times for certain procedures. *The completed matrix provides proof of the completed task.*

Procedure 13-4 Scheduling of Inpatient and Outpatient Admissions and Procedures

PURPOSE:
To assist patients in scheduling inpatient and outpatient admissions and procedures ordered by the physician.

EQUIPMENT/SUPPLIES:
Calendar
Black ink pen
Telephones
Referral slip
Patient's calendar or schedule (helpful, but not critical)

Physician requests/orders regarding procedures/admissions being scheduled

PROCEDURE STEPS:
1. In a private and quiet location, discuss with the patient the inpatient admission or outpatient procedure ordered by the physician. RATIONALE: Helps the patient identify the time necessary for this appointment and the reason for it.

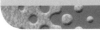

(continues)

Procedure 13-4 (continued)

2. If required, seek permission from the patient's insurance company for the procedure or admissions. RATIONALE: Clearly identifies for the patient who is responsible for the bill and how it is to be paid.

3. Produce a large, easily read calendar and check to see if the patient has one also. RATIONALE: Visualization of the calendar is easier in determining available time for the appointment. Patient's calendar further identifies available days and times for the appointment(s).

4. Place telephone call to the facility where the appointment is to be scheduled. Identify yourself, your physician, the clinic from where you are calling, and the reason for the call. RATIONALE: Alerts the receiver of the call that a physician's office is calling to schedule an appointment. NOTE: *The more familiar the medical assistant is with the specific procedure to be scheduled or a hospital admission, the easier it is to make certain the patient has all the information necessary. It can be helpful for medical assistants to discuss such arrangements with specialty clinics and hospitals.*

5. Identify any urgency. Request the next available appointment for the particular appointment to be scheduled and provide the patient's diagnosis. Identify any time that is not possible for the patient. RATIONALE: Tells the receiver how quickly an appointment is to be made, for what reason, and if any dates or times are not possible.

6. As a time is suggested, confer with the patient for an immediate response.

7. Once the appointment has been scheduled, provide receiver pertinent information related to the patient (e.g., full name, insurance information, Social Security number, telephone number). RATIONALE: Provides essential information to secure the appointment for the proper patient.

8. Request any special instructions or advanced data necessary for the patient. RATIONALE: Helps to assure that a smooth transition is made from the physician's office to the facility where the referral is made and provides the patient with any special instructions.

9. Complete the referral slip for the patient; send or fax a copy to the referral facility. RATIONALE: Assures that the patient, the referral facility, and the patient's chart have a copy of the reason for the appointment, any specific instructions, and the date and time of the appointment.

10. If an immediate hospital admission is to be made, provide the patient time at the telephone to call family members to make arrangements to receive personal items and any other arrangements necessitated by the appointment. RATIONALE: Provides patients a little time to notify a family member and make necessary arrangements.

11. Place a reminder notice to yourself on the calendar or in a tickler file. RATIONALE: To check to make certain the appointment was completed and a report is received from the appointment facility.

12. Document the referral in the patient's chart. A copy of the referral slip and all pertinent data are to be included. Document in the chart when the appointment is completed and a report is received from the referral facility. Date and initial.

DOCUMENTATION

11/30/20XX—10:45 AM Referral to Eastside Radiology for breast ultrasound made.
12/01/20XX—1 PM   Patient given instructions and copy of referral slip. Original referral slip sent to Eastside Radiology. C. Tamparo, CMA

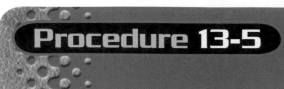

Procedure 13-5

Making an Appointment on the Telephone

PURPOSE:
To schedule an appointment entering information in the appointment schedule according to office policy.

EQUIPMENT/SUPPLIES:
Telephone
Black ink pen
Appointment book, computer screen, or appointment work sheet
Calendar

PROCEDURE STEPS:

1. *In a private and quiet location,* answer the ringing telephone before the third ring. Identify the facility and yourself. RATIONALE: Assures the patient calling that he or she has the correct number; sets the tone for the conversation. The private location assures that others will not hear any information said during the telephone call.

2. As the patient begins to speak, make notes on your personal log sheet of the patient's name and reason for the call. RATIONALE: Makes certain you are focusing on the call and will not have to ask the patient to repeat something you missed.

3. Determine if the patient is new or established, the physician to be seen, and the reason for the appointment. RATIONALE: Provides necessary information to determine when the patient should be seen and how much time will likely be necessary.

4. Discuss with the patient any special appointment needs, and search your appointment schedule (using book, computer, or appointment work-sheet) for an available time. A computer appointment schedule will automatically bring up the next available appointment slot that fits the need

of the patient. RATIONALE: Tells the patient that their needs and the needs of the clinic are essential to this conversation.

5. Once that patient has agreed to an appropriate time, enter the patient's name in the schedule. Enter last name first, followed by the first name, telephone number (home, work, or cell), and the chief complaint (reason for the visit). If using a manual system, write or print legibly with a black pen in the appointment book or worksheet so that any staff member needing the information will be able to read it. If using a computer system, check the data for accuracy as it is entered into the spaces provided. RATIONALE: Provides necessary information for staff to pull a record or to make a chart; chief complaint helps identify the length of time to allot for the appointment. The telephone number provides immediate information should there be a need to change the appointment without having to pull the chart.

6. Repeat the date and time for the appointment, using the patient's name. Provide any necessary instructions about coming to the facility. RATIONALE: Confirms the appointment date and time with the patient and gives them information about how to get to the facility.

7. End the call politely, perhaps saying, "Thank you for calling. We will see you at 3:45 PM Monday. Good-bye."

8. Make certain you transferred all necessary information from your telephone log to the appropriate appointment schedule. Draw a diagonal line through your notes on the log. This indicates you have completed the task.

Case Study 13-1

Rhoda Au has persistently canceled her appointments at Inner City Health Care; although she always reschedules, she has canceled her last four appointments. Today, she did not call to cancel nor did she show up for her fifth appointment. Walter Seals, CMA, who is responsible for scheduling and patient flow, is concerned that Rhoda is canceling because she is afraid to come in for some reason. Rhoda has been a patient for a few years now, and she was always responsible about keeping her appointments.

CASE STUDY REVIEW

1. From the point of view of the urgent care center, why should Walter be concerned that Rhoda is canceling appointments? What action might be taken?
2. From the patient's point of view, why should Walter be concerned?
3. How should Walter record these cancellations and no-shows?

Case Study 13-2

Audrey Jones, RMA, is a clinical medical assistant in Drs. Lewis and King's clinic. In the past three weeks, Audrey has been doing phone triage, primarily because the clinic has been so busy, the physicians believe triaging calls will help. In fact, Audrey discovered that the administrative medical assistant was doing triage quite well, but that there does not seem to be sufficient appointment slots to meet the patient demand.

CASE STUDY REVIEW

1. What might be done to determine if there is a better scheduling style to fit the current demands?
2. What happens when professional staff, physicians, and patients view this medical facility as "too busy"?
3. What are some solutions that you can identify?

SUMMARY

Today's ambulatory care setting needs to function efficiently to provide quality care, ensure adequate patient flow, and maintain positive patient relationships. Proper scheduling of patients and other visitors is key to an efficient operation, and the well-organized medical assistant will design a system that meets with both physician and patient satisfaction.

There are at least six common methods of scheduling; ambulatory care settings should use the one that is most appropriate to their patient population, practice areas, and physician preferences. Scheduling methods can and should be customized to the setting, for this usually provides the most adaptable, workable system.

Patient scheduling tools also vary and can be tailored to facility needs. All ambulatory care settings must carefully document appointments, cancellations, and no-shows. The goal is to use scheduling tools wisely and consistently in all scheduling activities while making the patient feel valued.

STUDY FOR SUCCESS

To reinforce your knowledge and skills of information presented in this chapter:

- ❑ Review the Key Terms
- ❑ Practice any Procedures
- ❑ Consider the Case Studies and discuss your conclusions
- ❑ Answer the Review Questions
  - ❑ Multiple Choice
  - ❑ Critical Thinking
- ❑ Navigate the Internet and complete the Web Activities
- ❑ Practice the StudyWARE activities on the textbook CD
- ❑ Apply your knowledge in the Student Workbook activities
- ❑ Complete the Web Tutor sections
- ❑ View and discuss the DVD situations

REVIEW QUESTIONS

Multiple Choice

1. Appointment scheduling should always be:
   a. recorded only in pencil
   b. current, accurate, and saved as documentation
   c. left on the front desk for patient viewing
   d. recorded only in red ink

2. Triaging:
   a. involves taking only emergencies
   b. is assessing the urgency of a call and need for appointment
   c. means sorting appointments by specialized procedure
   d. is only performed by physicians

3. Representatives from medical supply and drug companies:
   a. should only be seen as a last resort
   b. should not be scheduled, but seen only if the physician has time
   c. can provide a valuable service and should be scheduled for short visits
   d. have complex information to communicate and need one-hour appointments

4. The double-booking method:
   a. gives two or more patients the same appointment time
   b. keeps patients waiting unnecessarily
   c. is never the system of choice
   d. is purely for the physician's convenience

5. The stream method:
   a. gives patients appointments as they walk in
   b. schedules appointments at set times throughout the workday
   c. only works in single-physican offices
   d. refers to streamlining paperwork for each appointment

6. Daily appointment sheets:
   a. indicate when physicians and staff take lunch
   b. provide a permanent record for legal risk management and quality management
   c. are available only in computerized patient scheduling
   d. both a and b
7. Analyzing patient flow:
   a. can maximize an office's scheduling practice
   b. often reveals why patient flow is not efficient
   c. may indicate a change in pattern for patient scheduling
   d. all of the above
8. One principal above all else to be observed in scheduling is:
   a. always schedule in ink
   b. schedule for the patient's convenience
   c. be flexible and sensitive
   d. referral patients are first
9. If a patient must wait for an appointment:
   a. it is best to say nothing about the delay
   b. explain the delay and offer options when possible
   c. find ways to make the patient comfortable
   d. both b and c
10. Scheduling outpatient procedures is:
    a. best done by patients who understand their availability
    b. coordinated and completed by the physician's staff
    c. an important way to enhance patient satisfaction
    d. both b and c

Critical Thinking

1. Discuss the rationale and the procedure to follow for a canceled appointment and a no-show appointment.
2. Why is there no one best system of scheduling?
3. Form small discussion groups and develop solutions to the following problems by (i) defining the problem, (ii) describing the appropriate steps if required, and (iii) developing a possible solution.
   a. Lenore McDonnell has called to cancel her appointment for the third consecutive time. (Background: Her last blood pressure reading in the office was 195/115, and there is a known history of stroke in her family.)

b. Dr. Lewis is running an hour behind schedule. It is now 1:00 PM. He is now seeing a return patient. He has two new patients scheduled and has a surgery scheduled for 2:00 PM. (Background: Return patients require 30 minutes and new patients 60 minutes.)
   c. You are using the modified wave system. You have three appointments scheduled for 10:00 AM, one for 10:50 AM, and three for 11:00 AM. The office closes at 11:30 for lunch so Dr. King can speak at a hospital luncheon. A patient calls and insists to be seen on an emergency basis. (Background: Dr. King's partner is unavailable to cover for her.)
   d. Two patients are scheduled to be seen at 11:30. It is now 11:50, and Dr. Whitney has indicated that he will not be through with his current patient for another 20 minutes. (Background: Both patients waiting to see Dr. Whitney have nonemergency problems.)
4. For the following situations, briefly explain which type of scheduling system you would choose and why.
   a. A four-physician practice has only two physicians seeing patients at any one time. There are three medical assistants sharing front- and back-office duties for all of the physicians.
   b. An obstetrics practice specializes in problem pregnancies. There is one administrative and one clinical medical assistant.

WEB ACTIVITIES

1. Go to www.physicianpractice.com for any information you can find regarding online patient scheduling. Identify advantages and disadvantages of online scheduling.
2. Go to your favorite search engine and key in "patient scheduling." Numerous sites will appear. Many offer a free download to examine components. What particular components seem most helpful? How many are separate software pieces as compared with software in connection with total practice management? How many require specialized training? Recommend two or three packages to examine more closely.

THE DVD HOOK-UP

DVD Series	Program Number
Skills Based Series	**1**

Chapter/Scene Reference
• *Scheduling Patients over the Phone*
• *Strategies and Methods of Scheduling*

In this chapter, you learned about proper scheduling techniques. Just as phone procedures vary in a medical office, so do scheduling techniques.

In this DVD program, you observed the extern, Jamal, working with Anita. In the first scenario, Anita took a phone call from a new patient. Anita asked the new patient about his symptoms before asking about insurance information.

1. Why do you think that Anita asked the patient about his symptoms before finding out what type of insurance he had?
2. Why is it important to find out what type of insurance the patient has before he or she comes into the office?

3. What do you need to do when a physician tells you that he or she is unable to see patients on a certain date because of a conference?

DVD Journal Summary
Write a paragraph that summarizes what you learned from watching the designated scenes from today's DVD program. Think about your own experiences when you have been acutely ill. Does your medical office always fit you in on the day that you call? How do you feel when the office tells you they have no openings for two to three days? How do you feel when you have to wait longer than a half hour to see the physician?

REFERENCES/BIBLIOGRAPHY

Leibrock, C. (2000). *Design details for health*. New York: John Wiley & Sons.

Lewis, M. A., & Tamparo, C. D. (2002). *Medical law, ethics, and bioethics for ambulatory care* (4th ed.). Philadelphia: F.A. Davis.

CHAPTER 14

Medical Records Management

OUTLINE

KEY TERMS

Accession Record
Caption
Consecutive or Serial Filing
Cross-Reference
Indexing
Key Unit
Nonconsecutive Filing
Out Guide
Problem-Oriented Medical Record (POMR)
Purging
Shingling
SOAP
Source-Oriented Medical Record (SOMR)
Tickler File
Unit

FEATURED COMPETENCIES

CAAHEP—ENTRY-LEVEL COMPETENCIES

Administrative Competencies

- Perform clerical functions
- Organize a patient's medical record
- File medical records

Legal Concepts

- Identify and respond to issues of confidentiality
- Establish and maintain the medical record
- Document appropriately
- Demonstrate knowledge of federal and state health care legislation and regulations

Operational Functions

- Utilize computer software to maintain office systems

ABHES—ENTRY-LEVEL COMPETENCIES

Communication

- Receive, organize, prioritize, and transmit information expediently
- Application of electronic technology

Administrative Duties

- Perform basic secretarial skills
- Prepare and maintain medical records
- Apply computer concepts for office procedures
- File medical records

Legal Concepts

- Determine needs for documentation and reporting
- Document accurately
- Use appropriate guidelines when releasing records or information

246

OBJECTIVES

The student should strive to meet the following performance objectives and demonstrate an understanding of the facts and principles presented in this chapter through written and oral communication.

1. Define the key terms as presented in the glossary.
2. Discuss the ownership of medical records.
3. State the reasons for accurately maintaining ambulatory care office files.
4. Describe how information is released from the medical record.
5. Correct a medical record.
6. Recall eight common supplies used in medical records management.
7. Identify the rules described under Basic Rules for Filing.
8. Describe the five steps commonly used when filing any documentation.
9. State three advantages and three disadvantages of the manual medical record and the electronic medical record.
10. Name the two filing systems most often used in the ambulatory care setting.
11. State the purpose of cross-referencing.
12. Recall four common documents filed in the patient's medical record.
13. Describe electronic medical records and their usefulness to the ambulatory care setting.
14. Discuss confidentiality and privacy as related to medical records.

SCENARIO

Consider a situation that might arise at the multiphysician Inner City Health Care. Patient Juanita Hansen was seen on Tuesday morning by Dr. Whitney for acute stomach pain. She was given a thorough examination and sent for appropriate testing that afternoon. She was then scheduled to return to Inner City on Friday to see Dr. Whitney.

After she was seen Tuesday morning, Juanita received an upper and lower gastrointestinal series; the results were then sent to Dr. Whitney's office. However, because Karen Ritter, RMA, the medical assistant, could not locate Juanita's chart to file the test results, she just set them aside. Friday arrived and Juanita came back to Inner City for her appointment, anxious to know the results of her tests. Dr. Whitney found Juanita's chart, which was inadvertently left on his stack of dictation, and realized the patient's test results had not been filed.

This left Dr. Whitney with an anxious patient. Karen Ritter is off today, so the physician checks with the other medical assistants on duty. They have no knowledge of the test results. Two acts—not replacing the file, and not promptly filing Juanita's test results—cause undue stress for the physician, medical assistants, and the patient.

INTRODUCTION

A vital function of any medical facility is the maintenance of patient records identifying the care given. Medical assistants, both administrative and clinical, will spend a fair amount of time managing the patients' records. As seen in the scenario, a misplaced patient chart or a missing piece of important information causes stress to everyone involved and leaves the patient feeling that the staff is incompetent. Medical records potentially record all medical data about an individual from birth until death. It is seldom, however, in today's mobile society that a patient's record is that comprehensive. Patients are increasingly concerned about their medical records and the protection of their privacy. There are a number of statutes and agencies that support the protection of patients' medical information, but there are so many individuals who handle the information, perform tasks related to the patient, or need data for proper medical treatment, that patients have cause to be concerned.

OWNERSHIP OF MEDICAL RECORDS

State statutes have ruled that medical records are the property of those who create them. The information within the medical record, however, belongs to the patient, and that information is always to be protected with the utmost privacy and confidentiality. Patients may be allowed access to their medical records, ask for notes or information to be added to their files, and request certain information not be included in their files.

Physicians who involve their patients in their medical record keeping foster trust and respect with their patients. For example, a physician who enters patient data into the computerized patient record while sitting at a computer monitor in the examination room beside the patient has the opportunity to explain that the information is entered now so there is no room for error in reporting, or in the physician not accurately recalling the patient information if entered at a later time. A patient who asks a primary-care physician to put the pen aside while discussing possible depression symptoms is concerned about privacy, especially if the patient is the pediatrics department manager in the same large metropolitan medical center/hospital. The physician should realize that a discussion of how to keep this information confidential so that other employees are not aware of the patient's concern is in order.

THE IMPORTANCE OF MEDICAL RECORDS

The primary purposes of medical records in the ambulatory care setting are to:

1. Provide a base for managing patient care
2. Provide interoffice and intraoffice communication as necessary
3. Determine any patterns that surface to signal the physician of patient needs
4. Serve as a basis for legal information necessary to protect physicians, staff, and patients
5. Provide clinical data for research

Spotlight on Certification

RMA Content Outline
- Records management
- Charts

CMA Content Outline
- Maintaining confidentiality
- Documentation/reporting
- Releasing medical information
- Records management

CMAS Content Outline
- Medical Records Management

AUTHORIZATION TO RELEASE INFORMATION

It is recommended that before any information is released from the medical record, even if it is subpoenaed, the patient be notified and written approval received. Medical facilities will have appropriate forms for such release of information. The form should identify the reason for the release of information and what information is specifically requested. *Only* that information should be released. This does not include the release of information to a patient's chosen insurance carrier. A number of different methods exist to release that information. For some insurance carriers, the release is granted when the patient accepts the insurance coverage. For others, a yearly release form must be signed by the patient.

THE IMPORTANCE OF ACCURATE MEDICAL RECORDS

Accurate medical records are essential to patient care in any ambulatory care setting. Patient files are critical to the facility's smooth functioning and are important when referring the patient to outside specialists with whom the facility may need to coordinate care. Each treating physician must be aware of tests, procedures, and diagnoses. Maintaining a conscientious record of patient care is also absolutely essential in controlling the costs of medical care.

Medical records management is also important because of the legal issues that every medical office and health care professional must face today. The standard in court is that if there is no record of any piece of information related to a patient and that patient's care and treatment, then it did not happen. The question to ask yourself about any piece of information is: "Does this relate to the patient's care, and should it be in the chart?" To be prepared in the event of medical litigation, you must document all medical treatment. No matter how competently a physician has performed treatment, if a written record cannot prove how and what was done, there is no basis for a defense in a court of law.

Correcting Medical Records

The medical record must be readable and accurate; however, errors do occur and may not be discovered immediately. Any corrections necessary to a paper medical record should be corrected using the following method: draw a single line using a red ink pen through the error, make the correction, write "Corr." or "Correction" above the area corrected, and indicate your initials and the current date. The red line through the information indicates the "error" portion of the report. The words "Corr." or "Correction" by the correction indicates the change. The date and initials identify when the correction was made and by whom. Obliterations should never occur. When the medical record becomes the center of attention in malpractice litigation, forensic experts will be able to tell if a record has been tampered with or if information or pages have been added later. When not properly done, altered records become a detriment to a physician's defense in court. Refer to Procedure 14-3.

Errors discovered after the fact in an electronic medical record are corrected differently. Although it could be easy to do so, the error is *not corrected* by simple word processing. In a truly paperless office, a notation is entered at the place of the error, a line is drawn through the error (using the tracking device in the word processing software), and the correction is made immediately after the information lined out. "Corr." or "Correction" is indicated and your initials and the date added. The finished product will look almost exactly like a correction in a paper medical chart. See Procedure 14-4.

If any correction is necessary in a piece of information after either a paper chart or an electronic chart has been sent to another physician or facility, make a copy of the corrected information and send it to the physician or facility as quickly as possible.

MANUAL OR ELECTRONIC MEDICAL RECORDS

Today's world has a mixture of manual, or paper, medical records and the electronic form of medical records. Electronic medical records are widely seen in large medical clinics, in metropolitan clinics with hospitals, and in the hospital setting. Many ambulatory care settings, however, have not yet fully computerized their medical records. This is in part because of physicians' reluctance to let go of the paper medical record and the incredible expense of switching to computerized medical records. Also, there is the concern of how to transfer the current paper record to the computer record. Consider the following advantages and disadvantages of both records:

MANUAL MEDICAL RECORD

Advantages	Disadvantages
Currently established and understood	Can be used by only one person at a time
Easier to protect confidentiality	Easily misplaced or misfiled
No worry of computer malfunction	Equipment and storage space required

ELECTRONIC MEDICAL RECORD

Advantages	Disadvantages
Multiple users is possible	Needs protection to
Not easily misplaced or	prevent loss of data
misfiled	Expensive to establish
Patterns and data more	and maintain
easily accessed	May require on-site
Quickly available in	assistance
emergencies	
Office storage space not	
required	
Legible, organized patient	
documentation	
Improved medication	
management	

The medical record system must be one that fits the facility and satisfies the needs of the physicians. Usually, medical record systems are adapted for a particular facility using certain common components. Whatever system is used, the management of the medical records must provide easy retrieval of information. Files must be organized, data entered legibly, and all documentation complete and correct. Wording must be easily understood and grammatically correct. How corrections are made in the chart, how documents are removed or added to the chart, and the chart format must be predetermined and understood by all users of the information.

TYPES OF MEDICAL RECORDS

Just as the choice of a filing system is important to the efficient use of files, so too is the arrangement of materials within the charts. Again, the choice of method must be in accordance with how the information needs to be accessed and used for each individual office. No one method is correct. In the examples that follow, arrangement of materials is also discussed.

Problem-Oriented Medical Record

The **problem-oriented medical record (POMR)** type of record keeping uses a sheet, generally on the inside cover or other prominent location, which lists vital identification data, immunizations, allergies, medications, and problems. The problems are identified by a number that corresponds to the charting relevant to that problem number; that is, bronchitis #1; broken wrist #2; and so forth. If the patient returns in nine months with recurring bronchitis, the same number (#1) is used.

The patient chart is then further built by adding a numbered and titled page for each problem the patient experiences; for example, bronchitis #1; broken wrist #2.

Each problem is then followed with the **SOAP** approach for all progress notes:

S   Subjective impressions
O   Objective clinical evidence
A   Assessment or diagnosis
P   Plans for further studies, treatment, or management

This process makes the chart easier to review and helps in follow-up of all the patient's medical needs (Figure 14-1). The SOAP approach also allows medical personnel to be aware of the patient's current medications. Starting and resolution dates for each problem also are noted on the tracking sheet.

Internists, family practitioners, and pediatricians use the POMR system more commonly than do specialists because they see their patients for a variety of problems over a long span of time.

There are a number of medical supply companies that produce various formats for POMR charts. There are flip-up folder styles; book-style folders made of 125 lb. manila or white stock with twin prong fasteners are the most popular. Divider pages may come with tabs that are preprinted to your specific needs or have adhesive labels that can be printed on your inkjet or laser printer exactly as you want them. Sometimes, the inside front and back covers are printed with information to be filled in. These areas are often used to provide essential personal information such as name, address, telephone numbers, insurance information, and responsible party. In a prominent place, usually on the inside front cover, is the word "ALLERGIES" in big letters (often preprinted in red). Any allergies that patients have are listed here. Also prominently displayed should be any forms the patient has signed granting release of information, as well as any forms signed to comply with Health Insurance Portability and Accountability Act (HIPAA) regulations.

The problem list may be entered on a divider flap or on specially printed paper. Other dividers may be used for laboratory reports, progress notes, history and physicals, hospital admissions, and medications. Depending on the practice and the wishes of the physician, tab dividers are available for consultations, correspondence, insurance data, hospital notes, pathology reports, and electrocardiogram reports. The problem list is most likely the first divider used, followed by laboratory reports, and progress notes, usually in the SOAP format.

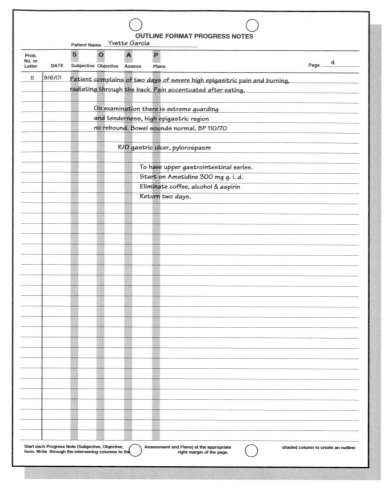

Figure 14-1 Example of SOAP progress notes. (Courtesy of Bibbero Systems, Inc., Petaluma, CA.)

Source-Oriented Medical Record

The **source-oriented medical record (SOMR)** groups information according to its source; for example, from laboratories, examinations, physician notes, consulting physicians, and other sources. Many offices use this method because it makes different types of information quickly accessible. A fastener folder is used that contains several partitions with their own fasteners. This allows for a separate section for laboratory reports, pathology, progress notes, physical examinations, and correspondence to be filed chronologically within each section. In the SOMR system, many physicians will use the SOAP method to record their chart notes.

The organization of the SOMR is quite similar to the POMR chart with the one exception that the SOMR does not have the problem list. Also, the SOMR may continually add sheets of identifying information with appropriate sections in the chart rather than transferring any data. Many electronic medical record software packages use either the POMR or the SOMR format and are easily adapted to a particular physician's practice.

Strict Chronological Arrangement

Using strict chronology, data are filed strictly with the most recently charted materials to the top of the folder. For instance, a patient is treated from 1994 to the present. To locate information recorded in 1997, it is necessary to flip through the chart until the material for the year 1997 is located. This method makes it difficult for a physician or medical assistant to quickly assess a patient's clinical picture. This type of arrangement may seem confusing, but it may fit a specialty office such as a dietitian, radiologist, or physical therapist where patients are usually seen on a short-term basis.

Shingling Medical Records

The **shingling** method is generally used to file laboratory reports. Many of these reports are smaller than the standard size sheets of paper. Shingling ensures that medical personnel have quick access to the most recent data. In addition, it keeps small pieces of paper from being misplaced or lost within the medical record. Simply put, the sheets of paper are "shingled" either up or across the page, the most recent report placed on top of the previous one. Special sheets with self-adhesive strips are available for this purpose.

To fully understand records management and proper filing techniques it is helpful to first look at the manual system. Computerized systems are designed to make the process easier to use, but the basic premises are the same.

EQUIPMENT AND SUPPLIES

There are three primary types of file cabinets used in medical offices: vertical, lateral, and movable file cabinets.

Vertical Files

Vertical files are cabinets that have pullout drawers where files are stored (Figure 14-2). Files are retrieved by lifting the appropriate file up and out. These may be used for business records and documents. The cabinet illustrated in Figure 14-2 includes a locking device.

The best vertical files have a center trough in the bottom of each drawer with a rod running through for holding divider guides. The rod and guides help in keeping file folders from slipping down underneath other file folders and getting misplaced or lost.

Open-Shelf Lateral Files

Open-shelf lateral file cabinets make quick retrieval of files possible (Figure 14-3). The records are retrieved by pulling them out laterally from the shelf. They are used most often with color-coded filing systems where visual inspection makes it possible to ensure files are kept in the proper order. It is necessary to be able to close and lock the open-shelf lateral files.

Movable File Units

Movable file units allow easy access to large record systems and require less space than vertical or lateral files. These units may be electrically powered to move on floor tracks or may be physically moved with an easy-to-turn handle mechanism. The movable shelving unit is electrically powered to open aisles for accessing files or to close aisles when those files do not need to be accessed. There are also movable file storage units that will automatically travel on a computer-controlled carousel track moving files around until the required section reaches the operator.

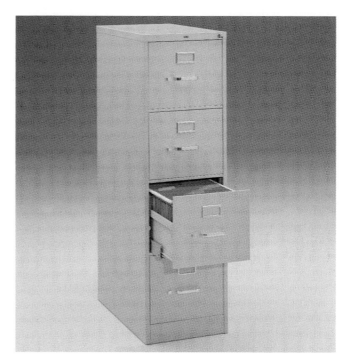

Figure 14-2   Vertical file cabinet. (Courtesy HON® Company.)

File Folders

File folders are designed for different types of labels. Extending along the top edge (the edge that will be visible when filing) are tabs that are cut in varying sizes and positions to allow for different methods of labeling. Figure 14-4 shows the types of cuts, or tabs, found on file folders.

Identification Labels

A variety of labels are used to display the information required to select the correct name or number designation for a particular file. The identification label is adhered

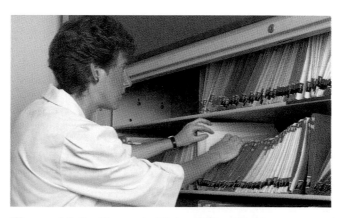

Figure 14-3   Open-shelf lateral file cabinet.

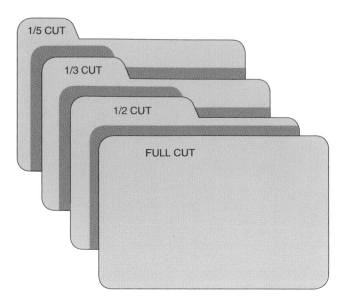

Figure 14-4 Types of cuts, or tabs, on file folders.

either along the top of the file folder (top tab) in vertical file cabinets or along the side of the file folder (side tab) in lateral file cabinets.

Guides and Positions

Guides are used to separate file folders. Guides are somewhat larger than file folders and are of heavier stock. Guides are described by the position of the tab, designated according to its location. For instance, a tab located at the far left would be in the first position, the next one to the right would be in the second position, and so forth. If using third-cut file folders, there are three positions of guides; if using fifth-cut file folders, there are five positions. Guides are used in vertical and lateral systems.

Captions. **Captions** are used to identify major sections of file folders by more manageable subunits (AA–AC, A, B, Office Supplies). Captions are marked on the tabs of the guides (Figure 14-5). These are denoted as single caption and double caption:

- *Single captions* contain just one letter, number, or unit:

   ○ A, B, C, D

   ○ Adams, Smith, Jones

- *Double captions* contain a double notation to denote a range of files:

   ○ Ab–Be, Co–Dy, Ho–Le

   ○ Appleston–Bertram, Cody–Devoe

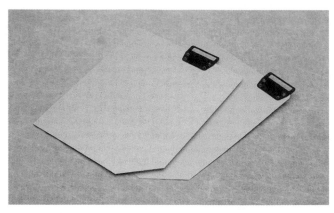

Figure 14-5 Guides separating file folders into subsections. Captions such as A,B,C (single captions) or Ab–Be, Co–Dy (double captions) are placed on the tabs of the guides to identify the sections.

Out Guides

Out guides or out sheets are devices to help in tracking charts. An out guide is a cardboard or plastic/paper sheet kept in place of the patient chart when charts are removed from the filing storage (Figure 14-6).

BASIC RULES FOR FILING

Regardless of the type of filing system used, alphabetizing is the key to organizing all files and charts. It is necessary to know more than just the alphabetic order of the letters A to Z. Thus, certain indexing rules have been developed by the Association of Medical Records Administrators (AMRA) to facilitate the alphabetic process in maintaining files in the medical office.

Indexing Units

There must be an organized method of identifying and separating items to be filed into small subunits. This is accomplished with the use of what we call **indexing** units. A unit identifies each part of a name. In this process, each **unit** is identified according to unit 1 (the **key unit**), unit 2, unit 3, and so forth, with each segment of the filing label identified. This process can be applied to individual

Critical Thinking

Now that you have read about types of charting systems and file folders, identify which type of cut on either the top or side of a folder you believe would be most convenient. Justify your response.

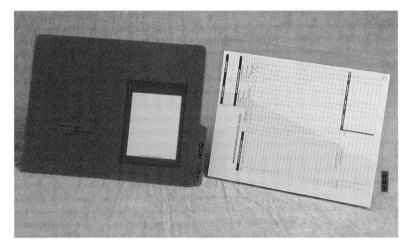

Figure 14-6 An out guide indicating the name of the person who has possession of the file should always be put in place of a patient's record when it is removed from the file.

names, organizations, or clinics. Accepted filing rules describe how to assign unit numbers to each element.

Example. Annette Barbara Samuels

Unit 1	Samuels
Unit 2	Annette
Unit 3	Barbara

 When working in a medical setting with patient charts, the patient's legal name is always used for the chart rather than a nickname or abbreviation. If the office has a practice of calling patients by preferred names, a note of name preferences and nicknames may be noted on the chart. However, the filing label should use the proper name.

Example. The following items to be filed would be assigned units as illustrated:

	Units Assigned		
	1	2	3
Cole Blanche Little	Little	Cole	Blanche
Wayne Lee Elder	Elder	Wayne	Lee
Kelso Medical Supply	Kelso	Medical	Supply

Filing Patient Charts

Rule 1. The names of individuals are assigned indexing units, respectively: last name (surname), first name, middle, and succeeding names.

	Units Assigned		
	1	2	3
Jaime Renae Carrera	Carrera	Jaime	Renae
Lee Allen Au	Au	Lee	Allen
Bill Hugo Schwartz	Schwartz	Bill	Hugo

Rule 2. Names that include a single letter are indexed as the legal name and are placed before full names beginning with the same letter. "Nothing comes before something."

	Units Assigned		
	1	2	3
J. Larson	Larson	J	—
James R. Larson	Larson	James	R

Rule 3. Foreign language prefixes are indexed as one unit with the unit that follows. Spacing, punctuation, and capitalization are ignored. Such prefixes include *d, da, de, de la, del, des, di, du, el, fitz, l, la, las, le, les, lu, m, mac, mc, o, saint, sainte, san, santa, sao, st, te, ten, ter, van, van de, van der,* and *von der* (*st, sainte,* and *saint* are indexed as written).

	Units Assigned		
	1	2	3
Gerald Steven St. Simon	Stsimon	Gerald	Steven
Carol Louise del Rio	Delrio	Carol	Louise

Rule 4. When titles are used, they are considered as separate indexing units. If the title appears with first and last names, the title is considered to be the last indexing unit. When dealing with patient charts, the first name always accompanies the title and last name.

	Units Assigned			
	1	2	3	4
Dr. Marlene Elaine Smith	Smith	Marlene	Elaine	Dr
Prof. Marcia Tai Lewis	Lewis	Marcia	Tai	Prof

Rule 5. Names that are hyphenated are considered as one unit.

	Units Assigned		
	1	2	3
Adele Marie Johnson-Smith	Johnsonsmith	Adele	Marie
Ray Steven Reynolds-Martin	Reynoldsmartin	Ray	Steven

Rule 6. When indexing names of married women, the name is indexed by the legal name. Remember that patient charts are legal documents, making this practice necessary (use cross-referencing as necessary).

	Units Assigned			
	1	2	3	4
Amy Sue Sung (Mrs. John)	Sung	Amy	Sue	Mrs John
Tami Jo Strizver (Mrs. Todd)	Strizver	Tami	Jo	Mrs Todd

Rule 7. Seniority and professional or academic degrees are the last indexing unit and are used only to distinguish identical names.

	Units Assigned			
	1	2	3	4
James Edward Brown, Jr.	Brown	James	Edward	Jr
James Edward Brown, Sr.	Brown	James	Edward	Sr

Rule 8. Mac and Mc are filed in their regular place alphabetically. Some clinics will provide a special guide for both Mac and Mc for ease in filing.

Maasch
Mabbott
MacDonald
Mazziotti
McAffe

Rule 9. Numeric units are broken down such that numeric seniority terms are filed before alphabetic terms.

	Edward Lee Kletka, IV
BEFORE	Edward Lee Kletka, Jr.
	George Lee Curtis, II
BEFORE	George Lee Curtis, Sr.

Filing Identical Names

When names are identical, the address may be used to order files. The address is indexed by:

First:	City
SECOND	STATE
Third	*Street Name*
Fourth:	**Address #**

Therefore, the following Acme Drug Supply files would be arranged from first to last as follows:

1. Acme Drug Supply, **839** *Kentucky Boulevard,* Crawford, MISSOURI
2. Acme Drug Supply, **683** *Wildflower Avenue,* Fairbanks, ALASKA
3. Acme Drug Supply, **1539** *Wildflower Avenue,* Fairbanks, ALASKA
4. Acme Drug Supply, **742** *Terminal Street West,* Fairbanks, ARIZONA
5. Acme Drug Supply, **731** *Terminal Street East,* New York, NEW YORK

Although this is the official indexing rule, most medical offices prefer alternative methods for filing identical charts. The primary consideration here is that patient addresses often change frequently. Therefore, preferred methods include date of birth or social security number.

STEPS FOR FILING MEDICAL DOCUMENTATION IN PATIENT FILES

Before a discussion of the common filing systems, it is helpful to review procedural steps that accurately and efficiently process data sheets, laboratory requests, dictation, and so forth from the time they are generated to the time the file is returned to the medical records section. Efficiently following these steps will save considerable time in the ambulatory care setting.

Inspect

Carefully inspect the report to identify the patient, subject, or file to whom the information belongs. Remove clips and staples. Make certain the information is complete.

Critical Thinking

Identify the steps you might take in "inspecting" the charts before filing. What would you do if you found something missing or an unsigned report?

Index

Use the indexing process to determine how the chart would be located, properly identifying indexing units and their order.

Code

Coding in medical records is the process of marking data to indicate how information is to be filed. If using a system other than a strict alphabetic system, determine the proper coding for the chart so it can be retrieved. Otherwise, identify the indexed units by underlining or highlighting. This makes refiling more effective and assures that the item will always be filed in the same place. If a cross-reference is required, identify the cross-reference by double underlining and placing an X nearby. This chapter includes detailed information on coding and cross-referencing.

Sort

If there are a number of reports/documents to be filed, sort them into units according to the captions on the charts. This will eliminate wasted time in working back and forth through the alphabet or numbers. Figure 14-7 shows a medical assistant using a desk sorter to put files and reports in alphabetic order.

File

The papers are placed in the proper charts and the charts returned to their proper place in the medical records section. Be alert to the labels and refile any information or charts that have been misfiled.

FILING TECHNIQUES AND COMMON FILING SYSTEMS

There are three major filing systems commonly used in the ambulatory care setting: alphabetic, numeric, and subject filing. The alphabet is intrinsic to all methods, and the basic rules for filing, covered previously, are used in all systems.

Color coding is used a high percentage of the time in all three systems to minimize filing errors. Another system, geographic, is seldom used in the ambulatory care

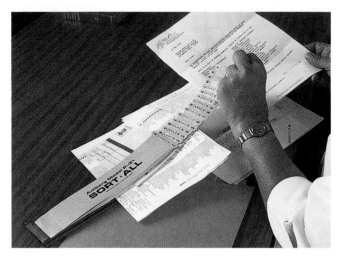

Figure 14-7 Medical assistant using a desk sorter to alphabetize reports to make filing easier.

setting unless there are multiple offices. Even then, a form of color coding may be used.

Color Coding

Color coding is a technique often used in the three major filing systems. Numerous color-coding systems are available. Patient charts most often use an alphabetic system of color coding, although color coding can be used in numeric filing as well. Smead Manufacturing, Kardex, Bibbero, and Colwell are all companies widely known in medical and dental fields for their color systems. Color coding may seem complicated at first, but once medical assistants understand the principles behind it and practice its application a number of times, the task becomes much easier, and there is immediate recognition if a chart is misfiled.

Color coding makes retrieval of files more efficient with the use of visible color differences that facilitate easier maintenance of the files. Color-coding filing systems also use an alphabetic system; after they are coded by color, that designation is used to order the files alphabetically.

Tab-Alpha System. The various forms of the Tab-Alpha system are designed primarily for filing systems that use vertical files where all individual charts are clearly visible in one unit.

Each alphabetic letter is assigned a different color. Each folder has a color-coded label. Only full-cut folders are used:

- Colored labels are applied over the edge of the full cut for the first two letters of the key indexing unit (Winston, Paul Lewis: WI).

- A third white label is placed over the tab edge, which contains all of the indexing units (Winston, Paul Lewis).

- In addition, some offices use a color-coded label to indicate the last year the patient was seen. This makes an efficient method for easily identifying active and inactive files.

- Any additional labels (e.g., allergies, last year seen, or industrial claim) are attached to the chart according to the office procedure.

Alpha-Z System. Forms of the Alpha-Z system are designed for use with either open lateral files or vertical drawer files (Figure 14-8A). Alphabetic letters are used as the primary guides. Breakdowns of alphabetic combinations are added as determined by the needs of a particular facility.

A combination of 13 colors is used in the Alpha-Z system with white letters on a solid colored background for the first half of the alphabet and white letters on a colored background with white stripes for the second half of the alphabet (Figure 14-8B).

The 13 colors used are shown in Table 14-1. Folders have three labels:

- The first label contains the typed name, a color block, and the letter of the alphabet for the first letter of the first indexing unit:

Winston, Lewis Paul YELLOW "W"

- The second and third labels are color-coded to correspond to the second and third letters of the first unit:

"I" on pink background and "N" on red-striped background

Customized Color-Coding Systems. Many offices use color systems to meet specific needs.

Colored File Folders by First Name. One method color codes the first letter of the first name. The folders then are filed alphabetically by last name.

Example. *A* is assigned red folders; *M* is assigned green folders; *S* is assigned blue folders

Michael Taylor	Green Folder
Annette Samuels	Red Folder
Susan Boyer	Blue Folder

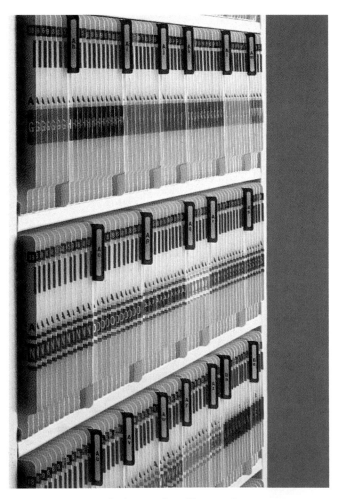

Figure 14-8A Color-coding filing system uses open-lateral shelving unit with color-coded files. (Courtesy Smead Manufacturing Company.)

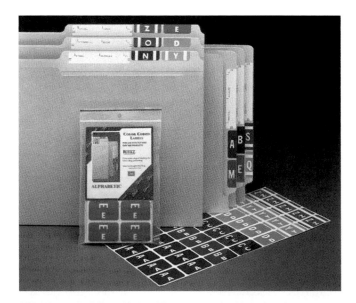

Figure 14-8B Alpha-Z color-coded labels shown on top- and side-cut files.

Many small medical offices use this system and find it quite effective. In the multiphysician urgent care center, this would be quite time-consuming when locating files for patients of all physicians.

Colored File Folders by Last Name. Another method using this system assigns colored folders according to the first letter of the last name. The folders are then filed alphabetically.

Example. *S* is assigned pink folders; *B* is assigned gray folders.

Bill Schwartz	Pink Folder
Corey Boyer	Gray Folder

TABLE 14-1	THIRTEEN COLORS ARE USED IN THE ALPHA-Z SYSTEM	
White Letter Colored Background	**White Letter Striped Colored Background**	**Color**
A	N	Red
B	O	Dark Blue
C	P	Dark Green
D	Q	Light Blue
E	R	Purple
F	S	Orange
G	T	Gray
H	U	Dark Brown
I	V	Pink
J	W	Yellow
K	X	Light Brown
L	Y	Lavender
M	Z	Light Green

This system makes it easy to spot folders that have been misfiled under an incorrect first letter, but it does not break it down further for misfilings within the first-letter guides.

Color-Coded Numbers. The color-coded number system is used in a numeric filing system and operates in the same way as alphabetic systems. Numbers from 0 to 9 are color coded. The appropriate colored numbers are then placed on the tabs of the patient's folder.

Alphabetic Filing

Strict alphabetic filing is one of the simplest filing methods, as files are strictly maintained by assigning a label to each file. The first letter of that label (e.g., Jones, Invoices, or Pharmacies) is then used to alphabetize the files from A to Z. When a limited number of files is accessed, this is an acceptable method of maintaining records. Also note that every filing system will utilize the alphabet somewhere.

Numeric Filing

Numeric filing is organized by number rather than by letter. A key benefit of numeric filing is that it preserves patient confidentiality because the individual's name is not obviously apparent on the file folder.

Numeric filing systems are either consecutive (serial) or nonconsecutive.

Consecutive or Serial. The **consecutive or serial filing** method is commonly used in handling invoices, sales orders, and requisitions. Each record is numbered and filed in ascending order.

Example. 576 93 or 57693

Unit 1	5
Unit 2	7
Unit 3	6
Unit 4	9
Unit 5	3

Nonconsecutive. The **nonconsecutive filing** system uses groups of two, three, or four or more digits (e.g., Social Security numbers). This system is often used in hospitals and large clinics. Numbers are grouped and arranged in ascending order using the digits to the far right or the terminal digits. Each group of numbers is considered a unit (one number). To file the terminal digit files in numerical order, begin with strictly the terminal digit unit.

Example. 2108 23 879

Unit 1	879
Unit 2	23
Unit 3	2108

Components of Numeric Filing. There are four essential components that are used with a numeric system, whether it is a manual or computerized system.

Serially Numbered Dividers with Guides. Consecutive numeric guides (5, 10, etc.; 50, 100, etc.) separate the individual file folders into smaller groups of files.

Miscellaneous (General) Numeric File Section. This is reserved for records that have not been assigned numbers. Patients should automatically be assigned a number on the first visit. However, there are occasions where patients cannot be assigned a number initially. The miscellaneous section is generally in front of all the numeric folders for ease of locating items. Files in the miscellaneous section are filed alphabetically by patient name. This is the best place for the miscellaneous file(s) for two reasons:

1. They do not have to be moved each time a numbered file is added to the back of the order.
2. In a large system of files, retrieval from the front is quick and easy.

Alphabetic Card File. This alphabetic file is necessary as a source to locate files or records. A card contains name, address, and file number (or an M if located in the mis-cellaneous section); any **cross-reference** is here rather than in the numeric files.

The alphabetic card file in a manual system would be equivalent to the computerized record of the patient and whatever number is assigned to him or her in that computer record. If using a computerized system, the program generally will automatically cross-reference the number with the alphabetic list that was generated with the initial entry. If laboratory data come into the office on Leo M. McKay, there would need to be a method to know where to locate his chart to file the report; that is, the alphabetic listing.

With a manual system, the alphabetic file is kept in an index card fashion. This file needs to contain the complete name and address (and any other information denoted by the office policy; e.g., insurance and emergency numbers).

Noted with this information there needs to be either an M for miscellaneous (for those items not assigned a number) or an assigned number (Figure 14-9A and B).

If a cross-reference is required, prepare a cross-reference card and include an X next to the file number (or M) to indicate this is the cross-reference card and not the primary location (see Figure 14-9C).

Accession Record. The **accession record** is a journal (or computer listing) where numbers are preassigned. Each new item to be assigned is written on the line next to the number (Figure 14-10). Each new entry for which a chart will be created must be assigned a number. A computerized system would have an accession record in its memory bank. See Procedure 14-1 for numeric filing steps.

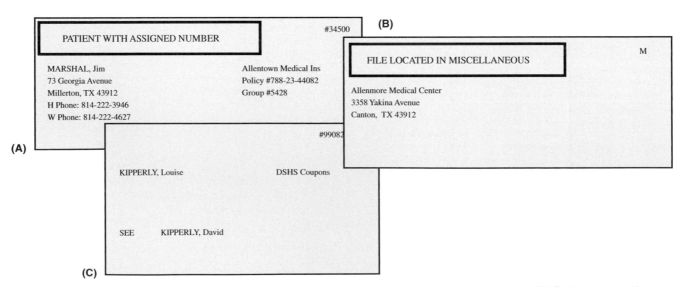

Figure 14-9 Card files used in numeric filing system: (A) Patient with an assigned number. (B) Patient record has not had a number assigned and is located in miscellaneous section. (C) Cross-reference card.

Subject Filing

There are many reasons why material would be filed using a system of subjects in a medical office. If physicians are doing research, they might wish to index research according to diseases. Subject files are convenient for locating frequently used services or for filing reference materials for patient needs. Insurance company information also might be filed by subject.

When using a subject filing system, scan the material to determine the subject or theme. As with color-coding and numeric filing, an alphabetic file is necessary. This can be either a subject list or an index card file listing the subjects. Also, as with numeric filing, all cross-reference cards are done only with alphabetic file listings.

Within the folders, material can be arranged either alphabetically or chronologically; keep in mind the objective for maintaining the particular files. For instance, if using subject indexing for research projects physicians have conducted, identify the subject category; then in the material, code an item for reference to that specific material. See Procedure 14-2 for subject filing steps.

Choosing a Filing System

To select a filing system, each office must decide what the primary objectives are with respect to storage of patient files, business records, and research files within the office. How will the charts be used primarily? Is there information that will need to be tracked by others not familiar with the records? It is often the case that more than one filing system will be used, such as alphabetic filing for patient charts, a numeric system for research subjects, and a subject system for miscellaneous correspondence.

The number of documents to be filed seems to be one primary determinant in selecting an alphabetic or numeric system. Alphabetic filing is quite manageable for many clinics. However, when the number of patients is quite large, a numeric system becomes practical because there are an infinite set of numbers available. With the numeric system, there is only one of each assigned designation. However, with an alphabetic system, there are a number of common names (e.g., Smith, Jones, Adams, and Johnson) that can have many multiples requiring additional sorting to narrow the search for the correct chart. In addition, with multiple charts of the same last name, the chances for misfiling increases.

 Confidentiality is another reason to select a numeric filing system. Confidentiality of charts is maintained more easily with numeric files because there is no visible name on the outside of the chart. In addition, numerically referenced records can be used in research activities where random sampling and anonymity are required.

 To make the medical facility HIPAA compliant when traditional paper-based or manual charts are used, you need to ensure that there is no patient-identifiable information on the outside of the chart. This includes the patient address or any other information that might be used to determine the identity of the patient, including Social Security numbers, birth dates, or phone numbers. Any information that reveals a health condition or payment status should also be removed from the outside of the chart. Recall earlier the example of locked storage cabinets for manual files. It should also be noted that the file cabinets are to be closed and locked when there is no one in the office; that includes lunchtime when the staff may be having lunch in the staff lounge.

FILING PROCEDURES

By adhering to some common principles in medical records management, any filing system will be more effective and enable the medical assistant to store, identify, retrieve, and maintain medical records efficiently.

Cross-Referencing

In running an efficient medical facility, files must be stored for quick and accurate retrieval. If there is any doubt as to where a particular file would be located,

#	File Name
800	CARRERA, Jaime
801	AU, Rhoda
802	TREMONT Drug Supply
803	
804	
805	
806	
807	

ACCESSION LOG BOOK

Figure 14-10 Accession record or log sequentially lists predetermined numbers to be used to assign to numeric records. The next number available in this system is 803.

cross-reference the file. Many offices fail to take the extra time it requires to do this. However, with the growing number of foreign names, hyphenated names, and step-families, it is well worth the effort. When the office receives a letter and a release of information form inquiring about medical facts on Mr. David Kipperly's four stepchildren who were involved in an accident, how will these files be located? If they are cross-referenced under the stepfather's name, this will be a relatively easy procedure. However, if the medical assistant is unfamiliar with the family (as in a larger urgent care center with a large volume of patients), this may become a time-consuming job. Another scenario might involve insurance information on Janet Morgan. A search of the records does not produce a file for any Janet Morgan. The reason for this is that Janet Morgan is married, and her chart has been filed under Janet Hill-Morgan. Time spent cross-referencing contributes to a more efficient method of retrieving information.

A cross-referencing system does not need to be elaborate. It is quite sufficient to use inserts with labels attached that are inserted in the appropriate place in the storage units. For instance, a plain piece of cardboard, rather than a file or chart, could be inserted for "Janet Morgan." This insert would simply have a label directing one to the location of the primary file.

The proper steps for cross-referencing, together with several examples where cross-referencing might be used, are discussed in the next section.

Steps for Cross-Referencing.

1. Identify the primary filing label.
2. Make a proper file to be used as the primary location for all medical records.
3. Identify one (or more) alternatives where one might find the file.
4. For the alternative filings, make a cross-reference sheet, card, or dummy chart that lists the primary reference and refers back to the location of the primary file.

Example. The patient, Jaime Renae Carrera, has made it known to the office that most of the correspondence received will refer to the name Renny Carrera, as this is his preference. The SEE reference will identify where the primary file is located.

PRIMARY FILE:	Carrera, Jaime Renae
X-REFERENCE FILE:	Carrera, Renny
	SEE Carrera, Jaime Renae

Rule 1. Married Women. The primary file would be the patient's legal name with the cross-reference being listed under her husband's name.

PRIMARY FILE:	Au, Rhoda A. (Mrs.)
	Lee Au
X-REFERENCE FILE:	Au, Mrs. Lee
	SEE Au, Rhoda A. (Mrs.)

Rule 2. Foreign Names. The primary file would be located under the patient's legal name. It is important, therefore, that you identify the first, middle, and surname (last name) when the patient comes for the first visit. Unless people are familiar with a particular group of names, the first, middle, and surnames are often confused with one another. Again, your experience will teach you which cross-references should be set up.

PRIMARY FILE:	Sing, Yange Teah
X-REFERENCE FILE:	Yange, Sing Teah
	SEE Sing, Yange Teah
X-REFERENCE FILE:	Teah, Yange Sing
	SEE Sing, Yange Teah

Rule 3. Hyphenated Names. With the proliferation of hyphenated names, it is common for materials to be listed under different combinations of the hyphenated name. For instance, a married woman may have records under her maiden name, her husband's surname, and her hyphenated name. Therefore, it is necessary to make two cross-references.

PRIMARY FILE:	Krenshaw-Skiple, Rose Marie
X-REFERENCE FILE:	Skiple, Rose Marie
	SEE Krenshaw-Skiple, Rose Marie
X-REFERENCE FILE:	Krenshaw, Rose Marie
	SEE Krenshaw-Skiple, Rose Marie

Rule 4. Multiple Listings. A great deal of correspondence is received with multiple listings of names. At times, the medical office may receive correspondence from only one of the involved parties. Rather than keep a separate file for each, maintain a primary file as listed on the letter and then

cross-reference file(s) for the individual names.

PRIMARY FILE:	Olsen, Piper, and Dillard Associates
X-REFERENCE FILE:	Piper, Richard C., M.D.
	SEE Olsen, Piper, and Dillard Associates
X-REFERENCE FILE:	Olsen, Francis William, M.D.
	SEE Olsen, Piper, and Dillard Associates
X-REFERENCE FILE:	Dillard, Thomas E., M.D.
	SEE Olsen, Piper, and Dillard Associates

Tickler Files

Sticky notes and writing notes on the calendar are popular methods of reminding office personnel to follow up with some required action. However, a well-organized, efficient office will maintain what is known as a **tickler file,** a method that serves as a reminder that some action needs to be taken at a date in the future.

Some systems have a calendar that pops up to allow reminders to be placed on the calendar. The computer system reminds you of the note when that particular day arrives. Some computer systems have built-in reminders that automatically give a reminder for such things as annual physical examinations, monthly blood pressure checks, medication checks, and anything else that might be beneficial to both patient and physician. Some systems automatically pick up these reminders from the progress notes that are a part of the electronic medical record.

Many computer systems today have provisions for establishing ticklers on files. However, a standard practice of using index cards for tickler files is easy to maintain (Figure 14-11).

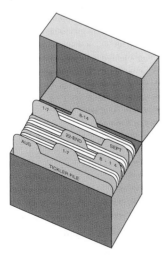

Figure 14-11 Tickler files should be reviewed daily or weekly to follow up on activities and actions that must be taken.

The tickler card should contain the following information:

- Patient name
- Tickler date (when action should be taken)
- Required action (e.g., schedule surgery or mail reminder)
- Additional relevant information (telephone number)

If action is to be taken with a patient or on behalf of the patient (e.g., scheduling a hospital admittance or sending a reminder of a checkup visit), place the information on the tickler card as soon as possible so this task is not forgotten.

When filing records, be sure to look for such words as "on _____ date we will," "pending action," or "follow-up," indicating that some course of action needs to be taken.

Release Marks

It is a good practice to use some type of release mark on every item that is filed (date stamp, initials, check mark). Ideally, the physician should initial the document after it has been read. Then, if action is required by the medical assistant, a release mark is in a consistently identified place on every document. If no action is required after the physician has signed or initialed it, place a release mark on the document. A release mark on every piece of correspondence serves as an excellent quality-control measure.

Checkout System

Many offices have developed dummy charts or cardboard files labeled "out sheets" or "out guides." Most of these guides are identified by an OUT label or metal holder, but they could be assigned a particular color; the key is that they stand out as different from the primary folders.

On the out guide, there should be a minimum of the following information:

- A record of when the chart was removed
- Where the chart can be located

Other information that is useful to note includes:

- Expected date of return
- Actual date the chart was returned

- Signature of the personnel checking out the record

- Notation on what section of the chart file was borrowed, such as a laboratory report or specialty examination

Some clinics prefer to have *temporary folders* rather than just an out guide. There are also out guides with pockets to file data in the absence of a chart. This allows for data storage on a temporary basis until the primary file is returned. The data can then be filed permanently when the primary folder is returned. If these folders are of a different color or have a different type of tab/label, they can be spotted easily so the staff can track the temporary files to be sure they do not become permanent folders.

Locating Missing Files or Data

Misfiling can occur for a number of reasons. When this situation occurs, a specific procedure must be established to conduct a search for the missing information. By systematically searching, the missing data usually can be located. This systematic search can be aided by making a mental note of the particular items that commonly are misplaced; that is, thin-paper laboratory reports, small laboratory slips, and look-alike names such as "Ward" filed under "Wart" or "Adam" filed under "Adams." Make a note of what was misfiled and where the information was located to more easily locate similar items in the future.

To locate missing pieces of information when the correct file is located but not the particular item within that file:

- Check all of the items within the file.

- Check other files with similar labels.

To locate missing files:

- Check the folders filed before and after the proper location of the misplaced file.

- Look at folders with similar labels.

- Check the physician's desk, the desk tray, and with other office personnel.

- If using a color-coding system, look for folders with the same coding as the misplaced file.

- If using a numeric system, look for possible transposition of combinations of numbers.

- Check for transposition of first and last names.

- Check for alternative spellings of names or look-alike names.

Misplaced files can be frustrating and time-consuming to locate. The best strategy is to check files for the proper filing order whenever returning or retrieving a file folder. When removing a file to answer a question, leave the file following it sticking out slightly to make its return easy and correct. Most importantly, when finished with a record, refile it immediately.

Filing Chart Data

Types of Reports. The patient's chart is the key source of information relating to treatment. There are a number of reports kept in the chart, all serving to provide a total picture of patient care. Following are the most common documents that will be part of the patient's medical record.

Clinical Notes. Clinical notes include documentation such as the medical history, the physical examination, and the follow-up notes. They track the patient's course of treatment.

Correspondence. Correspondence varies from office to office. Some offices file all types of correspondence together. Other offices file correspondence about the patient's treatment with the clinical notes.

Laboratory Reports. Included in laboratory reports are X-ray reports, CT scans, ultrasound reports, blood work, urinalysis, EEGs, ECGs, physical therapy–related reports, and pathology reports—information related to clinical data that assess the patient's condition.

Miscellaneous. The miscellaneous category includes insurance-related papers, requests for transfer of medical records, and personal notes from/to patients. In general, miscellaneous would encompass matters not related to direct treatment.

Retention and Purging

As information accumulates, it is necessary to maintain files by the process known as **purging.** Purging can involve several forms of action.

Record Purging. Record purging requires sorting through records and removing those not in active use. Each facility should establish a standard policy for control and processing of records.

 States have different time requirements for retention of various types of records that will take into account the Statute of Limitations (see Chapter 7). See Table 14-2 for general guidelines.

TABLE 14-2   RECORDS FOR RETENTION

Patient Index Files

These include appointment books or daily appointment sheets. They are kept for an indefinite period. They may be required for litigation or research.

Case Histories

The length of storage depends on state requirements and individual practice requirements. Product liability cases have deemed long-term storage of these records necessary (20+ years). The records of minors must be retained at least until the age of majority. The statute of limitations is a deciding factor as well, usually three to six years.

If records are to be destroyed because of death of physician or closure of a practice, the following procedure is required: Each patient should be notified of the circumstances and given the opportunity to have his or her records forwarded to another physician. After notification, the records must be retained for a "reasonable" period (determined by state regulations). A period of three to six months is generally determined to be a "reasonable" period. The records must be destroyed by burning or shredding to protect confidentiality.

Personal/Professional Records

Professional licenses should be stored permanently in a secure location.

Office Equipment Records

These records are generally kept until the warranties and depreciation are no longer valid. They should be kept in an easily accessible location if under maintenance contract.

Insurance Records

Professional liability policies are kept permanently. Other policies are kept in active files while in force.

Financial Records

Bank records are kept in active files for up to three years, and then placed in inactive storage. Tax records must be retained permanently.

Laboratory and X-ray Data

Originals should be retained permanently with the patient's case history.

As a way of controlling risk and practicing responsible risk management, many facilities are choosing to maintain large inactive files rather than destroy records. Some keep them on optical disks or microfiche (discussed later in this chapter). Check with the Medical Practice Act in your state to determine record-keeping requirements.

Active Files. Active files include records that need to be readily accessible for retrieval of information.

Inactive Files. Inactive files consist of records that need to be retained for possible retrieval of information. Files not currently being accessed for information would thus become inactive. Often, the type of practice will dictate the relevant time period when files are determined to be inactive (generally two to three years).

Closed Files. Closed files are those that are no longer required. Again, patient files are retained for significantly longer periods of time because of litigation and research considerations.

CORRESPONDENCE

Most ambulatory care settings process a considerable amount of correspondence not directly related to patient care. Such items include employment applications, letters from/to pharmaceutical representatives, advertisements for medical supplies, magazine subscription information, and letters to/from other physicians on a variety of subjects. This correspondence is processed using alphabetic filing rules. However, an additional step is necessary to determine whether the correspondence is incoming or outgoing. The correspondence must be filed under some aspect that will be distinctly identifiable; that is, what idea, subject, name would most likely be thought of if someone wanted to retrieve that correspondence or file additional relevant correspondence.

Filing Procedures for Correspondence

Once it is determined whether correspondence is incoming or outgoing, follow the basic rules for filing. In addition:

- Remove paper clips and staple items together.

- Inspect to see if the item is ready to be filed; that is, if any appropriate action has been taken. If not, take care of copies and enclosures, and then place notes in the tickler file for future action before proceeding with the indexing.

- On incoming correspondence, be sure the letterhead is related to the letter.

Example: A personal letter written by a patient on hotel stationery—index the signature on the letter.

Example: When both the company name and the signature are important, index the company name. A letter from Preston Industries written by the company president—index Preston Industries, not the president's name, which may change.

Example: If there is no letterhead and you have determined the material is not relevant to a patient, index the name on the signature line. A letter received from Carlton Fiske, RPT, advising your office of services his firm has to offer your patients—index Fiske.

- On outgoing correspondence, look at the inside address and the reference line.

Example: A letter to the District Court regarding Karen Ritter, an employee who is summoned to jury duty—index Karen Ritter rather than District Court.

Example: If the correspondence is relevant to a patient, index the patient's name. A letter RE: Wayne Elder—index under Elder.

Example: If the correspondence is not relevant to a patient, look to the inside address for the indexing information. A letter inquiring about cost estimates for redecorating the office reception room—index the firm in the inside address.

Example: When the inside address is relevant and contains both a company name and a person's name, index the company name. (This avoids the problem of personnel changes.) Cross-referencing would be done under the individual name. A letter to Marvin Fairchild, President of Brandex Pharmaceuticals—index Brandex Pharmaceuticals with a cross-reference for Morgan Fairchild, President, SEE Brandex Pharmaceuticals.

Example: If the letter is personal, the name of the person to whom the letter is written would be used for indexing purposes. Dr. Whitney writes a letter to Dr. Lewis, one of his colleagues, asking if he plans to attend an upcoming conference—index Dr. Lewis.

- On incoming or outgoing correspondence, code the indexing units of the designated label. If the correspondence is being cross-referenced, be sure to note the cross-referencing unit and place the X in a visible place. You may find that the body of the letter contains an important name or subject.

- Create a miscellaneous folder for items that do not have enough in number to warrant an individual folder. Items in the miscellaneous folder are filed alphabetically first, and then identical items are filed with the most recent piece on top. An individual folder is then created when enough pieces accumulate on a particular item.

COMPUTER APPLICATIONS

 Computers are playing an ever-increasing role in the management of records in the ambulatory care setting.

Electronic Medical Records

Total electronic automation in any medical facility is a major undertaking. It can be both frightening and exhilarating. Careful study of systems available, impact on physicians and staff, time necessary for moving from manual to electronic files, and cost involved should be measured against the benefits incurred. Will patients be served quicker and more efficiently? Will physicians and staff be able to spend more time with person-to-person care of patients? Will the cost savings offset the total cost involved? Is the move to a truly paperless office possible?

The electronic medical record is software that creates, stores, edits, and retrieves patient charts on a computer. Paper charts can be replaced by electronic charts. Although the costs are high, money can be saved in reduced transcription costs, labor costs, reduced copying expenses, and malpractice insurance costs.

Electronic automation in the medical facility is discussed in several other chapters (in particular, see Unit 5: Managing Facility Finances). For purposes of this chapter, and after reading about the fairly detailed "manual" records management tasks, consider the use of computers for electronic medical records.

Electronic medical records can be purchased as single-computer applications or as part of a larger "practice management" software package. Often, medical facilities will start with one aspect of a practice management software package (usually not electronic medical records), and then gradually add the other pieces. Electronic medical records are able to do all the following:

- Create and print customized encounter forms and superbills

- View patient records of all physician encounters and laboratory results, transcription notes, radiologic images, and so forth

- Utilize predefined templates to make examination notes, procedures, review of systems, and postoperative checks quicker and more efficient

- Indicate or choose medications (from a list of more than 80,000 medications), with specific instructions that can be electronically admitted into the chart and faxed to the pharmacy

- Flag any drug interaction, contraindications, or allergies related to the patient

- Provide physicians' pen units or small computers in which to enter data with a simple touch of the pen

- Provide immediate access of the patient record to physicians and necessary staff members

- Be easily retrieved and never lost or misplaced

- Eliminate the coding and filing of medical charts

- Store medical charts for as long as necessary in a small space on computer disks or CDs

- Reduce the amount of phone tag retrieving necessary information from a paper file

- Create reminders for follow-up as necessary

- Provide more efficient method of signing charts

- Can be e-mailed to a referring physician or easily printed, whether part of or the whole chart

Electronic medical records require that doctors use computers to open and view charts and write prescriptions. Progress notes can be created using clinical templates and a point-and-click form of entry. Commonly used clinical phrases can be dropped into the progress note with a push of a button. If physicians still prefer to dictate and have their notes transcribed, that can also be done. The transcribed and entered note will automatically update relevant information such as problem lists, vital signs, laboratory results, and so on. As voice recognition improves, it will become possible for the doctor to speak the entries normally keyed into the system.

Confidentiality is often mentioned as a concern in electronic medical records, but with network access limitations, system administrators can identify access and privileges according to the desired policy of the clinic. The electronic medical record is fully recognized as a legal document, is able to track any changes made, and can be presented to a court of law. Because a standard part of any electronic medical record installation is a system backup, you should never be without a medical chart even if the system goes down for a brief period.

Most medical assistants working in facilities that are fully computerized will say they hardly remember how they could function any differently. They also will report that moving from the manual to the electronic system

can be frustrating at times, but it is worth the effort in the long run.

Archival Storage

Most physicians preserve patient medical records for at least the life of their practice. This obviously is a space-consuming prospect, particularly in today's large practices. Computers are helping to solve this dilemma through electronic medical records and a process similar to microfiche and microfilm. Records can be copied with a laser beam onto what are called optical disks. This method not only eliminates the bulky storage problems encountered with traditional records, but records can be retrieved and viewed almost instantaneously on a computer screen.

Transfer of Data

 Electronic medical records are easily e-mailed in whole or in part. Computers are also streamlining transfer of records from one office or medical facility to another. Faxing is an everyday part of the medical office. Gone are the days when it took a physician's office days to obtain information vital to treating a patient. Within minutes, a patient's entire medical record can be sent electronically from one office to another. Scanners (optical character recognition) are devices that allow information to be converted to an image on the computer screen. For instance, a patient's entire medical record can be scanned by running this device over the pages; it is then recreated as a computer file exactly as it was in paper form.

Confidentiality

 Maintaining confidentiality is a major issue in using the computer and online devices for storage and transfer of medical information. Key considerations are:

- Maintaining confidentiality with transmission of data. A note that advises the receiver of the confidential nature of the material, instructions for return to the medical office if received in error, and a telephone number where you (the sender) can be advised of a transmission error are critical.

- Patient data should be sent electronically only when it is assured that the data are available for viewing only to the designated personnel.

- Precautions must be taken that the fax or computer receiving the information is in a location where the information will be accessed only by appropriate personnel.

- When using the computer to store and transfer data, consider how many personnel have access to that information. Security measures should be in place to limit access to only those with a legitimate reason for accessing the information.

Not enough emphasis can be placed on the confidentiality issue. Medical assistants employed in a medical facility will hear and see information that is completely private. It is never appropriate to discuss any of that information outside the clinic with any individual unless it is a person who needs that information for medical reasons. An appropriate situation in which information can be shared is when the name, address, and Social Security number or clinic number is given to the radiology department who will be performing the X-rays ordered by the

Critical Thinking

What might you say when you are working in a medical facility and another employee says to you, "Did you hear? John Clarkson, our mayor, came in today to be tested for STDs?"

physician. It is also unwise to discuss private information within the facility if it is not your concern, and especially if your voice might be overheard by someone waiting in an examination room, a patient using the restroom, or individuals in the reception area. If it is your nature to have difficulty keeping secrets, a career in medicine might not be your best choice.

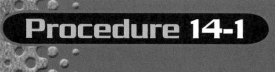

Procedure 14-1   Steps for Manual Filing with a Numeric System

PURPOSE:
To demonstrate an understanding of the principles of the numeric filing system.

EQUIPMENT/SUPPLIES:
Documents to be filed
Dividers with guides
Miscellaneous numeric file section
Alphabetic card file and cards
Accession journal if needed

PROCEDURE STEPS:
1. Inspect and index. RATIONALE: Assures that the information is ready for filing and determines how the chart will be located.
2. Code for filing units. Check the alphabetic card file for each piece to see if the card has already been prepared. RATONALE: Determines the number under which the chart will be filed.
3. Write the number in the upper right-hand corner if the piece has been assigned a number. RATIONALE: Tells you the number to be used in filing.
4. If no number is assigned (i.e., it has an M for miscellaneous), check the miscellaneous file. If

a miscellaneous item is ready to be assigned a number, make a card and note the number in the right-hand corner of the card file, cross out the M, and make a chart file. RATIONALE: Tells you if a number should be prepared because of numerous items in miscellaneous, or if the piece to be filed should stay in miscellaneous.
5. If there is no card, make up an alphabetic card including a complete name and address, and then write either M or assign a number. RATIONALE: Ensures that there is always an alphabetic card with necessary demographic information and an assigned number or M for each piece of information and chart.
6. Cross-reference if necessary and file the card properly. You are then ready to file the document in the appropriate file folder/chart. RATIONALE: Assures less likelihood of misfiling if necessary cross-references are prepared.
7. File in ascending order. RATIONALE: Establishes a pattern for filing.

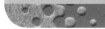

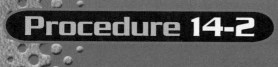

Procedure 14-2 — Steps for Manual Filing with a Subject Filing System

PURPOSE:
To demonstrate an understanding of the principles of the subject filing system.

EQUIPMENT/SUPPLIES:
Documents to be filed by subject
Subject index list or index card file listing subjects
Alphabetic card file and cards

PROCEDURE STEPS:
1. Review the item to find the subject. RATIONALE: Checks the item for the main topic of information to determine where piece will be filed.
2. Match the subject of the item with an appropriate category on the subject index list. RATIONALE: Saves you time so you do not create an unnecessary subject index list.
3. If the item contains information that may pertain to more than one subject, decide on the proper cross-reference. RATIONALE: Assures that any confusion will be checked with a cross-reference.
4. If the subject title is written on the material, underline it. RATIONALE: Readily identifies the subject used for filing.
5. If the subject title is not written on the item, write it clearly in the upper right-hand corner and underline (____) it. RATIONALE: Indicates the subject used for filing; consistently places the subject in the expected place.
6. Use a wavy (___) line for cross-referencing and an X as with alphabetic and numeric filing. RATIONALE: Clearly identifies any cross-referencing.
7. Underline the first indexing unit of the coded units. RATIONALE: Assures the correct order for filing.

Procedure 14-3 — Correcting a Paper Medical Record

PURPOSE:
To demonstrate appropriate method to correct an error in a medical chart.

EQUIPMENT/SUPPLIES:
Document containing error
Document containing correction
Red ink pen

PROCEDURE STEPS:
1. Review information on correcting medical records. RATIONALE: Assures you know the rules for correcting paper records.
2. Draw a single line through the error using a red ink pen. RATIONALE: Identifies the portion of the record in error.
3. Write in the correction. RATIONALE: Corrects the noted error.
4. Write "Corr." or "Correction" above the corrected information. RATIONALE: Identifies the information as a correction of an error.
5. Initial and date the correction. RATIONALE: Identifies the person who made the correction and the date it was made.

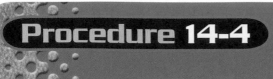

Procedure 14-4 Correcting an Electronic Medical Record

PURPOSE:
To demonstrate appropriate method of correcting errors in electronic medical record.

EQUIPMENT/SUPPLIES:
Computer with screen open to document containing error
Document containing correction

PROCEDURE STEPS:
1. Review information on correcting electronic medical records. RATIONALE: Assures you know the rules for making corrections in electronic medical records.
2. Set the computer software to "track" the area to be corrected. RATIONALE: Assures that any changes made in the document can be distinguished.

3. Using the dash key, line out the error. RATIONALE: Identifies the portion of the record in error. The line appears on the screen and will show when printed.
4. Key in the correction to be made right beside the error. RATIONALE: Corrects the noted error. The correction appears in a different color on the screen and when printed.
5. Key "Corr." or "Correction" after the corrected information. RATIONALE: Identifies the information as a correction of an error.
6. Initial and date the correction. RATIONALE: Identifies the person who made the correction and the date it was made.

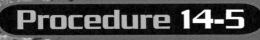

Procedure 14-5 Establishing a Paper Medical Chart for a New Patient

PURPOSE:
To demonstrate an understanding of the principles for establishing a paper medical chart.

EQUIPMENT/SUPPLIES:
File folder used in the facility (flip-up or book-style)
Divider pages used in the facility (SOAP, laboratory reports, HIPAA information sheets, and so forth)
Adhesive twin prong fasteners for divider pages
Twin hole punch for twin prong fasteners
Selected tabs to identify folder and divider pages
Demographic patient information completed before or at the first appointment

PROCEDURE STEPS:
1. Assemble all supplies at a desk or table. RATIONALE: Everything is in one place for efficient use.

2. Punch holes in the manila file folder and any necessary divider pages. RATIONALE: Creates holes for the twin prong fasteners.
3. Affix the adhesive twin prong fasteners. RATIONALE: Places fasteners as appropriate for material to be attached.
4. Assemble the divider pages dictated by the practice and the office policy in the proper location of the chart over the twin prong fasteners. RATIONALE: Assures that items are placed in the same place as all other charts in the facility.
5. Securely fasten twin prong fasteners over the divider pages. RATIONALE: Assures that no pages will fall out of the chart.
6. Index and code the patient's name according to the filing system to be used (i.e., alphabetic,

(continues)

Procedure 14-5 (continued)

numeric, or color). RATIONALE: Determines where the chart will be placed.

7. Affix appropriately labeled tabs to the folder cut. RATIONALE: Prepares the chart for patient information.

8. Transfer demographic data in black ink pen or affix the demographic divider sheet to the inside front cover of the chart. RATIONALE: Identifying patient information is readily available inside the chart cover.

9. Affix HIPAA required information to the chart, after it has been read and signed by the patient, as determined by office policy. RATIONALE: Assures that this task not omitted.

10. Place prepared chart in proper location for pickup by the physician or clinical medical assistant. RATIONALE: Signals to all staff that the chart is ready for the patient's visit.

Case Study 14-1

Karen Ritter, administrative medical assistant at Inner City Health Care, has been chiefly responsible for managing this urgent care center's medical records. However, because Karen is only a part-time employee, the office manager feels she needs to delegate some of the responsibility of maintaining all office files to Liz Corbin, a medical assistant who also works part-time. Karen knows the system well and had a hand in designing an effective numeric filing method that both ensures patient confidentiality and satisfies the needs of Inner City and its large volume of patients. Now she is trying to orient Liz, who has little experience with the filing system, to the intricacies of medical records management.

CASE STUDY REVIEW

1. What is a good starting point for Liz Corbin's education in medical records management?

2. What are the basic procedures for filing any piece of documentation that Liz needs to learn?

3. Under the direction of the office manager, Inner City is gradually shifting to a computerized system for all operations. Eventually, patient files will be computerized. What can Karen and Liz do to prepare for this eventuality?

Case Study 14-2

Dr. King is notorious for misplacing files. Often, Dr. King, who does not want to bother busy staff, walks to the lateral file shelves and removes a file or two. Likewise, he may decide to refile a chart that he has had on his desk. He has been known to take charts home when he wants to do some research.

CASE STUDY REVIEW

1. What might the staff do to ensure that Dr. King does not remove charts or refile them without proper use of out guides?

2. Devise a plan to give Dr. King the comfort he desires in the medical clinic where he is a founding partner, yet still protect the patients' charts and assure the staff of the charts' locations.

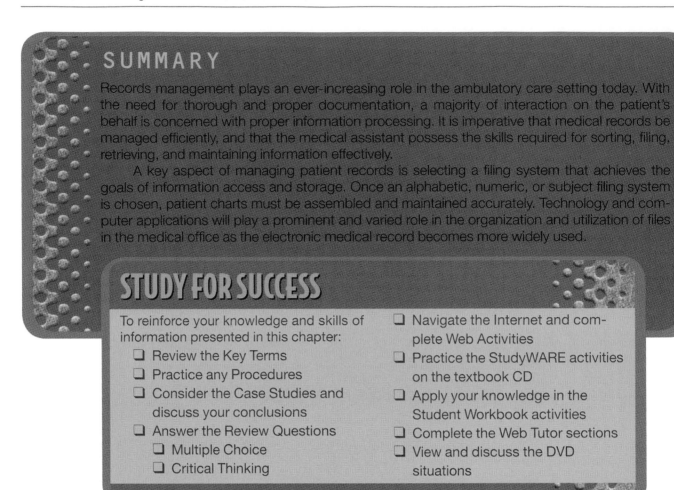

SUMMARY

Records management plays an ever-increasing role in the ambulatory care setting today. With the need for thorough and proper documentation, a majority of interaction on the patient's behalf is concerned with proper information processing. It is imperative that medical records be managed efficiently, and that the medical assistant possess the skills required for sorting, filing, retrieving, and maintaining information effectively.

A key aspect of managing patient records is selecting a filing system that achieves the goals of information access and storage. Once an alphabetic, numeric, or subject filing system is chosen, patient charts must be assembled and maintained accurately. Technology and computer applications will play a prominent and varied role in the organization and utilization of files in the medical office as the electronic medical record becomes more widely used.

STUDY FOR SUCCESS

To reinforce your knowledge and skills of information presented in this chapter:
- ❑ Review the Key Terms
- ❑ Practice any Procedures
- ❑ Consider the Case Studies and discuss your conclusions
- ❑ Answer the Review Questions
  - ❑ Multiple Choice
  - ❑ Critical Thinking
- ❑ Navigate the Internet and complete Web Activities
- ❑ Practice the StudyWARE activities on the textbook CD
- ❑ Apply your knowledge in the Student Workbook activities
- ❑ Complete the Web Tutor sections
- ❑ View and discuss the DVD situations

REVIEW QUESTIONS

Multiple Choice

1. Maintaining order in files by separating active from inactive files is:
   a. indexing
   b. coding
   c. purging
   d. alphabetizing
2. A system used as a reminder of action to be taken on a certain date is called:
   a. accession log
   b. tickler file or reminder note
   c. release mark
   d. purging system
3. To maintain an accurate filing system, select from the following list the tool used to ensure that records are tracked when borrowed:
   a. release mark
   b. out guide
   c. alphabetic card file
   d. cross-reference file

4. The correct indexing from first to last for assigning units to the name John Porter O'Keefe II would be:
   a. O'Keefe John Porter II
   b. John Porter O'Keefe II
   c. II O'Keefe John Porter
   d. the "II" would be disregarded
5. Of the four systems of filing, the best for every ambulatory care setting is:
   a. the numeric system
   b. the color-coding system
   c. the one that is customized to the needs of the office
   d. the alphabetic system
6. Medical records are the property of:
   a. the patients for whom the record is about
   b. insurance carriers who help to pay medical costs
   c. the physicians who create the record
   d. a and c

7. Corrections to medical records:
   a. are made by erasing the error and replacing it with the correction
   b. are made by placing a single line through the error and replacing it with the correction
   c. are never made to charts because of the legal nature of the information
   d. are made only by the physician
8. The first indexing unit for Jayne Carol Warden-Bloomberg is:
   a. Carol
   b. Jayne
   c. Warden
   d. Wardenbloomberg
9. When identical names are being indexed, the system most preferred in a medical office is:
   a. index the address
   b. index the telephone number
   c. index the birth date or Social Security number
   d. index a preassigned clinic number
10. The preferred order for steps in filing medical documentation is:
    a. code, index, sort, inspect, file
    b. inspect, code, index, sort, file
    c. sort, inspect, index, code, file
    d. inspect, index, code, sort, file

Critical Thinking

1. A patient's chart has been subpoenaed for pending malpractice litigation. In preparing the chart, you discover an error that was made when the results of the laboratory report were incorrectly documented in the chart. You have the original laboratory report. What should you do?
2. Identify how you would index and cross-reference the following medical chart:

Patient:	John Bryan Houk	
Mother:	Sara (Houk) Judson	(Assumed her maiden name following divorce)
Father:	Brett J. Houk	(Covers son on his medical insurance)

3. Research the Statute of Limitations in your state for medical records to determine how long a medical record should be kept. The statute will also tell you what triggers activity on a medical file that might dictate it be kept longer than normally indicated.
4. When determining the type of equipment to purchase for storage of medical records, identify a minimum of three indicators to keep in mind.
5. It has been said that filing records is the easiest task the medical assistant will perform; yet it is often the most difficult. What reasons can you give for this statement?

WEB ACTIVITIES

1. Using your favorite search engine, key in "medical record authorization for release of information." Are you able to find a site that has a sample blank form to be completed? Are there any surprises? For how long is the authorization valid?
2. Go to http://www.smead.com to view their many color-coded filing systems. Can color be used in both alphabetic and numeric filing? Now go to http://www.kardex.com to review their systems. Select a system and identify why it would be your choice for a medical clinic. What problems might occur with the self-adhesive products shown on these Web sites?
3. Search for information on electronic medical records. Identify the number of sites that come up. Select two or three sites that allow you to view or download a sample of the product software. Identify your likes and dislikes and give your rationale. What would influence you if you were helping to select electronic medical record software for a medical facility where you are employed?

THE DVD HOOK-UP

DVD Series	Program Number
Critical Thinking	**2**

Chapter/Scene Reference
• *Forms of Communication*

In this chapter, you learned about the importance of the medical record. Because the medical record is a legal document, you must take care in both the creation and use of the record.

In the designated DVD scene, you observed Paula giving a testimonial about the frustration that patients feel when they receive bills or other information with incorrect information. This can easily occur if the assistant is not detail oriented. You need to pay close attention to the exact spelling of the patient's name and make certain that you use correct numerals when entering a patient's phone number or address into the computer.

1. How would you feel if you received bills from your medical office with your name continually misspelled?

2. Would an error such as this cause you to question your medical care? Why?

DVD Journal Summary
Write a paragraph that summarizes what you learned from watching the designated scenes from today's DVD program. The computerized record is becoming much more common in today's medical office. Many medical assistants enter information directly into the patient's electronic chart while the patient is sitting in the examination room. Does your present typing speed allow you to be efficient when performing electronic charting? What will you do if the patient demands to see information in his or her electronic chart?

REFERENCES/BIBLIOGRAPHY

Fordney, M. T., French, L., & Follis, J. J. (2004). *Administrative medical assisting* (5th ed.). Clifton Park, NY: Thomson Delmar Learning.

Johnson, J. (1994). *Basic filing procedures for health information management*. Clifton Park, NY: Thomson Delmar Learning.

Lewis, M. A., & Tamparo, C. D. (2002). *Medical law ethics & bioethics for ambulatory care* (5th ed.). Philadelphia: F.A. Davis.

Malkin, J. (2002). *Medical and dental space planning* (3rd ed.). New York: John Wiley & Sons.

CHAPTER 15

Written Communications

KEY TERMS

Agenda
Blind Copy
Bond Paper
Clinical E-Mail
E-Mail
Form Letter
Full Block Letter
Keyed
Memorandum (Memo)
Minutes
Modified Block Letter, Indented
Modified Block Letter, Standard
Optical Character Reader (OCR)
Portfolio
Proofread
Simplified Letter
Uniform Resource Locators (URLs)
Watermark
ZIP+4

OBJECTIVES

The student should strive to meet the following performance objectives and demonstrate an understanding of the facts and principles presented in this chapter through written and oral communication.

1. Define the key terms as presented in the glossary.
2. Describe the impact of written communication in the ambulatory care setting.

(continues)

FEATURED
COMPETENCIES

**CAAHEP—ENTRY-LEVEL
COMPETENCIES**

Professional Communications

• Respond to and initiate
  written communications

**ABHES—ENTRY-LEVEL
COMPETENCIES**

Communication

• Use appropriate medical
  terminology

• Receive, organize, prioritize, and transmit information expediently

• Use correct grammar, spelling, and formatting techniques in written works

• Fundamental writing skills

• Professional components

Administrative duties

• Perform basic secretarial
  skills

OBJECTIVES (continued)

3. Identify the role of the medical assistant in producing written communications.

4. List the four major letter styles.

5. Compose and key letters using appropriate components of a business letter.

6. Identify various types of form letters that may be written by the medical assistant.

7. Proofread a letter for grammar, spelling, and content.

8. Use proper proofreading marks to correct a document.

9. Describe the various classifications of mail and determine when each class should be used.

10. Address envelopes to satisfy postal regulations.

11. Describe the use of new communication technology in the ambulatory care setting and discuss appropriate confidentiality issues.

12. Discuss legal and ethical issues relating to written communications, as well as HIPAA regulations.

SCENARIO

When they are produced with care, written communications can be a time-consuming part of the administrative medical assistant's day. This is why Marilyn Johnson, CMA, the office manager at Drs. Lewis and King's office, has compiled a style manual for the two-physician practice. Marilyn is clearly aware that professional looking and sounding letters send a message to all recipients. Yet, she wants to make correspondence writing and producing as efficient as possible; her style manual provides an easy-to-use resource for anyone in the office responsible for composing or sending written documents.

In her style manual, Marilyn has included examples of the "house" letter format, which is block style; a list of commonly used medical terms for easy spelling reference; answers to common questions staff have in regard to word usage; proofreader's marks; proper addressing procedures for envelopes and packages, depending on whether they are being sent by U.S. mail or by an alternative delivery method; and a quick list of the best ways to send various types of correspondence. Marilyn has also included a list of "Do Nots" to help her staff avoid mistakes in their written communications.

INTRODUCTION

One of the key responsibilities of the administrative medical assistant is written communication. All written material produced by the ambulatory care setting is critical, because it reflects positively or negatively on the professionalism of the office. Letters to patients, to referring physicians, to other health care organizations, and even interoffice correspondence should be thoughtfully composed, carefully produced according to the style selected by the office manager, and mailed and delivered in a way that is both time- and cost-efficient.

Written correspondence is important in conveying a professional image of the ambulatory care setting and impacts public relations either positively or negatively. It must also be remembered that written documents provide a permanent or legal record in the event of any litigation, and thus must be carefully and accurately worded.

In most ambulatory care settings, medical assistants will be responsible for creating many forms of written communications. Examples of these forms of communications include:

• Various types of letters, such as letters to order supplies and equipment, letters replying to various types of inquiries, collection letters, promotional letters

• Memoranda and interoffice communications

- *Referrals, consultation, and surgical report letters*
- *E-mail and fax correspondence*
- *Written instructions for patients*
- *Meeting agendas and minutes*
- *Promotional brochures*
- *Policy and procedure documents*

COMPOSING CORRESPONDENCE

The medical assistant must always remember that the quality of the correspondence reflects the standards of the medical office. It is important to also remember that there is a difference between social correspondence and business correspondence. Social correspondence tends to be lengthy and personal in nature, whereas business correspondence should be clear, concise, courteous, and accurate. It is best to keep business letters to one page in length whenever possible.

Writing Tips

Rosemary Fruehling, a writer and lecturer, states, "Business writing is good when it achieves the purpose the author intended." Practice and careful attention to detail are required to write effective business letters. Writing tips for consideration include:

- Follow the style and format determined by your physician–employer. Physicians often prefer a professional, formal style of letter composition.

- Think about key points to be addressed in the letter and organize them before beginning composition. The first paragraph should state the reason for writing and focus the reader's attention.

- Establish a tone of voice. Be personable and cordial in tone while remaining professional.

- Use only language that the reader will understand.

- Most sentences should be short and contain only one idea or thought.

Spelling

It is important that all correspondence contain no misspelled or incorrectly used words. When in doubt, always look the word up in a dictionary (Table 15-1). When checking spelling in a dictionary, develop the habit of reading the definition as well. This will help imprint the correct spelling and meaning of the word.

 Be careful about relying on the spell check function of your computer; many medical words are not formatted into the computer. The computer does not recognize if you have used the wrong word, only that the word is spelled incorrectly. For example, the words *to*, *too*, and *two* may all be spelled correctly but may be misused within the sentence structure.

TABLE 15-1	FREQUENTLY MISSPELLED WORDS
abscess	ischemia
aneurysm	larynx
arrhythmia	malaise
calcaneus	ophthalmology
cirrhosis	palliative
clavicle	parenteral
curettage	pharynx
hemorrhage	pneumonia
hemorrhoids	psychiatrist
homeostasis	pyrexia
humerus	rheumatic
ischium	roentgenology
ilium	sphygmomanometer
ileum	staphylococcus

TABLE 15-2	FREQUENTLY MISUSED WORDS	
advice	advise	
affect	effect	
capital	capitol	
coarse	course	
coma	comma	
command	commend	
complement	compliment	
comprehensible	comprehensive	
council	counsel	
conscience	conscious	
deposition	disposition	
device	devise	
elicit	illicit	
eligible	illegible	
elude	allude	
ensure	insure	assure
explicit	implicit	
farther	further	
heal	heel	
hear	here	
hole	whole	
knew	new	
know	no	
lean	lien	
patience	patient	
personal	personnel	
plain	plane	
precede	proceed	
principal	principle	
right	write	
stationary	stationery	
taught	taut	
their	there	they are
to	too	two
vain	vein	
weak	week	
weather	whether	
you	your	you are

It may be helpful to develop a list of frequently misused words in an alphabetized notebook, card index, or in a special file on your computer (Table 15-2). Several computer word processing software packages contain English/medical spell check features. A new word that is not currently identified in the spell check or medical check package may be added to the program.

Proofreading

Before presenting any correspondence to the physician for signature or mailing, the document should be **proofread**. Proofreading is the process of reading the document and checking for accuracy. Accuracy involves checking to be sure that the correct grammar, spelling, punctuation, and capitalization have been used and that the message is clear and concise and presented in a logical organization.

Proofreading marks most commonly used are shown in Figure 15-1. Standard proofreading marks used to indicate corrections hasten the editing process. Some proofreading tips that may be useful include:

- Proofread each document twice; once on the screen checking for obvious errors, and then as a hard copy to be sure everything is accurate and makes sense.

- Prepare the document, set it aside, and proofread a third time later. Inaccuracies or errors may "jump" out in a later review.

- Do not proofread when tired.

- If the document is long, proofread in several short intervals.

- Read a long document to another person and have him or her check sentence structure and content accuracy.

- Use a card or ruler as a guide to maintain your place within the document.

- Use a piece of colored clear plastic over the document to rest your eyes. This is especially helpful when proofing a long document.

COMPONENTS OF A BUSINESS LETTER

The following sections describe the components of most business letters. See Procedure 15-1, Preparing and Composing Business Correspondence Using All Components (Computerized Approach). Figure 15-2 graphically illustrates the placement of business letter components, Table 15-3 provides guidelines in preventing errors in letter placement, and Figure 15-3 illustrates how placement can be altered to suit letter size.

Date Line

The date is usually **keyed** on line 15 or two to three lines below the letterhead. Keying is when data are input by keystrokes on a computer. The date should be completely written out as January 15, 20XX rather than

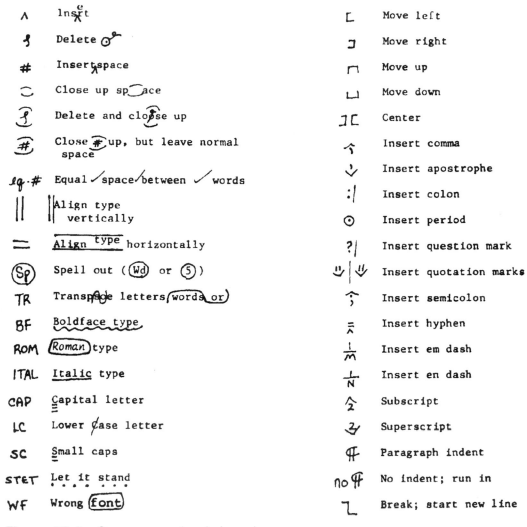

Figure 15-1 Common proofreader's marks.

1/15/20XX. (If military style is used, the format would be 01 JAN 20XX.)

Inside Address

The inside address is keyed flush with the left margin. This address may be two, three, or four lines. Some rural areas only require two lines. If the letter is addressed to a physician, the credentials appear after the name. Do not type Dr. John Jones, M.D. (Both Dr. and M.D. are titles; use one or the other.)

Salutation

The salutation is keyed flush with the left margin on the second line below the inside address. A colon follows the salutation. The formal salutation should refer to the receiver of the letter using title and last name (e.g., "Dear

Mr. Marshal:"). If the receiver and sender know each other well, the receiver's first name may be used (e.g., "Dear Jim:").

Subject Line

If used, the subject line is keyed on the second line below the salutation starting at the left margin. This may begin flush with the left margin, indented five spaces, or centered.

The patient's name or subject (meeting or topic) may be used on the subject line.

Body of Letter

The body of the letter should begin on the second line below the salutation unless a subject line is used that precedes two lines above the body. The body format will

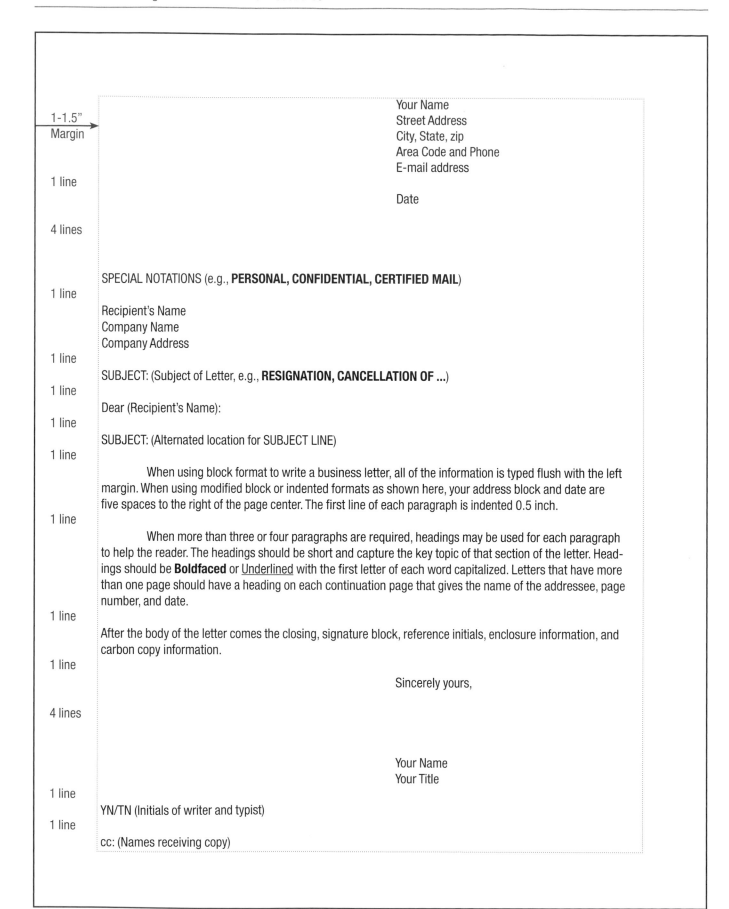

Figure 15-2 *Placement of business letter components.*

TABLE 15-3	**GUIDELINES IN LETTER PLACEMENT**

The following guidelines are helpful in preventing errors in placement:

1. An imaginary picture frame should surround the letter. Margins may be 1, 1.5, or 2 inches (Figure 15-2).
2. The last line of the letter should end no less than 1 inch from the bottom of the page.
3. Do not divide the last word on a page.
4. A minimum of three lines should be keyed on the second page of a letter. When dividing a paragraph at the bottom of a page, keep a minimum of two lines on the bottom of the page and two lines at the top of the next page.
5. If using a computer to prepare letters, it is easy to make adjustments to create a professional letter.
6. Single-space within paragraphs.
7. Double-space between paragraphs.

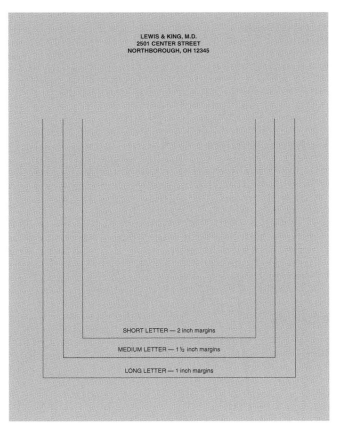

Figure 15-3 Letter length spacing.

depend on the style of letter used. Paragraphs will begin flush with the left margin in full block letter style, or they may be indented five spaces when using the modified block letter style.

Complimentary Closing

The complimentary closure begins on the second line below the body of the letter. The closure depends on the formality of the letter. Only the first letter of the first word of the complimentary closure is upper case.

The style used in the complimentary closure should correspond with the salutation.

Letter Style	Complimentary Closing
Formal	Respectfully yours or Respectfully
General	Very truly yours or Truly yours or Sincerely or Sincerely yours
Informal (used when reader and writer are on first-name basis)	Regards or Best wishes

Keyed Signature

A keyed signature is a professional courtesy to the reader. Often, a letter is received in which the signature of the sender is not legible. The keyed signature should be at least four lines below the complimentary closing. This space may be lengthened to six lines if you are keying a short letter.

Reference Initials

The keyed signature may be the only initials used if the same person composed and signed the letter. If reference initials are used, the name of the individual composing the letter should be in uppercase letters with the medical assistant's initials keyed in lowercase letters.

Example:

WL:jg or WL/jg

Enclosure Notation

The enclosure indication can be either one or two lines below the keyed reference initials.

The number of enclosures may be indicated using one of several methods:

- Enclosures
- Enc.
- 1 Enc.
- 2 Enclosures
- Enclosures (2)

Some enclosures should be identified specifically, that is, check for $84.

Enclosures also may be sent under separate cover. If this method is used, state that the enclosure is under separate cover. It may be written as Enclosure under separate cover: Sarah Jones's medical record.

Copy Notation

If copies of the letter are to be sent to other parties, the copy notation should be one or two lines below the reference initials. The notation "c" (copy) or "pc" (photocopy) should be followed by the name of the person receiving the copy. When more than one person is to receive a copy of the original letter, key "c:" by the first name. Align the other names under the first person identified alphabetically or by rank.

Example:

c: Joseph Brown, MD
        John Smith, MD

A **blind copy** notation "bcc:" may be used to send copies of the letter to individuals without the recipient's knowledge. This message is only keyed on the copy of the individual receiving the blind copy. The use of blind carbon copies has decreased and in some practices is no longer used.

Postscripts

Postscripts (abbreviated as P.S.) may be used to:

1. Express an afterthought
2. Identify a thought that has been intentionally deleted from the body of the letter
3. Make a strong significant point

Postscripts are keyed two spaces below reference initials and enclosures.

Continuation Page Heading

There are two methods used to begin the continuation page heading. There should be at least a 1-inch space at the top of each continuing page of the letter. Plain paper matching the color, weight, size, and quality of the letterhead should be used. The following are examples of appropriate continuation page headings.

Example:

(1 inch from top of page)
Jeremy Brown, MD   -2-   May 4, 20XX

or
Jeremy Brown, MD
Page 2
May 4, 20XX

LETTER STYLES

The administrative medical assistant may be responsible for creating a variety of letters that support the needs of the ambulatory care facility. Word processing software has business letter and memo templates useful in creating these documents.

One efficient approach to letter composition is to create a **portfolio** or database of frequently used **form letters.** Individualize letters by using the current date and the receiver's name and mailing address. When a form letter is carefully composed and produced, it may not be perceived as a form letter by the recipient.

With the physician–employer's permission, the medical assistant may sign certain letters, including most form letters. Form letters that may be written by the medical assistant include:

- Letters to thank referring physicians
- Letters emphasizing to patients criteria for care as directed by the physician
- Letters announcing new insurance or HMOs accepted
- Letters to order supplies or subscriptions
- Letters acknowledging speaking engagements
- Letters to announce vacation schedules or other office closures
- Letters to announce new staff
- Letters to remind patients of payment due or notification of collection procedures

Letters prepared for the physician's signature should be placed with an addressed envelope on the physician's desk for review and signature. Place the envelope flap over the letter and attach with a paper clip. Also include with the letter any enclosures for the physician's approval.

Four major styles of letters are used by medical and professional offices. These are:

1. Full block
2. Modified block, standard
3. Modified block, indented
4. Simplified

Full Block

The **full block letter** is most time-efficient for the ambulatory care setting because the medical assistant does not have to use excessive motion to tab indentions or to place address, complimentary close, or keyed signature. When using the full block style, all lines begin flush with the left margin. This style is suggested when desiring a contemporary-looking efficient letter.

Modified Block

In the **standard modified block** style letter, all lines begin at the left margin with the exception of the date line, complimentary closure, and keyed signature, which usually begin at the center position or a few spaces to the right of center. Figure 15-4 illustrates a modified block style letter without indention.

The assistant may choose to use the **indented modified block** style letter. In this format, paragraphs

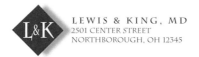

LEWIS & KING, MD
2501 CENTER STREET
NORTHBOROUGH, OH 12345

NORTHBOROUGH
FAMILY MEDICAL GROUP

January 12, 20XX (approximately 15th line)

Jeremy Brown, MD   (approximately 20th line)
111 S Main
Blossom, UT 10283-1120

Dear Dr. Brown:

Blossom Medical Society Meeting

Thank you for inviting me to speak at the Blossom Medical Society Meeting June 15, 20XX. As requested, my topic will describe the use of the MRI in assisting physicians to make a more accurate diagnosis without resorting to invasive procedures. The exact title of my speech will be sent by next Friday.

Please have your office manager send information regarding the number of participants expected, time of meeting, location, and any other details that will assist me in preparing my speech.

I will write or call if I have any additional questions.

Yours truly,

Winston Lewis, MD

Winston Lewis, MD

WL:jg

Enclosure: Handout on MRI

Figure 15-4   Sample standard modified block style letter; all elements start at left margin, except date, complimentary closing, and keyed signature.

Critical Thinking

This textbook identifies spacing for short, medium, and long letters generated in medical offices. What types of information or letters would be written using each type of spacing?

may be indented five spaces. Figure 15-5 illustrates a modified block style letter with indented paragraphs.

Simplified

The **simplified letter** style omits the salutation and complimentary closure. All lines are keyed (input by keystroke) flush with the left margin. The subject line

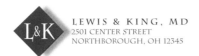

LEWIS & KING, MD
2501 CENTER STREET
NORTHBOROUGH, OH 12345

NORTHBOROUGH
FAMILY MEDICAL GROUP

January 12, 20XX (approximately 15th line)

Jeremy Brown, MD   (approximately 20th line)
111 S Main
Blossom, UT 10283-1120

Dear Dr. Brown:

Blossom Medical Society Meeting

Thank you for inviting me to speak at the Blossom Medical Society Meeting June 15, 20XX. As requested, my topic will describe the use of the MRI in assisting physicians to make a more accurate diagnosis without resorting to invasive procedures. The exact title of my speech will be sent by next Friday.

Please have your office manager send information regarding the number of participants expected, time of meeting, location, and any other details that will assist me in preparing my speech.

I will write or call if I have any additional questions.

Yours truly,

Winston Lewis, MD

Winston Lewis, MD

WL:jg

Enclosure: Handout on MRI

Figure 15-5 Sample modified block style letter with indented paragraphs; this format is the same as the standard modified except that the subject line and paragraphs are also indented.

is keyed in capital letters three lines below the inside address. The body of the letter begins three lines below the subject line. The signature line is keyed in all capital letters four lines below the body of the letter. The Administrative Management Society recommends this style of letter. However, in medical offices, this style is most often used when sending a form letter. Figure 15-6 illustrates a simplified style letter.

SUPPLIES FOR WRITTEN COMMUNICATION

Begin written communication at the computer workstation by checking to see that all supplies required to prepare the document are at hand. Check the computer settings and turn the printer on, making sure it is properly loaded with the correct letter stock. The paper

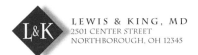

LEWIS & KING, MD
2501 CENTER STREET
NORTHBOROUGH, OH 12345

NORTHBOROUGH
FAMILY MEDICAL GROUP

January 12, 20XX (approximately 15th line)

Jeremy Brown, MD   (approximately 20th line)
111 S Main
Blossom, UT 10283-1120

   (triple-space)

BLOSSOM MEDICAL SOCIETY MEETING

   (triple-space)

Thank you for inviting me to speak at the Blossom Medical Society Meeting June 15, 20XX. As requested, my topic will describe the use of the MRI in assisting physicians to make a more accurate diagnosis without resorting to invasive procedures. The exact title of my speech will be sent by next Friday.

Please have your office manager send information regarding the number of participants expected, time of meeting, location, and any other details that will assist me in preparing my speech.

I will write or call if I have any additional questions.

Winston Lewis, MD   (4 line spaces)

WINSTON LEWIS, MD

WL:jg

Enclosure: Handout on MRI

Figure 15-6   The simplified style letter has no salutation or complimentary closing. The subject line and keyed signature are all upper case.

should be **bond,** of good quality, and at least 20 to 24 pound stock with a watermark. A **watermark** is legible when paper is held to the light. Choose a shade of white, cream, or gray.

Although colored paper may be more eye-catching, it does not display a professional image. Also, be sure that the paper stock is compatible with printers used in the ambulatory care center.

Letterhead

The letterhead style and design is usually chosen by the physician(s) and may include a specially designed logo for the practice. The physician/practice name, street address or post office box number, city, state, and zip code, and telephone number with area code are usually printed on the letterhead. Many offices also add their fax number and e-mail address. Letterhead information may be placed at either side or in the center of the paper.

Second Sheets

When an order is placed for letterhead, the medical assistant should order additional plain paper of the same stock as the letterhead to be used for second page sheets. The number of sheets will vary from office to office. If physicians normally dictate long letters, this must be taken into consideration when ordering quantities.

Printing Multipage Business Letters

Printing multipage business letters on letterhead stationery requires use of more than one tray in the printer, unless you want to collate the letterhead or hand feed it into the printer. The simplest procedure is to place the letterhead stationery into a tray other than the default tray. Then go to "File," "Page Setup," "Paper Source," and from the menu that appears, specify the tray containing the letterhead stationery. The menu lets you choose the tray for the first page and the tray for the rest of the document. Make sure that the "Apply To" box is set for "Whole Document."

Envelopes

The stock and quality of the envelopes should match the stationery used in the office. With the use of **ZIP+4** and City State Files, mail is processed more efficiently and effectively. The address should be standardized so it contains all delivery address elements. The correct name, city, state, and ZIP+4 codes must be used.

Example:

JEREMY BROWN MD
1111 S MAIN
BLOSSOM UT 10283-1120

If Dr. Brown uses a post office box for the delivery of his mail, that address should be used. The postal service delivers to the last line before the city, state, and zip code.

Example:

JEREMY BROWN MD
PO BOX 1453
BLOSSOM UT 10283-1120

Place the intended delivery address on the line immediately above the city, state, and ZIP+4 code. The other address may be placed on a separate line above the delivery line.

Example:

JEREMY BROWN MD
1111 S MAIN
PO BOX 1453
BLOSSOM UT 10283-1120
This letter would be received at the post office box, not the street address.

General Standards for Addressing Envelopes. For successful processing by **optical character readers (OCRs),** the U.S. Postal Service suggests that the address on letter mail needs to be machine-printed, with a uniform left margin. It should be formatted in a manner that allows an OCR to recognize the information and find a match in its address files.

A scanner reads the zip code on the bottom line and prints a bar code in the lower right corner of the envelope. Envelopes that are handwritten cannot be read by the OCR. These letters must wait for more costly and slower manual sorting.

To conform to standards, eliminate all punctuation in the envelope address with the exception of a hyphen in the ZIP+4 code. Leave a minimum of one space between the city name and two-character state abbreviations and the ZIP+4 code. The OCR can read a combination of uppercase and lowercase characters in addresses but prefers all uppercase characters. See Procedure 15-2.

Dark ink on a light background using uppercase letters is the suggested method in preparing a keyed address. There should be a uniform left margin on all lines of the address. An imaginary rectangle that extends ⅝ to 2¾ inches from the bottom of the envelope with 1 inch on each side should contain the address. The lower right edge should be kept free of any marks. This area will contain the bar code, whether it is preapplied or printed by an OCR. The bar code area is ⅝ inch from the bottom and 4½ inches from the right side of the envelope.

The U.S. Postal Service publishes several pamphlets and booklets that describe the format to be used when sending any mail. Check with the postal service regarding the latest publications. Service and deliverability will be improved if these standards are used.

Types of Envelopes. Number 6¾ and number 10 are the envelopes most often used. A window envelope may also be used, especially when mailing statements.

Number	Size
6¾	6½″ long × 3⅝″ wide
10	9½″ long × 4⅛″ wide
7	7½″ long × 3⅞″ wide

The address on the statement need only be keyed once. The entire address is capitalized with no punctuation. Only one space should be used between the state abbreviation and the zip code. When this statement is folded with the address in view, it may be inserted into a window envelope. Make certain that the entire address is visible through the window.

To prepare envelopes for mailing, lay all envelopes facing upward in a row with the flaps displayed. Moisten all the envelopes with a sponge. With the dominant hand, seal the flap; with the nondominant hand, push the envelope aside while the next flap is closed. Procedure 15-3 illustrates letter folding and placement of envelopes for closure. The use of premoistened or peel-off strips helps speed up the process.

Mail Merge

Mail Merge lets you create form letters, envelopes, or mailing labels using data from a data source. You would use this feature to send mailings to your client base, to a list of prospects, among others. It permits sending a form letter with envelopes to hundreds of recipients in a matter of minutes.

Critical Thinking

Using a computer and printer, correctly address a number 10 envelope to a physician following all of the U.S. postal regulations. Print the envelope.

The client names and addresses are first stored in a Mail Merge data source, which can be a table or database such as Microsoft Excel®. For Microsoft Word®, a Mail Merge data source can be created by selecting "Mail Merge" in the "Tools" menu, selecting "Mail Merge Helper," and following the instructions given in Helper. Almost all word processor programs let you carry out a mail merge with an external database. You will need to consult the program manual for details.

Separate fields are suggested in the database for first name, last name, title, address, city, state, and postal code. To preclude time-consuming changes, three fields should be used for address, to accommodate clients with complex addresses. If a field is not required, leave it blank.

The Mail Merge Helper will give you the choice of editing the main document. Compose the document you want to send, and for each field where you want a new name or address, select "Insert Merge Field," and then select the name of the field you want to insert. You are now ready to print the form letters. Select "Mail Merge-Mail Merge Helper" from the "Tools" menu and select "Printer" from the "Merge To" box. Your printer should show the documents in the queue. See Procedure 15-4 for step-by-step instructions related to mail merge.

OTHER TYPES OF CORRESPONDENCE

Other specialized types of correspondence the medical assistant may be involved in preparing include memoranda, meeting agendas, and meeting minutes.

Memoranda

A type of interoffice correspondence is the **memorandum,** or **memo** for short. The use of memos permits messages to be sent quickly and without labor-intensive preparation. The memo format may already be preformatted on your computer software. If not, it is easy to design your own memo format.

The side margins should be set for 1 inch. Begin to key the memo heading 2 inches from the top of the page (line 13). The heading includes the words *date, to, from,* and *subject,* which should be boldfaced and capitalized. The words should each be keyed on a separate line with a double space between each line. By setting a tab stop 10 spaces in from the left margin, you will be able to tab to each entry and clear the headings to add the appropriate information. Triple space after the entry for the subject heading.

The body of the memo may begin at the left margin or may be set 10 spaces in so that the text starts directly

DATE: August 25, 20XX (key heading 2 inches
                     from top of page, line 13)
TO: Staff of Doctors Lewis & King (embolden and
                     capitalize headings and double space
                     between them)
FROM: Walter Seals, Office Manager

SUBJECT: Vacation Schedule (triple space after the
                     subject)

Doctors Lewis & King will be on vacation January 1–15.
Please do not schedule appointments during that time for
either doctor. Office personnel should report to work as
usual. During this two-week period, we will be preparing
for the annual audit.

Figure 15-7 Sample memorandum.

AGENDA
STAFF MEETING
Tuesday, September 1, 20XX
Location–Conference Room

Reading and approval of last months' minutes
Reports
     Risk Management Committee
     Personnel
Unfinished business
     Purchase of new X-ray machine
New business
     Doctors Lewis & King vacation January 1–15
     Annual Audit
Date and time for next meeting
Adjournment

Figure 15-8 Sample meeting agenda.

beneath the typed headings. No salutation is required in a memo. Figure 15-7 provides a sample memo.

Meeting Agendas

Most meetings operate by following *Robert's Rules of Order, Newly Revised* as their parliamentary authority. The outlined order of business is as follows:

- Reading and approval of the minutes
- Reports of officers, boards, and standing committees
- Reports of special committees (ad hoc)
- Special orders
- Unfinished business and general orders
- New business
- Date and time of next scheduled meeting

The **agenda** lists the specific items that the group plans to discuss at the meeting under each of the above-mentioned divisions. The medical assistant preparing the agenda must determine the topics that are to be discussed. Copies of the agenda should be sent to each group member before the meeting date, and extra copies should be taken to the meeting for those who may have misplaced or forgotten to bring the agenda with them to the meeting. Figure 15-8 provides a sample meeting agenda.

Meeting Minutes

A written record of what transpired during a meeting is called the **minutes.** The minutes should record what business actions were taken during the meeting, who made each motion and what it was, who seconded the motion, any pertinent discussion, and whether the motion was passed.

The first paragraph of the minutes should contain the following information:

- Kind of meeting (regular, special, emergency)
- Name of the group or association
- Date, time, and place of the meeting
- Who officiated at the meeting and names of members present and absent
- If the previous meeting minutes were read and approved

The body of the minutes should include a paragraph discussing each subject matter or each item listed on the agenda. All motions should be recorded including the exact wording of the motion, the name of the person making the motion, the person seconding the motion, and if the motion passed or failed. If the meeting had a guest speaker, the speaker's name and title and the subject of the presentation may be included in the minutes.

STAFF MEETING MINUTES

The monthly staff meeting of Doctors Lewis & King was held Tuesday, September 1, 20XX, in the conference room. The meeting was called to order by Walter Seals, Office Manager. Those members present included: Dr. Lewis, Dr. King, Marilyn Johnson, Ellen Armstrong, Jane O'Hara, Wanda Slawson, and Bruce Goldman.

The previous meeting's minutes were read and approved as published.

Marilyn Johnson, the CMA heading the Risk Management Committee, reported that a thorough walk through of the clinic had taken place to assess for safety issues. It was determined that the pull cords on the blinds could pose a potential hazard to small children. Marilyn made a motion that the blinds be upgraded with new vinyl louvered blinds with the plastic rod-type louver adjuster. Wanda Slawson seconded the motion. After discussion, a unanimous vote was cast to replace the blinds at the earliest time possible.

Walter Seals, Human Resource Manager, announced that he would be posting an opening for a CMA to work in the lab. All staff personnel were asked to share information about this opening with professionals who might be interested in working with Doctors Lewis & King.

Discussion was presented by Doctors Lewis & King regarding the purchase of a new X-ray machine. A committee consisting of Wanda Slawson, Bruce Goldman, and Marilyn Johnson was appointed to investigate the specific needs of the clinic and to locate appropriate vendors. They will present their findings at the next scheduled staff meeting.

New Business items include the fact that Doctors Lewis & King will be on vacation January 1–15, 20XX. We are asked to not schedule appointments during that time.

Walter Seals discussed preparations for the annual audit during the vacation period of Doctors Lewis & King. He will provide a schedule and timeline at the next staff meeting.

The next scheduled meeting will be October 3 at 12:30 PM in the conference room.

The meeting adjourned at 1:45 PM.

Ellen Armstrong

Figure 15-9 Sample meeting minutes.

The last paragraph should contain the next meeting date, time, and place, and the time of adjournment for this meeting. The person recording the minutes should sign them, and a copy of all minutes should be maintained in a notebook designated for that purpose. Corporations are required to have regular meetings with recorded minutes for legal purposes. Figure 15-9 provides a sample of recorded minutes.

PROCESSING INCOMING AND OUTGOING MAIL

The management of written communications also involves developing procedures for sorting, distributing, and otherwise processing incoming mail. It also includes posting and shipping outgoing items by the most cost- and time-effective method.

Incoming Mail and Shipments

All mail should be sorted by type before opening. Incoming mail includes telegrams, faxes, certified or registered letters, personal letters, e-mail, checks from patients, insurance forms, invoices, medical journals, newspapers, magazines for the reception area, and advertisements regarding equipment and supplies.

Once it is categorized, incoming mail is directed to the appropriate personnel in the office. Checks from patients and invoices may be distributed to the bookkeeper, insurance forms to the insurance clerk, medical journals and advertisements can be placed on the physician's desk, and magazines and newspapers can be placed in the reception area. Personal or confidential letters should not be opened unless the medical assistant has been given this responsibility by the physician or office manager.

Use a letter opener to open all mail before taking out the contents and reading the document. After removing the contents:

- Stamp the date it was received in the office.

- If the address is not included on the letter, write the address on the letter, as identified on the envelope or on the bank check (if patient is making a payment).

- When a colored reply envelope is sent with the statement to the patient, payments returned in these envelopes can speed up the sorting process.

- Look into the envelope to make certain that all contents have been removed.

- Attach the letter to the envelope with a paper clip, preferably on the left side.

Reply promptly to all requests, answering letters according to date of arrival; emergency situations need to be managed immediately.

Outgoing Mail and Shipments

Before placing postage on outgoing mail, weigh the item to be mailed, using a manual or electronic scale. A manual scale will read ounces. The assistant will then affix the appropriate postage, either stamps or postal meter. An electronic scale will automatically display the correct postage. If your office has a postal meter, this should be used to expedite mail. Metered mail does not have to be canceled or postmarked at the post office.

A postage meter is leased or purchased from a manufacturing company recommended by the postal service.

Critical Thinking

For the next week, practice sorting and prioritizing your personal incoming mail. If you live with others, ask permission to sort their mail and deliver it to them. Follow procedures outlined in this chapter. Write a paragraph about what you have learned by completing this exercise and how this experience might translate to a medical facility.

However, the postage meter must be taken to the post office to purchase postage. The meter is locked for the amount of postage purchased. Ambulatory care centers that send a large volume of mail may purchase a postage meter. See Procedure 15-5 for preparing outgoing mail.

Postal Classes

Check with the local post office to determine anticipated delivery turnaround to specific destinations. Common postal classes include:

1. *First-class mail.* Correspondence and statements are usually sent first class. All single-piece letters weighing less than 11 ounces are included in first-class mail. A postal card may be sent via this method if the card is not larger than 4¼ by 6 inches. The card may not be smaller than 3½ by 5 inches. If the recipient has moved, first-class mail may be forwarded at no additional cost.
2. *Priority mail.* Mail weighing more than 11 ounces and up to 70 pounds may be sent via priority mail. Check your postal service for current cost. The fee is based on weight and destination. Use the free priority mail stickers available from your local post office.
3. *Second-class mail.* Only newspapers and periodicals that have been authorized second-class privileges are sent by this manner.
4. *Third-class mail (bulk mail).* Circulars, books, catalogs, and other printed material and merchandise weighing less than 16 ounces can be sent via this method. Regular and special bulk rates are available only to authorized mailers. A minimum of 200 pieces of mail is required for the bulk rate, and an annual fee must be paid to send via this classification. All mail must be sent from one post office.
5. *Fourth-class mail (parcel post).* Fourth-class mail must weigh more than 16 ounces (1 pound) and not more than 70 pounds.
6. *Certified mail.* The certified mail service provides proof that a letter has been received. For example, if a physician dismisses a patient from the practice because of noncompliance of orders, a letter should be sent by certified mail, return receipt requested. When the receipt of acceptance of the letter is returned to the office, make certain that this receipt is filed in the patient's medical record. This provides legal protection for the physician. Other examples of mail that should be certified include birth certificates, marriage licenses, and deeds to property.
7. *Registered mail.* When an item has an intrinsic (real) value, it should be sent via registered mail.

Receipts are provided to identify the individual who accepted this mail. The sender declares a value on the item. A signature is required before delivery is made. Examples of items that should be sent by registered mail include clothing and jewelry.

8. *Express mail.* Express mail service is available 7 days per week for mailing items up to 70 pounds and 108 inches in combined length and girth. Express mail may be sent for noon delivery on the next day between major business markets.

Formats for Efficient Processing

Certified, registered, and special delivery markings should be placed below the stamp or approximately nine lines from the right top edge of the envelope. "Personal" or "confidential" notation should be keyed in all caps three lines below the return address. Adherence to other regulations will ensure accurate, timely delivery.

ZIP+4. ZIP+4 consists of the basic five ZIP code digits followed by a hyphen and four additional digits. The use of ZIP+4 will expedite the delivery of mail. If the envelope has been prepared properly to be read through OCR,

the digits will be converted to a bar code. This piece of mail then goes to the bar code sorter, which rapidly sorts for the final destination.

Abbreviations. When addressing mail, use the abbreviations for states and U.S. possessions (Figure 15-10) and use official postal service abbreviations for street suffixes, directionals, and locators (Figure 15-11).

International Mail

Classes of international mail include letters and letter packages, postcards and postal cards, aerogrammes, printed matter, direct sacks of printed matter, matter for the blind, small packets, and parcel post. Special services such as insurance, recorded delivery, registered mail, restricted delivery, return receipt, special delivery, cash on delivery mail, and certified mail are also available. For the most current information on rates and services, inquire at the local postal service.

TECHNOLOGIES

 In recent years, many new technologies such as fax and e-mail have changed the way written communications are sent. See Chapters 11 and 12 for more information related to confidentiality and Health Insurance Portability and Accountability Act (HIPAA) requirements.

Facsimile (Fax)

A facsimile, or fax, is the transmission of a written document through a telephone line using a fax machine both at the sender's and receiver's end. A fax can be sent as

AL	Alabama	NE	Nebraska	
AK	Alaska	NV	Nevada	
AS	American Samoa	NH	New Hampshire	
AZ	Arizona	NJ	New Jersey	
AR	Arkansas	NM	New Mexico	
CA	California	NY	New York	
CO	Colorado	NC	North Carolina	
CT	Connecticut	ND	North Dakota	
DE	Delaware	MP	No. Mariana Islands	
DC	Dist. of Columbia	OH	Ohio	
FL	Florida	OK	Oklahoma	
GA	Georgia	OR	Oregon	
GU	Guam	PA	Pennsylvania	
HI	Hawaii	PR	Puerto Rico	
ID	Idaho	RI	Rhode Island	
IL	Illinois	SC	South Carolina	
IN	Indiana	SD	South Dakota	
IA	Iowa	TN	Tennessee	
KS	Kansas	TX	Texas	
KY	Kentucky	TT	Trust Territory	
LA	Louisiana	UT	Utah	
ME	Maine	VT	Vermont	
MD	Maryland	VI	Virgin Islands, U.S.	
MA	Massachusetts	VA	Virginia	
MI	Michigan	WA	Washington	
MN	Minnesota	WV	West Virginia	
MS	Mississippi	WI	Wisconsin	
MO	Missouri	WY	Wyoming	
MT	Montana			

Figure 15-10 Abbreviations for states, territories, and District of Columbia.

AVE	Avenue	PL	Place
BLVD	Boulevard	RD	Road
CT	Court	STA	Station
CTR	Center	ST	Street
CIR	Circle	TPKE	Turnpike
DR	Drive	VLY	Valley
EXPY	Expressway	APT	Apartment
HTS	Heights	RM	Room
HWY	Highway	STE	Suite
IS	Island	PLZ	Plaza
JCT	Junction		
LK	Lake	N	North
LN	Lane	E	East
MTN	Mountain	S	South
PKY	Parkway	W	West

Figure 15-11 Abbreviations for street suffixes, directionals, and locators.

TABLE 15-4	ADVANTAGES OF THE FAX
Speed	The document is transmitted immediately or within minutes of sending.
Cost	Cost of a fax is the approximate cost of the telephone call. For long-distance faxes, this can be many times less than the cost of an overnight service.
Patient Care	Patient care could be enhanced, especially in emergency situations where the receiver may need to make decisions based on information in the document.
Legality	The receiver has the "hard copy" document versus relying on verbal information if the information is needed immediately.

FACSIMILE (FAX) CONSIDERATIONS

- Before releasing medical records to other medical personnel, a signed form authorizing the release must be obtained from the patient or legal guardian.
- If it is not of utmost urgency to transmit data immediately, it should be sent by a more secure means such as carrier or mail.
- Faxed messages should be used only when the telecopiers are located in a secure area; i.e., physician offices or nursing stations rather than mail rooms or open areas, unless they are secured with passwords.
- Always use a cover sheet containing the warning: "The following material is strictly confidential; all persons are advised that they may be prosecuted under federal and state law for sharing this information with unauthorized individuals."
- Always recheck to be sure that the fax is being sent to the correct telephone number and that the number was entered correctly.
- After faxing, call the person who is receiving the fax and confirm that it was received.

Figure 15-12 Facsimile (fax) considerations.

easily as putting the document in the machine, similar to the way a document is put in a copy machine, and dialing the receiving telephone number. See Procedure 15-6. There are several advantages to using the fax machine compared with traditional postal or carrier services. These advantages are listed in Table 15-4.

 There are other issues involved in using the fax, especially when sending patient information. Figure 15-12 provides insight on several legal and confidentiality issues that should be considered before sending any communications via the fax. See Chapter 11 for additional guidelines related to fax use.

 HIPAA requires all medical practices to implement technical measures to protect against unauthorized access to protected health information (PHI) when it is transmitted over electronic telecommunications networks. Two security measures must be addressed: the integrity of the information transmitted, and the vulnerability of the information to unauthorized use or disclosure.

When information is transmitted over public networks, static and other less benign problems can introduce errors into the information. The security rule requires the implementation of security measures to verify the integrity of the information that is transmitted.

Information transmitted over public networks may be intercepted and used by unauthorized users. In some cases, the interception can be deliberate to access sensitive information. In other instances, the interception may be the result of error by the person making the transmission. For example, a person sending a fax dials the wrong number and sends information to an unintended recipient.

The security rule requires implementation of a mechanism to encrypt PHI when appropriate. Encryption requires the cooperation of both parties to the transaction, and the encryption methods are specified in any agreement between the parties.

Electronic Mail (E-Mail)

 Medical information previously communicated via mail, telephone, or fax may now be sent from computer to computer using **e-mail.** Just as business communication requires proper use of written language, so does e-mail.

Composing e-mail is similar to composing any written communication. Just as a letter or memo has a particular format, the e-mail transmission should also follow a format style. The subject line should be brief and clearly identify the content of the e-mail body.

If your message is in response to another piece of e-mail, your e-mail software will probably preface the subject line with *Re:* (for regarding). If your e-mail software does not do this, it would be polite to key in "RE:". If your message is time critical, starting with "URGENT" is appropriate. If you are referring to a previous e-mail, you should explicitly quote that document to provide context.

If a message is to be sent to several parties, individual e-mail messages may be sent to each, thereby protecting their privacy. In many instances, however, it is useful for parties involved in a group "conversation" to be aware of who the other participants are. In this case, all of the addresses may be included on the same e-mail message. Sending a "bcc," or blind copy, also protects the privacy of your e-mail because it does not show to whom else the message was sent.

The body of the message should contain short and clear sentences. In trying to be brief and to the point, however, it is important to not leave out important facts or information. Remember also that some e-mail software only understands plain text. Italics, bold, and color changes should be used sparingly. Some software will also recognize **URLs (Uniform Resource Locators,** or Web site addresses)** in the text and make them "live." Because different software recognizes different parts of the address, if you include a URL in your e-mail message, it is much safer to use the entire address, including the initial http://. See Figure 15-13 for additional e-mail etiquette.

The advantages of using e-mail as a means of communication include:

- Asynchronous communication—both parties need not be available at the same time for communication to take place

- Physicians and patients can prepare, leave, read, and respond to messages at times that are convenient

- Can be used to automate certain tasks such as sending out appointment reminders or reports of laboratory results

- Creates a documentation trail of interactions between physician and patient

- Some patients may be more forthcoming using e-mail than in face-to-face discussion

The disadvantages of e-mail communications include:

- Lack of real-time interaction and feedback (see Chapter 12 for more information related to instant messaging)

- Lack of body language or vocal inflection, which may lead to misunderstanding

- Reimbursement for the time spent responding to patient messages and receipt of messages from non-patients may not be defined

- May not be suitable for time-sensitive material because determination of when the message will be delivered or read cannot be assessed

LEGAL AND ETHICAL ISSUES

Written communication, no matter what form is used, must take into consideration legal and ethical issues. A copy of all written communication should be maintained in the patient chart or in office files should it be needed at a later date.

E-MAIL ETIQUETTE

Most organizations implement etiquette rules for the following reasons:
- Professionalism: Using correct grammar, spelling, and language conveys a professional image.
- Efficiency: E-mail is a more effective means of communication.
- Protection from liability: Appropriate, business-like language in all e-mail communications limits liability risks.

Remember that an e-mail message is not delivered with body language. A great deal of human communication comes from nonverbal signals such as facial expressions and tone of voice. These cues help make the message clearer. The following etiquette rules promote professionalism, efficiency, and protection from liability:
- Use proper structure and layout. Use short paragraphs and blank lines between each paragraph. When making points, number or bullet each point.
- Do not attach unnecessary files.
- When sending attachments is necessary, tell the recipient the format of the attachment. If a large attachment must be sent, call the recipient first to be sure his or her Internet service will accept it.
- Do not overuse the high priority option.
- Do not overuse Reply to All. Use this feature only when your message needs to be received by everyone. Do not copy a message or attachment without permission. You could be infringing on copyright laws.
- Use a meaningful subject. This helps the recipient focus immediately.
- As a courtesy to your recipient, include your name at the bottom of the message. The recipient may not know that the return address belongs to you.
- Do not write anything you would not say in public.
- Do not write in CAPITALS. If you write in capitals, it seems as if you are shouting.
- Do not send Flame e-mails; that is, insulting message designed to cause pain, as when someone "gets burned."

When confidential or privileged material is sent via e-mail, it should include a disclaimer stating that any review, retransmission, dissemination, or other use of the material is prohibited. It should also state that if the message is received in error, the recipient should contact the sender and delete the material from the computer.

Figure 15-13 E-mail etiquette.

It is important to include e-mail in your office's confidentiality policy. Review the section on confidentiality and HIPAA in Chapter 11. Confidentiality issues must be considered if the ambulatory care office sends or receives **clinical e-mail**

messages from a computer that can be used by more than one person. Many offices use a privacy disclaimer to establish boundaries and ground rules for e-mail messages. The following is an example of such a disclaimer:

 This message is a privileged and confidential clinical communication intended solely for the person to whom it is addressed. If you are not the intended recipient, please be advised that any disseminating, copying, or distributing of this message is strictly prohibited. If you received this message in error, please forward it back to the sender.

Clinical e-mail to or from patients should be treated the same as telephone messages or letters. That means that they should be printed out and filed in the chart. It is important to remember to file both the initial message and any reply.

Before your office begins to use clinical e-mail, a written agreement of understanding should be designed for signature by the patients. In addition to obtaining the patient's permission for you to use clinical e-mail, key elements to incorporate in such an agreement may include:

- E-mail will be exchanged with established patients only.

- E-mail from the patient will include the patient's full name and number.

- The physician is not responsible for e-mail that is not received or responded to in a timely manner.

- E-mail may not be private and confidential.

- E-mail may be read by others, intercepted, or misaddressed.

- E-mail will be filed in the chart.

- E-mail will not be permanently stored on the computer system.

- Urgent issues need to be handled by telephone or in person.

Examples of appropriate uses of e-mail in the ambulatory care setting include:

- Appointment requests

- Prescription refill requests

- Reminder notices

- Insurance or billing questions

- Managed care referrals

- Interoffice correspondence

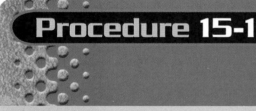

Procedure 15-1 — Preparing and Composing Business Correspondence Using All Components (Computerized Approach)

PURPOSE:
Prepare and compose a rough draft and final-copy letter using appropriate language and letter style to convey a clear and accurate message to the recipient.

EQUIPMENT/SUPPLIES:
Computer or word processor and printer
Printed letterhead and plain second sheet
Dictionary
Thesaurus
Medical dictionary
Style manual

PROCEDURE STEPS:
1. Organize key points to be addressed in a logical sequence. RATIONALE: To assist in writing an effective letter.
2. Go to "Page Setup" and set document margins, paper size and source, and the layout. Set the fonts to be used and paragraph parameters. Name and save the document. RATIONALE: Saves time and loss of formatting.
3. Compose a rough draft of the letter. With time and experience, these outlining steps may be

(continues)

Procedure 15-1 (continued)

eliminated before drafting the letter. RATIO-NALE: Business correspondence should be clear, concise, courteous, and accurate. A draft letter aids in checking that the letter is logical and achieves the intended purpose.

4. Use language that is easily understood. State the reason for the letter in the first paragraph and encourage action in the last paragraph. RATIO-NALE: For communication to take place, both parties must understand the message. The letter must be written so that the recipient understands the language and responds appropriately.

5. Read the draft for obvious errors in grammar, spelling, and punctuation. Use the appropriate reference material (dictionary, style manual, spell check, and so on) to check any inaccuracies. Read again for content. Is the message accurate, logical, and organized appropriately? Save the document again if any changes were made. Lay the letter aside and read it a third time at a later time. RATIONALE: Reading several times allows you to concentrate on different elements of the letter. Errors may jump out when reading for the third time.

6. Choose the letter format that is customary to the ambulatory care setting. Established templates saved on the computer or provided on computer software are time savers. RATIONALE: The letter style should be efficient to prepare and professional in appearance and content to represent the physician–employer in a professional manner.

7. Key in the date or use the computer's auto date feature on line 15 or two to three lines below the letterhead. RATIONALE: Using the component parts of a business letter ensures that the letter is professional in appearance and represents the physician–employer in a professional manner.

8. Key the recipient's name and address flush with the left margin beginning on line 20. RATIO-NALE: Using the component parts of a business letter ensures that the letter is professional in appearance and represents the physician–employer in a professional manner.

9. On the second line below the recipient's address, key the salutation flush with the left margin.

Follow the salutation with a colon unless you are using open punctuation. RATIONALE: Using the component parts of a business letter ensures that the letter is professional in appearance and represents the physician–employer in a professional manner.

10. Key the subject of the letter on the second line below the salutation flush with the left margin, if the subject line is being used. RATIONALE: Using the component parts of a business letter ensures that the letter is professional in appearance and represents the physician–employer in a professional manner.

11. Begin the body of the letter on the second line below the salutation or subject line. The body format will depend on the style of letter used. For example, if the full block format is used, paragraphs will begin flush with the left margin. Single-space within paragraphs; double-space between paragraphs. RATIONALE: Using the component parts of a business letter ensures that the letter is professional in appearance and represents the physician–employer in a professional manner.

12. Key the complimentary closure on the second line below the body of the letter. Capitalize only the first letter of the first word of the complimentary closure (e.g., Respectfully yours). RATIO-NALE: Using the component parts of a business letter ensures that the letter is professional in appearance and represents the physician–employer in a professional manner.

13. Key the signature four to six lines below the complimentary closing. RATIONALE: This ensures that the recipient will be able to determine who sent the letter.

14. If reference initials are used, key the initials two lines below the keyed signature (e.g., WL: jg). RATIONALE: Using the component parts of a business letter ensures that the letter is professional in appearance and represents the physician–employer in a professional manner.

15. Key the enclosure or carbon copy notation one or two lines below the reference initials. RATIO-NALE: Using the component parts of a business letter ensures that the letter is professional

(continues)

Procedure 15-1 (continued)

in appearance and represents the physician–employer in a professional manner.

16. Proofread the document and make corrections as necessary. RATIONALE: All information contained in the letter must be accurate and written in a clear and concise manner with logical organization. The grammar, spelling, punctuation, and capitalization must be correct to ensure a professional appearance and represent the physician–employer in a positive manner.

17. Save the document again and print two copies. RATIONALE: Document is saved on the computer, and a copy for signature and mailing is produced. A hard copy for the file is also established.

18. Prepare the envelope. Place the envelope flap over the letter and attach it with a paper clip. RATIONALE: Prepare the envelope using U.S. postal regulations to ensure delivery in a timely manner. Proofread to be sure the address is accurate to ensure deliverability. By placing the envelope flap over the letter and attaching it with a paper clip, the two will not become separated.

19. Place the letter on the physician's desk for review and signature. RATIONALE: The physician's signature signifies the letter is accurate, sends the intended message, and represents the office in a professional manner.

20. File a copy of the letter in an appropriate filing system. RATIONALE: May be needed in the future for reference or as documentation.

Procedure 15-2 Addressing Envelopes According to United States Postal Regulations

PURPOSE:
To address envelopes according to U.S. Postal Service regulations to ensure timely delivery.

EQUIPMENT/SUPPLIES:
Computer or word processor and printer with envelope tray
Envelopes
Address labels
U.S. Postal Service Publication 221, *Addressing for Success*

PROCEDURE STEPS:

1. Insert the envelope in the typewriter or select the envelope format from the software program. When using a word processor or computer, labels may be used rather than printing directly on the envelope. The label is then adhered to the envelope. Many printers have an envelope tray and software that will transfer the address from the letter to the envelope. This feature is a time saver because you only key the address once. RATIONALE: U.S. postal regulations suggest that the address on letter mail should be machine-printed, with a uniform left margin.

2. Visualize an imaginary rectangle on the envelope. The rectangle extends ⅝ inch to 2¾ inches from the bottom of the envelope, with 1 inch on each side. The address is placed within this rectangle (Figure 15-14). RATIONALE: U.S. postal regulations suggest that the address on letter mail should be machine-printed, with a uniform left margin.

(continues)

Procedure 15-2 (continued)

3. Key the address in uppercase letters. Be sure to maintain a uniform left margin on all lines. Eliminate all punctuation in the address except the hyphen in the ZIP+4 code. Leave a minimum of one space between the city name and the two-character state abbreviation and the ZIP+4 code. RATIONALE: A scanner reads the Zip code on the bottom line and prints a bar code in the lower right corner of the envelope. The OCR prefers all uppercase characters.

4. If you are not using preprinted envelopes, key the return address in uppercase letters in the upper left corner of the envelope. Include the name on the first line, address on the second line, and city, state, and ZIP+4 code on the third line. RATIONALE: The return address should be printed in the upper left corner of the envelope should the letter need to be returned to the sender for any reason.

5. Proofread the envelope and make corrections as necessary. RATIONALE: When all information is correct, processing will take place efficiently and correctly.

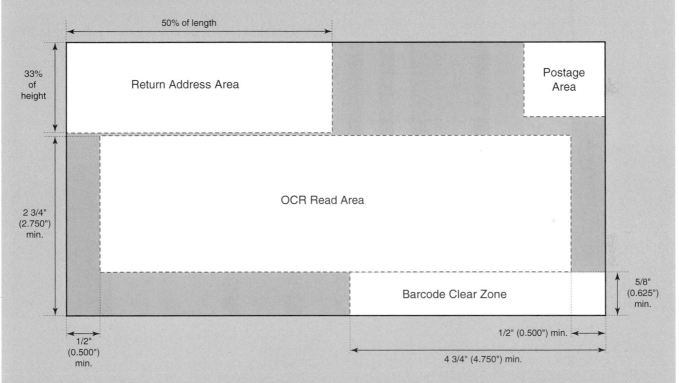

Figure 15-14 Designated zones for accurate reading of envelopes by optical character reader (OCR), the U.S. Postal Service's computerized scanner. (Courtesy United States Postal Service.)

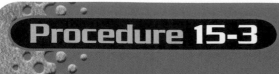

Procedure 15-3 — Folding Letters for Standard Envelopes

PURPOSE:
To fold and insert letters into envelopes so that the letters fit properly in the envelopes.

EQUIPMENT/SUPPLIES:
Letters to be mailed
Number 6¾ envelope
Number 10 envelope
Window envelope

PROCEDURE STEPS:
1. To fit a standard-size letter into a number 6¾ envelope, fold the letter up from the bottom, leaving ¼ to ½ inch at the top, and crease it. Then fold the letter from the right edge about one-third the width of the letter. Fold the left edge over to within ¼ to ½ inch of the right-edge crease. Insert the left creased edge first into the envelope (Figure 15-15A). RATIONALE: Ensures a proper fit of the letter into the envelope with a minimum of folds. The last crease made enters the envelope first. This enables the recipient to begin to read the letter with minimal effort.

2. To fit a standard-size letter into a number 10 envelope, fold the letter up about one-third the length of the sheet and crease it. Then fold the top of the letter down to within ¼ to ½ inch of the bottom crease, and crease the top. Insert the top creased edge first into the envelope (Figure 15-15B). RATIONALE: Ensures a proper fit of the letter into the envelope with a minimum of folds. The last crease made enters the envelope first. This enables the recipient to begin to read the letter with minimal effort.

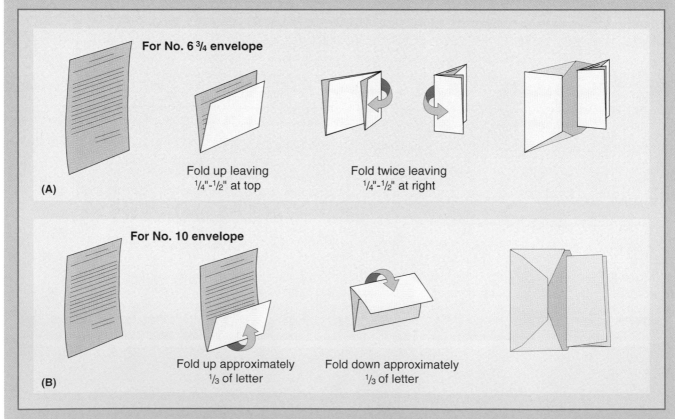

For No. 6 ³⁄₄ envelope

Fold up leaving ¹⁄₄"-¹⁄₂" at top

Fold twice leaving ¹⁄₄"-¹⁄₂" at right

(A)

For No. 10 envelope

Fold up approximately ¹⁄₃ of letter

Fold down approximately ¹⁄₃ of letter

(B)

Figure 15-15 Proper letter folding procedures for various envelope types (A–C) and bulk placement of envelopes for moistening before closure (D).

(continues)

Procedure 15-3 (continued)

3. To fit a standard-size letter into a window envelope, turn the letter over and fold the top of the letter up about one-third the length of the page so that the address is facing you. Then fold the bottom of the letter back to the first crease. Insert the letter into the envelope bottom first (Figure 15-15C). You should be able to read the entire address through the window. RATIONALE: Ensures that the entire address can be read through the window envelope and be delivered correctly.

4. Place envelopes as shown in Figure 15-15D to moisten before sealing. RATIONALE: Efficient method of sealing multiple letters for mailing.

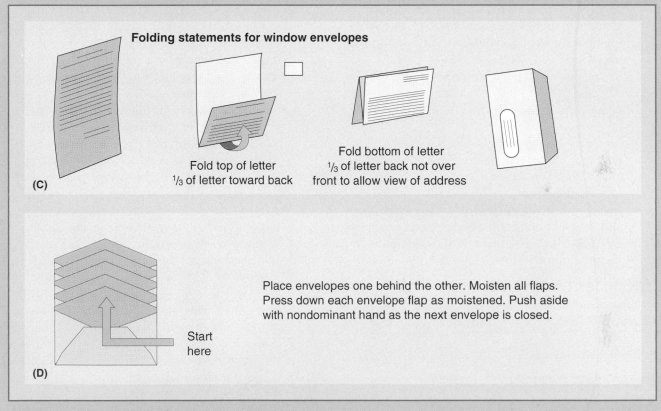

Folding statements for window envelopes

(C) Fold top of letter ⅓ of letter toward back

Fold bottom of letter ⅓ of letter back not over front to allow view of address

(D) Start here

Place envelopes one behind the other. Moisten all flaps. Press down each envelope flap as moistened. Push aside with nondominant hand as the next envelope is closed.

Figure 15-15 (continued)

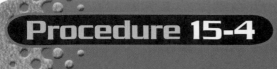

Procedure 15-4 — Creating a Mass Mailing Using Mail Merge

PURPOSE:

To create a mass mailing using the computer's Mail Merge Helper feature contained within Microsoft® Word. The procedure consists of four steps:

1. Create a generic main document to be sent to different addressees. RATIONALE: A clear and concise document is required that can be used to transmit your message for all addresses by changing only the name, address, and title within the document.
2. Development of a Data Source. RATIONALE: The data that are changed from addressee to addressee must be generated for insertion by the program.
3. Insertion of Merge Fields. RATIONALE: The program must have instruction as to where changeable or variable data are to be inserted into the document.
4. Merge the main document and variable data and send it to an output device such as a printer. RATIONALE: The program must be told how to output the final merged document.

EQUIPMENT/SUPPLIES:

Computer and printer
Composed correspondence keyed and saved as a Word document.
A developed data source

PROCEDURE STEPS:

1. Create main document:
   - The first step in creating a mass mailing is to compose and type the document in Microsoft® Word. At this step, identify each data field (name, address, and so forth) that will be variable to personalize the document for each addressee by inserting a readily identifiable character such as a "?" or "&." For use in Step 2, note the different unique data fields that are required.

2. Develop a Data Source:
   - Select "Tools" from the menu bar, and then select "Mail Merge" from the drop-down menu that appears.
   - Mail Merge Helper appears, displaying a screen that shows a checklist of actions required by you. You must first identify the type of main document being prepared. Select "Create" from item 1 on the screen and a drop-down menu will appear with several types of documents listed for selection. Select "Form Letter" for this exercise.
   - A new window immediately appears asking where to look for the main document. Because you have already typed the main document in the active window, click on "Active Window." You will notice that the screen displays your choices below the Create Button.
   - Go to item 2 on the screen and select "Get Data." A drop-down menu immediately appears listing several options. Select "Create Data."
   - A screen appears showing data field titles. It is possible to add additional fields or to eliminate some of the fields in the list. We will want to have three fields for complex addresses, so type into the upper left block entitled "Field Name" the word "Address3." Immediately, a new button appears below it saying "Add Field Name." Click this button; the name you just typed has been added to the existing list. If it is at the bottom of the list, move it to after "Address2" by first highlighting it and then moving it using the up and down arrows at the right of the screen.
   - All of the field names will not be needed, so delete work phone, home phone, country, and job title. Fields are deleted by first highlighting them, and then clicking the button "Remove Field Names." Check if everything is OK and click "OK."

(continues)

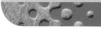

Procedure 15-4   (continued)

- A new screen appears and you are asked where to store your data file. Give it a name "Merge Data" and store it on your Desktop. You do this by left-clicking with your mouse on the arrow to the right of the "Save In" window. Click the arrow adjacent to select "Desktop." Click the "Save" button from the drop-down menu.
- A new screen now appears saying that no data are in your file and allowing you to edit your data. Select "Edit Data Source."
- A data form now appears with the field titles you previously selected and empty boxes are adjacent to each title. Fill in the boxes with the data you have made up for this problem. Any boxes where data do not exist should be left blank. After completing the first record (addressee), click the "Add New" button and a new blank form will appear. Continue until you have added data for at least three records. Click "OK" when finished.

3. Insert merge fields into the main document:
   - You should be back in your main document. You will now insert the field names in the appropriate locations you have marked in the original document with a "?" or "&" character. Insert your cursor and highlight one of the characters. Using your mouse, click on the toolbar entitled "Insert Merge Field." A drop-down menu will appear listing all of the field titles you selected while developing the data source in Step 2. Select the field appropriate to the location of your cursor and left-click. The field name will immediately appear in the main document with a double {{ on either end. Continue until you have replaced all of the characters with field names.
   - Check to make sure that the spacing and punctuation are correct. Each field name will be just as if you typed the actual data, with no additional spaces or commas.

4. Sending the merged document to the output device (printer):
   - Select "Tools," "Mail Merge," putting you back in Mail Merge Helper. Select "Merge" and a Merge To block appears. Select "Printer."
   - The printer screen appears. Make sure the printer connected to your computer is selected, the Page Range is set to "All," and the number of copies is set to 1. Click "OK." Three letters should print with the variable data you input to your data file.
   - If you have any errors in the data or in spacing, make the necessary changes. To edit your data file, get back to Mail Merge Helper and select "Edit Data Source," followed by clicking the file location suggested by a button that appears below the one you just clicked.
   - To move from record to record, use the arrows at the bottom of the screen. When you have finished editing, click "OK" and repeat printing as described earlier in this step.

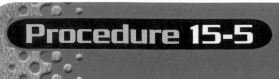

Procedure 15-5 Preparing Outgoing Mail According to United States Postal Regulations

PURPOSE:
To prepare outgoing mail for expeditious delivery.

EQUIPMENT/SUPPLIES:
Manual or electronic scale
Postage meter or stamps
Envelope or package to be mailed

PROCEDURE STEPS:
1. Sort the mail according to postal class. For example, all single-piece letters that weigh less than 11 ounces are included in first-class mail. Correspondence and statements are sent in this classification. RATIONALE: Sorting by postal class expedites processing at the post office.
2. Using the manual or electronic scale, weigh the item to be mailed. If you are using a manual scale, read the weight in ounces and compute the amount of postage due. If you are using an elec-tronic scale, the correct postage will be displayed on the scale. RATIONALE: Correct postage on each postal item is essential to ensure faster delivery service.
3. Using a postal meter or stamps, affix the appropriate postage to the piece to be mailed. Use of a postal meter expedites delivery of mail because metered mail does not have to be canceled or postmarked at the post office. RATIONALE: Correct postage on each postal item is essential to ensure faster delivery service.
4. Place the prepared mail in the area of the office designated for outgoing mail, or deliver the mail to the post office according to office policy. RATIONALE: Ensures that all mail going out is centrally located and that the postal worker can pick up outgoing and deliver incoming mail efficiently.

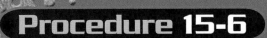

Procedure 15-6 Preparing, Sending, and Receiving a Fax

PURPOSE:
To send and receive information quickly and accurately by fax (facsimile).

EQUIPMENT/SUPPLIES:
Fax machine
Telephone

PROCEDURE STEPS:
To send a fax:
1. Prepare a cover sheet or use a preprinted cover sheet for the document to be faxed. Include the names of the sender and receiver, the number of pages being sent and whether this includes the cover sheet, and a short message if necessary. RATIONALE: A cover sheet aids in the correct delivery of a fax to the designated person. It also provides a disclaimer should the fax be received in error and what to do if it is misdelivered.
CAUTION: Fax machines may be located in areas where unauthorized personnel may see confidential material. Always include a notice of confidentiality on the cover sheet and always ask the receiver for permission to fax a confidential document.

(continues)

Procedure 15-6 (continued)

2. Place the document according to machine instructions. RATIONALE: Ensures that content will be read for transmission.
3. Dial the telephone or dedicated fax number of the receiver. If your fax machine has a display showing the number being faxed to, check to be sure the number you dialed is correct. Then press start. RATIONALE: Verify number to be sure fax is being transmitted to correct phone.
4. After the document passes through the fax machine, press the button requesting a receipt. Some fax machines automatically issue a report. RATIONALE: A receipt is your documentation of the date, time, and where the fax was sent.
5. Remove the document from the machine and, when necessary, call the recipient to be sure the fax was received. RATIONALE: Maintains confidentiality and verifies fax was received by intended recipient.

To receive a fax:

6. Be sure that the fax machine is turned on and that the telephone line to the machine is not being used. Most offices will have dedicated fax lines. RATIONALE: Enables you to receive a fax.
7. Remove the document from the machine after it is received and immediately deliver it to the addressee. RATIONALE: Maintains confidentiality and enables recipient to take action immediately if necessary.

Case Study 15-1

When she was assembling the style manual for all written communications generated by the office of Drs. Lewis and King, office manager Marilyn Johnson wanted it to be as comprehensive as possible. Therefore, she gathered research over a period of months, noting problems the office had experienced in written communications, such as letters going out without the physician's signature; she became familiar with proofreading devices that would ensure letter-perfect correspondence; she also developed source materials on the different classes of mail and the services of the U.S. Post Office.

CASE STUDY REVIEW

1. Marilyn is ready to outline the manual. Review the chapter information and create an outline indicating major topic headings for the Lewis and King style manual.
2. Because a few of the medical assistants are not comfortable with composing, what writing tips can Marilyn include to make them more confident?
3. Marilyn wants all letters to look alike. What information should she include to educate the manual users about the components of a standard letter?

Case Study 15-2

Drs. Lewis and King are considering adopting the use of clinical e-mail because many of their patients have home computers and use e-mail in their day-to-day communications. Office manager Marilyn Johnson is concerned about maintaining patient confidentiality and appropriate use of clinical e-mail. She has decided to develop a written agreement of understanding and plans to ask each patient to sign the agreement before transmission of any clinical e-mail is instituted. Marilyn also feels a privacy disclaimer could be of legal value to the office.

CASE STUDY REVIEW

1. Marilyn is developing the agreement of understanding. What are some key elements that should be included in the agreement?
2. Responding to patients using e-mail correspondence is different than social communication. What are some guidelines for e-mail correspondence that will be helpful to remember?
3. List several advantages and disadvantages to using e-mail in the ambulatory health care setting.

SUMMARY

Communication is vital in any ambulatory care setting, and the proper management of written communications ensures both a professional image and an efficient operation. Because of our ability to write letters, send reports, transcribe physician notes, and otherwise communicate with others, the quality of patient care is enhanced, because communication is at the core of much patient treatment.

As well as becoming knowledgeable about the techniques of written communication, it is important for the medical assistant to become comfortable with the act of composition and writing. Proper techniques in letter formatting and proofreading ensures quality control and the maintenance of high administrative standards. Ease in writing and communicating on paper ensures that information is accurate, reliable, and capable of being held up in a court of law if this becomes necessary.

The administrative medical assistant must be skilled in the use of technologies and understand and follow confidentiality and legal policies and procedures.

STUDY FOR SUCCESS

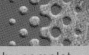

To reinforce your knowledge and skills of information presented in this chapter:
- ❑ Review the Key Terms
- ❑ Practice the Procedures
- ❑ Consider the Case Studies and discuss your conclusions
- ❑ Answer the Review Questions
  - ❑ Multiple Choice
  - ❑ Critical Thinking
- ❑ Navigate the Internet by completing the Web Activities
- ❑ Practice the StudyWARE activities on the textbook CD
- ❑ Apply your knowledge in the Student Workbook activities
- ❑ Complete the Web Tutor sections
- ❑ View and discuss the DVD situations

REVIEW QUESTIONS

Multiple Choice

1. When proofreading a letter, you should:
   a. never read it against the document
   b. always proof it only on the computer screen
   c. read long documents a section at a time
   d. always finish the job no matter how tired you may be
2. Form letters should be used:
   a. for all patients
   b. for all referring physicians
   c. only for pharmaceutical salespeople
   d. with individualized addressing when possible
3. Of the four major letter styles, which is the most contemporary?
   a. full block
   b. modified block, standard
   c. modified block, indented
   d. simplified
4. Form letters may be written for each of the following *except:*
   a. letters containing laboratory or diagnostic results
   b. letters announcing new insurance or HMOs accepted
   c. letters to announce new staff
   d. letters to order supplies or subscriptions
5. The subject line is keyed:
   a. on line 15 or two to three lines below the letterhead
   b. on the second line below the inside address
   c. four lines below the complimentary closing
   d. on the second line below the salutation
6. When keying a second page, all of the following apply *except:*
   a. always use a second-page heading
   b. when dividing a paragraph at the bottom of a page, keep one line on the bottom of the page and one line at the top of the next page
   c. a minimum of three lines should be keyed on the second page of a letter
   d. never use a letterhead page as a second page
7. After removing the contents from incoming mail, what should you do?
   a. stamp the date it was received in the office
   b. look in the envelope to make certain that all contents have been removed
   c. if the address is not included on the letter, write it on the letter as it appeared on the envelope
   d. all of the above
8. In the ambulatory care setting, the postal class likely to be used most frequently is:
   a. express
   b. first class
   c. bulk rate
   d. second class
9. The body of an e-mail communication should:
   a. contain short and clear sentences
   b. be written in italic, bold, and color for emphasis
   c. be brief and to the point but contain all pertinent information
   d. a and c only
10. To establish boundaries and ground rules for e-mail messages, many offices are developing:
    a. privacy disclaimers
    b. written agreements of understanding
    c. itineraries
    d. agendas

Critical Thinking

1. With a group of classmates, organize a spelling bee of commonly misspelled medical words. Include some English words that are often misspelled also. Conduct the spelling bee.
2. Practice how to compose business correspondence using all components. Procedure 15-1 will be a helpful guide. Print a draft copy of your letter and use common proofreader's marks to indicate any corrections.
3. Rekey the above letter and practice how to fold it correctly. Procedure 15-3 provides step-by-step instructions.
4. Practice how to address an envelope with all address elements in proper format for expeditious handling by the U.S. Postal Service. Procedure 15-2 provides step-by-step instructions for addressing envelopes. Now place your letter into the envelope correctly. Refer to Procedure 15-3 if you have forgotten how to insert the letter properly.
5. Discuss how to implement HIPAA requirements in the ambulatory care setting, addressing issues of unauthorized access to PHI when transmitted over electronic telecommunications networks (fax). Review Chapter 11 for additional information.
6. Discuss how legal and ethical issues impact the ambulatory care setting relative to clinical e-mail from a computer that can be used by more than one person in the office.

WEB ACTIVITIES

Use the Internet to research additional information pertaining to confidentiality and legal issues related to faxing medical records or using electronic mail to transmit medical information. Follow instructor's instructions on completing and turning in your results.

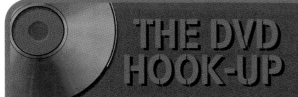

THE DVD HOOK-UP

DVD Series
Critical Thinking

Program Number
2

Chapter/Scene Reference
• *Forms of Communications (play only the portion on written communications.)*

In this chapter, you learned about the importance of written communications. Because of today's technology, there are fewer face-to-face communications with your patients, supervisors, and coworkers, and a great deal more written communication.

The designated DVD scene featured a testimonial from Carla. Carla stated that the majority of communication that takes place between the physician and other staff members is written; thus, much of how others will view you will depend on how well you communicate through writing.

1. Do you think that it is fair for others to judge you based on how well you write?
2. Describe how your writing skills may influence the outcome of a possible malpractice suit.

DVD Journal Summary

Write a paragraph that summarizes what you learned from watching the designated scene from today's DVD program. What are some areas that you need to work on to improve your written communication skills?

DOCUMENTATION

Clinically related e-mail to or from patients should be treated the same way as telephone messages or letters. That means they should be printed out and filed in the chart.

From: Elizabeth J. Parker
Sent: Tuesday, July 20, 20XX 8:55 AM
To: Dr. King [King@doctor.com]
Subject: Prescription refill

Please call in a prescription refill for my thyroid medication. The pharmacy is Inner City Pharmacy and the phone number is 890-271-2600. The prescription number is RX6437350 and I have enough pills for three days.

REFERENCES/BIBLIOGRAPHY

Humphrey, D. D. (2004) *Contemporary medical office procedures* (3rd ed.). Clifton Park, NY: Thomson Delmar Learning.

ingenix (2003, December). *HIPAA tool kit.* Salt Lake City, UT: St. Anthony's Publishing/Medicode.

Keir, L., Wise, B. A., & Krebs, C. (2003). *Medical assisting administrative and clinical competencies* (5th ed.). Clifton Park, NY: Thomson Delmar Learning.

Physicians Insurance 2000. (March/April 2000). *Physician's risk management update* (Vol. XI, No. 2.). Author.

Robert, H. M., III, Evans, W. J., Honemann, D. H., & Balch, T. J. (2000). *Robert's rules of order newly revised* (10th ed.). Cambridge, MA: Perseus Publishing.

OUTLINE

OBJECTIVES

The student should strive to meet the following performance objectives and demonstrate an understanding of the facts and principles presented in this chapter through written and oral communication.

1. Define the key terms as presented in the glossary.
2. Discuss the duties and responsibilities of the medical transcriptionist.
3. Differentiate among chart notes, history and physician examination reports, consultation reports, and medical correspondence.

(continues)

KEY TERMS

(continues)

KEY TERMS
(continued)

Microscopic Examination
Old Report or Aged Report
Operative Report (OR)
Pathology Report
Privileged
Progress Notes
Proofreading
Quality Assurance (QA)
Radiology Report
Review of Systems (ROS)
Risk Management
STAT Report
Transcriber
Turnaround Time
Waveform audio (WAV)

FEATURED COMPETENCIES

ABHES—ENTRY-LEVEL COMPETENCIES
Communication

- Use appropriate medical terminology
- Receive, organize, prioritize, and transmit information expediently
- Use correct grammar, spelling and formatting techniques in written works
- Application of electronic technology
- Fundamental writing skills

Administrative Duties

- Perform basic secretarial skills
- Apply computer concepts for office procedures
- Perform medical transcriptions

OBJECTIVES (continued)

4. List three examples of specialized reports and discuss what makes each different.
5. Describe turnaround time and its importance.
6. Recall a minimum of three formatting rules when preparing medical reports.
7. Discuss the role of the JCAHO as it relates to hospitals and physicians' offices owned by hospital organizations.
8. Discuss the proper ways to make corrections within medical reports.
9. Describe the process of flagging and its significance.
10. Discuss what is meant by the term *authentication* and identify three ways it may be done related to medical reports.
11. Identify four ways the medical transcriptionist can be compliant with the HIPAA.
12. Discuss risk management and its importance for the medical transcriptionist.
13. Review the ergonomics section in Chapter 11 and discuss how setting up an ergonomically friendly workstation may benefit the medical transcriptionist.
14. Describe two types of media used by modern transcribers.
15. Review the sections on facsimile machines in Chapters 11 and 15 and discuss important issues applicable to medical transcription.
16. Identify and describe the two major categories of attributes of the medical transcriptionist.
17. Discuss six categories of professionalism as they relate to medical transcription.
18. Compare and contrast the various types of work environments for the medical transcriptionist.
19. Briefly describe AAMT and its importance to medical transcription.
20. Describe the certification examination and who is eligible to sit for the examination.

SCENARIO

Inner City Health Care, a multispecialty clinic, employs two full-time medical transcriptionists. Marilyn Johnson, CMA, is the office manager and has former training and experience as a medical transcriptionist. This experience provides her with the basic understanding necessary to manage the medical transcription and medical records department of the clinic. Marilyn has involved the transcriptionists in the ergonomic set up of workstations and in the selection of state-of-the-art equipment and latest reference resources to create a safe work environment and one that encourages quality documents in a timely manner.

INTRODUCTION

Medical assistants and Certified Medical Administrative Specialists (CMAS) may also serve as transcriptionists in a medical setting. These individuals will need to be knowledgeable of the duties of transcriptionists, the proper format for medical reports, proofreading and error correction procedures, and confidentiality requirements. He or she may be responsible for coordinating with a contracted transcription service and possibly perform the **quality assurance (QA)** *and* **risk management** *tasks on completed work.*

DUTIES AND RESPONSIBILITIES FOR MEDICAL TRANSCRIPTIONISTS

The responsibility of the **medical transcriptionist (MT)** is to transform written or dictated medical information into an accurate, permanent record that is legible and uniform in format. The resulting medical record describes the encounter between the patient and health care provider and is extremely important from both a health care and legal standpoint.

The transcribed record is sometimes a matter of life and death to the patient. Diagnosis, laboratory test results, and prescribed drugs need to be accurately and completely transcribed as part of the permanent record to prevent incorrect diagnosis, drug interactions, and improper prescribing of medication.

The transcriptionist's job is anything but routine. He or she is part secretary, part editor, and part translator

Spotlight on Certification

RMA Content Outline
- Spelling
- Terminology
- Written communication
- Transcription and dictation
- Computers for medical office applications

CMA Content Outline
- Medical terminology
- Legislation
- Data entry
- Computer applications

CMAS Content Outline
- Medical Terminology
- Communications

and linguist all rolled into one career. The translator function may be the most challenging. Physicians and other medical professionals frequently speak in what is termed *Doctor Speak*. Just as Ebonics, the pseudo-language of the streets, is a plague in schools, so Doctor Speak plagues medical transcriptionists who must format, interpret, and edit, while maintaining a clear, legally correct record of what the physician or other medical personnel intend to place in the medical record.

 Medical records are documents governed by laws and may be subpoenaed for review by various courts. The medical report may play a major role in substantiating injury or malpractice claims. The transcriptionist should not only check the transcribed medical record for accuracy, but also have the QA or risk management administrator at the health care facility review the document before sending it to the originator for final approval and signature.

MEDICAL REPORTS

Medical reports become part of the patient's permanent medical record and are vital to continued patient care. Other physicians, attorneys, insurance companies, or the court may review the medical reports in part, or in their entirety. Therefore, the medical report must be neat, accurate, and complete. *Neat* refers to a medical report that is legible and assembled to permit easy access to information as needed. *Accurate* means that the dictation has been transcribed as dictated, and *complete* indicates that the document has been dated correctly and signed or initialed by the dictator.

Complete documentation of medical reports is also important for payment or reimbursement of services for which the physician expects to be paid. The billing and diagnosis codes reported on the health insurance claim form must be supported by the documentation contained within the medical report.

A new trend in transcription is the integration of digital images directly into the transcribed record. The response to inputting digital images (photographs, scans, and radiographs) has been positive from both the local health care community and patients themselves. This is attributed to easier understanding of a picture by patients and more precise presentation using both pictures and written text to medical professionals.

The tools required for integrating digital images into word processing programs is already available to most MTs in their current Microsoft Word® or Corel WordPerfect® software packages. They only have to obtain a disk containing digital images from their physician–employer. If the transcribed record is included in the computer-based electronic record, also known as the electronic chart, digital images can be attached allowing other clinicians to view, enlarge, and manipulate the images at will.

The transcribed medical report may be formatted in a variety of styles similar to business correspondence. Common transcribed reports include:

1. Chart notes and progress notes
2. History and physical examination report
3. Discharge summary
4. Operative report
5. Consultation report
6. Specialized reports
7. Correspondence

Hospitals and practices may require a specific format for reports different from those described in the following examples. A few helpful formatting rules are:

- Use section headings that clarify the report.

- Do not add sections left out by the dictator.

- Do not include unnecessary confidential information unless specifically instructed to do so.

- Note who dictated the report, if not the attending physician, and provide space for both to sign. The initials of the transcriptionist should be on the signature page.

- Use 1-inch margins all around, unless the document is to be filed in a chart that has a top opening, then use a 1.25-inch margin at the top only. If using sticky paper for chart notes, use 0.5-inch margins.

- Use paragraph format (see the following examples).

Chart Notes and Progress Notes

Chart notes, sometimes referred to as **progress notes,** are a concise description of the patient's encounter with the medical office. They are chronologically listed and may include in-person visits to the office, telephone and electronic mail (e-mail) inquiries. The present problem, the physician's physical findings, and the treatment plan should be identified within the chart note. Laboratory test results may be included also. The physician or office personnel may enter chart note information as informal handwritten notes, or keyed notes affixed to the appropriate space. All notes documented must include the date, time, and signature of person entering the data along with their credential. This information is pertinent for follow up questions or for litigation purposes. Figure 16-1 is a sample chart/progress note.

History and Physical Examination Reports

The **history and physical examination (H&P) report** documents information relating to the patient's main reason for treatment. The report is divided into two sections. The first is the history, which includes the **chief complaint (CC),** a description of symptoms, problems, or conditions that brought the patient to the office; **history of the present illness (HPI),** a chronological description of the development of the patient's illness; past medical and surgical history; family history; and social history.

The second section is the **review of systems (ROS)** and inquiry about the system directly related to the problems identified in the HPI. The physician determines the extent of the examination performed and documented based on the problems presented. The findings of the actual physical examination make up the documentation for the physical examination section of the report.

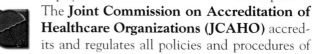 The **Joint Commission on Accreditation of Healthcare Organizations (JCAHO)** accredits and regulates all policies and procedures of hospitals and physicians' offices owned by hospital organizations. The JCAHO requires that hospitals provide H&P reports be filed in patient charts within 24 hours of admission. Occasionally, the patient will be seen in the physician's office and a decision is made to admit the patient to the hospital. In this case, the examination is performed in the office, but the report is dictated to the hospital that transcribes the document and files it within the patient's chart. The H&P format may also be used to

```
1/4/20XX                                    HANSEN, HENRY

RV following treatment for fx of the left wrist. The cast was removed
last week. The skin texture and turgor are returning to normal. Range
of motion has increased with physical therapy, and strength is slightly
improved at -4/5. PLAN: Continue whirlpool and ROM exercises. RV 4 weeks.
                                                                AE/rf
```

Figure 16-1 Sample chart/progress notes.

document a patient's annual physical examination in the office. Figure 16-2 is a sample H&P Report.

Discharge Summaries

The **discharge summary (DS)** documents the patient's history of hospital admissions. The DS includes the reason for hospital admission, a description of what transpired while the patient was in the hospital, the final diagnosis, follow-up instructions, discharge medications, patient's condition at discharge, and prognosis for recovery. The JCAHO requires that the completed DS be filed in the patient's chart within 72 hours of discharge from the hospital. Figure 16-3 shows a sample DS.

Operative Reports

The **operative report (OR)** chronicles the details of a surgical procedure performed in a hospital, outpatient surgical center, or clinic. The surgeon or assistant dictates the OR immediately after the operation. The OR describes the surgical procedure, preoperative and

---

HISTORY AND PHYSICAL EXAMINATION

PATIENT: Donald Waite
CHART #: 97223

HISTORY: The patient is a 72-year-old male who was admitted because of intermittent, moderately severe chest pain starting from the substernal region radiating to the back and to the left arm and associated with a choking sensation. The pain lasted from minutes to half an hour and was relieved by two nitroglycerin tablets.

This condition has been going on for the last two weeks. The patient has known arteriosclerotic heart disease and since his discharge in July 20XX, has been doing reasonably well on Procardia, nitrates, Persantine, and digoxin.

PAST HISTORY: The patient had a pacemaker implantation for sick sinus syndrome four years ago. He has a history of angina and myocardial infarction. He also has essential hypertension.

His past surgical history includes an appendectomy and bilateral herniorrhaphies. He has no allergies.

The patient still works as a projectionist in a movie house. He does not smoke but drinks occasionally. He denies any history of diabetes, liver, or kidney disease. There is no evidence of claudication. There is dyspnea on exertion and fatigability. GI is negative; GU is negative.

PHYSICAL EXAMINATION: The patient is out of distress right now. He has been given two injections of Demerol. Blood pressure is 120/68, ventricular rate is 72 per minute, and respiratory rate is 60 per minute. Color is good. Skin is warm. Examination of the head shows that right lenticular opacity is greater than the left. Neck veins are flat. There are no bruits. Carotids are brisk, and there is no evidence of thyroid enlargement. The heart is regular with no S3 gallops. There is a systolic ejection murmur at the base III/VI. The lungs are clear. The abdomen showed surgical scars. Extremities have no edema. Pulses are 2+, and there is no calf tenderness.

IMPRESSION: Unstable angina secondary to coronary artery disease with obstructive and mixed pattern spasm on an affixed lesion. Status postpacemaker implantation and degenerative joint disease with cervical degenerative arthritis.

Review of the EKG shows nonspecific ST-T wave changes in II, III, and aVF and in the anterolateral leads. Chest X-ray showed cardiomegaly, and the enzymes are pending.

RECOMMENDATIONS: The patient should be hospitalized in the coronary care unit and monitored. The nifedipine should be increased up to 60 mg—slowly. Continue Persantine. Continue transderm nitro—increase to 10. Monitor the blood level. Consider angiogram when he is stabilized.

Elizabeth M. King, MD

EMK/urs
d:11/2/XX
t: 11/2/XX

Figure 16-2   Sample history and physical examination.

PATIENT: Kelly Cohen
CHART #: 29324

ADMITTED: 9/26/XX
DISCHARGED: 11/19/XX

HISTORY/LAB: This infant was born on 09/26/XX to a 30-year-old, gravida II, para 1 female, with a last menstrual period of 3/22/XX estimated date of confinement 2/29/XX. The mother had been observed regularly during her pregnancy. However, she did develop preterm labor necessitating early hospitalization. At that time, the mother was placed on antibiotics and dexamethasone and delivered at approximately 26 weeks' gestation. At the time of delivery, the membranes ruptured spontaneously and fluid was clear. The infant had an Apgar score of 5 and 8 at 1 and 5 minutes, respectively. The infant required intubation in the delivery room and was then transferred to the NICU. On admission, weight was 1,159 grams, length 38.5 cm, head circumference 25.5 cm, chest circumference 26 cm. Assessment was 26 weeks' gestation.

COURSE/CONDITION ON DISCHARGE/DISPOSITION: At the time of admission the infant had respiratory distress, was intubated, and required Survanta. The infant was placed on IV fluid and antibiotics, and appropriate blood work was done. During the hospitalization, the infant improved with regard to the respiratory distress. However, the infant developed bronchopulmonary dysplasia, hyperbilirubinemia, and apnea of prematurity. The infant was placed on the appropriate medications and improved steadily. Her weight increased gradually. During the hospitalization, the infant was evaluated by Dr. Lally of Ophthalmology who will follow up on an outpatient basis.

The infant was discharged home on 11/20/XX. She had a hearing test, eye examination as stated, and was going to receive home physical therapy three times a week. She was on Fer In Sol drops and was feeding on Neosure and breast milk. The overall prognosis was guarded to good.

FINAL DIAGNOSIS: Preterm, 26-week female infant, appropriate for gestational age, apnea of prematurity, anemia, respiratory distress syndrome, bronchopulmonary dysplasia, hyperbilirubinemia, and presumed sepsis.

Elizabeth M. King, MD

EMK/vs
d:11/20/XX
t: 11/20/XX

Figure 16-3 Sample discharge summary.

postoperative diagnosis, and specimens removed, and it sometimes includes a sponge count and instrument inventory, an estimate of blood loss, and the condition of the patient on leaving the operating room. The report should also include the name of the primary surgeon and any assistants. The **authenticated** report should be filed in the chart as soon as possible after surgery so that others caring for the patient have needed information. Figure 16-4 shows a sample OR.

Consultation Reports

When one physician requests the services of another physician in the care and treatment of a patient, a **consultation report** is generated. The information may be disseminated in the form of a report or within the body of a letter. The contents of the consultation report/letter usually contain all of the elements of an H&P with a

focused history of the patient's illness and the body system directly related to the consultant's area of specialty. The consultant also includes within the report/letter the findings, supporting laboratory data, diagnosis, and suggested course of treatment. Figure 16-5 is a sample consultation.

SPECIALIZED REPORTS

The MT may be called on to prepare a variety of specialized reports. Following is an explanation of some of the specialized reports that may be encountered.

Pathology Reports

A **pathology report** is generated to describe the **gross** and **microscopic examinations** performed on organs, lesions, tissue samples, or body fluid removed during a surgical procedure. In some cases, the pathologist may

PATIENT: Joseph Oritz

DATE: 6/25/XX

SURGEON: Raja Rao

PREOPERATIVE DIAGNOSIS: Crohn's disease requiring central venous access for hyperalimentation.

POSTOPERATIVE DIAGNOSIS: Crohn's disease requiring central venous access for hyperalimentation.

OPERATION: Insertion of left-sided subclavian double-lumen central venous catheter.

ANESTHESIA: 1% lidocaine.

PROCEDURE: The patient was placed in the supine position with the neck extended to the right side. The left side of the chest was prepared and draped in the usual manner using Betadine solution. The subclavian vein on the left side was percutaneously and easily entered, and the guide wire was advanced into the superior vena cava. The double-lumen central venous catheter with VitaCuff was placed through the guide wire into the superior vena cava. Good blood flow was obtained. The catheter was sutured to the skin using 2-0 silk sutures and connected to IV solution.

A dry sterile dressing was applied.

The patient tolerated the procedure well.

_____

Juan Esposito, MD

JE/urs

d: 6/25/XX

t: 6/27/XX

Figure 16-4 Sample operative report.

examine the specimen before the patient is sutured to determine if a more extensive surgical procedure is required (i.e., malignant tumors).

Pathologists generally dictate the report in the present tense because they interpret the pathologic findings as they view the specimens. The report must be completed within 24 hours of receipt with a copy maintained by the laboratory and copies sent to each physician involved in the case. The original is maintained in the patient's chart. Figure 16-6 is a sample Pathology Report.

Radiology and Imaging Reports

A **radiology report** is a description of the findings and interpretations of the radiologist who studies the X-ray film taken of a patient. In some cases, a contrast medium may be administered either orally or by injection before the film is taken. A scan is a procedure that requires the use of radioactive isotopes.

When dictating, the radiologist may switch from present to past tense; that is, the procedure was performed in the past tense, and the findings are given in the present tense.

Stereoscopy and tomography are technologies that view structures within the body in dimensions or layers. Computed tomography (CT scan) uses radiography with computers to visualize a slice of the body part. Sonograms and echograms are another imaging technology that uses high-frequency sound waves to compose a picture of an area of the body. Magnetic resonance imaging (MRI) produces sectional images of the body without the use of radiology. New technologies create the need for understanding the imaging process and appropriate documentation of patient information.

When transcribing radiology or imaging reports, the date of service should be used rather than the date of dictation. Other details to be included within the report may include:

- Number and type of views taken

- Any special circumstances that could affect the examination

- Quality of the study (clear or blurry)

- Abnormal findings

- Normal findings

- Radiologist's impression, interpretation, diagnosis, and recommendations

- Signature of the radiologist

The report should be filed in the patient's chart within 24 hours of the procedure. Sufficient documentation must be in the report for the physician to use if he or she must prove that the study was medically necessary or if justification for reimbursement is required. Figure 16-7 is an example of a radiology report.

Autopsy Reports

An **autopsy report** may also be called an autopsy protocol, a necropsy report, or a medical examiner report. Autopsies are performed to determine the cause of death, or to ascertain and confirm presence of disease. It is important to understand that state law requires autopsies be performed in certain situations. For example, an autopsy report is required when someone dies suddenly,

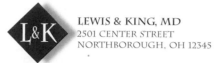

LEWIS & KING, MD
2501 CENTER STREET
NORTHBOROUGH, OH 12345

NORTHBOROUGH
FAMILY MEDICAL GROUP

January 4, 20XX

Margaret Holly, MD
Metroma Medical Center
900 Union Street, Suite 208
Metroma, MI 11666

RE: MARY O'KEEFE

Dear Dr. Holly:

Thank you for referring Mary O'Keefe to our clinic. She presented today stating that she recently relocated to Clinton with her husband and children to be closer to her parents. Mary has been experiencing symptoms suggestive of pregnancy and is here for evaluation. Over the past three weeks, she has noticed increased tenderness of her breasts, fatigue, and a feeling of being bloated. A home pregnancy test was positive.

Her past medical history is positive for the usual childhood diseases and the births of two children, following normal pregnancies. She has a negative past surgical history.

She has no allergies to medications and takes Tylenol for occasional headaches. She is married and has two children, ages 3 years and 12 months. She is employed part-time in an insurance office. She does not smoke or drink.

The family history is noncontributory.

On review of systems, her complaints are limited to those described above. She has had no nausea or vomiting, and no change in bowel habits. She has no dizziness, no fevers, and no urinary symptoms.

Physical examination revealed a 32-year-old white female in no acute distress. HEENT normocephalic, atraumatic. PERRLA, EOMI. The thyroid was not enlarged, and there was no cervical adenopathy. The lungs were clear. The heart had a regular rate and rhythm. The abdomen was soft and nontender. Bowel sounds were normal. The extremities revealed trace ankle edema. The neurological examination was within normal limits. Pelvic examination confirmed a gravid uterus, compatible with a very early pregnancy.

An abdominal ultrasound has been ordered and a beta HCG was drawn.

I believe Mary is pregnant and I will put her on our OB regimen starting with monthly visits. Thank you for your kind referral.

Sincerely,

Elizabeth M. King, MD

EMK/lmb

Figure 16-5 Sample consultation.

```
                    PATHOLOGY REPORT
PATHOLOGY NO.:    792 304
DATE:             12/20/XX
CHART NO.:        56 84 20
NAME:             Lee Allen Au          AGE: 15 Female
DEPARTMENT:       Surgery               MD: Dr. Raja Rao
TISSUE:           Appendix
HISTORY:          Right Lower Quadrant Pain
```

CLINICAL DIAGNOSIS: RLQ Pain

PATHOLOGICAL REPORT: The specimen is labeled appendix and is received in formalin. The specimen consists of an appendix that measures $6 \times 1 \times 0.5$ cm in greatest dimension. The serosa surface has some white fibrinoid material attached to it and on a cross section. Some purulent fibrinous material can also be seen. Representative sections are submitted in 1 cassette.

DIAGNOSIS: Acute suppurative appendicitis with periappendicitis and mesoappendicitis.

Thomas A. King, MD
Pathologist

TAK/rp

d: 12/20/XX
t: 12/20/XX

Figure 16-6 Sample pathology report.

MERCY MEDICAL CENTER
300 Main Street
Denver, CO 80201

RADIOLOGY #: 23445

PA & LATERAL CHEST   Date 10/07/XX

The pulmonary vessels are clearly outlined and are not distended. There are not any typical signs of redistribution. A few increased interstitial markings persist, but there are no typical acute Kerley B-lines. There may be a little residual pleural effusion at the costophrenic sinus and posterior gutters. Most of the pulmonary edema and effusion has otherwise cleared. The chest is not hyperexpanded. The thoracic vertebrae show spurring but no compression.

IMPRESSION:
1. No signs of elevated pulmonary venous pressure or frank failure at this time.
2. Residual pleural effusion is seen in the costophrenic sinus and posterior gutters, either residual or recent congestive failure.

BILATERAL MAMMOGRAMS   Date: 10/07/XX

Bilateral xeromammograms were obtained in both the mediolateral and craniocaudal projections. There is no previous exam for comparison. There is slight asymmetry of the ductal tissue in the lower outer quadrant of the right breast. There are no dominant masses, clusters of microcalcifications or pathologic skin changes identified.

IMPRESSION: Normal bilateral mammogram.

Renny Genray, MD
Radiologist

JOHN DOE, M.D.   SMITH, HARRIET #123456-7
Dictated by: Renny Genray, M.D.
D&T: 10/07/XX | 10/07/XX | RG/mt

RADIOLOGY REPORT

Figure 16-7 Sample radiology report.

when someone dies while unattended, or in the case of suspicion of crime.

When transcribing an autopsy report, more words should be spelled out and abbreviation use kept to a minimum, because these records may be entered into a court of law and must be accurate and clearly understood. Many states require that military time be used when documenting the time a body arrives at the coroner's office. Temporary anatomic diagnoses should be placed in the medical report within 72 hours and in the completed report within 60 days. Figure 16-8 is a sample autopsy report.

Correspondence

It is important for the MT to remember that medical correspondence also is considered medical documents and must be transcribed with the same care as any other medical report would. Review Chapter 15 for information regarding various styles and formats for business correspondence. Figure 16-9 is a sample of medical correspondence.

TURNAROUND TIME AND PRODUCTIVITY

Specific time limits are often established for completion of medical reports. **Turnaround time** indicates the specific time period in which a document is expected to

---

AUTOPSY REPORT

Patient Name:	George Matthews
Hospital No.:	11509
Necropsy No.:	98-A-19
Admitting Physician:	Joe Abbott, M.C.
Pathologist:	Loraine Muir, M.D.
Date of Death:	04/05/20XX, 9 PM
Date of Autopsy:	04/06/20XX, 8 AM
Admitting Diagnosis:	Adenocarcinoma, maxilla.
Prosector:	Keith Johnson, P.A.

FINAL ANATOMIC DIAGNOSIS

1. Old fibrotic myocardial infarction of the anterior and septal walls of the left ventricle with anterior ventricular aneurysm, 4.5 × 3.0 cm.
2. Patchy old fibrotic myocardial infarction of the lateral and posterior septal walls of the left ventricle.
3. Probable recent ischemic changes, especially of the anterior and septal walls of the left ventricle.
4. Severe calcified atherosclerotic coronary vascular disease with up to 95% stenosis of the right coronary artery (RCA), up to 70% stenosis of the left anterior descending (LAD) coronary artery, and greater than 95% stenosis of the left circumflex coronary artery (LCCA).
5. Bilateral arterionephrosclerosis.
6. Atherosclerotic vascular disease, aorta, moderate to severe; circle of Willis, moderate
7. Old infarct of right inner and inferior occipital lobe; small lacunar infarct, right caudate nucleus.
8. Bilateral pulmonary congestion, moderate.
9. Chronic passive congestion, liver, mild.
10. Simple cysts, right and left kidneys, up to 5.5 cm.
11. Diverticulum, 2.5 cm, duodenum.
12. Diverticulosis, sigmoid colon.
13. Status post partial left maxillectomy for adenocarcinoma, recent.

Elizabeth M. King, MD

EMK:xx

D:04/26/XX

T: 04/26/XX

Figure 16-8 Sample autopsy report.

---

be completed from the time it is received by the transcriptionist until it is returned to the physician to sign and made a part of the permanent medical record.

Turnaround times for hospital reports fall into three categories:

1. **STAT reports:** Laboratory reports are examples and should be complete within 12 hours or less.
2. **Current reports:** H&P reports are examples and should be complete within 24 hours or less.
3. **Old reports or aged reports:** DS reports are an example, except when the patient is being transferred to another facility. Old reports should be complete within 72 hours or less.

 Different facilities have different requirements; however, the transcriptionist or clinic personnel responsible for medical records should be aware that failure to meet deadlines could result in disciplinary or legal action. The reason for this stringent adherence to turnaround time is that STAT and current reports can influence timely treatment of the patient.

Workload, as well as productivity of the transcriptionist, affect turnaround time. When workload is too great to meet turnaround times, the medical records administrator must be notified immediately. Once a job has been accepted, the transcriptionist or transcription service is legally bound to meet the schedule short of a major catastrophe of the type legally considered to be an "act of nature."

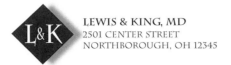

LEWIS & KING, MD
2501 CENTER STREET
NORTHBOROUGH, OH 12345

NORTHBOROUGH
FAMILY MEDICAL GROUP

January 4, 20XX

Susan Smith, Coordinator
Special Project Division
American Drug Company
90058 Northover Road
Welfond, PA 44578

Dear Ms. Smith:

It is my understanding that your department oversees the Aid for
Patients program, which provides Glucogenasin for indigent patients.
I am interested in learning more about this.

I have a 74-year-old female patient who would be greatly helped by this
medication. She suffers with hypertension, adult onset diabetes mellitus,
and moderate angina. Medication compliance has been a problem; however,
we feel that this new drug, with its q.d. dosage, will be easy for her
to deal with.

Any information you could forward would be appreciated.

Yours truly,

Winston Lewis, MD

WL/bk

Figure 16-9   Sample medical correspondence.

ACCURACY AND QUALITY ASSURANCE

Medical record documents are legal documents important to both the patient and the health care provider. As such, accuracy should have the greatest priority. Medical records departments should have an operational QA program in effect. A QA program establishes a process to provide accurate, complete, consistent health care documentation in a timely manner, whereas making every reasonable effort to resolve inconsistencies, inaccuracies, risk management issues, and other problems.

Errors and Proofreading

Proofreading is easier said than done and requires practice and diligence. More errors are missed while proofreading on the computer screen than using hard copy. The beginning MT should first proofread by listening to the tape while reading the document to establish that all dictated information has been transcribed. A second reading should be done to identify any misspelled words, incorrect grammar usage, punctuation errors, and inconsistencies in style and format. Many software programs help identify spelling and grammar errors; however, care should be taken to avoid using a contextually incorrect but properly spelled word (i.e., right/write, aural/oral, site/cite). Table 15-1 contains a list of frequently misspelled words that may be helpful to review.

The **American Association for Medical Transcription (AAMT)** recommends the following principles when reviewing a document:

- Compare the transcribed report against dictation. Do not just read the document.

- Use industry-specific standards for style, punctuation, and grammar (*AAMT Book of Style for Medical Transcription*).

- Consider risk management issues.

- Third parties, such as the QA person, proofing a document should provide feedback to the transcriptionist. Although 100% accuracy is desired, accuracy of audited documents should not be less than 98%. Accuracy less than this figure requires corrective action.

Common errors are usually in sentence structure, punctuation, and spelling. They are easily changed without altering the dictator's style or meaning. Sound-alike words are another area where errors occur. Be aware of

Critical Thinking

How will you determine which medication was prescribed for a patient: digitoxin or digoxin?

your personal errors and take steps to avoid them. Maintaining a personal journal provides a quick reference and allows you to see improvement in your proficiency.

Editing and Corrections

Editing is the process of reviewing the transcribed document for accuracy and clarity. It is important to remember that you must not change the dictator's style or meaning when editing. If the MT encounters a term that cannot be interpreted or something new that cannot be referenced, they should ask other MTs or QA personnel. If the question cannot be resolved, the document should be **flagged** to alert the dictator something needs to be corrected or resolved. The flagged message may indicate the doctor is cut off, what the term sounds like, or the message is incomprehensible. Provide as much information as you can to assist the dictator in recalling the dictated area in question.

Flagging procedures vary from one facility to another. In large facilities, flagged documents may be referred to QA personnel. The notation may be incorporated into the computerized document using a color-code approach with a flag message. The correct information can then be added to the document and the color coding removed. In-house flagging may simply consist of a sticky note or a preprinted flag attachment.

Up-to-date reference materials, adequate equipment, written procedures for dictating methods, **continuing education (CE),** an ergonomically and psychologically safe work environment, and supervision by qualified MTs are essential conditions for successful QA in medical transcription.

Errors that are made while keying a document should be corrected before printing the document. If an error is in handwritten chart notes or discovered after the document has been authenticated or signed by the dictator, draw a single line through the error and make the correction above or below the line. Identify the location of correct information as a cross-reference when possible. This procedure adds credibility to the record. Corrections into the medical report should always be made using red ink. Care should be taken not to obliterate the error, write over it, erase it, or try to fix it in any way. The person making the correction should date, initial,

DOCUMENTATION

8/28/XX Removed cast from right wrist and
instructed patient to make an appointment with PT. Radiology, BQL/CMA
9/12/XX

and identify his or her credential beside or just below the correction.

Authentication

In most cases, the physician dictating the information will sign or authenticate the document. There may be times when an attending physician or physician assistant will be responsible for dictating the material. Once the information has been transcribed, proofread, and sent to the physician, it should be read again for QA before the physician authenticates the document. His or her signature on the document indicates that the information was accurate and complete at the time of dictation.

When errors are found on self-adhesive typing strips, make the corrections as if the document had been handwritten. If the strip is not legible, or if it looks too messy once the corrections have been made, rekey a new strip and place it below the original. Be sure to identify it as "corrected for keying errors." The physician should sign the original and the corrected copy.

If the dictating physician is away from the office after dictating a report, and the report is urgent, the MT has two options: sign the physician's name with the MT's initials after it or send a photocopy of the report and state that a signed original will be forwarded on the physician's return. Office policy regarding this procedure must always be followed.

In today's technological world, electronic signatures have become a viable option. The electronic signature may be accomplished through several ways:

- Use of alphanumeric computer key entries as identification

- Use of an electronic writing device

- Use of a **biometric** system

Medicare and JCAHO guidelines require that the signature on medical reports, electronic or handwritten, be completed by the physician dictating the information and not delegated to anyone else. Federal law, state law, and JCAHO accreditation standards all address the issue of electronic signatures.

CONFIDENTIALITY

Confidentiality means treating the patient's medical information as private and not for publication. The patient has a right to privacy; therefore, medical information is **privileged.** Privileged information may only be communicated with the patient's permission or by court order. The MT must learn to follow the motto: *What you see here and what you hear here must stay here when you leave here.*

Health Insurance Portability and Accountability Act Regulations

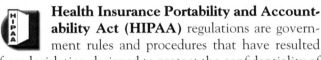

Health Insurance Portability and Accountability Act (HIPAA) regulations are government rules and procedures that have resulted from legislation designed to protect the confidentiality of patient information. This ranges from medical records to personal identification numbers that, if divulged, could result in identity theft.

The MT can meet most HIPAA regulations by adhering to the following simple rules:

- Do not divulge medical records you transcribe to anyone other than the dictator, your supervisor, or an authorized QA person. Files should not be discussed with the patient. Do not divulge files to an attorney or insurance representative without consulting with risk management personnel.

- Safeguard files in your possession. Take reasonable steps to keep files secure, such as keeping tapes and hard copy of reports in a locked file cabinet, using passwords for computer files, installing virus protection software, and using a firewall if appropriate. Do not carelessly carry files around on your person or in your car.

- Transmit files electronically only with the permission of your client or the dictating physician, and then agree on the proper procedures and protocols for transmission.

- Have a signed business associate agreement or similar document that defines the protocols you are expected to follow to protect patient confidentiality.

These general rules do not constitute legal advice; consult with appropriate legal counsel for specific questions.

Protocols

Protocols are the procedures your office or client has in place to ensure patient confidentiality. You are usually required to sign a **confidentiality agreement** stating that you will comply with the established procedures. Your contracts, together with the protocols, become a part of the institution's documentation demonstrating compliance with HIPAA regulations. The purpose of your signing a contract is to substantiate that you have received training and have been instructed in proper procedures to protect medical records.

Risk Management

 Risk management is defined by the AAMT as procedures and actions that identify, evaluate, reduce, and prevent the risk for injury and loss to patients, visitors, staff, and the legal entity; that is, corporation, partnership, or institution that employs the MT. From the MT's viewpoint, risk management involves protecting the confidentiality of the medical records and assuring the accuracy of those records. From the larger picture, risk management also involves workplace safety issues, civil rights issues, discrimination issues, environmental issues, compliance with governmental regulations for documentation related to billing and coding, and basically anything that could result in legal action being brought against the practice. Most institutions and clinics will have a person designated with the responsibility for risk management.

MTs are in an excellent position to assist the risk management officer, through their commitment to quality and their awareness of confidentiality procedures and possible medical errors indicated in the dictated data. Should a problem or error be detected that could be a risk management problem, the MT should immediately notify his or her superior, office manager, risk management officer, or the employer's or client's legal staff according to office policy.

 You will recall from Chapter 8 that ethics are not laws but rather standards of conduct. These standards vary from state to state, so you should research your specific state's standards. The AAMT adopted a Code of Ethics (see the AAMT Web site for the AAMT Code of Ethics available at: http://www.aamt.org/scriptcontent.rjobethics.cfm) for professional MTs who are employed in hospital settings or are self-employed. Medical Transcription Industry Alliance (MTIA) has established a Medical Transcription Industry Alliance Code of Ethics and Standards for MTs employed by transcription services. Take time to review these documents on the Internet (available at: http://www.mtia.com/about/pledge.html).

Although, in certain cases, the MT can be held financially responsible for errors and omissions, the MT usually is under the jurisdiction of *respondeat superior,* meaning that the physician–director or office manager is responsible for the wrongful acts of the MT working under their supervision. This is not meant to imply that MTs should not protect themselves by instituting some personal risk management such as carrying errors and omissions insurance. Insurance should be considered particularly if the MT is operating a home business and contracting transcription work.

EQUIPMENT AND FACILITIES

The transcriptionist uses most of the modern telecommunication tools that are available. The personal computer (PC), digital and magnetic tape dictation equipment, facsimile machine, photocopiers, and the telephone/cellular phone are all tools of the trade.

 Because the transcriptionist spends so much time keyboarding, special attention should be made to selecting ergonomically designed equipment for his or her office. Review the steps outlined in Chapter 11 to avoid eyestrain, repetitive wrist injuries, and back strain.

Computers and Software

 The PC running word processing software is the main instrument of the transcriptionist. See Chapter 11 for a detailed description of equipment and software. Also, a review of the section regarding patient confidentiality in the medical office will be beneficial at this time.

Dictation Equipment

Dictation equipment is the piece of equipment most used by the transcriptionist after the PC. The **transcriber** differs from a simple audio recorder in that it has independent controls for speed, tone, and volume. It can also be controlled to play, stop, rewind, and fast forward, with the play, rewind, and stop controls activated by a foot pedal. The unit usually has a feature that allows the machine to review a small segment of the tape or digital data after it has been stopped or rewound. Transcribers are equipped with headsets or earphones to minimize surrounding noise in the room where transcription is being performed.

Two types of media are used with modern transcribers: magnetic tape and digitally processed sound. **Magnetic tape** machines usually receive their input from the dictator by delivery of a magnetic tape directly to the transcriptionist or by recording the dictation over a telephone line to a magnetic tape in the office of the transcriptionist. **Digitally processed dictation** is similar to music downloaded over the Internet by your home PC. Digital files, using **waveform audio (WAV)** format or **digital speech standard (DSS)** format, are transferred from one computer to another over the Internet. This not only speeds up transfer of files, but also eliminates the cost of telephone time. This is an important consideration, especially when files are being sent from state to state or from one continent to another, which is an outsourcing practice used by many transcription services. Figure 16-10 shows a digital dictation machine.

Voice recognition systems are being used in an attempt to speed up transcription. The speaker's voice is converted into digital code not based on tone as with WAV files, but rather into alphanumeric characters that can be printed out. The major problem with this system is the difficulty in accounting for different accents, dialects, and dictating styles, not to mention Doctor Speak. Progress is being made in voice recognition software; however, it is still not economical for use in transcription because of the large amount of time spent in detecting and correcting transcription errors.

Today, more offices are becoming paperless by switching to an electronic medical records (EMR) system. The EMR system may be set up with screens for scheduling patient visits, ongoing screens containing data about the patient (i.e., allergies and history of complaints), H&P screen, diagnosis screen, prescription information screens, screens containing past laboratory values or for laboratory requests, and a screen for written instructions for the patient.

With the EMR system, each examination room has either a computer or a physician's handheld personal digital assistant (PDA). A template for the document, such as an H&P, comes up on the computer screen, and as the physician asks the patient questions related to the physical examination, the physician keys in the answers. Immediately after the examination, all areas of concern or change are entered into the document. If the patient is referred to a specialist within the physician's health maintenance organization (HMO), this information is readily available to them, and they can also enter their findings into the chart.

Once the physician has entered everything into the computer, the document is released for finalization by the MT. Careful review and editing for accuracy of grammar and spelling is completed, and any additional transcription is added to the document. See Chapters 11 and 14 for additional information about EMRs and PDAs.

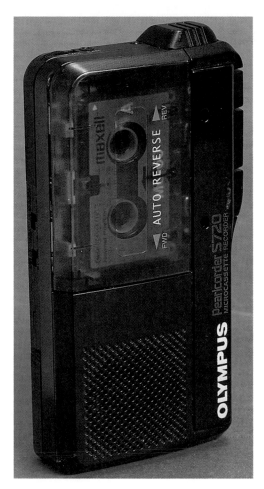

Figure 16-10 Example of a digital dictation machine.

Facsimile Machines

Facsimile (fax) machines are used in the medical community today to transmit various documents within the facility, to distant communities, and internationally. Notably, fax machines print on plain, thin paper or thermally treated paper. Exposure to sunlight quickly fades the printed material, and some paper does not produce clear images. A photocopy of important documents using bond paper will preserve the contents. It is a courtesy to send a hard copy of any important faxed document. Review Chapters 11 and 15 for additional information regarding fax machine use and confidentiality in the medical setting.

Photocopy Machines

Medical offices use photocopy machines in a variety of ways on a daily basis. A photocopy machine should be selected that will satisfy the office needs, produce copies that closely resemble the original, represent the office professionally, and be relatively maintenance free. When

Critical Thinking

How would you go about designing a medical transcription workstation that was ergonomic and compliant with HIPAA regulations?

disposing of unwanted or extra copies, remember confidentiality. Many offices shred unwanted pages to protect confidentiality and prevent litigation issues.

Ergonomics

See Chapter 11 for ergonomic considerations in designing office facilities for the medical transcriptionist.

MEDICAL TRANSCRIPTIONIST AS A CAREER

Medical transcription is a prosperous industry that offers the educated and experienced transcriptionist opportunities for employment around the world. Diverse work settings and a variety of specialty areas and complexity levels make medical transcription an engaging occupation. The MT career continues to evolve, offering the opportunity for continued learning experiences and self-actualization.

Attributes of the Medical Transcriptionist

The attributes of the medical transcriptionist may be broken into two major categories: personal attributes and acquired skills developed specific to the career itself. These two categories are key elements to being successful as an MT.

Personal attributes include the love of words. It is not uncommon to find medical transcriptionists working crossword puzzles and involved with various word games. They have an innate ability to listen closely to what others say and the skill for hearing and understanding different accents and languages. They enjoy detective work and are curious; if terminology is new to them, they use references to research and learn more. MTs are self-disciplined, detail-oriented, independent, and usually perfectionists. They are dedicated to professional development and enthusiastically committed to learning. They are not afraid to ask questions. They have a genuine caring attitude and an interest in patient care from a medical record point of view. MTs possess integrity and understand the importance and legal implications of medical confidentiality.

Medical transcriptionists must have excellent keyboarding skills. Entry-level positions may require 60 words per minute, whereas experienced MTs may transcribe more than 80 words per minute. Today's MT must be able to operate a variety of software programs efficiently and maintain continued learning as new programs are developed. Excellent language skills and above-average spelling skills are mandatory. It is recognized that the MT must understand the anatomy and physiology of the human body and have knowledge of surgical terms, equipment, instruments and anesthesia, and directional and body plane terms. A background in common laboratory tests; radiology techniques and terms; drug names and their uses, both brand and generic; common signs and symptoms of diseases; and treatment modalities is also required.

Job Description

The *AAMT Model Job Description* is a practical, useful compilation of the basic job responsibilities of a medical transcriptionist. It is designed to assist human resource managers, department managers, supervisors, and others in recruiting, supervising, and evaluating individuals in medical transcription positions. It is also useful for prospective medical transcriptionists as a checklist for employment readiness.

Employment Opportunities

Medical transcriptionists may seek employment in a variety of settings—hospitals, multispecialty clinics, dental specialties, transcription services, home-based offices, research facilities, radiology clinics, pathology laboratories, tumor boards or registries, law offices, or veterinary hospitals. MTs may work as employees, supervisors, managers, teachers, or may be self-employed or freelancers.

Hospitals, multispeciality clinics, and dental specialties generally offer competitive salary and benefit packages. Payment for professional membership and registration fees for CE opportunities may also be included in the benefits package. Some offices may also include money to purchase reference materials. A stable work schedule and job security are experienced for those who perform to their standard and have a positive work ethic.

 The disadvantages of working in hospital and multispeciality clinics are the inflexible work schedule, low wages, facility politics, and the prospects of a supervisor who is unfamiliar with the needs of transcriptionists. The impacts of managed care and its associated cost-cutting efforts lead more of these facilities to outsource their medical transcription needs.

Transcription service employees often enjoy competitive pay rates. They transcribe a variety of accounts (physician offices, specialty offices, and so on), so there is a vast difference in the complexity and length of the documents. The work environment is usually quite comfortable, and flexible scheduling is a primary advantage. Disadvantages may include the absence of immediate feedback concerning questions regarding dictation and compensation. Often, in these types of settings, compensation is based on production. If there is a lack of tapes available for transcription, or if the MT takes a day off, it will be reflected in the paycheck.

Transcription services often employ **home-based MTs** who transcribe exclusively for those employers. The employer may provide the equipment and the MT works directly under the supervision of the employer. The disadvantages of a home-based business include that larger facilities frequently outsource dictation that is difficult because of the specialty or it has been dictated by a foreign-speaking physician. It has been estimated that 7 of 10 dictating physicians are foreign-born today. If you do not have an ear and an aptitude for dialects, it may be impossible to service these accounts and maintain a livable wage.

The entrepreneurial MT may opt to establish a freelance business. **Freelance MTs** function as independent contractors. Often, they transcribe hospital overflow. The advantages of freelance are a sense of accomplishment and independence, and opportunity to work flexible hours. If you have been employed specifically for medical offices, clinics, or other specialties and feel well qualified, it is best to concentrate your independent transcription work within your field of expertise. Generally, independents are paid by production—by the line, page, or character count. Your earnings will probably be excellent *if* you are highly productive, transcribe accurately, and remain focused on building the business. The disadvantages of freelance include having to handle all areas of a business including bookkeeping, pickup of dictation and delivery of completed work, and finding other MTs to cover during illness, vacation, or overload periods. Be sure to check with your insurance agent to verify that office equipment and confidential information is covered by homeowners' insurance. Another disadvantage is the unpredictable income; income is dependent on someone else's need. Some freelance MTs feel isolated and never free to get away from their work.

Insurance companies and law offices also may employ MTs. In these environments, the MT analyzes discrepancies in health records and translates medical language in a chart into lay language for attorneys. Other opportunities for MTs include teaching within hospitals, community colleges, or vocational/technical schools;

preparing manuscripts for research documentation; or authoring textbooks for MTs.

Professionalism Related to Medical Transcription

 Professionalism as related to medical transcription has many requirements. Following is advice on how to maintain a professional attitude.

- *Display a professional manner and image.* Working as an MT requires one to bathe daily; hair should be clean and easy to manage, and dress should be appropriate to the surroundings. The MT should always respect others and use good communication skills.

- *Demonstrate initiative and responsibility.* Demonstrating initiative means being to work early enough to organize and begin the workday at the appointed time. All deadlines must be met or changes approved.

- *Work as a member of the health care team.* The MT is a member of the health care team and as such must sign a business associate agreement and a confidentiality agreement. They should report incidents of confidentiality discrepancies and any perceived medical procedural errors to appropriate risk management personnel.

- *Prioritize and perform multiple tasks.* The MT must prioritize the documents to be transcribed to satisfy turnaround time and maintain productivity standards.

- *Adapt to change.* From time to time the MT will have to adapt to change when new physician dictation is added. Each physician, clinic, and hospital may have different preferences in formatting styles, heading titles, and placement.

- *Enhance skills through CE.* New technology, breakthroughs in medicine, and new medications are recognized daily as researchers explore ways in which to treat disease and increase longevity. MTs must remain current with new medical developments to maintain their professionalism.

AAMT

The AAMT began in 1978 as a nonprofit organization incorporated in California. One of the greatest desires of AAMT's founders was that MTs be appropriately recognized for the important contribution they make in health care. As a direct result of AAMT's continued efforts to promote the profession, medical transcription is a respected profession, with practitioners recognized as medical language specialists.

AAMT Membership

AAMT offers individual membership for professional development, and corporate or institutional membership for visibility and promotion. Other types of membership include practitioner, associate, and student. Student membership is available to any person who is not working as a transcriptionist and is verified as being enrolled in a nine-month or two-semester (defined as 15–18 weeks) medical transcription program that includes a student–instructor relationship. Student application requirements include: (1) obtain a signed letter from your instructor on school letterhead, indicating enrollment date and length of the program; and (2) enclose the letter with an AAMT membership application and your annual payment of $50.

Certification for Medical Transcriptionists

 A qualified MT, described as one with a minimum of two years' experience in performing medical transcription in a variety of medical and surgical specialties, may apply for the certification examination through the **Medical Transcriptionist Certification Commission (MTCC).** The MTCC is the credentialing program of the AAMT. MTCC offers a voluntary two-part certification examination to individuals who wish to become **certified medical transcriptionists (CMTs).** For additional information regarding certification, visit AAMT's Web site at: http://www.aamt.org.

Case Study 16-1

Erin Saunders is a recent graduate from a reputable junior college offering a two-year program in medical transcription. Erin was an excellent student and graduated at the top of her class. She is investigating types of employment opportunities available and has put her résumé together. Erin's long-range goal is to become a CMT.

CASE STUDY REVIEW

1. List the types of work environments available for MTs and briefly describe the transcription with which each would be involved.
2. Review the CMT test content and determine which work environments would best prepare Erin for the examination. Provide the rationale for your decision.

Case Study 16-2

At the offices of Drs. Lewis and King, the MT has just completed the following content in a document: "This patient developed a persistent lesion on the inner aspect of the left upper lip. This lesion was at the junction of the vermilion and mucous membrane. A punch biopsy was obtained of this 1 cm lesion and was read as a probable verrucous squamous cell carcinoma of the lower lip."

CASE STUDY REVIEW

1. What inconsistencies, if any, do you find within this document?
2. What should the MT do to verify inconsistencies and inaccuracies?
3. How should these inconsistencies and inaccuracies be corrected?

SUMMARY

Medical transcription is a vital part of patient health care. Without appropriate medical documentation it is impossible to provide quality health care, to bill insurance carriers properly to ensure physicians are reimbursed for services rendered, and to support and protect the physician should records be subpoenaed. The MT must keep all patient information strictly confidential and may be asked to sign a confidentiality agreement. A breach of confidentiality is one of the few areas in which the MT can be held liable.

Professional MTs often become CMTs and recertify every three years. A current credential indicates the active involvement in CE activities that keep the transcriptionist knowledgeable of new technologies, techniques, procedures, and drugs being used. MTs will continue to be medical language specialists. Their role and job description may change, however, with the innovation and use of new technology.

STUDY FOR SUCCESS

To reinforce your knowledge and skills of information presented in this chapter:
- ❑ Review the Key Terms
- ❑ Consider the Case Studies and discuss your conclusions
- ❑ Answer the Review Questions
  - ❑ Multiple Choice
  - ❑ Critical Thinking
- ❑ Navigate the Internet by completing the Web Activities
- ❑ Practice the StudyWARE activities on the textbook CD
- ❑ Apply your knowledge in the Student Workbook activities
- ❑ Complete the Web Tutor sections

REVIEW QUESTIONS

Multiple Choice

1. Acquired skills developed specific to MTs include:
   a. minimum keyboarding speed of 60 words per minute
   b. love of words
   c. ability to listen and understand different accents and languages
   d. self-disciplined, detail-oriented, and independent
2. Turnaround time for most laboratory reports should be:
   a. STAT
   b. current
   c. within 12 hours
   d. both a and b
3. MTs with a question that cannot be resolved should:
   a. guess at what is being dictated
   b. edit the document and exclude what cannot be understood
   c. flag the document
   d. refuse to transcribe documents for that physician

4. QA measures documents for all of the following *except:*
   a. line length of document
   b. accuracy and completeness
   c. consistency in health care documentation
   d. timely preparation
5. The MT who is employed by a transcription service but works from the home is known as a(n):
   a. home-based MT
   b. freelance MT
   c. associate MT
   d. self-employed MT
6. Examples of ergonomics include all of the following *except:*
   a. glare screens
   b. lumbar cushions
   c. footrests
   d. straight, flat keyboards

7. The credentialing program of AAMT is known as the:
   a. JCAHO
   b. AAMA
   c. MTCC
   d. CSR

8. AAMT student membership is available to:
   a. anyone working as an MT who has completed training
   b. anyone not working as an MT and currently enrolled in a two-year program
   c. anyone not working as an MT and currently enrolled in a nine-month or two-semester student–instructor related course
   d. anyone not working as an MT and currently enrolled in a correspondence course

Critical Thinking

1. You have excellent keyboarding skills and understand word processing programs well. Your spelling and medical terminology skills, however, are poor. How will this impact your medical transcription productivity?
2. Discuss professionalism with a classmate as it relates to medical transcription. What if an MT you are working with does not exhibit these attributes? What might they do to demonstrate professionalism?
3. List a minimum of three HIPAA regulations that apply to medical transcription. What are the consequences of not being compliant?
4. Turnaround time is an important issue in medical transcription. What happens when the transcriptionist does not complete medical documents within the turnaround time limits? What steps could be taken to assure compliance with turnaround time?
5. What if a serious error is made when transcribing a discharge summary and the court subpoenas the document because of litigation? What legal responsibility does the transcriptionist have for the accuracy of the document?

WEB ACTIVITIES

1. Using the World Wide Web, locate the AAMT Web site (http://www.aamt.org) and search through the Web pages to locate the *Medical Transcriptionist Job Description* and *Statement on Quality Assurance for Medical Transcription*. Download these items.
   a. Study the differences between Professional Levels 1, 2, and 3 provided on the job description. Where do you fit? Where would you like to be in five years? What will you have to do to achieve your goals?
   b. Now read through the *Statement on Quality Assurance for Medical Transcription*.
   c. Write a summary report responding to the three questions related to the job description and the QA statement. Follow your instructor's directions related to this activity.

REFERENCES/BIBLIOGRAPHY

American Association for Medical Transcription. (1990). *AAMT model job description: Medical transcriptionist.* Modesto, CA: author.

Burns, L., & Maloney, F. (2003). *Medical transcription and terminology: An integrated approach* (2nd ed.). Clifton Park, NY: Thomson Delmar Learning.

ingenix. (2003, December). *HIPAA Tool Kit.* Salt Lake City, UT: St. Anthony Publishing/Medicode.

Novak, M. A., & Ireland, P. A. (1999). *Hillcrest medical center. Beginning medical transcription course* (5th ed.). Clifton Park, NY: Thomson Delmar Learning.

Tessier, C. (1995). *AAMT book of style for medical transcription.* Modesto, CA: author.

Tossey, K. L. (1998). The integration of digital photographs into medical transcription. *Journal of the American Association for Medical Transcription, 17*(6), 19–21.

UNIT 5
Managing Facility Finances

Daily Financial Practices

OUTLINE

KEY TERMS

Accounts Payable
Accounts Receivable
Adjustments
Balance
Cashier's Check
Certified Check
Credit
Day Sheet
Debit
Encounter Form
Guarantor
Ledger
Money Market Savings
  Account
Notary
Payee
Pegboard System
Petty Cash
Posting
Traveler's Check
Voucher Check

OBJECTIVES

The student should strive to meet the following performance objectives and demonstrate an understanding of the facts and principles presented in this chapter through written and oral communication.

1. Define the key terms as presented in the glossary.
2. Understand the importance of communication in regard to establishing patient fees.
3. Identify circumstances that require adjustment of fees.
4. Develop a knowledge of various credit arrangements for patient fees.
5. Differentiate between manual and computerized bookkeeping systems.
6. Describe the pegboard system.

(continues)

Perform Bookkeeping Procedures

- Prepare a bank deposit
- Post entries on a daysheet
- Perform accounts receivable procedures
- Post adjustments
- Process credit balance
- Process refunds
- Post NSF checks

Operational Functions

- Utilize computer software to maintain office systems

ABHES—ENTRY-LEVEL COMPETENCIES

Administrative Duties

- Apply computer concepts for office procedures
- Prepare a bank statement and deposit record
- Reconcile a bank statement
- Post entries on day sheet
- Process refunds
- Post NSF checks
- Use physician fee schedule

Financial Management

- Use manual and computerized bookkeeping
- Manage accounts payable and receivable
- Maintain records for accounting and banking purposes

OBJECTIVES (continued)

7. State the advantages and disadvantages of computerized systems for financial practices.
8. List six good working habits for financial records.
9. Describe the encounter form.
10. Identify the parts of the patient account or ledger.
11. Discuss preparation of patient receipts.
12. Describe month-end activities.
13. Demonstrate a knowledge of banking procedures, including types of accounts and services.
14. Show proficiency in preparing deposits and checks and reconciling accounts.
15. Explain the process of purchasing equipment and supplies for the ambulatory care setting.
16. Demonstrate proficiency in establishing and maintaining a petty cash system.

SCENARIO

At the offices of Drs. Lewis and King, many different types of patients are seen: most have some kind of insurance, either a traditional plan or an HMO-type plan, some are on Medicare, a few on Medicaid, and occasionally a patient does not have any insurance or any financial resources to pay for treatment. Whoever schedules the first patient appointment also opens a courteous discussion with the patient about physician fees and the patient's anticipated method of payment. Initiating this discussion of fees at the beginning of the physician–patient relationship keeps patients informed of their responsibility for payment and helps the medical assistants at Drs. Lewis and King's practice make any necessary credit arrangements with the patient before treatment begins.

INTRODUCTION

Ambulatory care settings are primarily designed to serve the patient. However, without sound financial practices, patient care will suffer and the practice will not thrive and grow. The health care industry has become more complex in recent years with the explosion of managed care. The impact of managed care affects not only the way patients receive treatment, but the manner in which the ambulatory care center is administered from a financial point of view.

The discussion of fees is only a small part of the ambulatory care setting's daily financial practices. Selecting an appropriate system for tracking patient accounts, overseeing banking procedures, managing the purchase of supplies, and establishing a petty cash system are all important to the smooth functioning of today's ambulatory care setting.

PATIENT FEES

Physicians receive education, training, and experience in diagnosing and treating the concerns of their patients. That is their major concern; therefore, the management of the business details usually is the responsibility of the medical assisting staff. Informing the patient about physician charges, collecting payments, making credit arrangements if necessary, and making certain patients and their physicians receive the full benefit of medical insurance becomes the responsibility of the medical office staff. An attitude that anticipates that the majority of patients pay their medical bills in a timely and responsible manner is helpful in completing this task.

Helping Patients Who Cannot Pay

There are times when patients may have difficulty paying their bills. The economy changes, and with its fluctuations, individuals lose their jobs and often their medical insurance. The majority of today's employment force does not recall a time without medical insurance when patients expected to pay the total fee for medical services. These same patients may not fully comprehend what medical services cost. They likely do not understand the explanation of benefits (EOB) from their insurance reports. There is also a growing number of "working poor" in our society, who may work two or more part-time jobs but never qualify for company insurance benefits and struggle daily to pay necessary bills. Some patients must decide whether to put food on the table or pay the doctor. Emergencies may deplete an individual's financial resources as well. These are the times when the office staff might make financial arrangements with patients allowing full payment for the services provided. Patients will appreciate the assistance, and the medical assistant can expect the patient to abide by the plan agreed on. Such an agreement also fosters a climate where patients are less likely to withdraw from any necessary medical treatment when their finances are low.

Determining Patient Fees

Physicians generally have placed a value on the services they provide. In today's managed care climate, ambulatory care settings have many different arrangements with patients, insurance carriers, and health maintenance organization (HMO)-type insurance contracts. Managed care contracts pay physicians predetermined fees for specific procedures and services. See Chapter 18 for further details on physicians' fees.

Discussion of Fees

The manner in which billing is done and fees established will vary depending on the type of medical facility, the needs of the practice, and the professional services rendered. Today, the fee for the visit is simply stated, and if a person does not have cash or a check, the option of credit or debit card payment is often provided. If a patient is a member of an HMO, the patient is expected to pay for any established co-payment amount.

Inherent to the total billing process is the necessity of informing patients of charges and exactly what portion of

Spotlight on Certification

RMA Content Outline
- Financial bookkeeping

CMA Content Outline
- Equipment and supply inventory
- Bookkeeping systems
- Accounting and banking procedures

CMAS Content Outline
- Fundamental Financial Management
- Patient Accounts
- Banking

Patient Education

One way to easily provide information to patients regarding fees is to include in the office brochure office policies regarding fees, insurance, co-payments, and how third-party payments are handled. If credit and debit cards are allowed, include that information as well.

the bill they are expected to pay. Ideally, the patient should be told the approximate cost of the procedures at the start of treatment. For Medicare and Medicaid patients, this must be in writing and should indicate the type of procedure(s), the total responsibility of the patient, and the reason why this is the patient's responsibility. This form is officially known by Medicare as an Advanced Beneficiary Notification (ABN), or by Medicaid as a waiver. These forms are the only legal means an office has to collect payment on charges not allowed by Medicare or Medicaid.

Charges for some daily routine visits may be submitted to an insurance carrier, and the office may not know what portion is covered until information is received from the carrier. The facility may contract with numerous insurance plans including private carriers and participation in these plans determines the amount the patient owes. Many misunderstandings will be prevented and subsequent collection of delinquent accounts expedited when the office staff is well informed about insurance reimbursement and carefully explains fees to the patients.

Adjustment of Fees

If an office accepts assignment with Medicare and Medicaid, they are mandated to charge every patient the same amount for similar services rendered. If an office then extends a professional courtesy, it is considered insurance fraud. The office would then be billing insurance an increased rate than what they charge others. Deductibles are to be collected from the patient as part of their premium expectation. Unless you follow government guidelines for establishing when a patient is financially unable to pay their portion of the bill, you cannot give discounts to patients for cash payments.

Adjustments may be made for patients with limited income. For example, for patients who recently lost a job or ran into unfortunate financial circumstances, the physician may write off a portion of the bill. This sum will be written off against the physician's income, and the patients do not pay that portion.

Adjustments also may occur with Medicare, Medicaid, Blue Shield, and private health insurance patients. Physicians who accept assignment in these programs agree to accept as payment in full what the insurer allows. For instance, a fee of $150 may be charged, but $95 is accepted as payment in full by the provider after deductibles and co-payments are satisfied. The remainder of the bill, $55, is written off so that the patient is not responsible for the nonallowed amount.

Medical assistants must be aware, however, of the pitfalls of adjusting or reducing fees. It is difficult to accept all hardship cases and still remain a viable practice. It is always a helpful resource to patients who cannot pay to be given the names and telephone numbers of local health care clinics that may be able to accept them as patients on a sliding scale or no-fee basis.

Refunds. On occasion, a refund will be necessary. It usually occurs when the insurance carrier pays more than anticipated. Notably, there are members of the older adult population who may still be a little uncomfortable with Medicare and are accustomed to paying for all their medical expenses out of pocket; therefore, they will pay their entire bill when the statement is received. When Medicare payments arrive, an overpayment is created. The financial transaction required is to prepare a check for the amount due to the patient and enter the transaction on the **day sheet** and patient account. In most cases, such a refund will bring the patient balance to zero.

CREDIT ARRANGEMENTS

If the patient will need to pay a substantial out-of-pocket amount, it is beneficial to make the patient aware of this and discuss different credit arrangements that can be made. Many ambulatory care settings will work out installment payments, usually without finance charges, to spread the cost of services over a pre-agreed period. This eases the financial burden on the patient and also makes it more likely that the office will be able to collect balance due.

Payment Planning

Medical assistants can help patients plan for anticipated medical expenses (having a baby, surgery, extensive therapy). When patient and physician know in advance that there will be costly medical expenses, the medical assistant should review the patient's insurance coverage. It is also helpful to prepare an estimate sheet, which will give the patient an idea of the cost of the medical services for the planned treatment. The estimate may also include the cost of anesthetist, consultants, and hospital charges.

Many ambulatory care settings accept credit and debit cards as a means of payment. Remember that this is strictly for the convenience of the patient, and physicians cannot increase their charges for patients who wish to use these cards even though the physician is charged a fee for this service. Credit and debit cards are convenient and assure payment; therefore, the practice may wish to encourage their use.

The one advantage to the ambulatory care setting that accepts credit cards is that monies for fees charged are usually available within 24 hours or so. Also, the physician is relieved of the responsibility of collection. However, credit card companies do assess a fee for every charge made, which the ambulatory care center must pay.

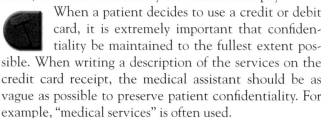 When a patient decides to use a credit or debit card, it is extremely important that confidentiality be maintained to the fullest extent possible. When writing a description of the services on the credit card receipt, the medical assistant should be as vague as possible to preserve patient confidentiality. For example, "medical services" is often used.

THE BOOKKEEPING FUNCTION

Daily financial management in the ambulatory care setting is important to the functioning of the office, because it directly affects overall accounting and bookkeeping procedures. Accounting generates financial information for the ambulatory care setting and is defined as a system of monitoring the financial status of a facility and the specific results of its activities. Accounting provides financial information for decision making (see Chapter 21). Bookkeeping, the actual daily recording of the accounts or transactions of the business, is a major part of this accounting process. This chapter deals with daily bookkeeping (or recording) functions necessary to manage the income and expenses of an ambulatory care setting.

Managing Patient Accounts

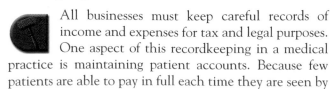 All businesses must keep careful records of income and expenses for tax and legal purposes. One aspect of this recordkeeping in a medical practice is maintaining patient accounts. Because few patients are able to pay in full each time they are seen by

the physician, it is necessary to maintain account records for each individual or family as opposed to simply keeping a record of cash received as is done in many other types of business. The money owed to the office by patients is known as **accounts receivable;** this must be carefully monitored to assure that the physician is paid for services provided in a timely manner, and that patients are properly credited for payments made.

There are various ways to track patients' balances. In this chapter, we discuss the two most common methods:

* The **pegboard system** (also known as the write-it-once method)

* Computerized systems

 Though most practices' financial records are fully automated, many probably started with some sort of manual system (generally pegboard). Converting from manual to computerized recordkeeping takes a great deal of time at the beginning, but it offers great versatility and reduces the need to record and re-record entries.

A well-prepared medical assistant will understand both the manual and computerized systems.

The Importance of Good Working Habits in Financial Transactions. In managing the day-to-day finances of the ambulatory care setting, always observe the following guidelines:

1. Always work with care and accuracy; it is extremely easy to transpose numbers (i.e., entering 23 instead of 32) or make other posting errors. A moment of carelessness can result in hours spent trying to find the mistake.
2. The work must be kept current or it may become an overwhelming chore.
3. Double-check all entries made for accuracy.

In a manual bookkeeping system, follow these additional rules:

* Use a consistent ink color; black or blue is preferred.

* Form your numbers and letters carefully, using neat and clear writing.

* Align your columns carefully, preferably using paper with grid lines.

* Write small enough to stay within the columns.

- Be careful when placing or carrying decimal points.

- Double-check all math.

- If a mistake is found, draw one line through the error and write "Corr." or "Correction" above it. Red ink may be used in correcting errors on a paper copy.

Pegboard System. A complete pegboard or write-it-once system consists of day sheets, ledger cards, **encounter forms** or charge slips, and receipt forms. The forms are designed to work together to simplify the task and to avoid costly and embarrassing mistakes in patient accounts. All forms will have matching columns that align and are held in place on the pegboard when the system is in use (Figure 17-1). The forms are on NCR© (no carbon required) paper, which permits entering of charges, credits, or adjustments, called **posting,** onto the day sheet, encounter form, or receipt and the patient's ledger card simultaneously. The day sheet provides complete and up-to-date information about accounts receivable status at a glance. Also, a pegboard system is relatively inexpensive.

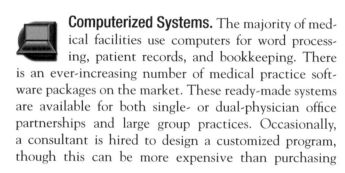

Computerized Systems. The majority of medical facilities use computers for word processing, patient records, and bookkeeping. There is an ever-increasing number of medical practice software packages on the market. These ready-made systems are available for both single- or dual-physician office partnerships and large group practices. Occasionally, a consultant is hired to design a customized program, though this can be more expensive than purchasing

mass-produced software. When selecting and using any computer system:

- Be sure the system will meet not only current needs, but future needs as well (some packages can be expanded to grow with the practice).

- Adopt a system that allows the practice to start with one component such as scheduling and add another component such as bookkeeping and medical records at a later date until the entire practice is computerized.

RECORDING PATIENT TRANSACTIONS

The administrative medical assistant is largely responsible for recording patient transactions for the practice. Bookkeeping activities are exact: They are either right or they are wrong, and in any forms of business, they have to be right to be correct and to be "in balance." In the pegboard or manual system, if an error is made during entry, it will carry through to all the other documents, thus compounding the error. In a computerized system, there is the old but

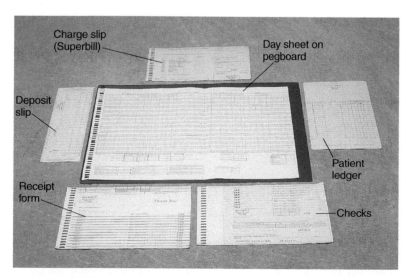

Figure 17-1 An example of the pegboard system and possible overlays.

true statement, "garbage in, garbage out." *All* entries must be correct; there is no room for just a "slight" mistake.

In one way or another, the forms and procedures discussed in the following sections are common elements to any system of bookkeeping for a medical practice.

Encounter Form

The encounter form is also known as the charge slip, superbill, or multipurpose billing form. It is used in both manual and computerized bookkeeping systems. It often is a three-part form that has the following functions:

1. Provides patients one copy with a record of account activity for the day (usually a pink form)
2. Provides a second copy of account activity for possible insurance submission (usually a yellow form)
3. Provides a third copy that serves the office's permanent copy of account activity (usually a white form)

The encounter forms can be custom designed to fit the particular practice, computer system, or pegboard. Information on the form includes the patient's name, address, account number, and necessary insurance information, as well as any previous balance. Often, the encounter form is attached to the patient's chart so the physician is able to indicate the day's activities and charges; the physician can also indicate a requested return visit. The encounter form also includes procedure and diagnosis codes. The most applicable procedure codes can be preselected and printed on the encounter form to fit the practice, with blank lines added for infrequently used procedures. Often, physicians use the form to check the appropriate procedures and diagnoses while with the patient. The encounter form also will carry the name, address, and telephone number of the practice and the attending physician's Identification Number.

Encounter forms are designed to fit over the pegs of pegboard system when a manual system is used. In a computerized system, an encounter form carrying the same information is prepared for the patient, printed, and attached to the patient file. Some computer systems automatically match the correct charge to the procedure code identified.

Patient Account or Ledger

The financial record of the patient is known as that patient's account. All the patient accounts with balances make up the accounts receivable. Patient accounts are recorded in an accounts receivable **ledger.** (Figure 17-2 illustrates a typewritten ledger.) The ledger, or record of services, lists payments and balances due. In family practice, each adult has his or her own ledger or account that carries insurance information, name of subscriber, and patient's relationship to the subscriber. A responsible party is identified for each minor or patient who does not have insurance, and that name also will appear at the top of that ledger. Charges for any members of the family seen in the office are entered on their own ledger. It is important that charges and credits be applied to the correct family member for insurance purposes and accurate bookkeeping practices.

In cases of divorced parents and blended families, the parent with physical custody of the child is considered to be **guarantor** and the one responsible for payment if the child is not insured with a contracted insurance carrier. This prevents the office staff from having to interpret divorce decrees and parenting plan documents. This information should be clearly identified and discussed with the parent when appointments are made.

In the manual system of bookkeeping, ledger cards are used. They have a minimum of three columns for entering figures:

1. **Debit** column is on the left and is used for entering charges and a brief description of services, including a procedure code.
2. **Credit** column is to the right of the debit column and is used for entering payments.
3. **Balance** column is at the far right and is used to record the difference between the debit and credit columns and shows any amount due.

Most ledger cards have space for another column called **adjustments,** which are used to indicate any insurance payments, personal discounts or write-offs, or any other adjustments that might need to be recorded.

The Identification Number is usually the physician's tax identification number or state license number. Either can be used for identification purposes for tax purposes. Physicians must submit an application to the Centers for Medicare and Medicaid Services to receive their own National Provider Identifier (NPI). This single identification number will eventually replace all other identifiers used by physicians for reimbursement and other transactions with private payers and the government. It is anticipated that all health plans will be required to have the NPI numbers of physicians in use by 2007. The NPI and its use is mandated by HIPAA regulations.

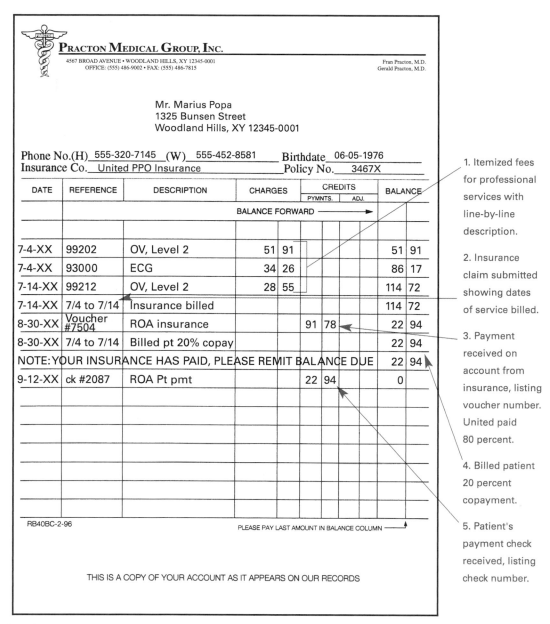

Figure 17-2 Typewritten ledger card illustrating posting of professional services, fees, payments, adjustments, and balance due.

The adjustment column is a credit column; therefore, entries here normally reduce the balance due. When making an adjustment intended to increase the balance, a negative entry (in parentheses) is made to show that you reverse the function when you balance. (Add instead of subtract the amount.) For example, Edith Leonard had surgery, and because of a hardship, the physician agreed to reduce the fee by half of the balance remaining after insurance has paid. At the time of surgery, a charge of $2,500 is entered on her ledger and the day sheet. Today, payment is received from her insurance company in the amount of $2,000, which would normally leave a balance

of $500. However, because the physician agreed to write off half of that amount ($250), you enter $250 in the adjustment column when posting the insurance payment. That amount is subtracted from the previous balance to get the new total of $250.

The ledger is placed under the charge slip or encounter form in a pegboard system and aligned before posting. Never post any patient entry in this manual system without the patient's ledger in place. This prevents recording information on the day sheet, and thus inadvertently omitting it from the patient's ledger. In the computerized system, a patient's account or ledger can be printed with the same information by just entering the patient's name and usually an identification number. Most facilities find that the computerized patient account ledger provides more room for helpful detail.

Day Sheet

All financial transactions for professional services are posted daily on a day sheet or daily ledger. This is an important part of the overall bookkeeping process, thus legibility and absolute accuracy are critical. At the close of each business day, the day sheet is balanced to provide a complete picture of all patient financial activity for that day. Those balances carryover from day to day to provide the accumulated data needed for month-end closing. If more than one day sheet is required to record all the transactions in the pegboard system, pages are numbered and the information is carried forward just as if it were a new day. There are a number of different styles for the day sheet; some provide a deposit portion to use as a deposit slip and a section used for business analysis. For example, if the physician wants to know the amount of income generated from laboratory services performed in the office, the totals can be obtained from the day sheet columns where only laboratory charges were posted. Over time, the laboratory income totals can be compared with the cost for running the laboratory.

The pegboard write-it-once section is where individual transactions are posted, using the ledger card and encounter form on top of the day sheet. The information in this section includes the date, patient name, description of transaction or service, charges, credits, and previous and current balances. At the bottom of the day sheet, transactions are totaled and balanced at the end of the day. This total section includes space to bring forward the previous page balance for a month-to-date total. These totals allow the physician and office manager to monitor totals that assist in predicting the financial status for the practice. The total accounts receivable figure shows how much is owed to the physician by all patients to date, allowing management to see the total outstanding balance at a glance. A major disadvantage to this system, as mentioned earlier, is that an error made in one place is going to carry through to all the other forms. When balancing this financial information, always use a calculator's print function to create a tape of the calculations. These tapes are an invaluable time saver if the initial balance is incorrect and you need to search for mistakes.

Daily sheets or ledgers in a computerized system require the same data. The patient's name, date, diagnosis, and services provided are posted. The computer system or database pulls up the correct charge and posts it to the patient account and the accounts receivable ledger. Any error made is quickly changed and corrected throughout. Totals are automatically created for the day-end total, month-end total, and cumulative total from the beginning of the year.

Receipts

Unlike encounter forms, receipt forms used for payments on accounts usually are not customized other than to have the name, address, and telephone number of the practice preprinted. The receipt form is used only when someone makes a payment on an account on a day when no services were rendered. In the pegboard system, this transaction is entered on the day sheet and the ledger card at the same time the receipt is filled out. When payments are received by mail, the same system is followed; however, there is no need to create a receipt. In a computerized system, the receipt is easily printed for the patient as soon as the information has been entered and the patient account updated. If the patient needs a receipt and the payment is not posted right away, a handwritten receipt is acceptable.

The physician may have charges created from emergency department visits, patient hospital visits, surgeries, visits in a convalescent nursing facility, or other out-of-office services. These charges are to be entered on the day sheet and the ledger or patient's account. Some physicians produce information manually in a pocket-size notebook, in a calendar, or on a personal handheld computer and give it to the medical assistant on their return to the office. The medical assistant then enters the data into the daily sheet and the patient's account. If the physician uses the handheld computer for the tracking and recording of office charges, the medical assistant can electronically download the billing information.

Month-End Activities

In the pegboard system, when the last day sheet for the month has been balanced, it is then necessary to verify that the month-end figures on the day sheet agree with patient accounts. Though this may be a time-consuming process in the manual system, it will find mistakes before they grow into major accounting or collection problems.

Reconciling the month-end sheet to the patient ledgers is accomplished by adding all the open balances on the ledgers and verifying that the total agrees with the end-of-month accounts receivable balance on the last day sheet of the month. When these figures agree, the accounts receivable balance is correct.

By following these procedures of "checks and balances," it is likely that all payments have been properly credited to patient accounts and deposited, and that all charges shown as outstanding on the day sheet agree with the outstanding balances of the individual patient accounts. If a payment is somehow misplaced, the deposits will not agree with the credits or with the patient ledgers and it will be known immediately that there is an error. Not only does this catch errors, it also eliminates the possibility of loss of a check or undetected theft of funds, because when a mistake is caught immediately, the payer can stop payment on the missing check or credit or debit card slip and a new payment can be made.

Computerized Patient Accounts

A software management program offers many advantages in managing patient accounts. The program automatically creates an encounter form the day before the patient is seen or when the receptionist prints out the schedule. After the physician's examination, the program calculates the charges for the monthly billing statement (Figure 17-3). The management program also creates and updates the patient account, adds new names to the list

Douglasville Medicine Associates
5076 Brand Blvd., Suite 401
Douglasville,NY 01234
Ph: (123) 456-7890
Fax: (123)456-7891
E-mail: admin@dfma.com
Web site: www.dfma.com

STATEMENT OF ACCOUNT

MANUEL RAMIREZ
1211 Gravel Way
Douglasville, NY 01234

Date: 1/3/20XX

Account No: RAM001

Date	Patient	Description of Service	Total Charges	Patient Payment	Insurance Payment	Adjust-ments	Dedu-ctible	Current Balance
18-Oct-XX	Manuel Ramirez	Established Patient - Level 3	$78.00	$0.00	$47.20	$19.00	$0	$11.80
29-Oct-XX	Manuel Ramirez	Colonscopy	$315.00	$0.00	$0.00	$0.00	$0	$315.00
29-Oct-XX	Manuel Ramirez	Established Patient - Level 5	$176.00	$0.00	$0.00	$0.00	$0	$176.00
		Totals:	$569.00	$0.00	$47.20	$19.00	$0	$502.80

0 to 30 Days Current	31 to 60 Days Past Due	61 to 90 Days Past Due	91+ Days Past Due	BALANCE DUE	
$0.00	$0.00	$502.80	$0.00		$502.80

Important Note:

Figure 17-3 Computerized patient statement.

of patients and to the daily log, and transfers data to produce insurance forms, statements, a list of checks received each day, and deposit slips. In addition, the program automatically ages accounts at each billing cycle and creates billing statements. As a result, when patient accounts are computerized, practice collections usually increase.

The computerized patient account contains personal information about each patient, including their name, address, and telephone number; the person responsible for payment; and all insurance carriers. The account also lists all previous office visits and the procedures, procedure codes, charges, payments, and adjustments for each visit. Most account management software can be customized to meet the special needs of the individual ambulatory care setting.

As billing information is entered from the encounter forms, the computer automatically updates the account by adding a description of each procedure and procedure code and each diagnosis and diagnosis code. The computer software automatically posts the charges and calculates the balance after credits and adjustments are entered.

Once charges and payments have been entered and the day has been closed, they are not easily removed or changed. This is an important software design because it ensures that monies are not removed from receivables credited to a previous month. This procedure would cause the practice year-end balance to be unresolved.

As useful and efficient as a computerized bookkeeping system can be, it is important to recognize that an inadequate manual system will not get better once computerized. Also, it takes time to move to a computerized system, train personnel, and enter existing patient data. Manual and computer systems may need to run concurrently for a month or two.

BANKING PROCEDURES

Understanding bank accounts and services, making deposits, preparing checks, and reconciling accounts are all a part of daily financial practices. Although many banking services are similar from one bank to another, it is a good idea for the medical assistant in charge of maintaining daily accounts to investigate the banking resources of the local community. In an effort to secure new business, many banks compete for customers by offering special services that can be of use to the ambulatory care setting.

Online Banking

Personal use of the Internet has changed banking and the services it provides. Online banking allows individuals to check account balances, transfer funds between accounts,

pay bills electronically, check credit card balances, view images of checks and deposits, and download account information 24 hours a day/7 days a week. Considerable time and expense can be saved with online banking, but there are also some cautions to observe. Any online banking should be completed only through the use of secure and unique passwords granted to only those individuals deemed necessary.

Types of Accounts

Checking and savings accounts are the two primary types of accounts.

Checking Accounts. The checking account is the primary account type the medical assistant will use in the ambulatory care setting. Today, there are many variations on checking accounts. In the event that the medical assistant is responsible for establishing a new account, it is worthwhile to investigate features of different checking accounts both within the same bank and at competing banks.

Some features that may differ include:

- Interest paid
- Monthly fees
- Check charges
- Automated teller machine (ATM) access and fees
- After hours deposit capabilities
- Initial deposit and balance requirements
- Overdraft protection
- Fees for checks
- Special services extended free of charge such as **notary,** cashier's checks, traveler's checks, and online banking.

When selecting an account, rather than choosing the account with the lowest fees, consider convenience, the relationship possible with a given bank, bank hours, number of bank locations, and other factors.

Savings Accounts. Savings accounts were initially distinguished from checking accounts because they paid interest on the money deposited. However, many checking accounts pay interest now as well. In either case, the interest is usually minimal on accounts that give immediate access to the deposit. **Money market savings accounts** may pay a higher rate of interest, although they require a higher initial deposit and maintenance

Critical Thinking

What factors make money market funds a good investment during one period, but provide little return for the investment at another time?

of a higher balance, usually around $2500. Access to the account may be limited. Savings accounts are useful when access to money is not needed frequently or when accumulating an amount necessary to invest for long-term goals.

Types of Checks

For the most part, the ambulatory care setting will use a standard business check. However, for special purposes, it is useful to understand the other check types available:

- A **cashier's check** is often used when a check must be guaranteed for the amount in which it is written. Because a cashier's check is the bank's own check drawn against the bank's accounts, the recipient has the assurance that the check will clear. Cashier's checks are obtained at the bank by paying the bank representative cash or sometimes a personal check for the amount of the cashier's check.

- A **certified check** is the depositor's own check that the bank has "certified" with a date and signature to indicate that the check is good for the amount in which it is written.

- Money orders are available from banks and the U.S. Postal Service. They are purchased with cash and are used in ways similar to cashier's checks. A few patients may use money orders to pay their bill.

- A **voucher check** is a type of check with a stub attached to it that can be used to indicate invoice dates, services provided, and so on. Many payroll checks are written on voucher checks; the voucher check is also frequently used in the ambulatory care setting for accounts payable.

- **Traveler's checks** are available in most banks and are convenient and safer to use than cash when traveling. They are written in specific denominations ($10, $20, $50) and require a signature when purchased and when used. However, many banks today will advise customers to use ATM machines for necessary cash when traveling to areas where ATM machines are readily available.

Deposits

Deposits are usually made daily because they serve as another proof of posting and because it is unwise to leave large sums of money in the office overnight. The office should have a rubber endorsement stamp from the bank; use it to immediately imprint the back of all checks received directly from patients and in the mail. Before depositing them, be sure all checks are stamped. Scanning or photocopying all checks before deposit is one way to ensure accuracy.

Because the endorsement transfers rights to whoever holds the check, it is important to take certain precautions. A blank endorsement consists of a signature only (whether in pen or with a stamp) and presents a danger in that, if the check is lost or stolen, someone else could endorse the check below the signature and cash it. A restrictive endorsement should be used on all checks received in the ambulatory care setting. Restrictive endorsements include the signature and the words "for deposit only" or "pay to the order of..." (include the name of bank and account number; in addition, all possible payees' names should be listed under the company name, with the practice address). This restricts the use of the check should it be lost or stolen.

Cash on Hand

There is the need in most medical practices to have cash available on a daily basis. If it is the practice to collect co-payments and any coinsurance at the time of service, some patients will pay in cash and need change. Cash is usually kept in a locked change drawer that will contain up to $150 in small bills at the beginning of each day. Any time a patient pays cash for their service, a receipt is to be written. Receipts are prenumbered, thus monitoring loss or theft. Cash amounts paid by patients must also be noted in their account or ledger. The terms *received on account (ROA) cash* is usually written in the description column. If payment is made by check, follow the same procedure except the word *check* is written instead of *cash*.

At the end of each day, the cash drawer is balanced. The amount of cash received will be noted on the deposit slip as "currency." The remaining amount in the cash drawer will be the same as the beginning amount. Also, the day's cash received must match the cash control on the daily sheet. It is a good idea for only one person to handle the cash in the cash drawer; thus, it is not necessary for more than one person to balance the cash drawer at the end of the day. The cash drawer is not to be confused with petty cash, which is discussed later in this chapter. Petty cash is used to purchase small items such as postage, office refreshments, and so on. Checks are always written for major purchases, with the cash drawer used only to accommodate patient needs when payment is made in cash.

Most business accounts use a deposit slip similar to the one in Figure 17-4. They are always filled out in duplicate or a copy is made—one copy to accompany the deposit, and one to be retained for office records. As shown, these deposit slips are longer than those generally used for personal accounts and have room for more entries and more information. If your manual day sheet has a built-in duplicate deposit slip, it will have been completed during posting.

A computerized system of financial records can provide deposit slips that may be used. The same procedure is followed as previously discussed. Procedure 17-3 outlines the steps in preparing a deposit.

Accepting Checks

When accepting checks from patients and other individuals, take a few minutes to inspect the check; this may eliminate checks returned from the bank for various reasons:

- Inspect the check for correct date, amount, and signature.

- Do not accept a third-party check (a check written to the patient from another person or company) unless it is from the insurance carrier.

- If a deposited check is returned marked "insufficient funds" (NSF), call the bank that returned it and verify availability of funds. If funds are available, immediately redeposit the check for processing. If the check is returned a second time marked NSF, it is necessary to perform two bookkeeping functions. First, deduct the amount from the checking account balance of the practice. Second, add the amount back into the amount due by the patient in his or her account balance by entering the amount in the paid column in parentheses and increase the balance by the same amount. Place a brief explanation in the description column. Follow the office procedure for notifying the patient that the check was returned. See Procedure 17-6.

Lost or Stolen Checks

In the event that a check is missing and is thought to be lost or stolen, report this to your bank immediately. In some cases, you may be advised to stop payment to prevent unauthorized cashing of the check. In other situations, the bank may place a warning on the account, advising bank representatives to be especially careful about checking signatures to detect any attempt at a forged signature.

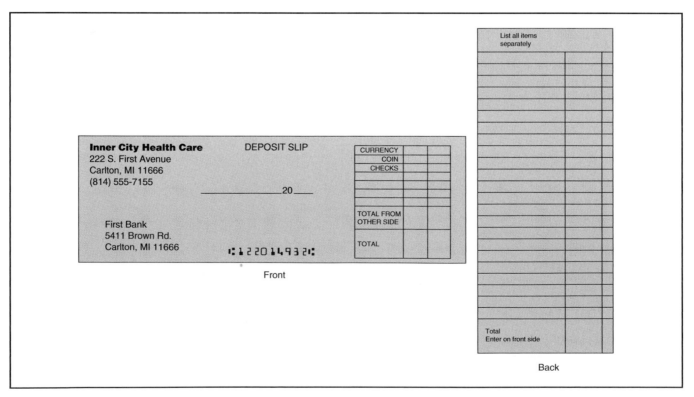

Figure 17-4 Sample deposit slip.

Writing and Recording Checks

Part of daily financial practices includes writing checks to pay bills **(accounts payable),** refunds of overpayment, and replenishment of petty cash. Writing the checks and paying the bills is usually done systematically. Chapter 21 discusses accounts payable and disbursement records in greater detail. It is important that checks be prepared electronically or written legibly to avoid bank errors. Checks should be dated and must include the name of the **payee** and the amount of payment entered both in figures and in words. It is also advisable that the "memo" line indicates what the check is for and includes any account or invoice number for reference. See Figure 17-5 for a sample of a properly completed check.

Rules for Preparing Checks. Follow these few rules to ensure that checks are properly prepared and recorded:

- Confirm that the numeric and written amounts agree.

- Confirm that everything is spelled correctly.

- Follow office procedure for having the physician or office manager approve all expenditures and sign all outgoing checks.

- Determine that the check has been signed by an individual with signature privileges.

- Confirm that it is payable to the correct payee and that the current date is used.

Reconciling a Bank Statement

Each month the bank will send a statement for the checking account (Figure 17-6). With online banking, a bank statement can be accessed electronically at any time. It also can be printed and used similar to a standard printed bank statement. The statement will show the account balance according to the bank's records, a listing of all checks that have cleared the bank, deposits received by the bank, and any service charges deducted from the account. It is necessary to reconcile the entries in the checkbook against this statement to be sure there are no errors either in the checkbook or in the bank's records. Your bank statement is another means of ensuring that the accounts receivable is accurate for the previous month. If you use an accounting software package, this will also have a computerized option for reconciling.

Procedure 17-4 details the steps involved in reconciling the statement.

PURCHASING SUPPLIES AND EQUIPMENT

It is important to ensure proper control over purchasing of supplies and equipment for several reasons:

1. To avoid purchase of unnecessary items
2. To avoid duplication of items purchased
3. To provide a system for payment of only those items properly ordered and received

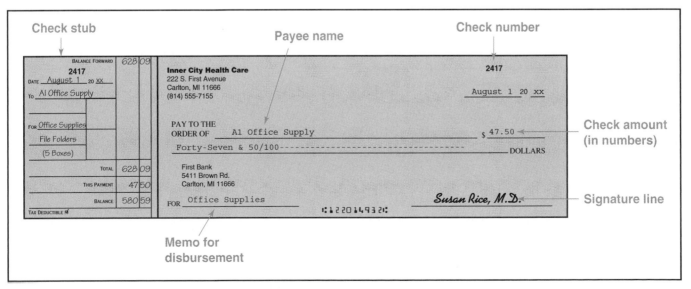

Figure 17-5 Sample of a properly completed check and check stub.

Summary of Account Balance   Closing Date 1/15/XX

Account # 1257-164013   Ending Balance $8,347.62

Beginning Balance $7,152.18
Total Deposits and Additions $8,643.86
Total Withdrawals $7,433.21
Service Charge $ 15.24

Number	Date	Amount	Number	Date	Amount
201	12/18/XX	173.82	234	1/4/XX	96.31
223*	12/18/XX	44.12	235	1/4/XX	73.48
224	12/20/XX	586.00	236	1/6/XX	325.40
225	12/21/XX	24.15	237	1/7/XX	40.00
226	12/22/XX	33.90	238	1/8/XX	66.77
228*	12/23/XX	1250.00	241*	1/9/XX	15.55
229	12/24/XX	11.75	242	1/10/XX	12.45
230	12/24/XX	19.02	243	1/10/XX	4441.25
231	1/2/XX	43.80	244	1/10/XX	64.55
232	1/3/XX	39.00			
233	1/4/XX	71.50			

*Denotes gap in check sequence

Date	Deposit Amount	Date	Deposit Amount
18-Dec	361.75	4-Jan	825.00
19-Dec	586.00	5-Jan	1286.71
20-Dec	918.21	7-Jan	608.00
21-Dec	201.00	8-Jan	811.15
2-Jan	475.00	9-Jan	1092.68
3-Jan	1478.36		

Front

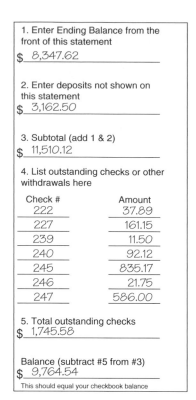

1. Enter Ending Balance from the front of this statement
$ 8,347.62

2. Enter deposits not shown on this statement
$ 3,162.50

3. Subtotal (add 1 & 2)
$ 11,510.12

4. List outstanding checks or other withdrawals here

Check #	Amount
222	37.89
227	161.15
239	11.50
240	92.12
245	835.17
246	21.75
247	586.00

5. Total outstanding checks
$ 1,745.58

Balance (subtract #5 from #3)
$ 9,764.54

This should equal your checkbook balance

Back

Figure 17-6   Sample bank statement.

To accomplish these things, you should follow the first rule of purchasing: nothing is ordered or paid for without a purchase order or purchase order number. A copy of the purchase order is sent to the supplier and a copy is retained by the office for verification of shipment and payment of invoice.

Preparing a Purchase Order

Purchase order forms are available from office supply companies or can be ordered from a printer and customized to the needs of the ambulatory care setting. As an alternative to ordering preprinted purchase order forms, the clinic staff may choose to create their own forms using Microsoft Excel® software. This enables the clinic to have electronic access to the form with imbedded formulas. Figure 17-7 shows a typical purchase order form properly completed, which is reviewed here section by section.

The purchase order form can vary greatly; some have more or less information. The form shown in Figure 17-7 contains the usual information required. The important thing is that the purchase order is used consistently.

- *Date*. Day purchase order is made.

- *Purchase order number*. A preprinted number that is used on invoices and statements from the supplier

and on the check used to pay the invoice. It is also important for tracking the status of the order. In smaller practices, the purchase order number may simply be the name of the person ordering with the date the order was placed immediately following.

- *Bill to address*. This is generally used when items are to be shipped to an address different from the address where the supplier will send the bill for goods or services.

- *Ship to address*. When items are to be sent by supplier, this must always be completed.

- *Vendor information*. The name and address of supplier where purchase order is to be sent.

- *Req. By*. States which individual or department has requested the item(s).

- *Buyer*. States the individual in the office who is authorized to issue a purchase order.

- *Terms*. Agreement between buyer and seller as to when payment is due.

- *QTY*. Quantity of item being ordered (number of units).

- *Item*. Vendor's catalogue part or item number.

PURCHASE ORDER

NO. 1742

Date:

Bill To: **Inner City Health Care** 222 S. First Avenue Carlton, MI 11666 (814) 555-7155	Ship To: **Inner City Health Care** 222 S. First Avenue Carlton, MI 11666 (814) 555-7155	Vendor: **AZ Medical Supply** 4721 E. Camelback Rd. Phoenix, AZ 85252 (602) 555-3246

REQ BY	BUYER	TERMS
Karen Ritter	Walter Seals	Net 30

QTY	ITEM	UNITS	DESCRIPTION	UNIT PR	TOTAL
10	427A	Box	Surgical Gloves - Sz 7	8.20	82.00
1	327DC	Case	2" gauze pads	54.30	54.30
5	1943C	Box	Tongue Depressors	5.40	27.00
15	7433	Ea	Examination Table paper (roll)	9.50	142.50
				SUBTOTAL	305.80
				TAX	25.98
				FREIGHT	Prepaid
				BAL DUE	331.78

Figure 17-7 Purchase order form.

- *Units.* How the item is sold—individually (ea.), by the box, case, or dozen. Many suppliers will not split units (i.e., sell less than a full case).

- *Description.* Brief description of item (helps as a cross-check for vendor in the event that an item number is entered incorrectly).

- *Unit price.* How much *one* unit (ea., box, case, dozen) costs.

- *Total.* Cost of one unit multiplied by the number of units being ordered.

- *Discount.* If any discount is allowed for quick and early payment, it is noted here. For instance, there might be a 10% discount for paying within 10 days. The discount amount is entered before the Total column is summed.

- *Subtotal.* Sum of the Total column.

- *Tax.* Sales tax required by the state.

- *Freight.* How much the customer must pay to have the order delivered (not always applicable).

- *Bal. Due.* The sum of the subtotal, tax, and freight charges; this is how much the office will be billed.

Verifying Goods Received

Proper purchasing procedure does not stop with the completion and mailing of the purchase order. When goods are received, it is necessary to verify that the correct items and quantities were shipped by the vendor. See Chapter 21 for discussion of accounts payable.

PETTY CASH

Petty cash is money kept in the office for minor, routine, or unexpected expenses such as postage-due mail or coffee supplies. Keep petty cash totally separate from the cash drawer that is used to make change for patients paying their co-payment. Keeping this cash on hand eliminates the necessity of the physician or office manager having to sign checks for such items. Petty cash is not used to pay bills or make large routine purchases.

The amount of cash on hand for this purpose is small, usually $75 to $100, and is usually kept in small denominations such as ones and fives and only a few tens. However, records must be as carefully maintained as for any other financial transactions and balanced each day before closing.

Establishing a Petty Cash Fund

If your office does not already have a petty cash fund or if you are in a new practice that has not yet established a fund, the physician or office manager will need to decide how much the fund should be and write a check to "Cash" for that amount.

Tracking, Balancing, and Replenishing Petty Cash

Tracking. Keep a supply of petty cash vouchers on hand to track how petty cash is used. When money is taken from petty cash, a voucher must always be completed and the receipt from the purchase attached. Vouchers and

receipts are kept in the petty cash box with the money until the fund is replenished.

Balancing and Replenishing. When the fund gets low, write another check to "Cash" to bring it back up to the original amount. To determine the amount of the check, it is necessary to first balance the account. After the account is balanced, list how funds were spent in such a way that the bookkeeper can disburse the check properly.

Procedure 17-5 outlines the steps involved in balancing a petty cash account.

DOCUMENTATION

Financial records of patients are to be kept separate from the patients' medical charts. Except for the attachment of the encounter form or superbill at the time of the visit, they rarely are seen together. Often, only the patient's medical chart is necessary for documentation; other times, only the financial information is necessary. This policy also serves as a reminder that the care given to patients has nothing to do with their ability to pay.

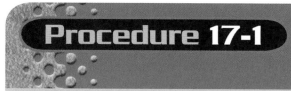

Procedure 17-1 Recording/Posting Patient Charges, Payments, and Adjustments

PURPOSE:
To record information including services rendered, fees charged, any adjustments made, and balances pertaining to a patient's visit to the physician and patient's account.

EQUIPMENT/SUPPLIES:
Calculator
Computer
Patient's account or ledger

PROCEDURE STEPS:
1. Check the patient's account before the patient's appointment to make certain it is up to date. The account will indicate any recent insurance payments, any amount received on the account, and any balance due. RATIONALE: Allows the medical office assistant to focus entirely on the patient at arrival time and gives a current picture of the patient's account.

(continues)

Procedure 17-1 (continued)

2. When the patient arrives, check for name, address, telephone number, and any changes in medical insurance. Make any changes in the account or on the ledger. RATIONALE: Assures that information is current and up to date.

3. On the encounter form or superbill, complete any necessary items such as the date of service and the responsible party's name. Then attach it to the patient's medical chart that is now ready for the clinical medical assistant to take with the patient to the examination room. RATIONALE: The encounter form allows physician to indicate appropriate procedure and diagnosis codes.

4. When the physician completes the treatment or examination, he or she will check the procedures and diagnosis on the encounter form. RATIONALE: Physician marks the appropriate codes and signs the encounter form, indicating it is correct. The physician or licensed caregiver is the only one authorized to select the appropriate procedure codes.

5. When the patient returns to the front desk, refer to the physician's fee schedule, enter the charge next to each procedure, and calculate the total. If the procedure description is not indicated, one is to be provided. A description is necessary for each service. Many computer systems will match the physician's fee to the procedure code and calculate the total. Make certain to enter the codes correctly. Check to see if the codes match the services provided. If they do not match, refer it back to the physician or licensed caregiver for correction. RATIONALE: Medical office staff and the patient can identify the charge to the particular service given and know that the coding and charges will match.

6. In the *manual pegboard system*, post each service or procedure as a charge or debit. Post any payments received today in the payment column as a credit. In the *computerized system*, the fee will automatically be entered as soon as the procedure code with matching description is entered.

Any payments received and entered will show as a credit. RATIONALE: Clearly indicates charges made and payments received, creating an updated account.

7. If any adjustment applies to the account, enter the amount in the adjustment column. If there is no adjustment column and the adjustment will *reduce* the bill, enter the amount in the payment column enclosed by parentheses. If the adjustment will *increase* the bill, place the amount in the charge column (no parentheses) with an explanation in the description column. In the *manual system*, the adjustment amount will be either added or subtracted from the totaled figures. The *computer system* automatically adds or subtracts the amount from the total when properly entered. RATIONALE: Adjustment is shown as separate from basic charge so that the physician's fee profile is unaffected.

8. In the *manual system*, determine current balance by adding credits and subtracting debits to the running balance and determine the amount in the current balance. Always use a calculator (one with a tape is recommended) to calculate and verify your mathematics. The *computer system* will create the totals for you. RATIONALE: Completes the recording of patient charges, payments, and adjustments.

9. If the recording is a payment from the patient, place a restrictive endorsement on the check. RATIONALE: Ensures that the check can only be cashed by the authorized party.

10. Enter the amount in the payment column. In the description column, identify as cash, check, or insurance payment. If payment is a check, enter the number of the check. RATIONALE: This information is necessary in making the bank deposit slip.

11. Place the cash or processed check in the appointed secure place awaiting deposit. RATIONALE: Keeps receivables together and ready for deposit.

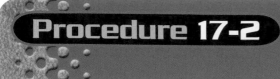

Balancing Day Sheets in a Manual System

PURPOSE:
To verify that all entries to the day sheet are correct and that the totals balance.

EQUIPMENT/SUPPLIES:
Day sheet
Calculator

PROCEDURE STEPS:

1. *Column totals.* The first step in balancing a day sheet is to total columns A, B_1, B_2, C, and D, and enter the total for each column in the boxes marked "Totals This Page." The column totals are then added to the figures entered in the "Previous Page" column boxes to arrive at the "Month to Date" totals, which provide the total charges, credits, and so forth entered from the first working day of the month to the present. RATIONALE: Establishes column totals.

2. *Proof of posting.* This box is used to verify that entries have been made correctly and that the column totals are accurate. *All figures entered here are taken from the "Totals This Page" column boxes.*

   a. Enter today's column D total, which shows the sum of all the previous balances entered when the transactions were posted.

   b. Added to this is the column A total of all charges for that day, to arrive at a subtotal and enter the amount where indicated in the box.

   c. Because columns B_1 and B_2 are both credit columns that reduce balances, they are added together entered in the box labeled "Less Cols B_1 and B_2"; the total of credits is subtracted from the subtotal. If all entries and addition are correct in the posting area, the result should equal the amount in column C and the transactions for that day are balanced. RATIONALE: Verifies entries have been made correctly and that the totals are accurate.

   Overview: When an individual transaction is entered, the patient's previous balance (D) is added to the charges for the day (A). If there are any payments or adjustments made at that time, they are entered in the B columns and subtracted from the A + D amount to achieve the new balance (C). Because each transaction is actually D + A − B = C, the column totals of D + A − B will always equal the C total.

	D		A		B		C
	10	+	5	−	2	=	13
	2	+	7	−	1	=	8
Column Totals	12	+	12	−	3	=	21

3. *Accounts Receivable (A/R) Control.* This box simply adds the previous day's A/R balance to the current day's totals to include the current day's business and arrive at the new A/R total.

   a. The column A and column B totals are carried straight across from the Proof of Posting box to the corresponding blanks in the A/R Control box.

   b. Add the amount already entered in the Previous Day's Total space to the Column A amount to arrive at a subtotal.

   c. Subtract the amount carried over from the "Less Columns B_1 and B_2" box to find the new A/R amount. RATIONALE: Determines new accounts receivable balance.

4. *A/R Proof* verifies, or proves, the A/R balance in the A/R Control box. *The figure entered on the first line of this box will not change during a calendar month* because it shows how much the A/R balance was on the first working day of the month. *All other figures entered will be taken from the "Month-To-Date" column boxes.*

   a. Enter the amount from column A (month-to-date) where shown.

   b. Add the column A amount to the "A/R 1st of Month" figure and enter the sum in the subtotal space.

   c. Enter the B_1 and B_2 month-to-date amounts and subtract from the subtotal. This amount goes in the Total A/R space.

(continues)

Procedure 17-2 (continued)

If all posting and addition are correct, the Total A/R amounts in the A/R Control and A/R Proof boxes will match and the day is balanced. RATIONALE: Verifies the accounts receivable balance in the accounts receivable control box.

5. *Deposit verification* involves totaling the columns in Section 2 and entering the sum of the columns in the space marked "Total Deposit." NOTE: The Total Deposit and the Total of Payments Received in column B₁ should match. RATIONALE: Verifies deposit total.

6. *Business Analysis Summary.* If this section is used, total each column in the summary section. NOTE: If the Business Analysis Summary is used to break out charges by type or by physician, the sum of the columns should equal today's column A total. If it is used to credit payments to different physicians, the sum of the columns will equal today's payment column. RATIONALE: The total deposit and the total of payments received in column B₁ should match to prove totals.

7. *After the day sheet is balanced,* there is one step remaining: the transfer of balances.
   a. Take out a new day sheet for the next day.
   b. Transfer the "Month-To-Date" column totals to the "Previous Page" columns boxes on the new sheet.
   c. Enter the Total A/R amount from the last day sheet in the "Previous Day's Total" space of the A/R Control box on the new day sheet.
   d. Enter the A/R 1st of Month Amount in the A/R Proof box on the new sheet. RATIONALE: Transfers balances to prepare a new day sheet for the next day's activities.

The new day sheet is now ready for posting.

Procedure 17-3   Preparing a Deposit

PURPOSE:
To create a deposit slip for the day's receipts.

EQUIPMENT/SUPPLIES:
New deposit slip
Check endorsement stamp
Calculator
Cash and checks received for the day

PROCEDURE STEPS:
1. Separate all checks from currency (paper money). RATIONALE: Each must be entered as a separate total.
2. Count all currency to be deposited and enter the amount in the space provided. Gather bills facing the same direction in order (i.e., 50s, 20s, 10s, and so on). RATIONALE: Follows bank procedure.
3. Count all coins to be deposited and enter the amount in the space provided. Coins may need to be wrapped. RATIONALE: Follows bank procedure.
4. On the back of the deposit slip list each check separately. Include the patient name in the left-hand column and enter the amount of the check in the right-hand column. RATIONALE: Follows bank procedure.
5. Total the checks listed and copy the total on the front where it is indicated to place the total from the other side. RATIONALE: Follows bank procedure.

(continues)

Procedure 17-3 (continued)

6. The sum of currency, coins, and checks should always equal the total in the Payments column on that day's day sheet. RATIONALE: Proof of accuracy.
7. Attach the top copy of the deposit slip to the deposit, leaving the carbon on the pad. RATIONALE: Provides the office and bank with record of deposit.
8. Enter the date and amount of the deposit in the space provided on the checkbook stubs. RATIONALE: Keeps checkbook register current with money in account.

9. Add the amount of the deposit to the checkbook balance. RATIONALE: Keeps checkbook register current with money in account.
10. Deposit at the bank, either in person or at the night deposit. In either case, be sure a record of deposit is received (it will be mailed if the night deposit is used). It is not recommended that deposits be made through ATMs; currency should never be deposited in an ATM. RATIONALE: Proof bank processed the deposit as indicated.

Procedure 17-4 Reconciling a Bank Statement

PURPOSE:
To verify that the balance listed in the checkbook agrees with the balance shown by the bank.

EQUIPMENT/SUPPLIES:
Checkbook
Bank statement
Calculator

PROCEDURE STEPS:
1. Make sure the balance in the checkbook is current (all deposits and checks entered have been added or subtracted). RATIONALE: Ensures totals are accurate.
2. If there is a service charge listed on the statement, subtract that amount from the last balance listed in the checkbook. RATIONALE: Reconciles current balance.
3. In the checkbook, check off each check listed on the statement and verify the amount against the check stub. RATIONALE: Verifies accuracy.
4. In the checkbook, check off each deposit listed on the statement. RATIONALE: Verifies accuracy.

5. The back of the statement contains a worksheet to be used for balancing.
6. Copy the ending balance from the front of the statement to the area indicated on the back.
7. Go through the check stubs and list on the back of the statement in the area provided any checks that have not cleared and any deposits that were not shown as received on the statement.
8. Total the checks not cleared on the statement worksheet.
9. Total the deposits not credited on the worksheet.
10. Add together the statement balance and the total of deposits not credited.
11. Subtract the total of checks not cleared. This amount should agree with the balance in the checkbook. If so, the checkbook is balanced and the statement should be filed in the appropriate place. RATIONALE: Following procedure steps 5 through 11 completes verification of accuracy.

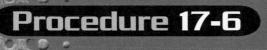

Procedure 17-5 Balancing Petty Cash

PURPOSE:
To verify that the amount of petty cash is consistent with the beginning amount less expenditures shown on receipts.

EQUIPMENT/SUPPLIES:
Petty cash box with cash balance
Vouchers
Calculator

PROCEDURE STEPS:
1. Count the money remaining in the box. RATIONALE: Verifies amount of cash and coin remaining in petty cash.
2. Total the amounts of all vouchers in the petty cash box. RATIONALE: Determines amount of expenditures.
3. Subtract the amount of receipts from the original amount in petty cash. This should equal the amount of cash remaining in the box. RATIO-

NALE: Proves that the amount of expenditures deducted from the beginning amount equals the amount left in the box.
4. When the cash has been balanced against the receipts, write a check *only for the amount that was used.* RATIONALE: Brings dollar amount back to original petty cash amount.

PETTY CASH CHECK DISBURSEMENT:
1. Sort all vouchers by account.
2. On a sheet of paper list the accounts involved.
3. Total vouchers for each account and record individual totals on the list.
4. Copy this list with its totals on the memo portion of the stub for the check written to replenish petty cash.
5. File the list with the vouchers and receipts attached, after noting the check number on the list.

Procedure 17-6 Recording a Nonsufficient Funds Check

PURPOSE:
To perform bookkeeping functions that keep account in proper balance.

EQUIPMENT/SUPPLIES:
The practice's account balance
Manual day sheet or computerized practice account
Manual ledger or computerized patient account
Nonsufficient funds (NSF) check

PROCEDURE STEPS:
1. Follow the office policy for notifying the patient of the returned check. RATIONALE: Policy may vary from clinic to clinic.
2. When the NSF check has been returned the second time, deduct the check amount from the account balance of the practice. RATIONALE:

The funds can no longer be counted as earnings received.
3. Add the amount of the NSF check back into the patient's computerized account or ledger. Place the amount in parentheses in the paid column and increase the total by the same amount. (In the *manual system,* the entry and math is performed by the medical assistant. In a *computerized system,* once the amount is entered as NSF, the computer correctly adds the amount in the patient's account and creates a new total.) RATIONALE: The amount is still owed by the patient, is not considered paid, and must be reflected in the amount due.
4. Place a brief explanation in the description of the column such as "NSF 12/09/XX."

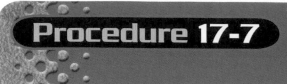

Procedure 17-7 Taking Inventory and Ordering Supplies

PURPOSE:
To perform an inventory of supplies used in the clinic and order needed supplies.

EQUIPMENT/SUPPLIES:
A computer
List of supplies kept in the clinic
3-ring binder
Clipboard
Paper/pen
Procedure manual

PROCEDURE STEPS:

1. Using a list of all supplies used in the various areas within the clinic, check the amounts needed on hand with the amounts currently on hand in each area. RATIONALE: This will give you the amount you will need to order to maintain required numbers of supplies on hand.

2. Check the clipboard for recently ordered supplies and remove them from the list of supplies needed. RATIONALE: This will prevent you from ordering supplies that have already been ordered but have not yet been received.

3. Write up purchase requisitions using a separate requisition for each supplier. RATIONALE: Each supplier needs a separate order sheet with costs and totals, and information specific to each supplier. This will also keep each order separate so accounts payable can be maintained properly.

4. On the purchase requisition, list the catalog number, the desciption of the item, the cost per container and the numbers of containers needed. RATIONALE: This will allow the supplier to see exactly what is being ordered. This step also allows for better tracking of supplies, especially if errors occur.

5. Then list the totals, add in the tax and shipping/handling. RATIONALE: Tax and handling is kept separate from the total cost of supplies so exact records can be maintained.

6. Give the completed requisition to the office manager (or person responsible for ordering supplies) keeping a copy in your inventory notebook noting the date. RATIONALE: Keeping a copy allows you to reference it readily should a question arise about the order.

Case Study 17-1

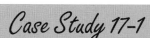

At the offices of Drs. Lewis and King, office manager Marilyn Johnson, CMA, is training a new administrative medical assistant in the practice's bookkeeping functions. The new medical assistant, Joann Crier, is a recent medical assistant graduate. This is her first position since graduating and earning her credentials. Joann has a basic interest in bookkeeping but wants Marilyn to instruct her, if possible, in the range of daily financial practices she may eventually be responsible for at Drs. Lewis and King's office.

CASE STUDY REVIEW

1. Suppose Marilyn were to give Joann a broad overview of every activity involved in Drs. Lewis and King's daily financial practices. What topic areas would she include?

2. Marilyn is knowledgeable about computerized bookkeeping systems. Joann is current in the use of computers as well. Drs. Lewis and King have asked Marilyn to investigate expanding the practice's computer system to include computerized medical records. How might Marilyn and Joann work together on this project?

3. Joann will be helping Marilyn with accounts payable. What does she need to know and what rules should she observe?

Case Study 17-2

Joann Crier has completed her three-month probation period with Drs. Lewis and King. She is doing quite well and has demonstrated skill in accurate financial documentation. She has been asked to take over reconciling the monthly bank statements and managing all the accounts payable, including getting the checks ready for the physician's signature. She has difficulty, however, completing these tasks until after hours when the office is closed and quiet. Marilyn Johnson has told her that it must be done within normal working hours unless special permission is granted.

CASE STUDY REVIEW

1. What suggestions can you make to Joann to allow her to complete these tasks during normal working hours?

2. What impact does the time of day, day(s) of the month, or place where the tasks are completed have on your suggestions?

3. Are there any circumstances you can identify when overtime might be warranted to allow Joann to complete the tasks after hours?

SUMMARY

In this chapter, we have discussed the daily financial duties in a medical office: patient bookkeeping, working with the checkbook, purchasing supplies and equiment, and petty cash. By becoming proficient in these functions, you will be prepared to handle the day-to-day financial aspects of any ambulatory care setting.

Patient bookkeeping involves not only a responsibility to the physician–employer (you are keeping track of income), but also to the patient, to be certain that charges for services rendered are correct and that payments are properly credited. The pegboard system is a comprehensive manual system to post and track these data. Computerized bookkeeping offers advantages of speed, high accuracy, and elimination of some routine tasks while providing the same important financial data.

It is also important to maintain a scrupulous accounts payable system to ensure that bills are paid on time and that payments are properly documented for tax purposes. To accomplish this, checks are prepared properly, prepared on time, and recorded to effectively track expenditures.

Whether working with a computerized system or a pegboard, accuracy is important at all times. To ensure maximum accuracy in all bookkeeping functions, observe a few rules: record all charges and receipts immediately; make deposits of checks and currency the same day they are received; always verify and recheck totals of all deposits and expenditures; stay current with all checking account duties such as account reconciliation; and be prompt with all accounts payable.

STUDY FOR SUCCESS

To reinforce your knowledge and skills of information presented in this chapter:
- ❏ Review the Key Terms
- ❏ Practice any Procedures
- ❏ Consider the Case Studies and discuss your conclusions
- ❏ Answer the Review Questions
  - ❏ Multiple Choice
  - ❏ Critical Thinking

- ❏ Navigate the Internet and complete the Web Activities
- ❏ Practice the StudyWARE activities on the textbook CD
- ❏ Apply your knowledge in the Student Workbook activities
- ❏ Complete the Web Tutor sections
- ❏ View and discuss the DVD situations

REVIEW QUESTIONS

Multiple Choice

1. "Usual" fee refers to:
   a. the fee based on the average charge for a specific procedure by all physicians practicing the same specialty in a defined geographic region
   b. the fee typically charged by a physician for certain procedures
   c. the midrange of fees charged for this procedure
   d. the fee based on the physician's decision

2. The use of debit/credit cards by patients to pay for services in ambulatory care settings is:
   a. never done
   b. unethical
   c. sure to compromise the integrity of the office
   d. a financial arrangement increasingly being used

3. The first section of the manual day sheet is used:
   a. to record deposits
   b. for business analysis
   c. to post individual transactions
   d. to total transactions

4. Good working habits for bookkeeping functions include:
   a. double-checking all entries for accuracy
   b. keeping the bookkeeping tasks current and up to date
   c. allowing the computer to create all the entries
   d. a and b

5. When moving from a manual to computerized bookkeeping system:
   a. expect to be up and running within a week
   b. the manual and computer systems may need to run concurrently for a month or two
   c. it is not necessary to understand manual bookkeeping systems
   d. accuracy will be assured in the computerized system

6. Encounter forms:
   a. may be ordered to fit the practice
   b. provide a separate ledger for each patient household
   c. list common services provided, procedural code, and diagnosis code
   d. a and c

7. Receipts:
   a. are used for payments on accounts
   b. are not given unless services are rendered the same day
   c. are mailed to patients when payment is made by mail
   d. are unnecessary, especially in the computerized system

8. When accepting checks from patients:
   a. Inspect for correct date, amount, and signature
   b. Immediately stamp with a restrictive endorsement
   c. Third-party checks are acceptable
   d. a and b

9. A check with an attached stub for recording information is called a:
   a. certified check
   b. cashier's check
   c. voucher check
   d. money order

10. It is important to ensure proper control over purchasing of supplies and equipment for the following reasons:
    a. to avoid purchase of unnecessary items
    b. to avoid duplication of items purchased
    c. to provide a system for payment of only those items properly ordered and received
    d. all of the above

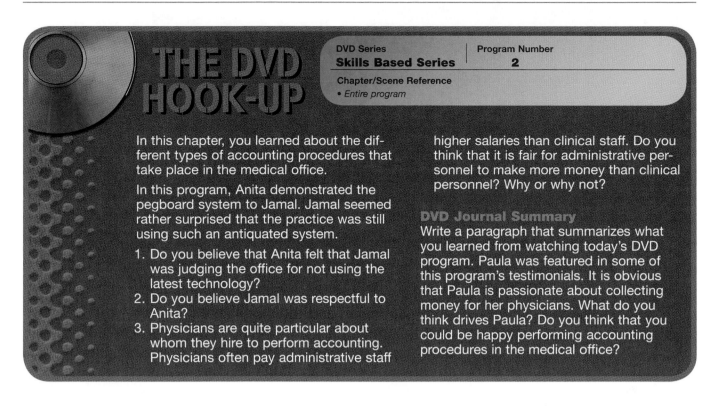

THE DVD HOOK-UP

In this chapter, you learned about the different types of accounting procedures that take place in the medical office.

In this program, Anita demonstrated the pegboard system to Jamal. Jamal seemed rather surprised that the practice was still using such an antiquated system.

1. Do you believe that Anita felt that Jamal was judging the office for not using the latest technology?
2. Do you believe Jamal was respectful to Anita?
3. Physicians are quite particular about whom they hire to perform accounting. Physicians often pay administrative staff higher salaries than clinical staff. Do you think that it is fair for administrative personnel to make more money than clinical personnel? Why or why not?

DVD Journal Summary

Write a paragraph that summarizes what you learned from watching today's DVD program. Paula was featured in some of this program's testimonials. It is obvious that Paula is passionate about collecting money for her physicians. What do you think drives Paula? Do you think that you could be happy performing accounting procedures in the medical office?

Critical Thinking

1. Discuss the types of checks identified in the text. Give an example of how each might be used or seen in the ambulatory care medical setting.
2. Check with a local bank or two to determine how after-hours deposits are made. Are any special supplies necessary? What is the bank's responsibility? What is the responsibility of the office staff?
3. When you reconcile the practice bank statement, you see that a check written almost 30 days ago to one of your supplier's has not been deposited. What course of action do you take, if any?
4. The manual bookkeeping system suggests that a consistent ink color always be used. What color would you choose? Why? Under what circumstances might it be appropriate to use pencil? When is red ink used? In this type of system, can the errors ever be erased? What do you do if an error is made?
5. Check for the current interest rates on both business regular savings and money market savings accounts. If you had $1,000 to keep in a liquid (quickly turned into cash) account for the practice, how much interest would you earn in one month through regular savings? Through money market savings?

WEB ACTIVITIES

1. Using your favorite search engine, search the Internet to determine how many medical or ambulatory care computerized bookkeeping systems might be available. A computerized system fairly close to the manual pegboard system is called Medi-Soft. What does your research tell you about their bar code data entry? Discuss the advantage or disadvantage of such an entry.
2. Research two other systems: MisysTiger and Soft-Aid. Identify key elements of each of these systems. Name a couple of reasons that it so difficult to select a particular system for a practice.
3. Browse the Colwell Professional Office Supply Web site (http://www.colwellsystems.com). This site provides many supplies necessary for bookkeeping systems. What do they offer as a product that could protect computer disks that will be generated by a computerized bookkeeping system? Describe what you are able to locate.

REFERENCES/BIBLIOGRAPHY

Fordney, M. T., French, L., & Follis, J. (2004). *Administrative medical assisting* (5th ed.). Clifton Park, NY: Thomson Delmar Learning.

CHAPTER 18

Medical Insurance

OUTLINE

OBJECTIVES

The student should strive to meet the following performance objectives and demonstrate an understanding of the facts and principles presented in this chapter through written and oral communication.

1. Define the key terms as presented in the glossary.
2. Define the terminology necessary to understand and submit medical insurance claims.
3. Recall at least five examples of medical insurance coverage and discuss their differences.
4. Recall the steps involved when screening patients for insurance.
5. Describe six primary managed care organization models.
6. Discuss the importance of obtaining referrals and pre-authorizations.

(continues)

KEY TERMS

(continues)

FEATURED
COMPETENCIES

CAAHEP—ENTRY-LEVEL
COMPETENCIES

Process Insurance Claims

- Apply managed care policies and procedures
- Apply third party guidelines
- Complete insurance claim
  forms

Legal Concepts

- Identify and respond to
  issues of confidentiality
- Perform within legal and
  ethical boundaries
- Document appropriately
- Demonstrate knowledge of
  federal and state health
  care legislation and
  regulations

Operational Functions

- Utilize computer software
  to maintain office
  systems

ABHES—ENTRY-LEVEL
COMPETENCIES

Professionalism

- Maintain confidentiality at
  all times
- Be cognizant of ethical
  boundaries
- Adapt to change

Communication

- Serve as liaison between
  physician and others
- Use appropriate medical
  terminology

(continues)

OBJECTIVES (continued)

7. Discuss legal and ethical issues related to medical insurance and
   the physician's office.
8. Discuss the impacts of HIPAA requirements related to insurance
   and the release of patient information.

SCENARIO

At Inner City Health Care, a multidoctor urgent care center in a large city, medical assistant Jane O'Hara, CMA, is responsible for all patient billing procedures. Inner City par-
ticipates in a number of insurance plans, so Jane must stay abreast of policy changes
regarding reimbursement, preauthorizations, and claims filing. She also tries to become
acquainted with the conditions of each patient's insurance coverage and helps patients
understand their responsibility, if any, for payment. Finally, Jane holds periodic meetings
with her assistants to update them; she continually stresses to them the importance of
timeliness in filing claims and the need for absolute accuracy in diagnosis and procedure codes, which must always reflect services actually performed.

FEATURED COMPETENCIES (continued)

- Receive, organize, prioritize, and transmit information expediently
- Application of electronic technology

Administrative Duties

- Perform basic secretarial skills
- Apply computer concepts for office procedures
- Apply managed care policies and procedures
- Obtain managed care referrals and pre-certification
- Complete insurance claim forms
- Use physician fee schedule

Legal Concepts

- Document accurately
- Use appropriate guidelines when releasing records or information
- Monitor legislation related to current healthcare issues and practices

Office Management

- Exercise efficient time management

Financial Management

- Analyze and use current third-party guidelines for reimbursement

In some ways, managed care coverage has simplified the patient's responsibility for payment, but it is more important than ever for the medical assistant to be accurate, timely, and conscientious in both filing insurance claim forms and understanding—and helping the patient to understand—the conditions of individual insurance policies.

The increasing complexity of health insurance today means that medical assistants must continually update their base of information. This chapter will provide the groundwork for understanding the role of insurance, its terminology, and its various forms, and it will give the medical assistant the confidence to take responsibility for claim filing in the ambulatory care setting.

UNDERSTANDING THE ROLE OF HEALTH INSURANCE

Health insurance was designed to help individuals and families compensate for the high costs of medical care. Medical care consists of the diagnosis of diseases/disorders and the care and treatment provided by the health care team of professionals to individuals who are ill or injured. Medical care, which also includes preventive services, is designed to help individuals avoid health or injury problems and is termed *health care*.

Health care insurance is a contract between an individual policyholder and a third-party or government program that reimburses the medical provider or the policyholder for medically necessary treatment or preventive care covered by that specific health care provider.

There is much discussion today about changes in the health care insurance industry. Foremost is the idea that

INTRODUCTION

An understanding of medical insurance and proper coding techniques is absolutely critical to the survival of the ambulatory care setting. In recent years, much has changed in medical insurance coverage: more patients are choosing health maintenance organizations (HMOs) and other managed care options, and even traditional insurance carriers such as Blue Cross and Blue Shield are modifying their insurance plans to include some aspect of managed benefits.

health care insurance should be available to all citizens of the United States. At this time, health insurance is usually tied to the employment package that covers the employee, and possibly the spouse and dependent children. One problem with work-related coverage is that some part-time employees are not eligible for health insurance, and thus often go uninsured. Another problem is if an employee takes a position elsewhere, medical benefits may not transfer equally. If a family member is ill with an ongoing disease such as cancer or diabetes mellitus, the new insurance policy may not cover that disease or condition for six months to one year. This is an **exclusion** known as a preexisting condition. Current changes in the law prevent insurance companies from penalizing a patient with a preexisting condition.

Another controversial aspect of health insurance is refusal to provide coverage for certain procedures because they are not sufficiently proven to be effective. In the early 1990s, bone marrow transplants were being performed on patients with breast cancer, at that time an experimental treatment for breast cancer. Because most insurance carriers will not extend coverage to experimental treatment, family and friends of patients often gathered for fund-raising drives to ensure that medical costs would be covered.

Not all insurance carriers cover the same exposures equally, and none of the carriers pays at the same rate. Similarly, not many of the carriers charge the same premiums to policyholders. Some insurance companies cover individuals, families, or employee groups through work or through groups such as American Association of Retired Persons (AARP). Some premiums reflect the insured person's past medical history and the company's exposure in covering the person. Premiums may be less if the insured person selects a higher annual deductible. Other premiums represent the rate that a group is able to obtain based on the group's claim history.

MEDICAL INSURANCE TERMINOLOGY

Before discussing the types of insurance coverage, one must understand the language used by the insurance industry. The terminology is specific in meaning and has been tested in courts of law to further define its meanings.

Terminology Specific to Insurance Policies

A policy is an agreement between the insurance company and the insured, or **beneficiary;** that is, the person covered under the terms of the policy. The insured

person may include as beneficiaries a spouse and dependent minor children; others may be included if related by blood and dependent on the insured for more than 50% of their support. The insurance carrier pays a percentage **(coinsurance)** of the cost of the services covered under the policy in exchange for a monthly premium or charge. This premium is paid by the insured or the employer, or it is shared by both.

At the inception or beginning of the policy, the insured is given an identification card, which must be presented before receiving medical treatment. This card contains the insured person's name, identification number, group number, and any co-payment amount or restrictions for treatment. The back of the insurance card contains an address where claims should be submitted and telephone numbers needed to receive prior authorization for treatment.

Deductible. The language of the policy spells out the terms of the coverage. Usually there is an annual **deductible,** or an amount of money that the insured must incur for medical services before the policy begins to pay. This deductible can range from $100 to $1,000, or an even greater amount depending on the language of the policy. The deductible must be met each year by medical charges that are incurred after the inception or anniversary date of the policy.

For instance, if Boris Bolski went to the physician on January 22 and incurred $258 in charges, but his policy did not go into effect until February 1, none of these charges would apply toward his deductible. If, however, he returned to the doctor on February 3 and incurred another $85, this amount could be applied against his deductible.

Coinsurance. After application of the deductible to the submitted bills, the insurance policy pays a percentage of the remaining amount. This percentage or coinsurance can vary from 50% to 100% depending on the language in a specific policy. Most traditional companies pay 80%.

Co-payment. Some insurance policies, especially **health maintenance organizations (HMOs)** and other managed care policies, require the patient to make a payment of a specified amount, for instance $5 or $10, at the time of treatment. This is usually done in place of a coinsurance being applied to the claim. This payment must be collected at the time of the office visit. Some policies have both a **co-payment** and a coinsurance clause.

Preexisting Condition. The earlier example of Boris Bolski presents another problem. If a person had an illness, disease, or injury before the inception of the insurance regardless of whether treatment was received, there is a good chance that most insurance policies will not cover any charges related to that specific illness, injury, or disease because it is considered a preexisting condition. Most policies have a specific waiting period before coverage is extended to those preexisting conditions. This waiting period can be a matter of months, years, or the lifetime of the policy. If the person had a previous insurance policy that was not as inclusive as the new policy, often the new policy would still consider this a preexisting condition and will deny payment until the waiting period is met. However, if the new policy has similar benefits and the person had no lapse in coverage, legally, the company must cover those conditions without applying a preexisting condition or waiting period to the policy.

Exclusions. Exclusions are noncovered services and are an important part of a policy. Some policies exclude elective procedures (procedures that are not medically necessary) such as cosmetic surgery, whereas other policies may allow some elective procedures. Other examples of exclusions or noncovered services might be preexisting conditions, dental services, chiropractic services, or routine eye examinations. Not every policy has the same exclusions.

Coordination of Benefits. When more than one policy covers an individual, the policy language provides for **coordination of benefits (COB).** This is determined by the policy language and coordinates payments between the policies so that the final total benefit is not greater than the original charge. Policy language again determines which of the two policies is primary or will pay first.

The employee's policy will pay first for the employee. For instance, if John O'Keefe is covered by an insurance policy where he works and is also covered by his wife's medical coverage, the policy Mr. O'Keefe gets from his employer will pay benefits first for him. The coverage under his spouse's policy will pay second because John is considered a dependent under that policy.

Whichever insurance is primary pays for their covered services up to the maximum allowed under the plan, less deductible and co-pay. The secondary insurance will coordinate the benefits and pay as appropriate, but never to exceed the total amount of the services. If the secondary insurance offers a COB, they will only consider the percentage paid as if they were primary; that is, Boris's $258 claim was allowed at 80% by both his primary and his secondary insurances. His primary insurance would pay $206.40, and if his secondary plan offered COB, they would pay 80% as well. Because $206.40 and $206.40 total $412.80, which is more than the total bill of $258, Boris's secondary insurance will pay the balance left by

the primary insurance, in this case, $51.60 (which may cover the co-pay, too). If Boris's secondary insurance does not offer COB, they would cover the same 80% the primary covered, and therefore would pay nothing. This is assuming that his deductibles have been satisfied.

The issue of which insurance is primary and which is secondary only applies when there are dependents covered under two policies. In this case, the **birthday rule** usually applies. When children of married parents are covered under both parents' policies, often, the birthday rule will be used to determine which policy is primary. This rule simply states that the policy of the parent with the birthday falling earlier in the year is primary. Thus, if the father's birthday is October 17 and the mother's birthday is May 12, the mother's policy will be primary. The year of the birth date is not relevant.

If the parents share the same birthday, then the policy with the earlier inception date is primary. If John and Mary both have birthdays on July 12, and the policy for John started August 1, 2004, and the policy for Mary started December 1, 2003, Mary's policy would be primary for their dependent children.

For children of divorced parents who are covered under both parents' policies, the policy of the custodial parent is usually primary unless divorce papers stipulate which parent is responsible.

Terminology Specific to Billing Insurance Carriers

There is specific terminology that one must understand when submitting insurance claims for medical benefits. Most ambulatory care settings will bill all appropriate insurance carriers to ascertain that the claim is made and the physician receives payment.

Many policies require **preauthorization** before certain procedures or before a visit can be made to a specialist or even a physical therapist. In these cases, the medical assistant must contact the insurance carrier with all of the diagnosis information and the proposed course of treatment. For instance, in a patient with a diagnosis of cholecystitis, preauthorization requires notification and approval before referring that patient to a surgeon for possible cholecystectomy. If this is not done, the surgery may not be covered.

A claim occurs when patients, having received treatment, wish to receive reimbursement under their insurance policies for charges for treatment. The patient (or the center's billing office) sends the claim to the insurance carrier for the amount of the treatment. This is done via a claim form, the most common of which is the CMS-1500 (12-90) (Figure 18-1). This form was formerly known as the HCFA-1500 and was managed by the

PLEASE
DO NOT
STAPLE
IN THIS
AREA

| | PICA | | | | | **HEALTH INSURANCE CLAIM FORM** | PICA | |

| 1. MEDICARE | MEDICAID | CHAMPUS | CHAMPVA | GROUP HEALTH PLAN | FECA BLK LUNG | OTHER | 1a. INSURED'S I.D. NUMBER | (FOR PROGRAM IN ITEM 1) |
| (Medicare #) | (Medicaid #) | (Sponsor's SSN) | (VA File #) | (SSN or ID) | (SSN) | (ID) | | |

2. PATIENT'S NAME (Last Name, First Name, Middle Initial)

3. PATIENT'S BIRTH DATE
MM   DD   YY   SEX   M   F

4. INSURED'S NAME (Last Name, First Name, Middle Initial)

5. PATIENT'S ADDRESS (No., Street)

6. PATIENT RELATIONSHIP TO INSURED
Self   Spouse   Child   Other

7. INSURED'S ADDRESS (No., Street)

CITY | STATE

8. PATIENT STATUS
Single   Married   Other
Employed   Full-Time Student   Part-Time Student

CITY | STATE

ZIP CODE | TELEPHONE (Include Area Code) ( )

ZIP CODE | TELEPHONE (INCLUDE AREA CODE) ( )

9. OTHER INSURED'S NAME (Last Name, First Name, Middle Initial)

10. IS PATIENT'S CONDITION RELATED TO:

11. INSURED'S POLICY GROUP OR FECA NUMBER

a. OTHER INSURED'S POLICY OR GROUP NUMBER

a. EMPLOYMENT? (CURRENT OR PREVIOUS)
YES   NO

a. INSURED'S DATE OF BIRTH
MM   DD   YY   SEX   M   F

b. OTHER INSURED'S DATE OF BIRTH
MM   DD   YY   SEX   M   F

b. AUTO ACCIDENT?   PLACE (State)
YES   NO

b. EMPLOYER'S NAME OR SCHOOL NAME

c. EMPLOYER'S NAME OR SCHOOL NAME

c. OTHER ACCIDENT?
YES   NO

c. INSURANCE PLAN NAME OR PROGRAM NAME

d. INSURANCE PLAN NAME OR PROGRAM NAME

10d. RESERVED FOR LOCAL USE

d. IS THERE ANOTHER HEALTH BENEFIT PLAN?
YES   NO   *If yes*, return to and complete item 9 a-d.

READ BACK OF FORM BEFORE COMPLETING & SIGNING THIS FORM.
12. PATIENT'S OR AUTHORIZED PERSON'S SIGNATURE I authorize the release of any medical or other information necessary to process this claim. I also request payment of government benefits either to myself or to the party who accepts assignment below.

SIGNED _____ DATE _____

13. INSURED'S OR AUTHORIZED PERSON'S SIGNATURE I authorize payment of medical benefits to the undersigned physician or supplier for services described below.

SIGNED _____

14. DATE OF CURRENT:
MM   DD   YY
ILLNESS (First symptom) OR INJURY (Accident) OR PREGNANCY(LMP)

15. IF PATIENT HAS HAD SAME OR SIMILAR ILLNESS. GIVE FIRST DATE   MM   DD   YY

16. DATES PATIENT UNABLE TO WORK IN CURRENT OCCUPATION
MM   DD   YY   MM   DD   YY
FROM   TO

17. NAME OF REFERRING PHYSICIAN OR OTHER SOURCE

17a. I.D. NUMBER OF REFERRING PHYSICIAN

18. HOSPITALIZATION DATES RELATED TO CURRENT SERVICES
MM   DD   YY   MM   DD   YY
FROM   TO

19. RESERVED FOR LOCAL USE

20. OUTSIDE LAB? $ CHARGES
YES   NO

21. DIAGNOSIS OR NATURE OF ILLNESS OR INJURY. (RELATE ITEMS 1,2,3 OR 4 TO ITEM 24E BY LINE)
1. |___.___| 3. |___.___|
2. |___.___| 4. |___.___|

22. MEDICAID RESUBMISSION CODE   ORIGINAL REF. NO.

23. PRIOR AUTHORIZATION NUMBER

24. A						B	C	D		E	F	G	H	I	J	K
DATE(S) OF SERVICE						Place of Service	Type of Service	PROCEDURES, SERVICES, OR SUPPLIES (Explain Unusual Circumstances)		DIAGNOSIS CODE	$ CHARGES	DAYS OR UNITS	EPSDT Family Plan	EMG	COB	RESERVED FOR LOCAL USE
From			To					CPT/HCPCS	MODIFIER							
MM	DD	YY	MM	DD	YY											
1																
2																
3																
4																
5																
6																

25. FEDERAL TAX I.D. NUMBER   SSN EIN

26. PATIENT'S ACCOUNT NO.

27. ACCEPT ASSIGNMENT? (For govt. claims, see back)
YES   NO

28. TOTAL CHARGE $

29. AMOUNT PAID $

30. BALANCE DUE $

31. SIGNATURE OF PHYSICIAN OR SUPPLIER INCLUDING DEGREES OR CREDENTIALS (I certify that the statements on the reverse apply to this bill and are made a part thereof.)

SIGNED _____ DATE _____

32. NAME AND ADDRESS OF FACILITY WHERE SERVICES WERE RENDERED (If other than home or office)

33. PHYSICIAN'S, SUPPLIER'S BILLING NAME, ADDRESS, ZIP CODE & PHONE #

PIN#   GRP#

(APPROVED BY AMA COUNCIL ON MEDICAL SERVICE 8/88)   *PLEASE PRINT OR TYPE*

APPROVED OMB-0938-0008 FORM CMS-1500 (12/90),   FORM RRB-1500,
APPROVED OMB-1215-0055 FORM OWCP-1500,   APPROVED OMB-0720-0001 (CHAMPUS)

CARRIER | PATIENT AND INSURED INFORMATION | PHYSICIAN OR SUPPLIER INFORMATION

Figure 18-1 CMS-1500 claim form (revised 12-90).

Health Care Financing Administration (HCFA). The **Centers for Medicare and Medicaid Services (CMS)** is a Federal agency within the U.S. Department of Health and Human Services (DHHS). This agency administers Medicare, Medicaid, and the State Children's Health Insurance Program (SCHIP), Health Insurance Portability and Accountability Act of 1996 (HIPAA), and Clinical Laboratory Improvement Act (CLIA).

The completed claim form is sent to the insurance carrier either by mail, electronically, or through a holding system that batches and transmits claims at timed daily intervals. The most common and expeditious method for submitting claims is electronically. Depending on the policy language and the **assignment of benefits,** payment is sent either directly to the physician (known as direct payment) or to the patient/insured but payable to both the insured and the physician (known as indirect payment).

TYPES OF MEDICAL INSURANCE COVERAGE

In today's health care environment, medical assistants will need to be aware of the different types of medical insurance policies.

Traditional Insurance

Traditional insurance provides coverage on a fee-for-service basis. There is usually a deductible and a co-payment or coinsurance amount. The health care provider submits bills to the insurance carrier, and after any deductible has been met, the health care provider or the patient, if the patient has already satisfied the bill, is paid in agreement with the terms of the insurance policy. The patient may be responsible for fees in excess of the contracted amount if the health care provider is not a preferred or participating provider. In the case of a preferred or participating provider, the health care provider has agreed to a discounted fee for different types of procedures performed on patients insured by the carrier. The provider then writes off the difference, and the patient is not responsible for that amount.

Traditional insurance is sometimes marketed as two types depending on the coverage. Basic insurance covers specific dollar amounts for physician's fees, hospital care, surgery, and anesthesia. Generally, they will not cover examinations to diagnose or treat fertility problems; but more carriers are covering routine physical and preventive care. Major medical insurance covers catastrophic expenses resulting from illness or injury.

Some traditional insurance carriers and most managed care insurance carriers require the patient to select

a **primary care physician** or **PCP.** The PCP becomes the first medical practitioner caring for the patient, also known as the gatekeeper, and is responsible for making referrals for further treatment by specialists or for hospital admission. The insurance carrier frequently will refuse payment for treatments not referred by the PCP.

Blue Cross and Blue Shield (BC/BS).

Whereas many traditional policies are offered by commercial carriers, the "Blues" are a well-known type of traditional, or independent, health insurance. Blue Cross was originally established to cover the cost of hospital admission and stay, radiology, and other basic coverage under the health plan. Blue Shield covered the major medical portion, picking up physicians' fees, medications, and other charges not covered on the basic portion of the plan. Today, both entities offer a full range of health care coverage. BC/BS plans are locally based in all 50 states, the District of Columbia, Canada, Puerto Rico, and Jamaica. They function independently in their own service area and are flexible enough to meet and satisfy the needs of the local community. They may be organized as not-for-profit corporations or as for-profit companies.

A BC/BS participating provider (PAR) chooses to sign a member contract and receives an incentive. PARs agree to accept the BC/BS reimbursement as payment in full for covered services because all PARs accept assignment. BC/BS agrees to reimburse providers directly and in a shorter turnaround time.

Each policyholder is given a card with the subscriber's name and a three-character letter prefix identification number. The letter prefix is important because it indicates under which BC/BS plan the person is insured. This identification number must be included on each claim form submitted to BC/BS; if it is not included, the claim will be denied.

Managed Care Insurance

Managed Care Insurance involves a **Managed Care Organization (MCO)** that assumes the responsibility for the health care needs of a group of enrollees. The MCO can be a health care plan, hospital, physician group, or health system. The MCO contracts with an insurance carrier, or is itself the carrier, to take care of the medical needs of the enrolled group for a fixed fee per enrollee for a fixed period, usually a calendar year. This payment system is called **capitation.** If the medical costs exceed the fixed fee, the MCO/provider loses income; conversely, if the costs are less than the fixed fee, the MCO/provider makes a profit. An MCO relies on as large an enrollee base as possible to average the cost of medical care.

MCOs were established in an attempt to curb medical costs and provide for more efficient use of medical resources. Almost all MCOs use PCPs as case managers or utilization management services to control what medical resources are used for each patient and to strictly control treatment plans and discharge planning. This policy has led to disputes over quality of care, and many states have enacted laws requiring external quality reviews by independent organizations. The quality-control programs include government oversight, patient satisfaction surveys, review of grievances, measurement of the health status of the enrolled group, and reviews by accreditation agencies. Medicare has established measurable standards for MCOs through its program, Quality Improvement System for Managed Care (QISMC). The federal government requires physicians to disclose incentive packages with MCOs to avoid conflict of interests resulting in reduced level of care solely for the purpose of reducing costs or treatment, thus recognizing a profit at the expense of patient care.

Six models exist for managed cared organizations. They are:

1. **Exclusive Provider Organizations (EPOs).** Enrollees must obtain their medical services from a network of physicians or health care facilities that are under exclusive contract to the EPO. The state insurance commissioner regulates EPOs.

2. **Integrated delivery systems (IDSs).** Enrollees obtain medical services from an affiliated group of service providers. The service providers consist of private practices and hospitals that share practice management and services to reduce overhead. An IDS may also be called one of the following: integrated service network, delivery system, horizontally integrated system, vertically integrated system or plan, health delivery network, and accountable health plan.

3. HMO. Enrollees obtain medical services from a network of providers who agree to fixed fees for services but are not under exclusive contract to the insurance carrier.

4. **Point-of-Service (POS) Plan.** The enrollee has the freedom of obtaining medical services from an HMO provider or by self-referral to non-HMO providers. In the case of self-referral, the enrollee will have to pay greater deductibles and coinsurance charges.

5. **Preferred Provider Organization (PPO).** Enrollees obtain services from a network of physicians and hospitals that have contracted their services at a discounted fee to an insurance company on a nonexclusive basis.

6. **Triple Option Plan.** Enrollees have the option of traditional, HMO, or PPO health plans.

See Table 18-1 for differences between traditional and managed care policies.

Medicare Insurance

Medicare Insurance is the largest medical insurance program in the United States. Most individuals 65 years and older, individuals with a disability that keeps them from working, and individuals with chronic kidney disease are eligible for Medicare. The two most common parts to Medicare coverage are: **Medicare Part A** and **Medicare Part B.**

Medicare Part A covers hospital admission and stay, home health care, and hospice care. It has a substantial deductible and a limit to the number of hospital days per stay and the total number of hospitalizations per year. Medicare Part A pays only a portion of a patient's hospital expenses, and the patient's out-of-pocket expenses are calculated on a benefit period basis. A benefit period begins with the first day of hospital stay and ends when the patient has been out of the hospital for 60 consecutive days. Many individuals subscribe to supplemental insurance (called Medigap policies) to cover the substantial deductible.

Individuals not yet 65 years old who already receive retirement benefits from Social Security, the Railroad Retirement Board, or disability are automatically enrolled in Part A and Part B effective the month of their 65th birthday. Three months before their 65th birthday, or the 24th month of disability, individuals are sent an initial enrollment package containing information about Medicare and a Medicare card. If both Medicare Parts A and B

TABLE 18-1   DIFFERENCES BETWEEN TRADITIONAL AND MANAGED CARE POLICIES

Traditional	Managed Care
Usually can go outside physician network	Usually must stay inside physician network
Coinsurance	Co-pay each visit
Annual deductible	No annual deductible
Illness or injury only	Preventive treatment, as well as illness and injury
Premium paid monthly to company by employer or subscriber	Premium paid monthly to company by employer or subscriber
M.D. paid by fee for service	Physician paid by capitation

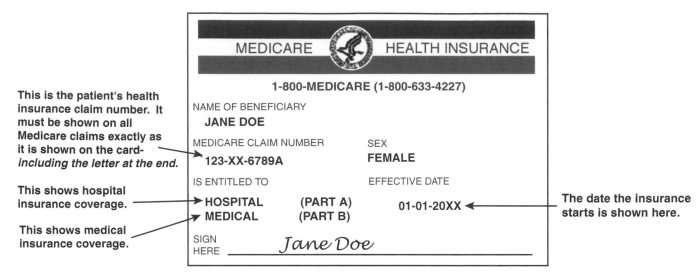

This is the patient's health insurance claim number. It must be shown on all Medicare claims exactly as it is shown on the card—*including the letter at the end.*

This shows hospital insurance coverage.

This shows medical insurance coverage.

The date the insurance starts is shown here.

MEDICARE   HEALTH INSURANCE

1-800-MEDICARE (1-800-633-4227)

NAME OF BENEFICIARY
JANE DOE

MEDICARE CLAIM NUMBER   SEX
123-XX-6789A   **FEMALE**

IS ENTITLED TO   EFFECTIVE DATE
HOSPITAL   (PART A)   01-01-20XX
MEDICAL   (PART B)

SIGN
HERE   *Jane Doe*

Figure 18-2   Medicare health insurance card.

are desired, they simply sign the Medicare card and keep it in a safe place for use when needed. Figure 18-2 shows a sample Medicare card.

Medicare Part B covers outpatient expenses that include physicians' fees, physical therapy, laboratory tests, radiologic studies, ambulance services, and charges for durable medical equipment. Durable medical equipment includes items such as canes, crutches, walkers, commode chairs, blood glucose monitors, and so on. Part B does not cover medications *except* certain diabetic testing supplies.

Currently, the patient must pay an annual deductible of $110 before Medicare Part B will begin to pay its share of the bills. Medicare then reimburses 80% of the Medicare fee schedule for medical care and 100% for laboratory fees. Medicare's fee schedule was adopted in 1992 and is based on the **resource-based relative value scale (RBRVS).** The RBRVS was developed using values for each medical and surgical procedure based on work, prac-

tice, and malpractice expenses and factoring for regional differences.

Example #1 shows how the Medicare worksheet would look if there were no exclusions or deductions.

Example #1:	
Office visit	$ 75.00
Return visit	+ 50.00
Total Charges	$125.00
Less deductible	−110.00
Subtotal	$ 15.00
Apply 80% coinsurance	× 80%
Insurance Payment	$ 12.00
Patient Owes	$ 3.00

Medical service providers can elect to accept Medicare fee schedules and be a PAR, or they may accept assignment on a case-by-case basis as a nonparticipating provider (non-PAR). Billing of Medicare is done through the regional carrier that is selected by a competitive bidding process. Medical providers are required to bill Medicare as a service to the patient. The regional carrier will file claims with supplemental insurers for PARs, but non-PARs must file claims with the supplemental insurer. The patient cannot be billed for the difference between the charged fee and the Medicare allowed fee. Physicians can drop out of Medicare and enter into a contract with their Medicare patients that allows them to charge what they wish for services, but they must not bill Medicare for any services for the

Critical Thinking

A patient has an office visit and is seen by the physician. The charge for the visit is $125. An insurance claim form is submitted to the local Medicare **fiscal intermediary** to apply against the deductible. At the next visit, the bill is $75. This bill also is submitted to Medicare. How much of the bill will insurance pay after the deductible has been subtracted? How much does the patient owe?

next two years, except in cases of emergency or urgent care. See Example #2.

Example #2:

	Total Charges	Allowed Charges
Office visit	$ 75.00	$ 70.00
Return visit	+ 50.00	+ 45.00
Total Charges	$125.00	$115.00
Less deductible	−110.00	−110.00
Subtotal	$ 15.00	$ 5.00
Apply 80% coinsurance	× 80%	× 80%
Insurance Payment	$ 12.00	$ 4.00
Patient Owes	$ 3.00	$ 1.00*

*(or $11.00 if physician does not accept assignment)

A Medicare + Choice Program (Medicare Part C) was instituted in 1997 and allows a choice of managed care programs. Individuals with Medicare Part C have cards identifying their status. The medical office should always ask to see the patient's Medicare card to verify coverage and effective dates. The type of plan coverage affects billing procedures.

Medicare Supplemental Insurance

Medicare Supplemental Insurance is a secondary insurance that covers Medicare deductibles, coinsurance requirements, and additional procedures not covered by Medicare. It is purchased by the patient through an insurance carrier or is provided as part of an employee retirement package. Supplemental **Medigap policies** are filed with the carrier by the Medicare regional carrier. The regional carrier is not required to file claims for employee retirement plan supplemental packages on behalf of the patient. Supplemental insurance frequently

requires the patient to seek treatment with specific providers and hospitals. Different programs have different coverage, which is dependent on the carrier and state requirements and should be determined when scheduling an appointment.

Medicaid Insurance

Medicaid Insurance covers medical care for certain qualifying low-income individuals. It is funded by the federal government and is administered by each state's department of Supplemental Security Income (SSI). Pregnant single women with income below the poverty level; those who cannot work because of emotional, mental, or physical difficulties; and people who are on Aid to Families with Dependent Children qualify for this program. Recipients will have an identification card for the program. Not all physicians accept Medicaid patients. When referring a patient to a specialist or another provider, it is wise to ascertain whether that provider accepts Medicaid patients. A referral form prepared by the PCP or referring physician usually is required.

Because Medicaid is always secondary to any supplemental insurance, billings to Medicaid are considered only after all other insurance payments have been made. When a person has both Medicare and Medicaid, charges are submitted first to Medicare and last to Medicaid.

 Both Medicare and Medicaid are federal programs, and errors in billing could be construed as fraud, for which there are criminal penalties. It is therefore imperative that all billing practices conform to the legal requirements of these programs.

TRICARE

TRICARE, formerly the Civilian Health and Medical Program for Uniformed Services (CHAMPUS), is medical insurance for dependents of active-duty military personnel, retired military personnel, dependents of retired military personnel, and dependents of personnel who died while on active duty. Three TRICARE options are available: HMO type, PPO type, and fee for service. All military clinics and hospitals are part of the TRICARE program and offer high-quality health care at lower rates to their subscribers.

Qualifying subscribers must be listed in the Defense Department's Defense Enrollment Eligible Reporting System (DEERS). The patient will have an identification card for the program. TRICARE claims are submitted to a regional TRICARE contractor similar to the Medicare regional carrier. A referral generally is required. There are 11 TRICARE regions (see Figure 18-3).

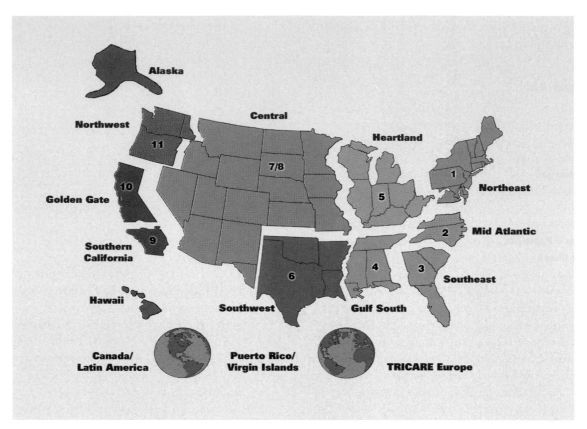

Figure 18-3 TRICARE regional map.

Civilian Health and Medical Program of the Veterans Administration

Civilian Health and Medical Program of the Veterans Administration (CHAMPVA) is medical insurance for spouses and unmarried dependent children of a veteran with permanent total disability resulting from a service-related injury and also the surviving spouse and children of a veteran who died of a service-related disability. The patient will have an identification card for the program. The program is administered by the Health Administration Center in Denver, Colorado.

Workers' Compensation Insurance

Workers' Compensation Insurance is medical and paycheck insurance for workers who sustain injuries associated with their employment. In some instances, the insurance covers family members in the case of death of the worker. The employer usually pays the premium to the state or an insurance carrier designated by the state. Some large employers assume the insurance risk and are self-insured. Federal and state laws define minimum standards for Workers' Compensation programs.

Workers' Compensation covers 100% of associated medical expenses. Claims are filed with the insurance carrier. Although most workers are insured under state programs, federal programs exist for the following specific groups:

- Office Workers' Compensation Programs (OWCP)
- Energy Workers' Occupational Illness Compensation Program
- Federal Black Lung Program
- Federal Employees' Compensation Act Program (FECA)
- Longshore and Harbor Workers' Compensation Program
- Mine Safety and Health Administration (MSHA)

Self-Insurance

Large companies, nonprofit organizations, and governments frequently use **self-insurance** to reduce costs and gain more control of their finances. Each self-insured plan will differ in coverage and claim filing requirements. The plan administrator should be contacted before scheduling a patient appointment.

SCREENING FOR INSURANCE

It is the responsibility of the medical assistant to screen all new patients for their insurance. New patients should be asked to arrive 15 to 20 minutes earlier than their appointment time to complete a patient registration form. The form requests vital information that enables the medical office to contact the patient, process their billing and insurance claims, know who to contact in case of emergency, authorize payment of insurance benefits, and record method of payment. Commercial forms are available for purchase or may be designed by office management personnel for this purpose.

The medical assistant will want to review each section of the patient registration form to verify that all information is complete and legible. Many offices make a photocopy of the patient's driver's license and attach it to the registration form. This procedure helps in identifying the correct person through photo identification should it be necessary. It is important to verify the spelling of all patient names: first, middle, and last.

Ask the patient to show their health insurance card and verify the effective date and pertinent information. Most offices will make a photocopy of both sides of the card to maintain in the patient's chart. In most cases, the back of the card contains information about any deductible, co-payment, and preapproval requirements, as well as the insurance company's name, address, and telephone number. It also shows any special claim submission instructions.

Each time a patient checks in, the medical assistant should ask questions to verify the following insurance information:

- Confirm the patient's current address.
- Confirm the patient's insurance carrier and plan.
- Ask for the patient's insurance card and verify information and effective dates.
- Determine if the insurance carrier covers the procedure.
- Determine that the patient's PCP is performing the procedure.
- Confirm whether a referral is required and whether an authorization number or authorization code is required. Confirm evidence of qualifying has been secured.
- Establish proof of eligibility.

When screening patients for insurance, it is important to understand the philosophy of the medical office. Some may see patients regardless of ability to pay; responsible medical assistants will investigate all avenues for reimbursement first. Some situations may include the patient who is eligible for Medicaid but has not yet applied, or the patient who has applied for Medicaid but has not yet received notification of qualification. See Procedure 18-1 for screening for insurance steps.

The medical assistant should investigate and verify that all avenues have been taken to achieve the proof of eligibility that the office will need to receive reimbursement from Medicaid. This may include calling the Medicaid office to verify eligibility, or going online and printing a proof of eligibility directly from the Medicaid system. This electronic data exchange system is called an envoy. Proof of eligibility cards are distributed to recipients and are in effect for at least one year. However, the most common avenue to ensure that services will be reimbursed is not to see any patient that does not have proof of Medicaid coverage. Medicaid sends their eligibility Medical Assistance Identification (MAID) (medical coupons) to the patient the first day of the month. This coupon guarantees the ambulatory care center payment for the services provided. Unless it is an emergency, some offices will not schedule Medicaid patients before the fifth of each month. This allows ample time for the beneficiary to receive the medical coupon. If the patient presents for their appointment without a medical coupon, and proof of eligibility cannot be determined elsewhere, it is common practice to have that patient reschedule the appointment. The exception would be in the instance of an emergency.

Medical assistants with responsibility for billing are one key to the success of a thriving ambulatory care center. Billing the insurance carriers promptly, completing claim forms properly, billing patients as needed, and keeping track of aging accounts will do much to ensure there is a flow of adequate income. In all insurance matters, be available to patients with questions regarding their insurance or accounts, because a friendly attitude helps patients feel positive about the care they receive and establishes a long-term relationship.

REFERRALS AND AUTHORIZATIONS

When their PCP refers a patient to a specialist, the term **referral** is used by managed care facilities. Referrals may be denied because of incomplete information contained on the referral form or because a medical necessity was not established. Referrals are generally categorized as one of three types:

- *Regular:* usually takes 3 to 10 working days to review procedures and approve
- *Urgent:* usually takes about 24 hours for approval
- *STAT:* may be approved via telephone after faxing the information to the utilization review department

The most common referral used by managed care plans is the regular referral. The Member Services department must be contacted to check the status of a referral. It is important to never tell the patient that the referral has been approved until you have obtained a hard copy of the *authorization* (a managed care term for approved referrals).

Preauthorizations or *precertification* are terms used to determine whether a service or procedure is covered and if the insurance plan approves it as medically necessary. Preauthorization is required for some services, hospital admissions, inpatient and outpatient surgeries, and most elective procedures. Once approved, an authorization number will be provided. The patient also receives a letter containing the authorization number and the approved services. The patient must take this letter with them and present it to the specialist's office on the day the service is provided.

When questions arise regarding preauthorization, precertification, or referral procedures, the medical assistant should call the plan's contact number for specific information. Many offices find it helpful to maintain a reference log regarding these requirements. Information to maintain includes:

- Name of the insurance plan
- Address and telephone number
- Name and telephone number of contact person or the person with whom you spoke
- Co-payment amount and deductible information
- Inpatient and outpatient surgery benefits
- Preauthorization requirements, second-opinion options
- Participating hospitals, radiology service providers, laboratories, and physicians

The authorization number and referral numbers are entered in Box 23 of the CMS-1500 form when billing for services.

DETERMINING FEE SCHEDULES

A physician charges for services using a variety of means for computing a fee schedule. Although all of the fee computation plans vary and give somewhat different results, they all have common elements. For example,

- *The overhead or practice expenses for the clinic or office.* This category includes rental of the physical building or office space and equipment; utilities; cost of medical supplies inventory; and salaries of nurses, medical assistants, bookkeepers, and other personnel who are paid on a salary or contract basis. It also includes cost of employee benefits such as retirement plans, sick leave, and vacation time.
- *The cost of medical malpractice insurance.* This is separated from general insurance, which is included in the preceding category, because of the significant portion of the fee attributed to this item and because it varies greatly for different types of services. OB/GYN procedures are probably the greatest for the entire medical community, including surgical procedures.
- *Hourly rate for the services provided by the physician.* This rate varies depending on the skill and training required for the procedure, the cost of living in the area, and the rate charged by other physicians in the area. (The law of supply and demand applies here as in any other economic arena.) Surgeons charge a greater rate than physicians in general practice, rates are greater in a metropolitan area than in a rural area, and experience level commands greater rates.

All of these cost elements are derived on an hourly basis. The sum of the above elements combined with the time required is used to arrive at the fee schedule for a procedure or service.

The advent of insurance plans, Medicare, and managed care plans has resulted in specific formulas being developed and accepted by the different plans to establish a fee schedule acceptable to the carrier. Several of the fee schedule systems in common usage are discussed in the following sections. All of them, however, incorporate the preceding three elements (practice expenses, malpractice expenses, and physician's experience).

Usual, Customary, and Reasonable Fees

Usual, Customary, and Reasonable (UCR) Fee Schedule is a fee system that defines allowable charges that will be accepted by insurance carriers. The actual rate may vary from one carrier to another, but the process is the same.

- Usual fee is the physician's average fee for a service or procedure. This fee is based on the economic analysis of the practice described earlier in this section.

- Customary fee is the average or range of fees within the geographic area that an insurance carrier will accept. It is frequently tied to a national average for a similar metropolitan or rural setting.

- Reasonable fee is the generally accepted fee for services or procedures that are extraordinarily difficult or complicated and require more time and effort by the physician.

An example of the operation of the UCR system is as follows: An insurance carrier operating on the UCR fee schedule may have determined a customary fee range for a new patient office visit with history and physical examination to be $140 to $225 for that region. If the amount billed by the physician were $160, the physician would be reimbursed for the service in full. Had the physician billed $250, the reimbursement would be $225, and the physician would have to write off the $25 nonallowed charge. Physicians who participate in UCR systems cannot bill the patient for the nonallowable charge.

Resource-Based Relative Value Scale (RBRVS)

Medicare has used the RBRVS since 1992. Under this system, physician's services are reimbursed based on relative value units (RVUs). Each service, procedure, or medication is assigned a code compiled from the *Current Procedural Terminology* (CPT) manual issued by the American Medical Association for procedures and the *International Classification of Diseases, 9th Revision, Clinical Modification* (ICD-9-CM) manual for diagnoses issued by the World

Health Organization. Medicare then issues three RVUs for each code in the *Medicare Fee Schedule* (MFS) manual issued each year on April 15. The RVUs are for physicians' work, practice expenses, and malpractice expenses. A geographic practice cost index (GPCI) related to the geographic area where the physician is located is issued for each RVU category. The GPCI is based on zip code for the address of the practice or wherever the service is performed. The payment for service is then established from the sum of the geographically adjusted RVUs multiplied by a nationally uniform conversion factor for services. The complex formula calculation is shown in Table 18-2.

Hospital Inpatient Prospective Payment System (IPPS)

The IPPS is a reimbursement system for hospitals based on similar diagnostically related groups (DRGs) of inpatients discharged. Rather than the traditional method of payment based on actual costs incurred in providing care, DRGs are based on an average cost for treatment of a patient's condition. The hospital is reimbursed for each discharge according to a predetermined rate for each DRG.

Hospital Outpatient Prospective Payment System (OPPS)

OPPS is a reimbursement system for hospital outpatients based on Ambulatory Payment Classifications (APCs), which group services according to similar clinical characteristics. Payments are established for each APC, and the hospital is reimbursed for each patient.

Capitation

Capitation is a payment system used primarily by managed care organizations. A fixed dollar amount is reimbursed to the provider for patients enrolled during a specific period.

TABLE 18-2	MEDICARE FORMULA FOR PAYMENT OF SERVICES				
Code	**Description of Procedure**	**Factor**	**Work**	**Overhead**	**Malpractice**
38206	Stem Cell Collection	RVU	1.5	0.67	0.06
		GPCI 2004	1.005	1.100	0.803
RVU Conversion Factor for 2004 is $37.34.					
Medicare Allowable =	[1.5 × 1.005 + work RVU × GPCI	0.67 × 1.100 + OH RVU × GPCI	0.06 × 0.803] × Malpractice RVU × GPCI	$37.34 = 2004 Factor	$85.61*

*Represents figures for a Seattle, Washington practice.

Critical Thinking

The purpose of this exercise is to understand how to determine the physician's fee by two different methods:
(1) RVU calculations, and (2) looking up in tables provided by the regional Medicare carrier. Determination of
RVU values and procedure code used in this exercise is explained in Chapter 19. Use the following factors to calculate the physician's fee billed to Medicare.

METHOD 1

Factor Procedure Code 11401	Work	Practice or Facility Overhead	Malpractice	Conversion Factor
RVU*	1.23	1.03	0.11	37.34
GCPI†	1.005	1.1	0.803	—

*Procedure performed in a facility.
†Values of GCPI for King County, Seattle, Washington 2004.

METHOD 2

Using the Internet, locate the Medicare regional carrier for the State of Washington following this procedure:

- Go to Medicare home page at http://www.medicare.gov.
- Select Medicare Billing, then select File a Claim.
- Select Helpful Contacts (from step 2).
- Select Carrier (Part B) (from step 1).
- Select state/territory: Washington.
- Go to the home page of the regional carrier: http://www.noridianmedicare.com.
- Enter as Provider.
- Accept proprietary agreement.
- Select from Current Publication Physician's Fee Schedule.
- Select year 2004.
- Select state Washington.
- Select King County—PDF Format.
- Look up Physician's Fee corresponding to Procedure Code 11401.

The fee generated by Method 2 should be the same as the fee calculated using Method 1.

The payment per patient is independent of services or
procedures provided to a patient. To be financially responsible, this system requires enrollment of a large number
of patients, so that a few patients do not unduly skew an
average cost. This type of system requires extensive practice of preventative medicine to be cost effective.

LEGAL AND ETHICAL ISSUES

Most Medicare claims are now submitted electronically,
and private payers in growing numbers are also using electronic claims submission. In a computerized system, everything related to billing and reimbursement is computerized
and transmitted electronically. If the office is participating
in CMA's Electronic Data Interchange (EDI), they will be
assigned a unique identifier number that constitutes their
legal electronic signature. Be cautious with this electronic
signature, because the office is responsible for any and all
claims made with it. The Health Insurance Portability and

Accountability Act (HIPAA) of 1996 (specifically title II,
subtitle F) regulates the security and privacy of transmitted health care information. Review HIPAA's regulations
in Chapters 11 and 15.

 Many legal and ethical issues related to insurance issues face the medical assistant on a daily
basis; therefore, it is important that each patient
be treated equally and fairly. As mentioned in Chapter
4, it is critical that patients not be stereotyped, regardless of whether they have multiple insurance plans or are
not covered by any insurance plan at all. Every patient
must be cared for objectively, with respect, and in a professional manner.

 Medical personnel are bound by law to maintain the confidentiality of all medical information and must be able to recognize information
that is protected by privacy rules and understand how it is
to be handled. Protected health information (PHI) may
be considered "individually identifiable health informa-

tion." This includes information that describes the health status of an individual, including basic demographics and the use of medical services, as well as information that either identifies, or can be used to identify, an individual. Medical personnel must remember that informed consent is not consent to use and disclose personal information.

HIPAA Implications

 HIPAA privacy requirements specifically address issues of confidentiality. These requirements include:

- Providing the patient with a notice of privacy practices form that outlines a provider's privacy practices, and obtaining the patient's acknowledgment of receipt of the notice

- Obtaining a patient's specific authorization to use or disclose personal information for purposes that are not covered by the consent

- Providing the patient, on request, with an accounting of disclosures of PHI

- Giving the patient access to his or her PHI and providing an opportunity to amend the information

Insurance Fraud and Abuse

 Insurance **fraud** and **abuse** are legal and ethical issues that must also be addressed. HIPAA defines fraud as "an intentional deception or misrepresentation that someone makes, knowing it is false, that could result in an unauthorized payment." Regardless of whether the attempt is successful, the act itself is considered fraud. Examples of fraudulent insurance activities include but are not limited to:

- Coding to a higher level of service to increase revenue

- Misrepresenting the diagnosis to justify payment

- Billing for services, equipment, or procedures that were never provided

- Receiving rebates or any type of compensation for referrals

Insurance abuse involves activities that are inconsistent with accepted business practices. Some examples of abuse include but are not limited to:

- Overcharging for services, equipment, or procedures

- Improper billing practices

- Violating participating provider agreements with insurance companies

Heavy penalties, including a $10,000 fine per claim form plus three times the fraudulent claim amount, may be sanctioned on individuals who knowingly and willfully misrepresent information submitted on insurance claim forms to gain greater payments or benefits.

To protect yourself and the medical practice from committing insurance fraud and abuse, you should begin by identifying risk areas based on errors in the past history of billing and insurance claims processing. Practice internal audits to monitor compliance with written protocols. Participate in seminars and in-service programs to keep current with coding and billing practices. Be sure to use only the current year's coding manuals to ensure accuracy. Code only what is documented in the medical record, and ask for clarification when needed.

 HIPAA regulations apply to PHI that is created, transmitted, received, or stored in an electronic form. The federal regulation uses the phrase "electronic PHI." Four legal obligations defined by the security rule under federal law for medical practices that are covered entities include:

- Ensure the confidentiality, integrity, and availability of electronic PHI.

- Protect against any reasonably anticipated threats or hazards to the security or integrity of such information.

- Protect against any reasonably anticipated uses or disclosures of such information that are not permitted or required by law.

- Ensure compliance with this subpart by its workforce.

One technical exception is verbal information that is transmitted in a telephone call or printed information that is faxed over a telephone line. In both cases, the information is being transmitted electronically, but it was not in electronic form before being transmitted. If the information transmitted by voice or fax was produced from information that was stored electronically, it is subject to the security rule. The security rule establishes obligations for medical practices that include:

- Complying with the security standards, including all "required" implementation specifications and all "addressable" implementation specifications to the extent that they apply to the medical practice.

- Reviewing and modifying security measures as needed to ensure the continued "reasonable and appropriate" protection of electronic PHI.

- Including provisions in business associate contracts that ensure the security of electronic PHI the business associate creates, receives, maintains, or transmits on behalf of the provider.

- Implementing reasonable and appropriate policies and procedures to comply with the standards, implementation specifications, and other requirements of the security rule.

- Documenting the policies and procedures implemented to comply with the security requirements—

including any action, activity, or assessment the standards require to be documented.

DOCUMENTATION

An auditor should check claim forms, whether submitted electronically or by hard copy, to see that they are completed correctly. Include all pertinent dates and diagnostic and procedural coding information necessary for insurance payers to generate reimbursement. Auditors will look specifically for any indicators of insurance fraud and abuse.

Procedure 18-1   Screening for Insurance

PURPOSE:
To verify insurance coverage and obtain vital information required for processing and billing insurance claim forms.

EQUIPMENT/SUPPLIES:
Patient registration forms
Clipboard and black ink pen
Patient's chart

PROCEDURE STEPS:

1. When scheduling the first appointment, ask the patient to bring his or her insurance card and to arrive 15 to 20 minutes before the appointment time to complete the patient registration form. RATIONALE: The insurance card is required to verify effective dates and pertinent information relative to insurance coverage. The registration form also requests vital information necessary for patient care and insurance billing.

2. When the patient turns in the completed registration form, review it immediately to be sure that all information has been collected and that it is legible. RATIONALE: It is important that all information has been included on the registration form and that the medical assistant can read it clearly when processing the insurance claim forms. If information is omitted from the claim form or is incorrect, the insurance carrier may deny the claim.

3. Ask the patient for his or her insurance card and make a photocopy of both sides of the card to be maintained in the patient's chart. RATIONALE: The insurance card provides vital information, including correct spelling of patient's name, insurance plan numbers, effective dates, telephone numbers to call regarding referrals and preauthorizations, and information about any deductible and co-payment.

4. Verify proof of eligibility for Medicaid patients. The patient should have his or her proof of eligibility card with him or her, or you may need to make a telephone call directly to Medicaid or use the online electronic data exchange system to determine proof of eligibility. RATIONALE: This information is required for Medicaid reimbursement.

5. Each time a patient checks in, whether established or new, the following information should be verified:
   - Address. Confirm the patient's current address and telephone number. RATIONALE: Patients may have moved and may not realize they had not reported their new address and telephone number to the office.
   - Verify insurance coverage. RATIONALE: This information is required for correct claims processing and billing procedures.

(continues)

Procedure 18-1 (continued)

- Ask for the patient's insurance card and verify information and effective dates. Also be sure that a copy of the card has been photocopied and is maintained in the patient's chart. RATIONALE: This is a means of keeping insurance records current for billing purposes.
- Determine if the insurance carrier covers the procedure. RATIONALE: If the carrier does not cover the procedure, reimbursement will need to come from a third party or the patient.
- Determine that the patient's PCP is performing the procedure. RATIONALE: This information is needed for reimbursement purposes.
- Determine if a referral is required and if an authorization number or code is needed. RATIONALE: Reimbursement by the carrier cannot take place without the proper documentation and authorization number.
- Confirm that evidence of qualifying has been secured. RATIONALE: Proof of eligibility must be verified for reimbursement from Medicaid.

Procedure 18-2   Obtaining Referrals and Authorizations

PURPOSE:

To ascertain coverage by the insurance carrier for specific medical services, hospital admissions, inpatient or outpatient surgeries, elective procedures, or when the PCP elects to refer the patient to another physician.

EQUIPMENT/SUPPLIES:

Patient's medical chart and copy of his or her insurance card
Name and telephone number of the contact person for the carrier
Completed referral form
Telephone/Fax machine
Pen/Pencil

PROCEDURE STEPS:

1. Collect all necessary documents and equipment (patient's chart/record, insurance carrier's information and telephone number). RATIONALE: Allows for efficient use of time in acquiring the referral or authorization.
2. Determine the service or procedure requiring preauthorization. You will also need to know the name and telephone number of the specialist involved, and the reason the request is being sought. RATIONALE: This information is required to complete the referral form to obtain authorization from the patient's insurance carrier.
3. Complete the referral form, being sure to include all pertinent information. RATIONALE: The request may be denied if all information has not been included.
4. Proofread the completed form. RATIONALE: Because of the importance of this step, accuracy is critical.
5. Fax the completed form to the insurance carrier. RATIONALE: It appraises the carrier of the patient's medical condition, requests preauthorization for treatment, requests a verification or authorization number, and confirms the treatment plan.
6. Maintain a completed copy of the referral form in the patient's chart. RATIONALE: The form can be accessed in the future should questions arise.
7. Maintain a copy of the authorization number or code in the patient's chart. RATIONALE: For future reference or in case the patient should misplace his or her copy of the number.

Case Study 18-1

Jane O'Hara, CMA, is responsible for all patient insurance billing procedures. Jane has the following information:

	Total Charges	Allowed Charges
Office visit	$85.00	$80.00
Return visit	$65.00	$55.00

Deductible has not been satisfied.

CASE STUDY REVIEW

1. Calculate the correct billing if the physician accepts assignment.
2. Calculate the correct billing if the physician does not accept assignment.

DOCUMENTATION

Documentation must support all claims submitted. Failure to document a service translates into nonperformance of that service, from the perspectives of quality patient care, legal safeguards, and reimbursement issues. In other words, a deed not documented is a deed not done.

Case Study 18-2

Preauthorization or precertification is encountered daily by Jane O'Hara at Inner City Health Care's multi-doctor urgent care center.

CASE STUDY REVIEW

1. How can Jane explain the rationale for these procedures to her patients?
2. What steps must Jane take to secure preauthorization or precertification?

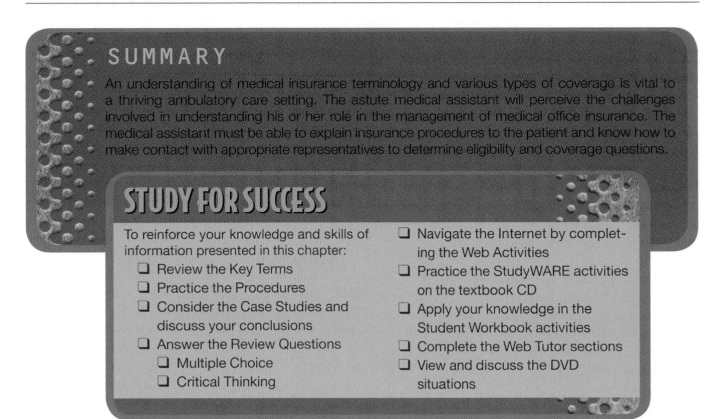

SUMMARY

An understanding of medical insurance terminology and various types of coverage is vital to a thriving ambulatory care setting. The astute medical assistant will perceive the challenges involved in understanding his or her role in the management of medical office insurance. The medical assistant must be able to explain insurance procedures to the patient and know how to make contact with appropriate representatives to determine eligibility and coverage questions.

STUDY FOR SUCCESS

To reinforce your knowledge and skills of information presented in this chapter:
- ❏ Review the Key Terms
- ❏ Practice the Procedures
- ❏ Consider the Case Studies and discuss your conclusions
- ❏ Answer the Review Questions
  - ❏ Multiple Choice
  - ❏ Critical Thinking

- ❏ Navigate the Internet by completing the Web Activities
- ❏ Practice the StudyWARE activities on the textbook CD
- ❏ Apply your knowledge in the Student Workbook activities
- ❏ Complete the Web Tutor sections
- ❏ View and discuss the DVD situations

REVIEW QUESTIONS

Multiple Choice

1. The most common avenue to ensure that services will be reimbursed is:
   a. not see any patient that does not have proof of Medicaid coverage
   b. complete an envoy
   c. go online and print a proof of eligibility directly from the system
   d. ask patients if they are covered
2. The most common insurance claim form is the:
   a. UB92 form
   b. ICD-9-CM
   c. CMS-1500 form
   d. CPT
3. Medicare:
   a. was created by Title 19 of the Social Security Act
   b. covers most persons 65 years and older
   c. is designed to cover prescriptions
   d. is handled separately by each state
4. If the charge is $150 and the deductible has not been met, Medicare will pay:
   a. $20
   b. $40
   c. $120
   d. 80 percent of UCR after $110 deductible

5. There are _____ primary MCO models operating across the country.
   a. four
   b. three
   c. six
   d. eight
6. Medicaid insurance:
   a. is funded by the federal government and administered by each state's department of SSI
   b. requires a Medigap policy
   c. consists of two parts, Part A and Part B
   d. requires PARs to accept assignment
7. BC/BS:
   a. are locally based in all 50 states in the United States
   b. operate like MCOs
   c. recognize Medicare Part B
   d. are part of CHAMPVA
8. TRICARE:
   a. is part of CHAMPVA
   b. is part of OWCP, MSHA, and FECA programs
   c. is a self-insurance program
   d. was formerly the Civilian Health and Medical Program for Uniformed Services

Critical Thinking

1. When children of married parents are covered under both parents' policies, how is the birthday rule used to determine which policy is primary?

2. Your Medicare patient has an office visit of $150 and a follow-up visit of $75. Your physician–employer does not accept assignment. Because this is the patient's first visit of the year, the deductible has not been satisfied. How will you determine the amount owed by the patient?

3. You are the medical assistant working the front desk and one of your responsibilities is to screen patients for insurance. What questions will you ask when collecting these data, and how will you word each question so that accurate information is received from the patient?

4. An established patient is seen by the doctor today, who determines that a liver scan is necessary to determine a diagnosis. You must ascertain if this procedure is a covered benefit, determine what the payment rate will be by the carrier, and secure preapproval if necessary. How will you go about collecting this information?

5. You must establish proof of eligibility for a patient. How will you go about doing this?

REFERENCES/BIBLIOGRAPHY

Fordney, M. T., French, L. L., Follis, J. J. (2004). *Administrative medical assisting* (5th ed.). Clifton Park, NY: Thomson Delmar Learning.

ingenix. (2003, December). *HIPAA tool kit.* Salt Lake City, UT: St. Anthony Publishing/Medicode.

Johnson, S. L. (2000). *Understanding medical coding: A comprehensive guide.* Clifton Park, NY: Thomson Delmar Learning.

Rowell, J. C., & Green, M. A. (2004). *Understanding medical insurance: A guide to professional billing* (7th ed.). Clifton Park, NY: Thomson Delmar Learning.

THE DVD HOOK-UP

DVD Series **Critical Thinking**	Program Number **5**

Chapter/Scene Reference
- *Introduction to Insurance and Coding*
- *Insurance and HIPAA*
- *Insurance Company Requirements*

In this chapter, you learned about the many types of insurance plans and the importance of gathering the proper information so that you can get reimbursed for services rendered.

In one of today's featured scenes, you observed Sandy telling her office manager and coworkers about an encounter that happened earlier in the week with a patient named Mr. Dickerson. Mr. Dickerson would not give Sandy a copy of his insurance card. Sandy sensed that the patient was trying to hide something and told him that he needed to be honest with her so that she could fully assist him. The patient shared that he recently lost his job and applied for Medicaid. Sandy looked up his information in the computer and was able to assist him.

1. What do you think about Sandy's communications skills?
2. Did Sandy appear to be empathetic even though she was direct?
3. Were you empathetic of Mr. Dickerson's dilemma?

DVD Journal Summary
Write a paragraph that summarizes what you learned from watching the designated scenes from today's DVD program. Working on the administrative side of the office is not always easy. Patients are attentive to their medical bills and may get upset when insurance does not cover particular services. What approach will you take to calm a frustrated patient who is upset because his or her blood work is not covered by Medicare?

CHAPTER 19

Medical Insurance Coding

OUTLINE

OBJECTIVES

The student should strive to meet the following performance objectives and demonstrate an understanding of the facts and principles presented in this chapter through written and oral communication.

1. Understand the process of procedure and diagnosis coding.
2. Code a sample claim form.

(continues)

FEATURED COMPETENCIES

CAAHEP—ENTRY-LEVEL COMPETENCIES

Process Insurance Claims

- Apply managed care policies and procedures
- Apply third-party guidelines
- Perform procedural coding
- Perform diagnostic coding
- Complete insurance claim forms

Legal Concepts

- Identify and respond to issues of confidentiality
- Perform within legal and ethical boundaries
- Document appropriately
- Demonstrate knowledge of federal and state health care legislation and regulations

Operational Functions

- Utilize computer software to maintain office systems

ABHES—ENTRY-LEVEL COMPETENCIES

Professionalism

- Maintain confidentiality at all times
- Be cognizant of ethical boundaries
- Adapt to change

Communication

- Serve as liaison between physician and others
- Use appropriate medical terminology
- Receive, organize, prioritize, and transmit information expediently
- Application of electronic technology

(continues)

374

OBJECTIVES (continued)

3. Explain the difference between the CMS-1500 and the UB92 forms.
4. Describe the way computers have altered the claims process.
5. Discuss why claims follow-up is important to the ambulatory care setting.
6. Discuss legal and ethical issues related to coding and insurance claims processing.

SCENARIO

At Inner City Health Care, a multidoctor urgent care center in a large city, medical assistant Jane O'Hara, CMA, is responsible for all patient billing procedures. Jane and her assistants must be acquainted with the requirements of each patient's insurance coverage and help patients understand their responsibility, if any, for payment. Finally, Jane holds periodic meetings with her assistants to update them; she continually stresses to them the importance of timeliness in filing claims and the need for absolute accuracy in diagnosis and procedure coding, which must always reflect services actually performed and, documented within the patient's chart.

FEATURED COMPETENCIES (continued)

Administrative Duties

- Perform basic secretarial skills
- Prepare and maintain medical records
- Apply computer concepts for office procedures
- Apply managed care policies and procedures
- Perform diagnostic coding
- Complete insurance claim forms
- Use physician fee schedule

Legal Concepts

- Document accurately
- Use appropriate guidelines when releasing records or information
- Monitor legislation related to current healthcare issues and practices

Office Management

- Exercise efficient time management

Financial Management

- Implement current procedural terminology and ICD-9-CM coding
- Analyze and use current third-party guidelines for reimbursement

INTRODUCTION

Coding is the basis for the information on the claim form. Medical coding is mandatory for the accurate transmission of procedures and diagnosis information between health care providers and various agencies that compile health care statistics and the insurance companies that act as third-party payers for health care services rendered to patients. To code accurately, the medical assistant must have a good understanding of medi- *cal terminology, especially of those medical specialties found in the ambulatory care setting.*

 The use of computers to generate the insurance claim form and to transmit the form to the third-party payer is commonplace today. Computers are able to compute and compare numbers only. Letters that are in a sequence, such as the alphabet, are able to be compared as to their relativity to each other. For instance, A comes before B in the alphabet, thus a computer can compare those two values. For that reason, all charges, patient accounts, insurances, diagnoses and procedures, and even various categories are assigned letters or numbers (alphanumeric). The letters/ numbers assigned to diagnoses and procedures (services) are called insurance codes. People whose jobs are to check accuracy of insurance codes and assign billing parameters (such as code modifiers) are called medical coders. (See Professional Coding Opportunities section at the end of this chapter for more information).

INSURANCE CODING SYSTEMS OVERVIEW

The process of translating written or spoken description of diseases, injuries, medical procedures, services, and supplies into numeric or alphanumeric format is called coding. The following coding systems are used within the United States and throughout most of the world:

- **Current Procedures Terminology (CPT)** system has been developed by the American Medical Association (AMA) to convert commonly accepted descriptions of medical procedures into a five-digit numeric code with two-digit numeric modifiers when required. This system is used to code medical procedures.

- Medicare has developed a supplement to the CPT system for procedures that are not defined with sufficient specificity. This system uses a five-digit alphanumeric code with an additional two-digit modifier if required.

- ***International Classification of Diseases, 9th Revision, Clinical Modification (ICD-9-CM)*** system has been developed by the World Health Organization (WHO) to classify all known diseases to assist in maintaining statistical records of morbidity (sickness) and mortality (death). Although not originally designed as a reimbursement system, it has been adopted in the United States for this purpose. This system is used for both diagnostic and procedure coding. The current ICD-9-CM code consists of a three-digit code with one or two numeric modifiers. The modifiers are separated from the three-digit code by a decimal point. The document is revised periodically and is updated yearly. The book is in its ninth revision. As of January 2005 the 10th revision is in final draft. Implementation will be based on the process for adoption of standards under HIPAA 1996. A two-year implementation window will be provided once the final notice to implement has been published in the Federal Register. The ninth revision is designated ICD-9-CM. The 10th revision will feature an increase in code digits from 4 or 5 to either 6 or 7 digits to accommodate growth in medical knowledge. The code in the 10th edition will also consist of alphanumeric digits.

Accuracy in coding is important. Imprecise coding can affect how quickly the physician is reimbursed and also the amount of the reimbursement. Codes must be appropriate to the documentation. Insurance carriers always **down-code** if documentation or codes are ambiguous and reimburse the physician for the lowest possible fee. Following are the three primary reasons why down-coding happens:

- The coding system used on the claim form does not match the coding system used by the insurance carrier. The carrier's computer will convert the submitted claim code to the closest recognized code. In most cases, the reimbursement amount will be less.

- If a Workers' Compensation claims examiner has to convert a CPT code to a relative value scale (RVS) code, the examiner will select the lowest-paying code. When billing Workers' Compensation, always use the RVS system used by that carrier and match the code to the best description of the CPT code.

- When attached documentation does not match the written description of the procedure, the reimbursement will always be the lowest paying code that fits the written description.

Up-coding, also known as code creep, over-coding, or overbilling, occurs when the insurance carrier is deliberately billed a higher rate service than what was performed to obtain greater reimbursements. Computer software programs have been developed to detect this practice easily. Often, complete audits are performed to assess the extent of up-coding practices. Sanctions and penalties are imposed on offenders.

 The Medicare program, in particular, often uses CPT codes, which are **bundled codes.** A bundled code is a grouping of several services that are directly related to a specific procedure and are paid

as one. For example, surgical dressings or reading test results may be bundled into evaluation and management codes. **Unbundling** refers to separating the components of a procedure and reporting them as billable codes with charges to increase reimbursement rates. This procedure may also be termed *fragmentation, exploding,* or *à la carte medicine.* This practice is considered fraud and may lead to audit, sanctions, and penalties.

CODING OF MEDICAL PROCEDURES

 When billing, medical assistants are expected to adhere to ethical standards and legal practices. All codes reported must be supported by documentation in the patient chart. Understanding medical terminology, anatomy, physiology, and procedures are critical to coding accuracy. It is also important to maintain coding skills by attending Continuing Education activities that discuss changes in codes and present guidelines and regulation requirements necessary for accurate coding. Networking with other medical coders is also a valuable method of staying current with what is happening in this profession.

CPT Manual Organization and Use

The CPT manual, issued every October, is used to code medical procedures and services of all kinds—office, hospital, nursing facility, and home services. The current volume, which is the fourth edition, is divided into seven sections that are discussed in the following paragraphs.

Evaluation and Management

The Evaluation and Management section takes every possible combination of visits into consideration and assigns each its own number. For instance, Mary O'Keefe, a new patient, is seen for a period of 45 minutes during which the physician takes a detailed history, examines the patient, and makes a medical decision of moderate

 Under HIPAA, a code set is any set of codes used for encoding data elements that may include but is not limited to the following medical categories: tables of terms, medical concepts, medical diagnoses, and medical procedures. Nonmedical code sets may be used to define state abbreviations, provider specialty, and remittance remarks to explain adjustments on a remittance.

complexity. The CPT code for this visit (99204) is found by looking under office services, new patient, time and service provided. In another instance, Abigail Johnson, an established patient, is seen in the hospital for several days. These visits (99231, 99232, or 99233) would be found under hospital services, subsequent hospital care, and the time and service provided. Codes for any type of evaluation or management are found in this section. In many offices, the physician will determine the level or charge for visits; however, the medical assistant must be familiar with all of the codes to make certain that billings are correct and that codes match the physician's documentation.

Anesthesia

The Anesthesia section includes all codes for anesthesia required for any procedure. The codes begin with the head and continue down the body to the legs and feet, concluding with anesthesia for radiologic procedures. If you want to find the correct code for anesthesia during a total hip replacement, you will find "Anesthesia" in the index, look for "hip" and refer to the codes listed: 01200–01214. When you refer back to the Anesthesia section, you find:

01200	Anesthesia for all closed procedures involving hip joint
01202	Anesthesia for arthroscopic procedures of hip joint
01210	Anesthesia for open procedures involving hip joint; not otherwise specified
01212	hip disarticulation
01214	total hip replacement or revision

As you read through the codes, you see that the correct code is 01214.

Surgery

The section on Surgery divides codes according to system. It begins with the skin, subcutaneous and areolar tissues, and continues through subsequent systems ending with ocular and auditory systems. The codes are very specific. For instance, a simple laceration repair is found as:

12001*	Simple repair of superficial wounds of scalp, neck, axillae, external genitalia, trunk and/or extremities (including hands and feet): 2.5 cm or less
12002*	2.6 cm to 7.5 cm
12004*	7.6 cm to 12.5 cm
12005	12.6 cm to 20.0 cm
12006	20.1 cm to 30.0 cm
12007	over 30.0 cm

Thus, the exact length of the laceration and complexity of repair can be found and coded correctly on the claim form. The asterisk signifies a surgical procedure for which a charge is made that does not include preoperative or postoperative visits.

Radiology, Nuclear Medicine, and Diagnostic Ultrasound

Coding in the Radiology section covers each procedure done and each specific alteration to the procedure. For instance,

75889	Hepatic venography, wedged or free, with hemodynamic evaluation, radiological supervision, and interpretation
75891	Hepatic venography, wedged or free, without hemodynamic evaluation, radiological supervision, and interpretation

Radiologic procedures are not often done in the physician's office, although they may be in larger urgent care centers. Occasionally, chest X-rays are done or, in an orthopedic specialty, many skeletal X-rays may be done. More often, though, radiologic studies are ordered by the physician through a local facility that bills the insurance company directly, using the diagnosis the physician has provided.

Pathology and Laboratory

The Pathology and Laboratory section includes every test and combination of laboratory tests that can be ordered, as well as a section on surgical pathology. This latter section includes specimens sent for examination, such as Pap smears, analysis of biopsy tissue from surgical sites, and tissue typing. Following is an example of a laboratory procedure code for hepatitis B that illustrates the complete selection of tests that may be ordered:

87340	Hepatitis B surface antigen (HBsAg)
86704	Hepatitis B core antibody (HBcAb); IgG and IgM
86705	IgM antibody
86706	Hepatitis B surface antibody (HBsAb)
87350	Hepatitis Be antigen (HBeAg)
86707	Hepatitis Be antibody (HBeAb)

The medical assistant should be aware of laboratory codes, because when a laboratory test is ordered, the laboratory may call to clarify the order. If the coding is correct, the laboratory should have no questions.

For surgical pathology, the codes are different. The level of examination for the item determines the code. The physician usually determines these levels or the charge for these services.

Medicine

The section of the CPT entitled Medicine includes codings for immunizations, injections, dialysis, allergen immunotherapy, and chemotherapy, as well as ophthalmologic, cardiovascular, pulmonary, and neurological procedures, to name a few. As in the earlier sections, there is a comprehensive breakdown of each procedure. Under Cardiography, for example:

93000	Electrocardiogram, routine ECG with at least 12 leads; with interpretation and report
93005	tracing only, without interpretation and report
93010	interpretation and report only

Under Chemotherapy Administration:

96408	Chemotherapy administration, intravenous, push technique
96410	infusion technique, up to one hour
+96412	infusion technique, one to eight hours, each additional hour
96414	infusion technique, initiation of prolonged infusion (more than eight hours), requiring the use of a portable or implantable pump

The plus symbol before the CPT code indicates that the procedure is an add-on to a previously described procedure. For example, 96410 would be used to describe the service and the time administered up to one hour. Anything longer than one hour would be listed as +96412 for each additional hour administration took place.

Index

The final portion of the CPT is a comprehensive index listing every procedure alphabetically. The proper use of the CPT involves looking for the procedure in the index, and then checking the number given to determine the precise code.

Each code found in the CPT has five numeric digits. Note that there are no letter codes and no decimal points in these codes. Each five-digit code stands for a specific procedure not duplicated elsewhere.

Modifiers

Occasionally, a service or procedure needs to be modified. In that case, there are two-digit alphanumeric modifiers that can be applied to the five-digit code. These modifiers can indicate unusual procedural services (-22), bilateral procedure (-50), multiple procedures (-51), two surgeons (-62), surgical team (-66), or repeat procedure by same physician (-76). When any of these or other modifiers are used and a full five-digit code for the modifier is desired, use 099 before the modifier code. Thus, they become 09922, 09950, 09962, and so on. The modifiers are delineated in the front of each section of the CPT to alert the coder to modifiers available for that section.

If more than two modifiers are needed for a procedure, use (-99) before any other modifier. Thus, if a procedure required a modifier of -22 and -51, code -99 before the other modifiers. For instance, "33411 Replacement, aortic valve; with aortic annulus enlargement, noncoro-

Critical Thinking

In which code book would you look to find the code for upper gastrointestinal endoscopy, simple primary examination (e.g, with small-diameter flexible endoscope) (separate procedure)? Which code did you select?

nary cusp," becomes 33411-99. This can also be written 33411 and 09999, indicating multiple modifiers.

See Procedure 19-1 for instruction in CPT coding.

MEDICARE SUPPLEMENTS TO THE CPT CODING SYSTEM

In 1983, Medicare created **HCPCS** (pronounced "hick picks"), the **Healthcare Common Procedure Coding System.** These codes are used as supplements to the basic CPT system and are required when reporting services and procedures provided to Medicare and Medicaid beneficiaries (patients). HCPCS uses the basic system (Level I) with two additional levels (II and III) as required. Level II provides codes to enable the provider to report nonphysician services such as durable medical equipment, supplies and medications (particularly injectable drugs), and ambulance services. Two-digit alphanumeric or letter modifiers are used in Level II codes to provide greater detail on procedures and medical supplies. (Note: The use of CPT code 99070 defining supplies and materials provided by the physician over and above those normally included in the office visit should be avoided, and Level II codes, which are more detailed, should be used.) Level III codes are defined by the Medicare regional Part B carriers. Local codes are five-digit alphanumeric codes and use letters S and W through Z.

CODING OF MEDICAL DIAGNOSES

The ICD-9-CM is published annually, available October 1, by the National Center for Health Statistics (NCHS) and Centers for Medicare and Medicaid (CMS).

ICD-9-CM Resource Manual Organization and Use

The ICD-9-CM was created by the WHO to provide a diagnostic coding system for the compilation and reporting of morbidity and mortality statistics for ICD-9-CM reimbursement purposes in the United States. A quarterly publication, *Coding Clinic for ICD-9-CM*, is available as the official guideline for ICD-9-CM. A similar publication should be available when the 10th revision is adopted. The guidelines given are applicable to all settings; physician's office and hospital inpatient, outpatient, and clinical settings.

ICD-9-CM is broken into three volumes:

- *Volume I*, also known as the Tabular List, lists all diagnostic codes in numeric order.

- *Volume II* is an alphabetic listing of all known diagnoses (Index to Diseases). It includes symptoms, accidents and their causes, and concurrent diagnosis. Volume II also contains a table of drugs and chemicals, a neoplasm table, and a list of external causes for injuries. Volume II is the recommended starting point to identify diagnostic codes.

- *Volume III* lists procedures in tabular form. It is not extensively used in the United States, where the procedure codes of the CPT are more commonly used. Information in Volume III can, however, be helpful in identifying a procedure in the CPT.

Step 1 in coding a diagnosis is to enter Volume II using the main reason or condition (main term) that brought the patient into the medical facility. This could be a "soreness in the throat" or a "broken leg," among other symptoms. The lookup entry (main term) in Volume II would never include the anatomical term of "throat" or "leg," but would list "sore" or "fracture." The main term is shown in boldface type in the upper left of the page in the margin. Information in parentheses following the main term is called a nonessential modifier. The presence or absence of nonessential modifiers does not affect the code assignment.

Step 2 is to identify subterms that further identify the condition. Subterms are indented two spaces from the main term identified in step 1. Sometimes there is too much information to fit on the subterm line and it will be included on a carryover line that is indented two spaces from the subterm line.

Step 3 consists of selecting the main or subterm that matches the diagnosis and obtaining the code. The code is then entered into the tabular list of Volume I (Classification of Diseases and Injuries) to verify that it identifies the proper diagnosis. The tabular listing is broken into 17 chapters that are grouped according to cause or body system. Sometimes the code identified from Volume II will not be found in the tabular list of Volume I because of space constraints. When this occurs, the code identified from Volume II should be checked; if found to be correct, that code should be used. Alternatively, sometimes more specific identification is provided in the tabular index in the form of fourth or fifth digits. When a more specific code is found, it should be used.

External Cause Codes

When the cause of a patient's visit is not due to a disease, but rather to an injury or poisoning, an additional code is required to identify the reason for the visit or the cause of the injury. These codes are called **E Codes** and are found

Critical Thinking

In which code book would you look to determine the code for hypoparathyroidism that is induced surgically? Which code did you select?

in Volume II. In the case of the broken leg, listed earlier, if the patient had fallen from a ladder, the code would be E881.0; if the patient had fallen from a scaffold, the code would be E881.1. Diagnosis codes are quite precise.

Supplementary Health Factor Codes

When the patient comes to the medical facility for a reason other than sickness or injury, a supplementary health factor code is used. These are called **V Codes.** Had the patient simply come in for a test, such as a TB skin test, a supplementary health factor code would be required. In this case the V Code from Volume II would be V47.1, Screening for Pulmonary Tuberculosis.

M Codes

M Codes (morphology codes) are used primarily with cancer registries. They are used to further identify behavior and the cell type of a neoplasm. This code is used in conjunction with neoplasm codes for the main classification.

Code References

Sometimes a diagnostic code will have a notation attached to it, NEC or NOS. NEC means "not elsewhere classified" and is used if there is not enough information to find a more specific code. NOS means "not otherwise specified."

See Procedure 19-2 for instruction in ICD-9-CM coding.

CODING ACCURACY

The more accurate the coding on the claim form, the less chance there is for error, the more quickly the physician is reimbursed, and the better the chance that the physician's reimbursement will reflect the actual charge. Many insurance carriers keep a fee profile of each physician's charges. This profile reflects the amount of each charge for each service and can affect the physician's reimbursement for those services.

Do not guess when coding. The coding that is used becomes a permanent part of the patient's medical record with the insurance carrier. If an incorrect code is used, that coded diagnosis will stay with

Critical Thinking

The physician operates as part of a clinic in an integrated medical facility with radiology, laboratory, and surgical facilities in the same building. The clinic is located in Philadelphia, Pennsylvania, with the physician operating as a participating physician in the Medicare System.

A healthy, 65-year-old man presents at the clinic with a chief complaint of a badly bruised left hand and an apparent dislocation of the metacarpophalangeal joint. He had been putting up Christmas lights at his home using a 20-foot aluminum ladder. The ladder had fallen, striking his left thumb as he tried to catch the ladder. He is an established patient.

The physician orders anteroposterior, lateral, and oblique radiographs of the hand to rule out fractures. The radiographs show no evidence of fractures. The diagnosis is dislocation of the metacarpophalangeal joint. The joint is bruised and extremely painful. The procedure performed is a closed treatment of the metacarpophalangeal dislocation with manipulation and requires anesthesia.

Determine the diagnostic and procedures codes. Should you consider E codes? Why or why not? Determine the physician's fee to be billed to Medicare.

that patient. This can be a difficult problem for insured persons if they change insurance carriers or if other health problems occur.

Consider a patient with hip pain. She has a history of ovarian cancer for which she has had radiology treatments. The hip pain is thought to be possible metastases from the original cancer site. When ruling out this possibility, the physician indicates the following code for the claim form:

198.89 Secondary malignant neoplasm of other specified sites: hip.

When the pain is finally discovered to be arthritis and it is determined that the patient needs a hip replacement, the insurance carrier denies coverage for this operation for the following reason: The patient's condition is terminal, and the company does not want her to spend her last months having surgery and recovering from surgery when she is already in poor health. And, of course, there is the cost factor to consider in the eyes of the insurance carrier.

Incorrect coding can be a problem with ruling out a diagnosis. For instance, a patient presents many symptoms of peptic ulcer disease. Do not immediately code that patient as having that disease until the diagnosis is confirmed. Instead, code the symptoms. When the tests come back and a specific diagnosis of peptic ulcer can be made, then code the disease as:

533.70 chronic without mention of hemorrhage or perforation without mention of obstruction.

When coding:

* Be as precise as possible.
* Do not guess.
* Do not code what is not there.

CODING THE CLAIM FORM

For the insurance company to understand what is being billed, the claim form is completed by the medical assistant or billing clerk in the ambulatory care setting. The physician completes an **encounter form** at the time of the visit. This encounter form (Figure 19-1) includes the date of service, the visit or consultation code, diagnoses for this visit, procedures done and laboratory tests ordered, and, if necessary, the date the patient is to return. This information is then translated onto the claim form.

The **CMS-1500** is the claim form accepted by most insurance carriers. This form is prepared using words and CPT codes for procedures performed and ICD-9-CM codes for diagnoses. Keep in mind that the codes must correlate; for instance, if a person had an ICD-9-CM diagnosis code of earache, otitis media, or 382.9, and the CPT procedure code indicated was 69090, ear piercing, the insurance company would question the claim and reject it for payment. The person completing the claim form must be *as precise as possible*. If the coding is wrong, the claim will be denied and the physician will not receive payment. Coding must correlate with the physician's note in the chart; otherwise, fraud is committed.

Coding the claim form is a precise way to communicate with the insurance carrier. Coding indicates the complexity of the visit, the diagnosis for the visit, and the specific procedures performed during the visit. This results in little confusion, and a minimum of communication is needed between the carrier and the physician's office because all information is contained in the codes.

For instance, Leo McKay, a regular patient, is seen for an extended visit to determine the cause of his abdominal pain. Symptoms include diarrhea, fever, nausea, and anorexia. An abdominal ultrasound is ordered, as well as laboratory tests, and the results are unknown at the time

of the insurance billing. The visit lasts 30 minutes and includes a full physical examination and a history of the present illness.

The CPT procedure coding for this visit is 99214, which reflects the examination and time spent with the patient, the history taken of this illness, and a medical decision of moderate complexity.

The ICD-9-CM diagnosis coding for abdominal pain is 789.0, for diarrhea 787.91, for nausea 787.02, and for anorexia 783.0. The claim form is submitted to the insurance carrier with these codes, and even though they are all symptoms, the claim will be paid because the visit and the tests ordered interrelate.

When the test results are known, they show a positive diagnosis of Giardia lamblia. The diagnosis code is changed to 007.1. Any further charges sent to the insurance carrier while Leo McKay is being treated for this problem are coded 007.1. The symptom codes from the first submission are dropped.

THIRD-PARTY GUIDELINES

Because patient information is easily accessed through medical charts, computerized databases, and the human factor, security and confidentiality measures must be in place in medical offices. When patients schedule an appointment and are seen by the physician, they enter into a contract for specific services. The first party is the person receiving the contracted service. The second party is the person or organization providing the service. A third party is one that is not involved in the patient–provider relationship but rather with reimbursement procedures.

 The patient has a right to expect that his or her health information will not be disseminated to others without written permission to do so. Confidentiality issues involve restricting the health information to only those individuals who need to know. Compliance with Health Insurance Portability and Accountability Act (HIPAA) of 1996 regulations is one way to safeguard protected health information (PHI). Chapters 11, 12, 13, 14, 15, and 18 all place emphasis on HIPAA as it relates to PHI. You may want to review those chapter sections again.

 Authorization to release necessary medical information to payers, such as insurance carriers, must be obtained from the patient, the parent, or the guardian *before* any information is released. A breach of confidentiality is the release of unauthorized PHI to a third party. One way to prevent this when processing insurance claims forms is to ask the patient, parent, or guardian to sign an "Authorization to Release Medical Information" statement *before* the claim form is

Tom Smith, M.D.		
OTOLARYNGOLOGY		*Yorktown Medical Group*
Name:	MR#:	DOB:
Address:	Ins. #:	Copay:
Phone #:	Referring MD:	Balance Due:
Date of Service:		

Evaluation and Management

FEE

* P R O C E D U R E S *

FEE

[ ] 99203	office/outpatient visit, new	
[ ] 99212	office/outpatient visit, est., limited	
[ ] 99213	office/outpatient visit, est., intermediate	
[ ] 99214	office/outpatient visit, est., extended	
[ ] 99261	follow-up inpatient consult	
[ ] 99271	confirmatory consultation	
[ ] 99284	emergency dept visit	
[ ] 99341	home visit, new patient	
[ ] ____	Other	

Medicine

[ ] 92552	pure tone audiometry, air	
[ ] 92553	audiometry, air & bone	
[ ] 92553	audiometry, air & bone	
[ ] 92557	comprehensive hearing test	
[ ] 92567	tympanometry	
[ ] 92568	acoustic reflex testing	
[ ] 92569	acoustic reflex decay test	
[ ] 99050	medical services after hrs	
[ ] 99052	medical services at night	
[ ] 99054	medical servcs, unusual hrs	
[ ] ____	Other	

Surgery

[ ] 21315	treatment of nose fracture, w/o stabilliza	
[ ] 21320	treatment of nose fracture, with stabiliza	

[ ] 30100	intranasal biopsy	
[ ] 30110	removal of nose polyp(s)	
[ ] 30200	injection treatment of nose	
[ ] 30300	remove nasal foreign body	
[ ] 30560	release of nasal adhesions	
[ ] 30901	control of nosebleed, simple	
[ ] 30903	control of nosebleed, complex	
[ ] 30905	control of nosebleed, posterior	
[ ] 30906	repeat control of nosebleed	
[ ] 31000	irrigation, maxillary sinus	
[ ] 31254	revision of ethmoid sinus	
[ ] 31287	nasal/sinus endoscopy, surg	
[ ] 31511	remove foreign body, larynx	
[ ] 31575	diagnostic laryngoscopy	
[ ] 38505	needle biopsy, lymph nodes	
[ ] 40490	biopsy of lip	
[ ] 42100	biopsy roof of mouth	
[ ] 42330	removal of salivary stone	
[ ] 42400	biopsy of salivary gland	
[ ] 42650	dilation of salivary duct	
[ ] 42700	drainage of tonsil abscess	
[ ] 42720	drainage of throat abscess	
[ ] 42804	biopsy of upper nose/throat	
[ ] 60100	biopsy of thyroid	
[ ] 69210	remove impacted ear wax	

* D I A G N O S I S *

Digestive System

[ ] 527.2	sialoadenitis
[ ] 527.6	salivary gland mucocele
[ ] 528.2	oral aphthae
[ ] 528.9	oral soft tissue dis nec
[ ] ____	Other

Injury and Poisoning

[ ] 802.0	nasal bone fx-closed
[ ] 873.43	open wound of lip
[ ] 873.64	opn wnd tongue/mouth flr
[ ] 910.0	abrasion head
[ ] 931	foreign body in ear
[ ] 932	foreign body in nose
[ ] ____	Other

Musculoskeletal System

[ ] 738.0	acq nose deformity
[ ] 738.7	cauliflower ear
[ ] ____	Other

Neoplasms

[ ] 210.4	benign neo mouth nec/nos
[ ] 225.1	benign neo cranial nerve
[ ] ____	Other

Nervous System and Sense Organs

[ ] 380.11	acute infection of pinna
[ ] 380.14	malignant otitis externa
[ ] 380.15	chr mycot otitis externa
[ ] 380.22	acute otitis externa nec
[ ] 380.23	chr otitis externa nec
[ ] 380.31	hematoma auricle/pinna

[ ] 380.4	impacted cerumen
[ ] 380.81	exostosis ext ear canal
[ ] 381.01	ac serous otitis media
[ ] 381.10	chr serous om simp/nos
[ ] 381.81	dysfunct eustachian tube
[ ] 382.00	ac supp otitis media nos
[ ] 382.01	ac supp om w drum rupt
[ ] 384.21	cent perf tympanic memb
[ ] 384.23	marginal perf tymp nec
[ ] 384.25	total perf tympanic memb
[ ] 385.33	cholestma mid ear/mstoid
[ ] 386.01	meniere dis cochlvestib
[ ] 386.04	inactive meniere's dis
[ ] 386.10	peripheral vertigo nos
[ ] 386.11	benign parxy smal vertigo
[ ] 386.35	viral labyrinthitis
[ ] 387.0	otoscler-oval wnd nonobl
[ ] 388.2	sudden hearing loss nos
[ ] 388.31	subjective tinnitus
[ ] 388.72	referred pain of ear
[ ] 389.01	conduc hear loss ext ear
[ ] 389.02	conduct hear loss tympan
[ ] 389.03	conduc hear loss mid ear
[ ] 389.10	sensomeur hear loss nos
[ ] 389.2	mixed hearing loss
[ ] ____	Other

Respiratory System

[ ] 461.0	ac maxillary sinusitis
[ ] 461.1	ac frontal sinusitis

[ ] 461.2	ac ethmoidal sinusitis
[ ] 461.3	ac sphenoidal sinusitis
[ ] 461.8	other acute sinusitis
[ ] 463	acute tonsillitis
[ ] 465.9	acute uri nos
[ ] 470	deviated nasal septum
[ ] 471.0	polyp of nasal cavity
[ ] 471.8	nasal sinus polyp nec
[ ] 471.8	nasal sinus polyp nec
[ ] 472.0	chronic rhinitis
[ ] 472.2	chronic nasopharyngitis
[ ] 473.0	chr maxillary sinusitis
[ ] 473.1	chr frontal sinusitis
[ ] 473.2	chr ethmoidal sinusitis
[ ] 473.3	chr sphenoidal sinusitis
[ ] 473.8	chronic sinusitis nec
[ ] 474.00	chronic tonsillitis
[ ] 477.9	allergic rhinitis nos
[ ] 478.0	hypertrph nasal turbinat
[ ] 478.1	nasal & sinus dis nec
[ ] ____	Other

Symptoms, Signs, and Ill-Defined Conditions

[ ] 784.7	epistaxis
[ ] ____	Other

Skin and Subcutaneous Tissue

[ ] 680.0	carbuncle of face
[ ] 701.4	keloid scar
[ ] ____	Other

Figure 19-1   Sample encounter form. The physician marks the procedures performed (CPT codes) and the diagnosis (ICD-9-CM codes).

completed. The CMS-1500 form provides space for this signature in Block 12.

Some medical offices, especially those who send claim forms electronically, will develop their own specialized "Authorization for Release of Medical Information" form. The customized form must contain the specific name of the insurance company and be signed by the patient, parent, or guardian. This form is generally valid for one year. The insurance company may request a copy of the signed form. When completing the CMS-1500, Block 12 may contain the words "SIGNATURE ON FILE," or the abbreviation SOF.

There are three authorization exceptions allowed by the federal government. The first two exceptions apply to Medicaid and Workers' Compensation. In these instances, the patient becomes a third-party beneficiary in the contract between the health care provider and the government agency sponsoring the insurance program. Providers agree to accept the program's payment as payment in full, and the patient may only be billed if the payer does not cover services rendered or if the patient is ineligible for benefits. The third exception is related to hospital admission. The patient must sign a release of medical information *before* being seen by the provider or receiving treatment in a hospital.

Most states have specific laws related to release of medical information regarding mental health services and federally assisted alcohol and drug abuse programs. Patients being screened for HIV infection or AIDS must sign an additional authorization statement *before* information may be released regarding their status. See Procedure 19-3 for specific steps involved in authorization to release PHI to third-party payers.

COMPLETING THE CMS-1500 (12-90)

The **CMS-1500 (12-90)** (Figure 19-2) has been adopted by insurance carriers as the only acceptable form on which to submit insurance claims. However, each insurance carrier has its own thoughts on how the form should be completed and no two companies agree entirely on the information required, the boxes checked, and the rationale about what information goes in which boxes.

To illustrate the completion of a claim form, a fictitious insurance carrier will be used. Insurance carriers often change their rules and regulations for submitting claims constantly. To avoid out-of-date material, we sent this claim for payment to How Much Insurance Company. Using the example given of Leo McKay in the coding section, the CMS-1500 in Figure 19-3 shows the properly completed claim form.

Remember, many insurance carriers will require some of the boxes to be filled in and others left blank. The billing person for the medical office will need to comply with the current requirements of the insurance carrier that is being billed. There is no right or wrong answer for every insurance carrier. If there is a question about billing, check with that carrier about their requirements.

The CMS-1500 claim form contains all of the identification information that the carrier will need to process or analyze the claim for payment. The top right-hand space, identified as CARRIER, provides space for the carrier's name and address to be keyed in. When ordering CMS-1500 forms for the medical office, they may be ordered plain or with a bar code. The bar code includes the carrier's name and address so that it may be scanned and would not require the same information to be rekeyed in the right-hand space. See Procedure 19-4 for instructions for completing a Medicare claim form. Before completing claims for carriers other than Medicare, the medical assistant should verify with a carrier's representative exactly which blocks are required for that particular carrier.

Uniform Bill 92 Form

The **Uniform Bill 92 (UB92)** form (Figure 19-4) is used for filing inpatient admissions, outpatient and emergency department services and procedures, home health care, hospice, and long-term care benefits under a health plan.

Although medical assistants in ambulatory care facilities will not typically encounter hospital billing forms such as the UB92, many medical assistants are now finding opportunities as claims processing specialists in hospital, nursing facility, and clinic billing offices. As a claims processing specialist, skills are transferable to anywhere in the United States and are interchangeable between provider specialties and insurance carriers. The UB92 claim form is the standard form used for inpatient and outpatient services by acute care hospitals; psychiatric, drug, and alcohol facilities; clinical and laboratory services; walk-in centers; nursing facilities; subacute facilities; home health care agencies; and emergency departments.

Using the Computer to Complete Forms

The CMS-1500 claim form is designed to accommodate optical scanning of paper claims. A scanner is used to convert printed or handwritten characters into text that can be viewed by the optical character reader (OCR). This technology greatly increases claims processing productivity with some claims being paid within 7 to 10 days.

Practice management software may require data be entered using uppercase and lowercase letters and other data be entered without regard to OCR guidelines. The computer program converts the data to the OCR format when the claim is printed or electronically transmitted to

PLEASE
DO NOT
STAPLE
IN THIS
AREA

CARRIER →

HEALTH INSURANCE CLAIM FORM

PICA

PICA

1. MEDICARE MEDICAID CHAMPUS CHAMPVA GROUP HEALTH PLAN (SSN or ID) FECA BLK LUNG (SSN) OTHER
(Medicare #) (Medicaid #) (Sponsor's SSN) (VA File #) (ID)

1a. INSURED'S I.D. NUMBER   (FOR PROGRAM IN ITEM 1)

2. PATIENT'S NAME (Last Name, First Name, Middle Initial)

3. PATIENT'S BIRTH DATE MM DD YY   SEX M F

4. INSURED'S NAME (Last Name, First Name, Middle Initial)

5. PATIENT'S ADDRESS (No., Street)

6. PATIENT RELATIONSHIP TO INSURED
Self Spouse Child Other

7. INSURED'S ADDRESS (No., Street)

CITY   STATE

8. PATIENT STATUS
Single Married Other
Employed Full-Time Student Part-Time Student

CITY   STATE

ZIP CODE   TELEPHONE (Include Area Code) (   )

ZIP CODE   TELEPHONE (INCLUDE AREA CODE) (   )

9. OTHER INSURED'S NAME (Last Name, First Name, Middle Initial)

10. IS PATIENT'S CONDITION RELATED TO:

11. INSURED'S POLICY GROUP OR FECA NUMBER

a. OTHER INSURED'S POLICY OR GROUP NUMBER

a. EMPLOYMENT? (CURRENT OR PREVIOUS)
YES NO

a. INSURED'S DATE OF BIRTH MM DD YY   SEX M F

b. OTHER INSURED'S DATE OF BIRTH MM DD YY   SEX M F

b. AUTO ACCIDENT?   PLACE (State)
YES NO

b. EMPLOYER'S NAME OR SCHOOL NAME

c. EMPLOYER'S NAME OR SCHOOL NAME

c. OTHER ACCIDENT?
YES NO

c. INSURANCE PLAN NAME OR PROGRAM NAME

d. INSURANCE PLAN NAME OR PROGRAM NAME

10d. RESERVED FOR LOCAL USE

d. IS THERE ANOTHER HEALTH BENEFIT PLAN?
YES NO *If yes,* return to and complete item 9 a-d.

READ BACK OF FORM BEFORE COMPLETING & SIGNING THIS FORM.

12. PATIENT'S OR AUTHORIZED PERSON'S SIGNATURE I authorize the release of any medical or other information necessary to process this claim. I also request payment of government benefits either to myself or to the party who accepts assignment below.

SIGNED _____   DATE _____

13. INSURED'S OR AUTHORIZED PERSON'S SIGNATURE I authorize payment of medical benefits to the undersigned physician or supplier for services described below.

SIGNED _____

PATIENT AND INSURED INFORMATION →

14. DATE OF CURRENT: MM DD YY   ILLNESS (First symptom) OR INJURY (Accident) OR PREGNANCY(LMP)

15. IF PATIENT HAS HAD SAME OR SIMILAR ILLNESS. GIVE FIRST DATE MM DD YY

16. DATES PATIENT UNABLE TO WORK IN CURRENT OCCUPATION MM DD YY FROM   TO MM DD YY

17. NAME OF REFERRING PHYSICIAN OR OTHER SOURCE

17a. I.D. NUMBER OF REFERRING PHYSICIAN

18. HOSPITALIZATION DATES RELATED TO CURRENT SERVICES MM DD YY FROM   TO MM DD YY

19. RESERVED FOR LOCAL USE

20. OUTSIDE LAB? $ CHARGES
YES NO

21. DIAGNOSIS OR NATURE OF ILLNESS OR INJURY. (RELATE ITEMS 1,2,3 OR 4 TO ITEM 24E BY LINE)

1. _____ . ___   3. _____ . ___

2. _____ . ___   4. _____ . ___

22. MEDICAID RESUBMISSION CODE   ORIGINAL REF. NO.

23. PRIOR AUTHORIZATION NUMBER

24. A DATE(S) OF SERVICE						B Place of Service	C Type of Service	D PROCEDURES, SERVICES, OR SUPPLIES (Explain Unusual Circumstances)		E DIAGNOSIS CODE	F $ CHARGES	G DAYS OR UNITS	H EPSDT Family Plan	I EMG	J COB	K RESERVED FOR LOCAL USE
From MM	DD	YY	To MM	DD	YY			CPT/HCPCS	MODIFIER							
1																
2																
3																
4																
5																
6																

25. FEDERAL TAX I.D. NUMBER SSN EIN

26. PATIENT'S ACCOUNT NO.

27. ACCEPT ASSIGNMENT? (For govt. claims, see back) YES NO

28. TOTAL CHARGE $

29. AMOUNT PAID $

30. BALANCE DUE $

31. SIGNATURE OF PHYSICIAN OR SUPPLIER INCLUDING DEGREES OR CREDENTIALS (I certify that the statements on the reverse apply to this bill and are made a part thereof.)

SIGNED _____   DATE _____

32. NAME AND ADDRESS OF FACILITY WHERE SERVICES WERE RENDERED (If other than home or office)

33. PHYSICIAN'S, SUPPLIER'S BILLING NAME, ADDRESS, ZIP CODE & PHONE #

PIN#   GRP#

PHYSICIAN OR SUPPLIER INFORMATION →

(APPROVED BY AMA COUNCIL ON MEDICAL SERVICE 8/88)   *PLEASE PRINT OR TYPE*

APPROVED OMB-0938-0008 FORM CMS-1500 (12/90), FORM RRB-1500,
APPROVED OMB-1215-0055 FORM OWCP-1500, APPROVED OMB-0720-0001 (CHAMPUS)

Figure 19-2 CMS-1500 health insurance claim form.

PLEASE
DO NOT
STAPLE
IN THIS
AREA

(SAMPLE ONLY - NOT APPROVED FOR USE)

CARRIER

□□ PICA

UNDERSTANDING HEALTH INSURANCE CLAIM FORM   PICA □□□

1. MEDICARE MEDICAID CHAMPUS CHAMPVA GROUP FECA OTHER	1a. INSURED'S I.D. NUMBER (FOR PROGRAM IN ITEM 1)
□ (Medicare #) □ (Medicaid #) □ (Sponsor's SSN) □ (VA File #) HEALTH PLAN BLK LUNG □ (SSN or ID) □ (SSN) ☒ (ID)	555-55-5555

2. PATIENT'S NAME (Last Name, First Name, Middle Initial)	3. PATIENT'S BIRTH DATE SEX	4. INSURED'S NAME (Last Name, First Name, Middle Initial)
MCKAY, LEO M	MM DD YY 04 01 1935 M ☒ F □	MCKAY, LEO M

5. PATIENT'S ADDRESS (No. Street)	6. PATIENT RELATIONSHIP TO INSURED	7. INSURED'S ADDRESS (No. Street)
123 W FIRST STREET	Self ☒ Spouse □ Child □ Other □	SAME

CITY STATE	8. PATIENT STATUS	CITY STATE
ANYWHERE PA	Single ☒ Married □ Other □	

ZIP CODE TELEPHONE (Include Area Code)		ZIP CODE TELEPHONE (INCLUDE AREA CODE)
11666 (814) 555 5555	Employed □ Full-Time Student □ Part-Time Student □	( )

9. OTHER INSURED'S NAME (Last Name, First Name, Middle Initial)	10. IS PATIENT'S CONDITION RELATED TO:	11. INSURED'S POLICY GROUP OR FECA NUMBER
		1122334

a. OTHER INSURED'S POLICY OR GROUP NUMBER	a. EMPLOYMENT? (CURRENT OR PREVIOUS) □ YES ☒ NO	a. INSURED'S DATE OF BIRTH SEX MM DD YY M □ F □

b. OTHER INSURED'S DATE OF BIRTH SEX MM DD YY M □ F □	b. AUTO ACCIDENT? PLACE (State) □ YES ☒ NO	b. EMPLOYER'S NAME OR SCHOOL NAME ABC MANUFACTURING COMPANY

c. EMPLOYER'S NAME OR SCHOOL NAME	c. OTHER ACCIDENT □ YES ☒ NO	c. INSURANCE PLAN NAME OR PROGRAM NAME HOW MUCH INSURANCE COMPANY

d. INSURANCE PLAN NAME OR PROGRAM NAME	10d. RESERVED FOR LOCAL USE	d. IS THERE ANOTHER HEALTH BENEFIT PLAN □ YES ☒ NO If yes, return to and complete item 9a-d

READ BACK OF FORM BEFORE COMPLETING & SIGNING THIS FORM.
12. PATIENT'S OR AUTHORIZED PERSON'S SIGNATURE I authorize the release of any medical or other information necessary to process this claim. I also request payment of government benefits either to myself or to the party who accepts assignemnt below.
SIGNED SIGNATURE ON FILE   DATE 01/14/XXXX

13. INSURED'S OR AUTHORIZED PERSON'S SIGNATURE I authorize payment of medical benefits to the undersigned physcian or supplier for services described below
SIGNED SIGNATURE ON FILE

14. DATE OF CURRENT: ILLNESS (First symptom) OR MM DD YY INJURY (Accident) OR 01 10 YYYY PREGNANCY (LMP)	15. IF PATIENT HAS HAD SAME OR SIMILAR ILLNESS GIVE FIRST DATE MM DD YY	16. DATES PATIENT UNABLE TO WORK IN CURRENT OCCUPATION MM DD YY MM DD YY FROM TO

17. NAME OF REFERRING PHYSICIAN OR OTHER SOURCE	17a. I.D. NUMBER OF REFERRING PHYSICIAN	18. HOSPITALIZATION DATES RELATED TO CURRENT CONDITION MM DD YY MM DD YY FROM TO

19. RESERVED FOR LOCAL USE		20. OUTSIDE LAB $ CHARGES ☒ YES □ NO

21. DIAGNOSIS OR NATURE OF ILLNESS OR INJURY. (RELATE ITEMS 1,2,3, OR 4 TO ITEM 24E BY LINE)
1. 789.0   3. 783.0
2. 558.9   4. ___.___

22. MEDICAID RESUBMISSION CODE   ORIGINAL REF NO.

23. PRIOR AUTHORIZATION NUMBER

24. A DATE(S) OF SERVICE From To MM DD YY MM DD YY	B Place of Service	C Type of Service	D PROCEDURES, SERVICES OR SUPPLIES (Explain Unusual Circumstances) CPT/HCPCS MODIFIER	E DIAGNOSIS CODE	F $ CHARGES	G DAYS OR UNITS	H EPSDT Family Plan	I EMG	J COB	K RESERVED FOR LOCAL USE
01 10 YYYY	3		99214	1,2,3	85 00	1				
01 10 YYYY	3		82270	1,2	13 00	1				

25. FEDERAL TAX ID SSN EIN	26. PATIENT'S ACCOUNT NO.	27. ACCEPT ASSIGNMENT? (For govt. claims, see back) □ YES ☒ NO	28. TOTAL CHARGE $ 98 00	29. AMOUNT PAID $	30. BALANCE DUE $ 98 00
91-1234432 □ ☒	MCK111				

31. SIGNATURE OF PHYSICIAN OR SUPPLIER INCLUDING DEGREES OR CREDENTIALS (I certify that the statements made on the reverse are this bill and are made a part thereof.) MARK WOO MD (814)555-1155 SIGNED DATE 01/14/YYYY	32. NAME AND ADDRESS OF FACILITY WHERE SERVICES WERE RENDERED (if other than home or office)	33. PHYSICIAN'S SUPPLIER'S BILLING NAME, ADDRESS, ZIP CODE & PHONE # INNER CITY HEALTH CARE 222 S FIRST AV Carlton, MI 11666 PIN# 10004086 GRP#

(SAMPLE ONLY - NOT APPROVED FOR USE)   PLEASE PRINT OR TYPE   SAMPLE FORM 1500 SAMPLE FORM 1500

Figure 19-3 Completed CMS-1500 claim form.

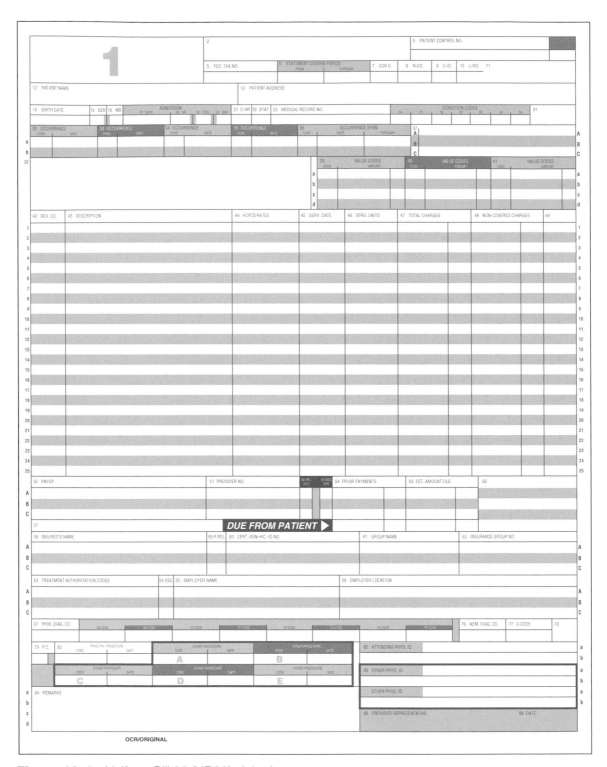

Figure 19-4 Uniform Bill 92 (UB92) claim form.

the carrier. Always use the software program's test pattern program to verify alignment of forms. Be sure the Xs are completely within the designated boxes. You may need to check this alignment each time a new batch of claims is inserted into the printer.

While completing the claim form on the computer, remember not to interchange a zero (0) with the alpha character (o). A substitute space should be used in place of the following keystrokes:

- Dollar sign or decimal in all charges or totals
- Decimal point in a diagnosis code number
- Dash in front of a procedure code modifier

- Parentheses surrounding the area code in a telephone number

- Hyphens in Social Security Numbers

When a fee is expressed in whole dollars, always enter two zeros in the cent column. Birth dates should be entered using eight digits (MM/DD/YYYY). Two-digit code numbers are used for months (i.e., January 01, February 02, and so on). If the day of the month number is less than 10, add a zero before the day (i.e., 03 for the third day of the month, and so forth).

Common Errors in Completing Claim Forms

Once the claim form has been completed, it should be proofread for accuracy and to make certain that all information has been filled in correctly. The following list provides common errors:

- Eliminate typographic errors. Check all numbers carefully to be sure they have not been transposed or entered incorrectly.

- Eliminate incorrect information. The name of the patient and the name of the policyholder must be the same.

- Verify that all blanks have been completed accurately. Specifically check that units of service are entered, hospital admission and discharge date are included, and procedure service date is provided.

- Verify that each procedure links correctly with the correct diagnosis (Block 24E).

- Verify that the procedure was medically necessary.

- Include the patient's name and policy identification information on each page of all attachments.

- Do not use staples, because the form cannot feed through the OCR if it is defaced or creased.

- Verify that the printer alignment was properly set and that all claim information is contained within its proper field.

- Be sure the claim form is signed appropriately.

MANAGING THE CLAIMS PROCESS

Once the claim form has been coded, a series of events take place: The medical assistant, who may have used a referral number generated by a point-of-service device, enters the claim into the office register of submitted claims; the insurance carrier processes the claim; an explanation of benefits is sent to the insured person; and, if necessary, follow-up procedures are instituted if payment is not received from the carrier within a specified time period. Each of these events is discussed in detail in the following sections.

Documentation of Referrals

 Many insurance plans require that a referral be preapproved by the plan before scheduling an appointment with other than the primary care physician. This is particularly true for managed care plans. The medical assistant working in both the primary care facility and specialist facility must make sure that when an approval is required, the necessary authorization has been obtained and referral number recorded in the patient's file. The referral number must be submitted as part of the claim submitted to the carrier by the specialist.

Point-of-Service Device

 An electronic device now available to some health care providers is a **point-of-service (POS) device.** This device provides immediate and direct access to patient eligibility information and managed care functions through an electronic network connecting the medical office and the health plan's computer.

The POS is a small card-swipe box similar in design and function to a credit card terminal (Figure 19-5). It allows medical office personnel to:

- Record a patient visit

- Check eligibility for patients in the health plan

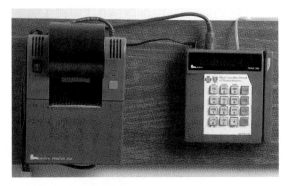

Figure 19-5 Point-of-service device allows direct communication between medical offices and the health care plan's computer. (Right) To enter information, the patient's insurance card is swiped through the machine, or the patient's identification number is entered on the keypad together with specific transaction code numbers. (Left) Responses from the plan's computer are printed directly in the medical office.

- Enter referrals for patients in managed care plans

- Verify referral information

- Check authorization status

- Enter inpatient authorization requests

- Enter outpatient authorization requests

 After the information is input by the medical assistant, the POS communicates with the health plan's computer system. The computer then returns an acknowledgment to the medical office confirming the transaction or giving an error message code. For example, when visits are recorded accurately, a reference number is generated that is used as the medical office's confirmation that the transaction is complete. On successful entry of a referral, a referral number is generated. Specialists may use this number on claims they submit for services they render under the referral.

Maintaining a Claims Registry

When claim forms are sent to the appropriate insurance carrier, it is wise and necessary for the medical office personnel to keep a diary or register of submitted claims (Figure 19-6). This **claim register** should include the patient's name, the insured's name if it is different from the patient's name, the dates of service for which the claim is being made, the amount of the claim, and the date the claim is submitted. When payment is received, the date of payment should be entered. When aging and reconciling accounts, the bookkeeper then can check the diary to note where the claim is in the process.

Following Up on Claims

Occasionally, claims may be denied because the claim form was not properly coded. However, if there is no pay-ment from the carrier and no other notification after a period of four to six weeks, it is necessary to follow up on the claim. The claim register will enable the office to keep track of the progress of claims.

To follow up, a toll-free number is provided by most carriers. The necessary information to have before making the call includes a copy of the claim form and the patient's name and insurance identification number. The carrier should be able to give the status of the claim. If payment is delayed, the carrier should be able to give the date when it can be expected. It is possible that payment was sent to the insured person, in which case a statement should be sent to the patient. If there is a problem with the claim, the medical assistant may need to investigate the cause of the error and submit a revised claim.

See Chapter 20 for information on billing and collection procedures.

THE INSURANCE CARRIER'S ROLE

On receipt of the claim form, the claims processor at the insurance carrier checks the codes to confirm that the procedures and accompanying diagnoses agree. The processor then analyzes the information to confirm that:

1. The coverage was in force at the time of treatment
2. The physician has contracted with the insurance carrier
3. There are no exclusions or restrictions on the policy for payment of that diagnosis
4. There are no preexisting condition restrictions
5. The diagnosis and procedures done are medically necessary and reasonable

The processor also checks to make sure that the billed amount falls within the usual, customary, and reasonable fee that the insurance carrier has developed for that specific procedure.

Explanation of Benefits

On completion of the processing of the claim, the insurance company sends an **Explanation of Benefits (EOB)** to the insured person. This form includes the dates; charges; amounts applied toward the deductible; amounts not covered either because of an exclusion or excess over the usual, customary, and reasonable charge; and the amount the company is paying for this claim. Some Explanation of Benefits forms even serve as a "bill" or "notice" in that they indicate the amount the insured must forward to the physician for payment of the account in full.

Date	Patient Name	Insured Name	Insurance Company	Dates Billed	Total Charges	Amount Received
1-18-__	McKay, Leo	—	How Much Ins Co.	1-10-__	98.00	

Figure 19-6 Example of claim register used to track insurance claims.

LEGAL AND ETHICAL ISSUES

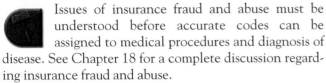

Issues of insurance fraud and abuse must be understood before accurate codes can be assigned to medical procedures and diagnosis of disease. See Chapter 18 for a complete discussion regarding insurance fraud and abuse.

Coding errors pose another type of legal and ethical issue. The Omnibus Budget Reconciliation Acts of 1986 and 1987 state that physicians can be assessed civil penalties if they "know of or should know that claims filed with Medicare or Medicaid on their behalf are not true and accurate representations of the items or services actually provided." This means that physicians can be held responsible not only for negligent mistakes they make, but also for mistakes made on their behalf by their medical assistants who complete insurance claim forms. The penalties assessed are usually in the form of a monetary fine and may also involve exclusion from Medicare and Medicaid programs for a period.

Compliance Programs

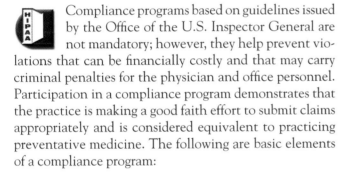

Compliance programs based on guidelines issued by the Office of the U.S. Inspector General are not mandatory; however, they help prevent violations that can be financially costly and that may carry criminal penalties for the physician and office personnel. Participation in a compliance program demonstrates that the practice is making a good faith effort to submit claims appropriately and is considered equivalent to practicing preventative medicine. The following are basic elements of a compliance program:

1. Have a designated compliance officer.
2. Develop and use written standards and procedures for coding.
3. Develop a plan for communicating coding standards and procedures.
4. Train personnel in standards and procedures.
5. Conduct periodic audits.
6. Respond to detected violations and notify appropriate government agencies.
7. Make personnel aware that they have an ethical duty to report suspected or observed fraudulent or erroneous coding practices so that they can be corrected. Publicize and enforce disciplinary standards on coding violations.

HIPAA Considerations

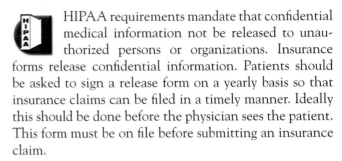

HIPAA requirements mandate that confidential medical information not be released to unauthorized persons or organizations. Insurance forms release confidential information. Patients should be asked to sign a release form on a yearly basis so that insurance claims can be filed in a timely manner. Ideally this should be done before the physician sees the patient. This form must be on file before submitting an insurance claim.

PROFESSIONAL CODING OPPORTUNITIES

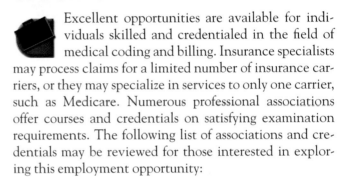

Excellent opportunities are available for individuals skilled and credentialed in the field of medical coding and billing. Insurance specialists may process claims for a limited number of insurance carriers, or they may specialize in services to only one carrier, such as Medicare. Numerous professional associations offer courses and credentials on satisfying examination requirements. The following list of associations and credentials may be reviewed for those interested in exploring this employment opportunity:

- American Academy of Professional Coders (AAPC; http://www.aapc.com): Certified Professional Coder Apprentice (CPC-A), Certified Professional Coder—Hospital Apprentice (CPC-HA), Certified Professional Coder (CPC), Certified Professional Coder—Hospital (CPC-H)

- American Health Information Management Association (AHIMA; http://ahima.org): Certified Coding Associate (CCA), Certified Coding Specialist (CCS), Certified Coding Specialist—Physician-Based (CCS-P)

- National Electronic Billers Alliance (NEBA; http://nebazone.com).

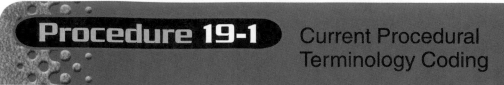

Procedure 19-1 — Current Procedural Terminology Coding

PURPOSE:
To convert commonly accepted descriptions of medical procedures (services) and visits of all types—office, hospital, nursing facility, home services—into a five-digit numeric code with two-digit numeric modifiers when required.

EQUIPMENT/SUPPLIES:
CPT code book for the current year
Copy of the encounter form and access to the patient's chart
Pencil and paper

CASE SCENARIO
Mary O'Keefe, a new patient, is seen for 10 minutes, during which the physician takes a focused history and completes a problem-focused examination. A routine urinalysis, nonautomated and without microscopy, is performed and a straightforward medical decision is made. Mary's preliminary diagnosis is painful urination. The urinalysis confirms a urinary tract infection. The physician writes her a prescription for an antibiotic and asks her to make an appointment in 10 days for another urinalysis to confirm the infection has cleared.

PROCEDURE STEPS:
1. Using the CPT code book, look in the Evaluation and Management section, Office or Other Outpatient Services, New Patient. Carefully read through the options until the code matching the described scenario has been found. RATIONALE: This section of the CPT code book provides codes used to report evaluation and management services provided in the physician's office or in an outpatient or other ambulatory care facility. You should have selected 99201.
2. Continue with the CPT code book, turn to the Index again, and look up Urinalysis, Routine. The code given is 81002. RATIONALE: This provides you with a code to investigate and determine its appropriateness.
3. Continue in the CPT code book and turn to the Pathology and Laboratory section. Follow the codes until you locate code 81002. Be sure the description provided there matches what the physician has documented in the patient's chart. RATIONALE: To verify that the code is correct and matches documentation.

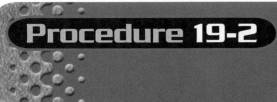

Procedure 19-2 International Classification of Diseases, 9th Revision, Clinical Modification Coding

PURPOSE:
The ICD-9-CM code books provide a diagnostic coding system for the compilation and reporting of morbidity and mortality statistics for reimbursement purposes.

EQUIPMENT/SUPPLIES:
Volumes 1 and 2 of the ICD-9-CM code books for the current year
Copy of the encounter form and access to the patient's chart
Pencil and paper

CASE SCENARIO
Mary O'Keefe, a new patient, presents at the office today reporting painful, frequent urination. She is seen for 10 minutes, during which the physician takes a focused history and completes a problem-focused examination. A routine urinalysis, nonautomated and without microscopy, is performed and a straightforward medical decision is made. Mary's preliminary diagnosis is painful urination. The urinalysis confirms a urinary tract infection. The physician writes her a prescription for an antibiotic and asks her to make an appointment in 10 days for another urinalysis to confirm the infection has cleared.

PROCEDURE STEPS:
1. Using Volume II, the alphanumeric Index to Diseases, of the ICD-9-CM code book, look up the main symptom or condition that brought the patient to the facility or the specific diagnosis confirmed by test results. In this case, the laboratory results confirmed a urinary tract infection. Code 599.0 RATIONALE: Use alphanumeric Volume II first to close in on the section of Volume I for specificity. Note: Enter the Tabular List, Volume I, with the first three digits of the code determined (599).
2. Using Volume I, look up code 599. Read through all of the 599 listings to determine the appropriate code having the highest level of specificity. RATIONALE: To establish the most accurate code: urinary tract infection, site not specified. 599.0 .

Procedure 19-3   Applying Third-Party Guidelines

PURPOSE:
To obtain written authorization to release necessary medical information to third-party payers.

EQUIPMENT/SUPPLIES:
Patient chart
CMS-1500 claim form

PROCEDURE STEPS:

1. When the patient signs in at the reception desk, check his or her chart to ascertain whether an "Authorization to Release Medical Informa-

tion" form has been signed and is currently valid. RATIONALE: PHI cannot be released without written authorization from the patient.

2. If there is no record of SIGNATURE ON FILE, have the patient sign Block 12 of the CMS-1500 claim form or the offices' customized "AUTHORIZATION TO RELEASE MEDICAL INFORMATION" form. RATIONALE: PHI cannot be released without written authorization from the patient.

1. MEDICARE	MEDICAID	CHAMPUS	CHAMPVA	GROUP HEALTH PLAN	FECA BLK LUNG	OTHER
(Medicare #)	(Medicaid #)	(Sponsor's SSN)	(VA File #)	(SSN or ID)	(SSN)	(ID)

2. PATIENT'S NAME (Last Name, First Name, Middle Initial)	3. PATIENT'S BIRTH DATE MM DD YY SEX M F
5. PATIENT'S ADDRESS (No., Street)	6. PATIENT RELATIONSHIP TO INSURED Self Spouse Child Other
CITY STATE	8. PATIENT STATUS Single Married Other
ZIP CODE TELEPHONE (Include Area Code) ( )	Employed Full-Time Student Part-Time Student
9. OTHER INSURED'S NAME (Last Name, First Name, Middle Initial)	10. IS PATIENT'S CONDITION RELATED TO:
a. OTHER INSURED'S POLICY OR GROUP NUMBER	a. EMPLOYMENT? (CURRENT OR PREVIOUS) YES NO
b. OTHER INSURED'S DATE OF BIRTH MM DD YY SEX M F	b. AUTO ACCIDENT? PLACE (State) YES NO
c. EMPLOYER'S NAME OR SCHOOL NAME	c. OTHER ACCIDENT? YES NO
d. INSURANCE PLAN NAME OR PROGRAM NAME	10d. RESERVED FOR LOCAL USE

READ BACK OF FORM BEFORE COMPLETING & SIGNING THIS FORM.

12. PATIENT'S OR AUTHORIZED PERSON'S SIGNATURE   I authorize the release of any medical or other information necessary to process this claim. I also request payment of government benefits either to myself or to the party who accepts assignment below.

SIGNED _____   DATE _____

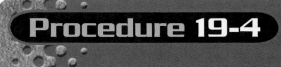

Procedure 19-4 Completing a Medicare CMS-1500 Claim Form

PURPOSE:
To complete the CMS-1500 insurance claim form for Medicare for reimbursement.

EQUIPMENT/SUPPLIES:
Patient information
Patient account or ledger card
Copy of patient's insurance card
Insurance claim form
Computer and printer

PROCEDURE STEPS:
1. The top right-hand space of the CMS-1500 claim form, identified as CARRIER, provides space for the carrier's name and address to be keyed in. If the CMS-1500 claim form has been ordered with a bar code, this information has already been imprinted within the bar code; therefore, it is not necessary to rekey the information. RATIONALE: The claims processor must know who the claim is from.

PLEASE DO NOT STAPLE IN THIS AREA		HEALTH INSURANCE CLAIM FORM	CARRIER

2. The PATIENT AND INSURED INFORMATION section asks for specific information related to the patient and his or her health insurance plan. The following is required information for Medicare in the PATIENT INFORMATION section. Complete each block as directed. RATIONALE: These blocks must be accurately completed or the claim may be denied.

1. MEDICARE (Medicare #)	MEDICAID (Medicaid #)	CHAMPUS (Sponsor's SSN)	CHAMPVA (VA File #)	GROUP HEALTH PLAN (SSN or ID)	FECA BLK LUNG (SSN)	OTHER (ID)
2. PATIENT'S NAME (Last Name, First Name, Middle Initial)				3. PATIENT'S BIRTH DATE MM DD YY SEX M F		
5. PATIENT'S ADDRESS (No., Street)				6. PATIENT RELATIONSHIP TO INSURED Self Spouse Child Other		
CITY		STATE		8. PATIENT STATUS Single Married Other		
ZIP CODE	TELEPHONE (Include Area Code) ( )			Employed Full-Time Student Part-Time Student		
9. OTHER INSURED'S NAME (Last Name, First Name, Middle Initial)				10. IS PATIENT'S CONDITION RELATED TO:		
a. OTHER INSURED'S POLICY OR GROUP NUMBER				a. EMPLOYMENT? (CURRENT OR PREVIOUS) YES NO		
b. OTHER INSURED'S DATE OF BIRTH MM DD YY SEX M F				b. AUTO ACCIDENT? PLACE (State) YES NO		
c. EMPLOYER'S NAME OR SCHOOL NAME				c. OTHER ACCIDENT? YES NO		
d. INSURANCE PLAN NAME OR PROGRAM NAME				10d. RESERVED FOR LOCAL USE		
READ BACK OF FORM BEFORE COMPLETING & SIGNING THIS FORM. 12. PATIENT'S OR AUTHORIZED PERSON'S SIGNATURE I authorize the release of any medical or other information necessary to process this claim. I also request payment of government benefits either to myself or to the party who accepts assignment below. SIGNED _____				DATE _____		

Block 1   Indicate the appropriate health insurance coverage applicable to this claim; for example, if a Medicare claim is being filed, check (X) the Medicare box.

Block 2   Enter the patient's last name, first name, and middle initial, if any, exactly as it appears on his or her insurance card.

(continues)

Procedure 19-4 (continued)

Block 3 — Enter the patient's 8-digit birth date (e.g., 08/22/1988). Place an *X* in the correct sex box.

Block 5 — Enter the patient's mailing address and telephone number.

Block 6 — Check the appropriate box for the patient's relationship to insured person when Block 4 is completed.

Block 8 — Check the appropriate box for the patient's marital status and whether employed or a student.

Blocks 9, 9a, 9b, 9c, and 9d — These blocks are completed if the patient has Medigap coverage.

Block 10 — Check the appropriate box indicating whether employment, auto liability, or other accident involvement applies to one or more of the services described in Block 24. Enter the state postal abbreviation. RATIONALE: Any block checked "yes" indicates there may be other insurance primary to Medicare. Identify primary insurance information in Block 11.

Block 10d — This block is used exclusively for Medicaid (MCD) information. If the patient is entitled to Medicaid, enter the patient's Medicaid number preceded by MCD.

Block 12 — The patient or authorized representative must sign and date the form unless the signature is on file. If the patient is physically or mentally unable to sign, a representative may sign on the patient's behalf. In this event, the statement's signature line must indicate the patient's name followed by "by" the representative's name, address, relationship to the patient, and reason the patient cannot sign. The authorization is effective indefinitely unless patient or the patient's representative revokes this arrangement. RATIONALE: The patient's signature authorizes release of medical information necessary to process the claim. It also authorizes payment of benefits to the provider of service or supplier when the provider of service or supplier accepts assignment on the claim.

3. Complete information regarding the insured person is requested in the INSURED INFORMATION section.

1a. INSURED'S I.D. NUMBER	(FOR PROGRAM IN ITEM 1)
4. INSURED'S NAME (Last Name, First Name, Middle Initial)	
7. INSURED'S ADDRESS (No., Street)	
CITY	STATE
ZIP CODE	TELEPHONE (INCLUDE AREA CODE) ( )
11. INSURED'S POLICY GROUP OR FECA NUMBER	
a. INSURED'S DATE OF BIRTH MM DD YY	SEX M F
b. EMPLOYER'S NAME OR SCHOOL NAME	
c. INSURANCE PLAN NAME OR PROGRAM NAME	
d. IS THERE ANOTHER HEALTH BENEFIT PLAN? YES NO *If yes*, return to and complete item 9 a-d.	
13. INSURED'S OR AUTHORIZED PERSON'S SIGNATURE I authorize payment of medical benefits to the undersigned physician or supplier for services described below. SIGNED _____	

PATIENT AND INSURED INFORMATION

Block 1a — Enter the patient's Health Insurance Claim Number (HICN) regardless of whether Medicare is the primary or secondary insurer.

Block 4 — If there is insurance primary to Medicare, either through the patient's or spouse's employment or any other source, list the name of the insured person in this block. When the insured person and the patient are the same, enter the word "Same". If Medicare is primary, leave blank.

(continues)

Procedure 19-4 (continued)

Block 7
Enter the insured person's address and telephone number. When the address is the same as the patient's, enter the word "Same". Complete this block only when Blocks 4, 6, and 11 are completed.

Block 11
If there is insurance primary to Medicare, enter the insured person's policy or group number.

Block 11a
Enter the insured person's 8-digit birth date and sex if different from Block 3.

Block 11b
Enter employer's name, if applicable.

Block 11c
Enter the 9-digit payer identification (ID) number of the primary insurer. If a payer ID number does not exist, enter the complete primary payer's program or plan name.

Block 11d
Leave blank. Not required by Medicare.

Block 13
RATIONALE: The signature here authorizes payment of mandated Medigap benefits to the participating physician or supplier if required Medigap information is included in Block 9. The patient or his or her authorized representative signs this block, or the signature must be on file as a separate Medigap authorization. The Medigap assignment on file in the participating provider of service's or supplier's office must be specific to the insurer. It may state that the authorization applies to all occasions of service until it is revoked.

4. The PHYSICIAN OR SUPPLIER INFORMATION section related to diagnosis and procedure coding is completed next. Following is an example of those blocks.

(continues)

Procedure 19-4 (continued)

Block 14   Enter patient's date of current illness, injury, or pregnancy.

Block 15   Leave blank. Not required by Medicare.

Block 17   Enter the name of the referring or ordering physician if the service or item was ordered or referred by a physician.

Block 17a   Enter the CMS-assigned Unique Physician Identification Number (UPIN) of the referring/ordering physician listed in Block 17.

Block 19   Enter the date the patient was last seen and the UPIN of his or her attending physician when an independent physical or occupational therapist submits claims or a physician providing routine foot care submits claims. For physical or occupational therapists, entering this information certifies that the required physician certification (or recertification) is being kept on file.

Block 21   Enter the patient's diagnosis/condition code. Use an ICD-9-CM code number and code to the highest level of specificity for the date of service. Enter up to four codes in priority order.

Block 24a   Enter date for each procedure, service, or supply. When "from" and "to" dates are shown for a series of identical services, enter the number of days or units in column G. This is a required field.

Block 24b   Enter the appropriate place of service code(s). Identify the location, using a place of service code, for each item used or service performed. This is a required field.

Place of service codes commonly used (but not limited to) include the following:
11   Office
12   Home

21   Inpatient hospitalization
22   Outpatient hospitalization
23   Emergency department—hospital
24   Ambulatory surgical center
25   Birthing center
31   Skilled nursing facility
32   Nursing facility
33   Custodial care facility
36   Military hospital or clinic

Block 24c   Medicare providers are not required to complete this block.

Block 24d   Enter the procedures, services, or supplies using CPT codes.

Block 24e   Enter the diagnostic code reference number as shown in Block 21 to relate the date of service and the procedures performed to the primary diagnosis. Enter only one reference number per line item. This is a required field.

Block 25   Enter the provider of service or supplier federal tax ID (Employer Identification Number) or Social Security number.

Block 26   Enter the patient's account number assigned by the provider's of services or supplier's accounting system. This field is optional to assist the provider in patient identification.

Block 27   Check the appropriate box related to accepting assignment.

Block 31   Enter the signature of provider of service or supplier, or his or her representative, and the date the form was signed. The claim can be processed without a signature if the signature is on file or a computer-generated signature is used. This is a required field.

Block 32   Enter the name, address, and zip code of the facility rendering service.

(continues)

Procedure 19-4 (continued)

5. The last section of the claim form to be completed is the PHYSICIAN OR SUPPLIER INFORMATION section regarding billing.

| 16. DATES PATIENT UNABLE TO WORK IN CURRENT OCCUPATION |
| MM DD YY   MM DD YY |
| FROM   TO |

| 18. HOSPITALIZATION DATES RELATED TO CURRENT SERVICES |
| MM DD YY   MM DD YY |
| FROM   TO |

| 20. OUTSIDE LAB? $ CHARGES |
| YES   NO |

| 22. MEDICAID RESUBMISSION CODE   ORIGINAL REF. NO. |

| 23. PRIOR AUTHORIZATION NUMBER |

F	G	H	I	J	K
$ CHARGES	DAYS OR UNITS	EPSDT Family Plan	EMG	COB	RESERVED FOR LOCAL USE

| 28. TOTAL CHARGE | 29. AMOUNT PAID | 30. BALANCE DUE |
| $ | $ | $ |

| 33. PHYSICIAN'S, SUPPLIER'S BILLING NAME, ADDRESS, ZIP CODE & PHONE # |
| |
| PIN#   GRP# |

PHYSICIAN OR SUPPLIER INFORMATION

Block 16 If the patient is employed and is unable to work in his or her current occupation, enter the date when patient is unable to work. RATIONALE: An entry in this field may indicate employment-related insurance coverage.

Block 18 Enter the date when a medical service is furnished as a result of, or subsequent to, a related hospitalization.

Block 20 Complete this block when billing for diagnostic tests subject to purchase price limitations. Enter the purchase price under charges if the "yes" block is checked. When the "yes" block is checked, Block 32 must also be completed.

Block 22 Leave blank. Not required by Medicare.

Block 23 Enter the prior authorization number for those procedures requiring prior approval.

Block 24f Enter the charge for each listed service.

Block 24g Enter the number of days or units. This field is commonly used for multiple visits, units of supplies, anesthesia minutes, or oxygen volume. If only one service is performed, the numeral 1 must be entered.

Block 24h Leave blank. Not required by Medicare.

Block 24i Leave blank. Not required by Medicare.

Block 24j Leave blank. Not required by Medicare.

Block 24k Enter the personal identification number (PIN) of the performing provider of service or supplier if the provider is a member of a group practice.

Block 28 Enter the total charges for the services (total of all charges in Block 24f).

Block 29 Enter the total amount the patient paid on the covered services only.

Block 30 Leave blank. Not required by Medicare.

Block 33 Enter the provider's of services or supplier's billing name, address, zip code, and telephone number. This is a required field. Enter the National Provider Identifier (NPI) for the performing provider. (Refer to Chapter 17 for details regarding NPI.)

Case Study 19–1

Leo McKay, an established patient at Inner City Health Care, schedules a visit, reporting nausea and severe abdominal pain. Dr. Mark Woo spends 30 minutes taking a history and doing an examination. He suspects an ulcer and orders laboratory tests (CBC complete, guaiac, lipid panel, and UA) to be done in the office and sends Mr. McKay for an upper GI series. Mr. McKay returns in 10 days to learn that the test results show a duodenal ulcer.

CASE STUDY REVIEW

1. What would the proper diagnosis codes be for Mr. McKay?
2. What would the proper procedure codes be for Mr. McKay?
3. In coding the claim form for Mr. McKay's visit, what ethical principle and legal principle should guide the medical assistant?

Case Study 19–2

Abigail Johnson, an established patient of Dr. Lewis, presents today with a chief complaint of abnormal weight gain. After her 45-minute appointment with the physician during which a detailed history, examination, and moderate complexity decision was made, a diagnosis of obesity of endocrine origin was determined.

CASE STUDY REVIEW

1. What is the proper CPT code for the visit?
2. What is the proper diagnosis code for Abigail Johnson?
3. What coding rules should be followed to ensure accuracy and correctness?

SUMMARY

Much material has been covered in this chapter. Remember, you can be the person to make a difference in insurance billing. By checking and double-checking your work, you make certain that the physician's time is being billed at the appropriate rate, that all procedures are billed with the proper diagnoses and CPT codes, and that the billing is sent to the correct insurance carrier. It takes much less time to double-check work once and have it correct *before* it is sent out than to send it out with errors that cause difficulty in the future.

An understanding of medical insurance coverages and coding procedures is vital to a thriving ambulatory care setting. The astute medical assistant will perceive the challenges involved in proper coding techniques and will understand his or her role in the management of the physician's office.

STUDY FOR SUCCESS

To reinforce your knowledge and skills of information presented in this chapter:

- ❏ Review the Key Terms
- ❏ Practice the Procedures
- ❏ Consider the Case Studies and discuss your conclusions
- ❏ Answer the Review Questions
  - ❏ Multiple Choice
  - ❏ Critical Thinking
- ❏ Navigate the Internet by completing the Web Activities
- ❏ Practice the StudyWARE activities on the textbook CD
- ❏ Apply your knowledge in the Student Workbook activities
- ❏ Complete the Web Tutor sections
- ❏ View and discuss the DVD situations

REVIEW QUESTIONS

Multiple Choice

1. CPT codes:
   a. are for diagnosis coding
   b. have five digits and may have two-digit modifiers
   c. have three-digit codes with a decimal point and one to two additional digits
   d. are updated semiannually

2. When coding a diagnosis, go first to:
   a. CPT
   b. Volume I of ICD-9-CM
   c. Volume II of ICD-9-CM
   d. E codes in ICD-9-CM

3. Level II of HCPCS:
   a. provides codes to enable the provider to report nonphysician services
   b. is the same as the regular CPT system
   c. is assigned by the fiscal intermediary
   d. uses the letter codes W, X, Y, and Z

4. The ICD-9-CM codes:
   a. were developed by the AMA as uniform descriptions of medical, surgical, and diagnostic services
   b. are divided into seven sections
   c. use modifiers
   d. code every disease, illness, condition, injury, and cause of injury known

5. Most insurance carriers accept which claim form?
   a. UB92
   b. CMS-1500
   c. CPT
   d. HCFA-1450

6. Claim registers are used to:
   a. anticipate claims to be sent to insurance companies for processing
   b. check how many claims are sent to Medicare
   c. monitor claims that have been sent to insurance companies for processing
   d. help in aging accounts

7. Insurance abuse:
   a. is the unauthorized release of confidential patient information to a third party
   b. is an intentional deception or misrepresentation that an individual makes, knowing it to be false, which could result in some unauthorized benefit
   c. refers to incidents or practices of providers, physicians, or suppliers of services and equipment that are inconsistent with accepted sound medical, business, or fiscal practices
   d. is impacted by the Omnibus Budget Reconciliation Acts of 1986 and 1987
8. Fraud is defined as:
   a. knowingly and willingly executing or attempting to execute a scheme to defraud any health care benefit
   b. is impacted by the Omnibus Budget Reconciliation Acts of 1986 and 1987
   c. is the unauthorized release of confidential patient information
   d. includes performing medical procedures that are not necessary

Critical Thinking

1. Electronic claims filing is mandatory for Medicare. Karen recently graduated from an accredited medical assisting program and is employed in the insurance department of a busy medical practice. She has asked her supervisor how she can gain more knowledge in coding and electronic billing procedures and how she might decrease the number of rejected claims. How would you respond to her if you were the supervisor?
2. The supervisor has given Karen a number of rejected claim forms and asks her to determine why the claims were denied and to maintain a log of these reasons to be discussed at the next staff meeting. How should Karen proceed with this assignment?
3. Karen finds that many claim forms were rejected because important information has been omitted. How might Karen suggest correction for these omissions?
4. The policy at Inner City Health Care is to request that the patient assign benefits by signing Block 13 of the CMS-1500 claim form if they do not pay for services on the day rendered. One of the patients is hesitant to comply with this policy. How should Karen explain this policy to the patient?
5. How might a compliance program benefit Inner City Health Care and what basic elements should it address?

WEB ACTIVITIES

 Use the Internet to search for current information on fraud and insurance abuse in Medicare billing. Document your findings following instructor guidelines.

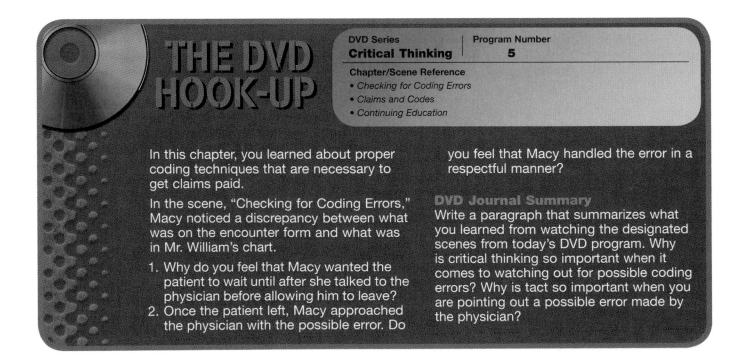

THE DVD HOOK-UP

DVD Series	Program Number
Critical Thinking	**5**

Chapter/Scene Reference
- *Checking for Coding Errors*
- *Claims and Codes*
- *Continuing Education*

In this chapter, you learned about proper coding techniques that are necessary to get claims paid.

In the scene, "Checking for Coding Errors," Macy noticed a discrepancy between what was on the encounter form and what was in Mr. William's chart.

1. Why do you feel that Macy wanted the patient to wait until after she talked to the physician before allowing him to leave?
2. Once the patient left, Macy approached the physician with the possible error. Do you feel that Macy handled the error in a respectful manner?

DVD Journal Summary

Write a paragraph that summarizes what you learned from watching the designated scenes from today's DVD program. Why is critical thinking so important when it comes to watching out for possible coding errors? Why is tact so important when you are pointing out a possible error made by the physician?

REFERENCES/BIBLIOGRAPHY

American Medical Association. (2005). *Current procedural terminology.* Chicago: American Medical Association.

American Medical Association. (Oct. 2005). *International classification of diseases, clinical modifications* (2nd ed., 9th rev.). Chicago: American Medical Association.

Fordney, M. T., French, L. L., & Follis, J. J. (2004). *Administrative medical assisting* (5th ed.). Clifton Park, NY: Thomson Delmar Learning.

ingenix. (2003, December). *HIPAA Tool Kit.* Salt Lake City, UT. St. Anthony Publishing/Medicode.

Johnson, S. L. (2000). *Understanding medical coding: A complete guide.* Clifton Park, NY: Thomson Delmar Learning.

Office of Inspector General, U.S. Department of Health and Human Services. (2000). *Compliance program guide for individual and small group physician practices.* Retrieved from http://oig.hhs.gov/modcomp/webcpg.txt. Accessed April 16, 2005.

Rowell, J. C. and Green, M. A. (2004). *Understanding medical insurance: A guide to professional billing* (7th ed.). Clifton Park, NY: Thomson Delmar Learning.

CHAPTER 20

Billing and Collections

OBJECTIVES

The student should strive to meet the following performance objectives and demonstrate an understanding of the facts and principles presented in this chapter through written and oral communication.

1. Define the key terms as presented in the glossary.
2. Analyze the importance of billing and collections to the ambulatory care setting.
3. Describe the advantages of billing at least the co-payment and co-insurance at time of service.
4. Discuss the Truth-in-Lending Act.
5. Compare manual billing and computerized billing.
6. Recall the components of a complete statement.
7. Differentiate between monthly and cycle billing.
8. Explain the process of aging accounts.
9. Analyze the importance of correct manner in telephone collections.

(continues)

SCENARIO

At Drs. Lewis & King, patient billing is typically done at time of service, and a charge slip noting date, description of charges, and fees is given to the patient on leaving the office. Office policy states that, if possible, patients should pay their part of the fee, or their co-pay, at time of service. Marilyn Johnson, the office manager, has found that this is the most efficient way to ensure timely payment and eliminates the need to mail a separate statement. However, the office is flexible and, if the patient cannot pay all or part of the charge at the visit, Marilyn works out a payment schedule that is acceptable to both office and patient.

- Application of electronic technology

Administrative Duties

- Apply computer concepts for office procedures
- Post collection agency payments

Legal Concepts

- Determine needs for documentation and reporting

Instructing

- Orient patients to policies and procedures

Financial Management

- Use manual and computerized bookkeeping systems
- Manage accounts payable and receivable
- Maintain records for accounting and banking purposes

INTRODUCTION

In the ambulatory care setting, patient billing is a critical administrative function that helps to maintain a healthy, viable practice. Timeliness is essential in billing, because the ambulatory care setting depends on its accounts receivable to pay its bills in a responsible manner. Billing need not be a complex activity, but it must be completely accurate. In offices still using pegboard accounting, billing and collection procedures are done manually, often using the patient's ledger card as the basis for the statement. If the office is computerized, patient bills and collection notices are typically computer generated.

The best method of patient billing and collections is a method that is customized to the practice and that regards the patient as a consumer who should be respected. Patients appreciate knowing in advance what charges and fees to expect. Many offices include these in their informational brochures or post them in a prominent place in the office.

Spotlight on Certification

RMA Content Outline
- Financial bookkeeping

CMA Content Outline
- Professional communication and behavior
- Legislation
- Bookkeeping systems
- Accounting and banking procedures

CMAS Content Outline
- Fundamental Financial Management
- Patient Accounts

BILLING PROCEDURES

The ambulatory care setting's cash flow and collection process are dependent on up-to-date and accurate billing techniques. The financial status of the practice is reflected in monthly statements indicating unpaid patient balances, which, if they persist, are reviewed for appropriate action, including referral to a collection agency. Copies of all billing forms will be retained in the patient account record.

Timeliness and accuracy have a significant influence on prompt payment and how soon collection of the patient account will be finalized. In other words, billing performance can be measured by the time it takes to generate and submit a complete statement, that is, a statement with full documentation. If an office is experiencing problems generating patient bills, a billing timeliness analysis worksheet can be constructed to identify internal delays that affect how quickly an account is billed, and thus paid. By focusing on inefficiencies in the revenue cycle, processes may be identified that need to be streamlined. For example, the date of service and insurance verification, the date the bill was generated, and the date the bill was submitted to the patient or third party can determine the efficiency of the billing process.

A billing efficiency report is another instrument that may be used to monitor efficiency. This report lists the previous month's billing backlog, which is added to the number of new accounts. The number of processed accounts is then subtracted. The weekly number of accounts that were rebilled also is noted, and the amount of time billing personnel spent on billing accounts is recorded. Production efficiency is calculated from these data. Inherent to this system is the careful monitoring of follow-up bills: whether they were paid, if the insurance was paid, and assessment of the patient's responsibility for payment.

CREDIT AND COLLECTION POLICIES

It is important that patients understand the billing policy and are educated about their accounts, how they are paid, and what their responsibility is toward payment. This is most easily accomplished in a patient-information brochure identifying all aspects of the medical practice, including how bills are paid. The office staff also must have a well-defined office policy related to patient billing and collecting.

Even uncomplicated patient billing should be done according to credit and collection policies established by the physician–employers of the ambulatory care setting. Having a formalized policy makes decision making easier and gives the medical assistant responsible for billing and collections authority to act. For example, some questions the physicians and office manager may want to address include:

- When will payment be due from the patient?

- What kind of payment arrangements can be made if the patient does not pay at time of service?

- At what point should a patient be reminded of an overdue bill?

- How is that reminder initially managed: by telephone, note on statement, or letter?

- At what point will a patient bill be considered delinquent?

Patient Education

Patients appreciate knowing their responsibility in terms of payment. Whoever schedules the first appointment with a new patient should diplomatically inform the patient of office policy on payment of fees. If the patient anticipates a problem in paying promptly, a schedule can be worked out that is agreeable to both parties.

- Will a collection agency be used? Who decides?

- If exceptions to office policy are to be made, who makes these exceptions and what steps are taken?

By answering these and other questions, a straightforward credit and collection policy can be devised that is a guide to both patients and the medical assistant in charge of billing.

PAYMENT AT TIME OF SERVICE

The best opportunity for collection is at the time of service. This process begins with the medical assistant who schedules appointments. Make certain all patients have the information they need. After determining the urgency and reason for the appointment, collecting information regarding a chief complaint, and assigning a time for the appointment, it is appropriate to discuss the financial concerns of patients. See Procedure 20-1. Patients may be shy in asking certain questions, but they have questions about most all of the following issues:

- Whether the physicians contract with their insurance carrier

- How payment is made if insurance does not cover certain procedures

- Can they be billed for co-payments and coinsurance

- How payment is made for services if they have no insurance

- An approximate cost of a particular service

Do not tell a patient, "We do not take your insurance." It is much better to make a statement such as, "Our physicians are not contract providers for that insurance. However, we can work with you on a fee-for-service basis and help make finances workable for you." The atmosphere has now been created to assure prompt collection and increased cash flow for the practice. To accommodate patients, offices now increasingly accept debit and credit card payments. Remember, also, that if your facility does use a sign-in method as patients arrive (see Chapter 14), then the all-important personal contact may be missed. With that missed opportunity also goes the opportunity to discuss finances.

Most of the insurance contracts require the physician–provider to bill the insurance company *before* billing the patient, except for the co-payment. It is critical to abide by each contract to protect the provider. If the patient is a member of a health maintenance organization (HMO) and the ambulatory care center is a participating provider, it is bound to the terms of that agreement. If not restricted by the insurance contract, be certain to explain to patients at the time of service that any payment made will be adjusted according to their insurance and the terms of that policy. Also remember that all patients must be treated the same and charged the same for services.

TRUTH-IN-LENDING ACT

In those situations where a payment schedule is arranged, office policy will dictate if any interest is charged. Although it is not illegal to charge interest on patient accounts, many physicians still prefer not to assign any interest on installment payments or past-due accounts.

CAPITAL AREA HEALTH CARE
839 Sycamore Park
Boise, ID 83725
(208) 863-4210

FEDERAL TRUTH-IN-LENDING STATEMENT
For Professional Services

Patient _____ Cari R. Jacobson _____

Address _____ 913 Swanson Street _____

_____ Boise, ID 61820 _____

Parent _____

1. Cost of services rendered	$1,500.00
2. Down Payment	225.00
3. Unpaid Balance	1,275.00
4. Amount Financed	1,275.00
5. Finance Charge	-0-
6. Annual Percentage Rate of Finance Charge	-0-
7. Total of Payments (4 + 5 above)	1,275.00
8. Total Amount After Payments	1,500.00

Total payment due is payable to __Dr. Leslie Swaggert__ at above address in _5_ monthly installments of $ _255_ . The first installment is payable on __August 1 20XX__ , and each subsequent payment is due on the same day of each consecutive month until paid in full.

__07-24-XX__ _____
Date of Agreement   Signature of Patient;
                            Parent if Patient is Minor

Figure 20-1 Truth-in-Lending Act document shows installment and interest agreement.

For installment payments (such as prenatal care or surgery), administrative medical assistants need to know the conditions of the **Truth-in Lending Act,** Regulation Z of the Consumer Protection Act of 1967 (see Chapter 7). If there is bilateral agreement between physicians and their patients for payment of medical services in more than four installments, that agreement must be in writing and must provide information on any finance charge. The information must be in writing even if there are no finance charges made. See Figure 20-1. The patient is given the original copy of the disclosure statement; a second copy is kept in the office.

COMPONENTS OF A COMPLETE STATEMENT

Once a patient has been accepted for treatment, it is important to maintain accurate and timely records of his or her account and payment history. That information is just as vital to the healthy management of the practice as the patient's medical chart. Invoice patient services promptly according to the office policy, send statements regularly, and make certain they are complete and accurate. Statements to patients must be professional looking, neat, inclusive of all services and charges, and easily understood. Procedure and diagnosis codes are necessary for insurance and reimbursement, but they usually mean nothing to patients. Make certain patients can understand the terminology used to explain the procedures they received.

Billing may occur in a number of different ways, with the computer-generated statement being the most widely used. As mentioned in Chapter 17, an encounter form may be used as the statement, especially if payment is made at the time of the service (Figure 20-2). Typewritten statements will likely use the continuous-form billing statement that is printed on a roll with perforated edges for separation. Photocopied statements are often used with a pegboard system. The ledger cards are coordinated with the same size copy paper. These photocopied ledgers are placed in a window envelope so that the address on the ledger card shows through the window.

If the statement is to be mailed, an enclosed self-addressed envelope is appreciated by the patient and may result in a faster turnaround of payment. Stamp the words "Address Service Requested" on the envelope just below the return address. When this statement is stamped on the envelope, a valuable tool in collections is available at minimum cost. If the statement cannot be delivered as addressed (the patient has moved or "skipped" and has left no forwarding address), the post office researches this information and returns

DATE	PATIENT	SERVICE CODE	FEES CHARGE	PAID	ADJ.	BALANCE DUE	PREVIOUS BALANCE	NAME	RECEIPT NO.
				CREDITS					

THIS IS YOUR RECEIPT _____ ▲

AND/OR A STATEMENT OF YOUR ACCOUNT TO DATE _____ ▲

		PATIENTS NAME	☐ M ☐ F

ADDRESS

CITY	STATE	ZIP

OFFICE VISITS AND PROCEDURES

99211	EST PT - MINIMAL OV	1				HOSPITAL VISIT	14	
99212	EST PT - BRIEF OV	2				EMERGENCY	15	
99213	EST PT - INTERMEDIATE OV	3				CONSULTATION	16	
99214	EST PT - EXTENDED OV	4		93000		EKG	17	
99215	EST PT - COMPREHENSIVE OV	5		93224		ELECTROCARDIOGRAPHIC MONITORING	18	
99201	NEW PT - BRIEF OV	6		93307		ECHOCARDIOGRAPHY	19	
99202	NEW PT - INTERMEDIATE OV	7		85025		CBC	20	
99203	NEW PT - EXTENDED OV	8		81000		URINALYSIS WITH MICROSCOPY	21	
99204	NEW PT - COMPLEX OV	9		36415		ROUTINE VENIPUNCTURE	22	
99205	NEW PT - COMPREHENSIVE OF	10		71020		RADIOLOGY EXAM-CHEST-2 VIEWS	23	
99238	HOSPITAL DISCHARGE	11		30300		REMOVE FOR. BODY-INTRANASAL	24	
99025	NEW PT - SURGERY PROC. PRIMARY	12					25	
	NURSING HOME VISIT	13					26	

RELATIONSHIP   BIRTHDATE

SUBSCRIBER OR POLICY HOLDER

☐ MEDICARE ☐ MEDICAID ☐ BLUE SHIELD ☐ 65-SP.

INSURANCE CARRIER

AGREEMENT #

GROUP #

D - OTHER SERVICES

AUTHORIZATION TO RELEASE INFORMATION: I HEREBY AUTHORIZE THE UNDERSIGNED PHYSICIAN TO RELEASE ANY INFORMATION ACQUIRED IN THE COURSE OF MY EXAMINATION OR TREATMENT.
SIGNED (PATIENT, OR PARENT IF MINOR)

_____ DATE _____

NEXT   AT   AM
APPOINTMENT   PM

RETURN _____ DAYS _____ WEEKS _____ MONTHS

PLACE OF SERVICE   ☐ OFFICE ☐ OTHER _____

DIAGNOSIS OR SYMPTOMS _____

DOCTOR'S SIGNATURE _____

CAPITAL AREA HEALTH CARE
839 SYCAMORE PARK
BOISE, ID 83725
(208) 863-4210

03626

Figure 20-2 Sample encounter form (charge slip) shown is a multipurpose form used to document information for insurance claims as well as to provide the patient with a receipt and documentation of procedures, diagnoses and fees. It can be used as the patient's first bill.

the envelope to you with a yellow sticker providing the new address and any other updated information. If the patient has ordered that mail be forwarded, the post office will forward the statement to the patient and send the medical facility a form with the new address. There is an approximate charge of 60 cents.

A well-prepared patient statement should contain not only information for the patient, but information needed to process medical insurance claims as well. The following information should be included:

- Patient's name and address
- Patient's insurance carrier and identification number
- Date and place of service
- Description of service and fee for each service
- Accurate procedure and diagnosis codes for insurance processing (see Chapters 18 and 19)
- Physician's signature and identification code

- Ambulatory care center name, address, telephone number, fax number, and Web site when applicable

Computerized Statements

 If the ambulatory care setting uses a computer system of bookkeeping, then statements will be computer generated. Typically, the medical assistant issues instructions to search the patient database for outstanding balances and directs the computer to print statements.

During this process, the computer program will also "age" accounts (see Aging Accounts section later in this chapter) and print collection letters (already in the database) for overdue accounts.

MONTHLY AND CYCLE BILLING

The billing schedule is often determined by the size of the medical practice. Monthly billing is a system in which all accounts are billed at the same time each

---

Sample of Cycle Billing

1. Divide the alphabet into four sections: A–F, G–L, M–R, S–Z.
2. Prepare statements for patients whose last names begin with A through F on Wednesday and mail them on Thursday of Week 1.
3. Prepare statements for patients whose last names begin with G through L on Wednesday and mail them on Thursday of Week 2.
4. Prepare statements for patients whose last names begin with M through R on Wednesday and mail them on Thursday of Week 3.
5. Prepare statements for patients whose last names begin with S through Z on Wednesday and mail them on Thursday of Week 4.

Figure 20-3 Typical schedule for cycle billing system.

month. In a smaller ambulatory care setting, monthly billing may be the most efficient method. Cycle billing staggers bills during the month and is a flexible system for larger practices.

Monthly Billing

In a monthly billing system, one or two days are devoted to billing and mailing all statements. Typically, statements should leave the office on the 25th of the month to be received by the first of the month. The major disadvantage of monthly billing is that a medical assistant may neglect other activities during this time-consuming period. To avoid these problems, billing statements may be prepared intermittently over a one- or two-week period and stored until the mailing date. To avoid confusion caused by delays in mailing, a message to "Disregard if payment has already been made" should be printed on the form. Patients become annoyed and the practice appears disorganized if a statement arrives several days after payment has been made.

Cycle Billing

In a cycle billing system, all accounts usually are divided alphabetically into groups, with each group billed at a different time. In this way, office personnel with numerous bills to process each month will be able to handle them in a more efficient manner. Statements are prepared on the same schedule each month. They can be mailed as they are completed, or held and mailed at one time. A typical cycle billing schedule is shown in Figure 20-3. The system can be varied to suit the needs of the individual practice.

PAST-DUE ACCOUNTS

As efficient and effective as the billing process may be, there will still be collections on some accounts. The most common reasons for past-due accounts include:

- *Inability to pay.* People may have financial hardships from time to time. Refer to Chapter 17.
- *Negligence.* People may forget to make a payment because they have been away or dealing with a family emergency.
- *Unwillingness to pay.* When a patient complains about a charge or refuses to pay, it may have nothing to do with finances. Often, they are dissatisfied with the care or treatment they have received. These patients should be referred to the physician or office manager for immediate attention.
- *Third-Party Payers.* Past-due accounts may result because of inaccurate or insufficient insurance information. Claims can be rejected because of many varied reasons, and time limits must be observed.
- *Minors.* Minors who are not legally emancipated may seek and receive treatment, but they are not responsible for paying the bill (see Chapter 7). If the medical practice treats minors who are not emancipated, an office policy should determine how minors pay for their services. Many facilities ask for cash at the time of the service. Emancipated minors are responsible for their bills.

COLLECTION PROCESS

The process of collecting delinquent accounts begins with first establishing how much has been owed and for how long.

Ideally, collection of accounts receivable should be prompt and conducted in a timely fashion. Management consultants recommend collecting at least a portion of the fees at the time of service and that a **collection ratio** of 90% or better should be maintained. Another important factor is the **accounts receivable ratio** that measures the speed with which outstanding accounts are paid. The desirable accounts receivable ratio is less than two months for collection of accounts receivable.

Collection Ratio

A collection ratio is a method used to gauge the effectiveness of the ambulatory care setting's billing practices. This ratio shows the status of collections and the possible losses in the medical facility. It is a good idea to obtain the ratio monthly, quarterly, and yearly. Typically, the collection ratio is calculated by dividing the total collections by the net charges (gross charges minus adjustments). This yields a percentage that is referred to as the collection ratio. See the following example:

$$\frac{\text{Total Amount Collected this Month}}{\text{Total Monthly Charges Minus Adjustments}} = \text{Monthly Collection Ratio}$$

$$\frac{\$11,374}{\$14,650} = .7695 \text{ or } 77\%$$

In this sample, you can determine that more time and energy needs to be spent in collecting accounts. The practice is losing almost 25% of its income potential. Not only is the income potential being lost, the ability to invest that income is also lost, making the potential loss even greater.

Accounts Receivable Ratio

An accounts receivables ratio indicates how quickly outstanding accounts are paid. It can also be a measure of how effective the collections are. To calculate the accounts receivable ratio, divide the current accounts receivable balance by the average monthly gross charges. This yields the typical turnaround for collecting accounts receivable. See the following example:

$$\frac{\text{Current Accounts Receivable}}{\text{Average Monthly Gross Charges}} = \text{Accounts Receivable Ratio}$$

$$\frac{\$102,048}{\$18,220} = 5.6$$

Because the goal of the accounts receivable ratio is payment in less than two months, you can quickly observe that this practice is close to a half year behind in collections. See Chapter 21 for additional information on accounts receivable and collection ratios.

The longer an office puts off attempting to collect delinquent accounts, the less chance there is of receiving payment. Statistics show that the value of the dollar decreases rapidly in the collection process. The more time and energy you put into collections, the less value you receive in return. That is, you may manage to collect the full amount due, but when you consider the time and expense involved, it may not have been worth the effort and expense. Therefore, the value of the debt to be received after successful collection must be considered when determining how aggressive to be in debt collections.

AGING ACCOUNTS

Account aging is a method of identifying how long an account has been overdue. This means that past-due accounts are identified according to the length of time they have been unpaid. When using a pegboard bookkeeping system, color-coded strips are attached to the ledger cards to show the age of an account, or the cards can be stored behind a color-coded divider in a separate file labeled "Unpaid." For example, a red strip might be used for accounts one month overdue, a blue strip for accounts two months overdue, and other colors for additional months overdue. A written code such as "OD3/2/23" should be written on the ledger card to indicate when the overdue notice was mailed, meaning "Overdue notice No. 3 mailed on February 23."

Depending on the type of patient served, different aging systems are used. In a computerized billing system, the accounts are automatically aged, and the aging schedule or process is shown on the computerized ledger.

Computerized Aging

Aging accounts using a computerized system is simple. Before printing billing statements, the medical assistant keys the appropriate commands to age the accounts. The program can age accounts according to several criteria: for example, by past due balance, zero balance, or credit balance accounts. Accounts can also be aged by government agency category or by insurance carrier. All Medicare or Medicaid accounts might be aged separately from other accounts. Sorting out Medicare and Medicaid accounts may also be done when computing the accounts receivable ratio and the collection ratio.

The computer can also generate and print an accounts receivable report showing each overdue account, the balance overdue, and a breakdown showing how long the account has been overdue. This breakdown is usually divided into accounts 0 to 30 days overdue, 31 to 60 days overdue, 61 to 90 days overdue, and 90 days or more overdue. Additional reports can be generated from the accounts receivable report. For example, the office staff may wish to reprint a report showing accounts that have been delinquent for more than 90 days or accounts that are delinquent by more than a certain dollar amount.

COLLECTION TECHNIQUES

Ambulatory care settings use both telephone and written communications in their collection techniques. Although both have some measure of effectiveness, some practices prefer to call the patient with a past-due account before officially initiating collection proceedings. The patient may have misplaced the statement, forgotten a payment, or been away on an extended vacation; a quick telephone call can often resolve the situation without the time and expense involved in collections. Also, the patient usually appreciates the courtesy and personal approach. See Figure 20-4 for a sample collections policy.

Correspondence to Insurance Carriers

Many patients have some form of medical insurance. Make it a practice to send each computer claim within

---

SAMPLE COLLECTION POLICY SCHEDULE

- Encounter form (if used) given to patient at time of visit
- Itemized statement sent no later than the end of that month
- Itemized statement with overdue notice no later than the end of the second month
- Telephone call reminding the patient of the bill. "We've sent two statements and we haven't received payment. Do you need more information from us?" Offer help at this point in establishing a payment schedule, and seek to get a commitment from the patient.
- If a financial schedule is to be established, prepare it and mail to the patient within a day of the phone conversation. Follow up on that commitment within 15 days. The follow up message may be a thank you for sending the first payment. Carefully monitor payments and their timeliness.
- If no payment schedule is made by the patient, send a letter stating the amount due before the account is past due three months. Discuss with office manager and/or physician regarding the merit of continued collection at this time.
- If collections are to continue, notify the patient one more time of their responsibility and ask for payment.
- If no payment is received, send a letter stating that "Your account has been turned over to a collection agency" if outside collectors are used. Make no more phone calls.*

*Some physicians send a letter of discharge to patients at this time via certified mail. (See Chapter 7.)

Figure 20-4 Sample collection schedule.

two days or less of the patient account data being entered into the computer. Batches of claims to insurance carriers should be forwarded at the end of each day. In the era of electronic claims processing, much time is saved in not having to prepare hard copies of the forms for mailing. Electronic claims transmission (ECT; also known as electronic medic claims, or EMC, and electronic claims submission, or ECS) dictates that the practice's computer system must be able to communicate with the insurance carrier's computer. This paperless process yields less errors than the manual process because ECT software includes some built-in checks to determine any invalid codes, sex or age conflicts, and correct procedure and diagnostic code linkages to the services provided. Sending insurance claims via the paper process will take more time to process, and the turnaround time for payment is also longer. Most claim departments of insurance carriers and government agencies employ large numbers of employees who have varying levels of experience. Payment can be delayed because of an overburdened claim department, a form that has been lost in transit, a misfiled form, an inexperienced employee, or numerous other reasons.

The medical assistant should maintain an up-to-date claims register or insurance-pending report and take firm control of the practice's collection procedures to ensure that claims are paid promptly.

This claim register or insurance-pending report may be a part of the computerized billing system. If so, the printout will show how much the practice charged insurance carriers and how much was received. This clearly shows which carriers are slower than others and where other problems might arise. For any claim pending more than 45 days, it is a good idea to make a call to the carrier to find out whether the claim has been received, where it is in the process, and whether the office staff might have done something to delay the process. Such phone calls can become carefully cultivated personal contacts with insurance representatives to pave the way for cooperation in the future.

In offices where the medical assistant files claims for patients, a follow-up collection policy is important to maintain strong cash flow. When carriers do not pay in full or question or deny a claim, the medical assistant should determine the nature of the problem and rebill or appeal the decision, whichever action is appropriate.

Telephone Collections

The medical assistant is likely to use the telephone for collection procedures. Telephoning is often an effective measure, because a patient may respond to a call more so than a bill received in the mail.

A successful telephone collection call is enhanced by keeping to the facts and being tactful, pleasant, and diplomatic. When making calls to patients regarding past-due accounts, there are some things to keep in mind to maintain the desired relationship with patients. Always remain courteous and respectful. Do not treat patients with suspicion or threats. Remember, the health profession is dedicated to helping people; avoid antagonizing patients.

Most people do not let their bills become past due on purpose or out of spite. Keep this in mind when making calls. Work with patients to encourage and enable them to pay any fees they owe.

 Certain legal rules and ethical guidelines govern telephone collections, such as:

- When making collection calls, callers must identify themselves and ascertain that they are talking to the person who is responsible for the account.

- A collection call could be embarrassing to the patient; therefore, it should not be made to the patient's place of employment.

- In most states, a debtor may be contacted only between 8 AM and 8 PM.

- Do not make telephone calls at odd hours or make repeated calls to the debtor's friends, employers, or relatives.

- If a contact must be made to the debtor's place of business, do not reveal to any third party the nature of the call. Patients have a right to confidentiality and privacy.

- Do not threaten to turn the person's account over to collection agencies.

Violating these rules makes the caller vulnerable to charges of harassment under the **Fair Debt Collection Practice Act.** See additional information at http://ftc.gov/os/statutes/fdcpa.

When collecting by telephone, it is helpful to keep complete, accurate records of the process indicating who said what and how much was promised as payment. If, after two weeks nothing has been resolved as a result of the calls, then another course of action may be the solution, especially for large sums of money owed. Collection letters may be the solution.

Collection Letters

Collection letters are sent to encourage patients to pay overdue balances. After two statements are mailed to patients and the charge slip has brought no response, the ambulatory care setting begins sending collection letters.

Lack of payment from a patient may not be considered serious until after 60 days. When the patient fails to respond to the encounter form, to the statement, or to a 60-day statement with an "Overdue" remark, a series of collection letters begins. One typical collection letter series is shown in Figure 20-5 A through C. Collection letters and notes are kept seperate from a patient's chart.

USE OF AN OUTSIDE COLLECTION AGENCY

Occasionally, the ambulatory care setting may turn over highly delinquent accounts to an outside collection agency. Discretion is always advised here, however, because the expense of collection may not justify the fees to be collected. For unpaid accounts with large balances, however, this is often a viable solution.

One service of the collection agency is to provide an intercept letter. For a nominal fee, this may be sent from the agency as the last resort before the account is turned over to collection. This communication alerts patients to the fact that if a response is not received, their account will go to collection. This often is the only action needed for the patient to pay the outstanding bill. Another service of a credit bureau or collection agency is to provide credit ratings of patients at the physician's request. Physicians who pay for this service are able to monitor patients' ability to pay their bills, as well as to trace a "skip," someone who leaves with an outstanding bill and no forwarding address.

When selecting a collection agency, be certain to hire one that is compatible with the medical office's philosophy. Questions that might be asked of potential collection agencies include the following:

- Does the agency handle only medical and dental accounts?

- What methods are used to make collections?

- Is the agency fee a flat charge per account or a percentage of the account recovered?

- How promptly does the agency settle accounts?

- Will the agency supply a list of satisfied customers or references?

- What ability does the medical practice have to end the agency's collection efforts?

Once a collection agency has been selected, carefully follow their instructions about any contact patients

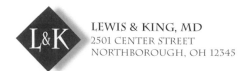

June 14, 20XX

Mr. John O'Keefe
12 Gravers Lane
Northborough, OH 12345

Dear Mr. O'Keefe:

Your account with our office is three months past due, and you have not responded to our previous requests for payment. Please pay your balance of $852 at this time, or contact us with a plan for payment.

Please call me at 312-824-6925 if you have a question about your account or a plan for payment. Otherwise, we expect your payment immediately.

Sincerely,

Marilyn Johnson
Office Manager

NORTHBOROUGH
FAMILY MEDICAL GROUP

(A)

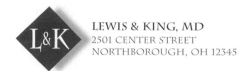

July 15, 20XX

Mr. John O'Keefe
12 Gravers Lane
Northborough, OH 12345

Dear Mr. O'Keefe:

Your son, Chris, was seriously ill in March when he came to Dr. King for treatment. Dr. King was pleased to use her experience and education to treat Chris, and it was in this same spirit of cooperation that we believed you would pay your account within a reasonable amount of time.

Four months have passed and you have still not remitted the $852 outstanding balance on your account. We cannot continue to keep your unpaid account on our books. If you are experiencing financial difficulties, please call the office so we can arrange a payment schedule that is agreeable to both of us.

Sincerely,

Marilyn Johnson
Office Manager

NORTHBOROUGH
FAMILY MEDICAL GROUP

(B)

Figure 20-5 Sample collection letters: (A) First letter. (B) Second letter.

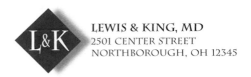

LEWIS & KING, MD
2501 CENTER STREET
NORTHBOROUGH, OH 12345

August 17, 20XX

CERTIFIED MAIL

Mr. John O'Keefe
12 Gravers Lane
Northborough, OH 12345

Dear Mr. O'Keefe:

This is our final attempt to collect your account of $852, which is five months past due. You have ignored all our previous letters [or letters and phone calls], so we have no alternative but to turn over your account to a collection company.

Your account is being assigned to Ambler Medical Collection Service, which will pursue whatever legal means is necessary to collect this debt. If you contact me at 312-824-6925 within seven days, we can prevent the account from this assignment and resolve the balance.

Sincerely,

Marilyn Johnson
Office Manager

NORTHBOROUGH
FAMILY MEDICAL GROUP

(C)

Figure 20-5 (continued) (C) Third letter.

make to the medical office regarding their account and any other guidelines in their contract with the practice. Keep a record of accounts given to the agency, as well as their rate of return. Hopefully, the agency will be able to motivate patients to pay for the health care services they have received while still maintaining the practice's good reputation and increasing your profit margin. Medical collections lets your patients know that the practice is serious about collecting past-due accounts.

There is often a question about how payments from collection agencies are posted. This is one purpose of the adjustment column. Place the amount received in the adjustment column because it is a subtraction from the amount due. If there is no adjustment column, put the amount in the charge column and put red parentheses around it or circle in red so the amount is actually subtracted from the balance. The remaining balance after collections is paid is written off. See Procedure 20-3.

USE OF SMALL CLAIMS COURT

 In certain circumstances, the ambulatory care center may consider bringing a case to small claims court. Typically, small claims courts handle cases that involve only limited amounts of debt (these vary from state to state), they usually do not permit representation by an attorney, and they are generally efficient and streamlined in their proceedings. Nonetheless, preparing for small claims courts and taking time to appear will require a certain investment of staff. It is also important to note that, if the court finds in the medical office's favor, the medical office still must collect the money from the defendant. An account assigned to a collection agency cannot be filed in small claims court.

SPECIAL COLLECTION SITUATIONS

In patient billing and collections, a number of special situations may arise.

Bankruptcy

If a patient has declared bankruptcy, statements may no longer be sent nor any attempt be made to collect delinquent accounts. A patient declaring bankruptcy usually does so under Chapter 7 or Chapter 13 bankruptcy law. In Chapter 7 bankruptcy, a patient declares bankruptcy to all debtors and is allowed to clear all debts and start fresh. The physician's office should file a proof-of-claim form and provide a copy of the patient's outstanding account to the bankruptcy court. In Chapter 13, also known as "wage-earner's bankruptcy," patients (wage-earners) are protected from bill collectors and are allowed to pay their bills over time. The court determines a monthly amount that the debtor can pay, collects that sum, and parcels it out to the creditors over a period as long as five years. The physician must file a claim as directed by the debtor's attorney to collect any fees outstanding. Because a physician's fee is an unsecured debt, it is one of the last to be paid. Bankruptcy laws are federal and are subject to the Federal Wage Garnishment Law of attaching property to satisfy debt.

Estates

Collection of fees when a patient has died must be directed to the executor of the estate or the one responsible for overseeing the estate. Some general guidelines to follow include:

- Show courtesy by not sending a statement in the first week or so after a death.

- Prepare an itemized statement of the deceased patient's account. (In some cases, a special form is required for this.)

- Mail the account information via certified mail with a return receipt requested to the administrator of the estate. The name can be obtained by calling the probate department of the superior court.

- If there is no known or identified administrator, send a copy of the itemized statement to the "Estate of (name of patient)" to the patient's last known address. Often, there is a family member who has assumed the responsibility for paying the patient's account balances.

- If unsure of how to proceed, contact the office's attorney or the clerk of the **probate court** for advice.

Tracing "Skips"

 As noted earlier in this chapter, a "skip" is a patient who has apparently moved with no forwarding address. If a statement is returned to your office marked "no forwarding address," first determine if there were any internal errors in addressing the envelope. If the address is determined to be correct, the medical assistant may try to call the patient with the number on the patient ledger; it is possible that the patient

has retained the same number, or there may be a new number given. If the medical assistant is unable to secure a telephone number, the office needs to decide whether to pursue the unpaid debt. This will depend on office policy and the amount that is owed. If it is decided to pursue an unpaid account, it could be turned over to a collection agency. If the medical assistant attempts to trace the skip by calling employers or relatives, it is important not to violate any laws in doing so and maintain the patient's confidentiality.

STATUTE OF LIMITATIONS

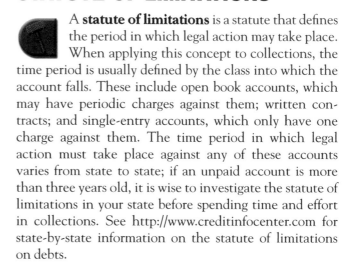 A **statute of limitations** is a statute that defines the period in which legal action may take place. When applying this concept to collections, the time period is usually defined by the class into which the account falls. These include open book accounts, which may have periodic charges against them; written contracts; and single-entry accounts, which only have one charge against them. The time period in which legal action must take place against any of these accounts varies from state to state; if an unpaid account is more than three years old, it is wise to investigate the statute of limitations in your state before spending time and effort in collections. See http://www.creditinfocenter.com for state-by-state information on the statute of limitations on debts.

MAINTAIN A PROFESSIONAL ATTITUDE

Collecting past-due accounts is one of the most difficult tasks delegated to medical assistants. Not everyone is able to perform the task. Placing calls can be discouraging, especially if the results seem less than anticipated. Not all accounts can be collected. Identify these accounts early, write them off, and save the medical practice time and money. Keep your emotions out of the process. Rely only on your information, the aged account, and the realization that the office policy is well thought out and provides a win-win solution for both the patient and the physician as much as possible. When dealing with a "true deadbeat" who has no intention of paying the bill, be proud of your physician's attention to that patient's need, but discuss with the physician the possibility of discharging the patient. Staff may need additional training and education from time to time to update skills on patient service and how to maintain goodwill during the collection process.

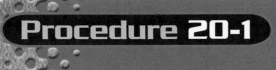

Procedure 20-1 Explaining Fees in the First Telephone Interview

PURPOSE:
To establish rapport with patients, to discuss physicians' fees, and to identify the patient's responsibility before the first visit.

EQUIPMENT/SUPPLIES:
Physician's fee schedule
Appointment schedule
Telephone

PROCEDURE STEPS:
1. Place the physicians' fee schedule and the appointment schedule close to the telephone. RATIONALE: The office staff that is prepared does not have to search for something vital to the phone conversation.
2. Answer the phone before the third ring. Identify the name of the clinic and yourself. RATIONALE: The person calling feels attended to and knows the call has been correctly placed.
3. Offer assistance; for example, a comment such as "How can I help you?" RATIONALE: Sets the tone for the patient to continue with the request.
4. After the patient is identified as a new patient and the nature of the visit is determined appropriate, discuss possible dates for the appointment. A statement such as, "Our next available appointment is Thursday at 11:30 AM Can you make it then?" is a good way to begin.

5. Tell the patient that you will be discussing clinic policies briefly now and will mail the Patient Information Brochure before the appointment. RATIONALE: The patient brochure details some of the information discussed in the telephone conversation and further verifies the clinic's policies.
6. Ask about medical insurance. Get the identification number, the name of the subscriber, employer, and a telephone number of the insurance carrier if possible. RATIONALE: This allows you to check for any preauthorization required and for the currency of the plan.
7. Explain that the clinic policy will require any co-payment and coinsurance to be paid at the time of the visit. RATIONALE: Establishes patient's financial responsibility immediately.
8. Check to see if the patient has transportation and knows how to get to the clinic; and provide directions if necessary. RATIONALE: Ensures that there is no confusion about location and accessibility.
9. Request that the patient arrive about 15 minutes before the appointment to complete some forms. RATIONALE: Ensures that the patient has time to complete information and can ask any questions that might occur.
10. After closing the telephone interview, promptly mail the Patient Information Brochure.

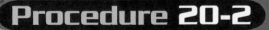

Procedure 20-2 Prepare Itemized Patient Accounts for Billing

PURPOSE:
To notify patients of the fees for services rendered and collect on those accounts.

EQUIPMENT/SUPPLIES:
Computer or typewriter
Calculator

Patient account or ledger cards
Billing statement forms

PROCEDURE STEPS:
1. Gather all accounts and ledgers with outstanding balances. RATIONALE: Everything in one place saves time and energy.

(continues)

Procedure 20-2 (continued)

2. Separate any accounts that are labeled as overdue. RATIONALE: Individual decisions on these accounts are necessary before taking action.

For each account, perform the following:

a. Verify the name and address of the patient and the person responsible for payment.

b. Place current date on the statement.

c. Scan the account information for any possible errors.

d. Itemize the procedures in terms patients understand and indicate charges.

e. Identify and subtract any payments (copayment, coinsurance, down payment) that have been made.

f. Use the calculator to verify the unpaid balance that is carried forward and is due. (For the d, e, & f items, the process is the same in the manual system as in the computer system; however, in the computer system, explanations and totals are calculated for the user.)

3. Discuss with the office manager any action to be taken on past-due accounts. Follow through with those instructions. RATIONALE: More than one person is involved in the collection process.

4. Place statements in envelopes and mail. RATIONALE: Ensures timely delivery of statements.

Procedure 20-3 Post/Record Adjustments and Refunds, including Collection Agency Payments

PURPOSE:

To keep track of financial adjustments.

EQUIPMENT/SUPPLIES:

Computerized or manual bookkeeping system
Patient's account
Black, blue, and red ink pen for use in manual bookkeeping system
Checkbook

PROCEDURE STEPS:

1. With the daily schedule of services/charges before you (either the manual daily sheet or the computerized equivalent), enter amount received from the collection agency on a patient's account and a note such as "Payment from ABC Collection Agency" in the explanation section. RATIONALE: Indicates funds received on a collection contract.

2. Record the amount received and the explanation in the patient's account as well. The amount received is *subtracted* from the account balance. The balance amount of the account is placed in the "adjustment" column. If there is no adjustment column, put the amount in the charge column with parentheses around it or circle the amount in red. These data are

copied to the patient's account in the write-it-once system or are automatically drawn into the patient's account in the computerized system. RATIONALE: Demonstrates the activity and amount from the collection agency on a patient's account in the patient account documents.

3. Subtract the amount paid by the collection agency from the total charges to create the new balance. RATIONALE: Clearly indicates what portion of the account the patient has paid and the amount that is not collectible.

4. The difference between the amount owed and the amount paid is entered as a negative adjustment on the day sheet. This balance will either be refunded or written off as uncollectible. Either way, indicate a zero balance on the patient's account in the day sheet. RATIONALE: At the end of the year, the uncollectible totals can be obtained indicating the amount of uncollected charges for the practice's income tax preparation.

5. Proceed to write a check for any overpayment: Determine who should receive the refund. Write a check for the amount. Post the amount as a refund on the patient's account. Attach a check to the patient's account and forward to the physician or office manager for signature.

Procedure 20-3 (continued)

RATIONALE: Sometimes the patient receives the refund, sometimes the insurance company is due a refund and so forth. Attaching the check to the patient's account allows the physician or office manager to look at the account before signing a refund check.

Case Study 20-1

For patient accounts more than 60 days overdue, the offices of Drs. Lewis and King begin a series of collection proceedings to attempt to collect the monies. Initially, they place a telephone call to the patient to determine whether a billing problem might be present that can be clarified over the telephone. If they cannot reach the patient, or the patient does not respond to the call, then collections begin. Marilyn has assigned this function of the billing process to Ellen Armstrong, because Ellen has a warm telephone manner and is good with patients.

CASE STUDY REVIEW

1. Why is Ellen's telephone manner of importance in the collection process?
2. In addition to telephone collections, what patient letters might Ellen send?
3. Ellen has come across an account that is delinquent and discovers that the patient has declared bankruptcy. What can Ellen do now?

Case Study 20-2

Morgan Bryant is the custodial parent and single mother of her five-year-old son, Custer, who has been a patient in the Valley Pediatric Clinic since his birth. Custer's father's insurance covered his medical expenses. During a separation and the resulting divorce, the medical bills continued to go to Custer's father. Morgan comes to the reception desk to discuss the collections letter she received. Her parenting plan requires her former husband to provide medical coverage for their son. However, it appears he canceled his policy coverage on his son four months ago and Morgan did not know until she received the letter. Morgan is in tears.

CASE STUDY REVIEW

1. What is the first step the receptionist should take?
2. Is there anything the clinic staff might have done differently in collecting this account?
3. What might be done for Morgan now? Are there resources Morgan might need to know about?

SUMMARY

Billing and collection activities in the ambulatory care setting are intricately linked to daily financial practices and claims processing, and the medical assistant responsible for billing should also be well aware of these other functions. Billing need not entail a complex or elaborate system, but whether accomplished by manual or computer methodology, it needs to be precise, professional, and comprehensive, as all communications with patients should be. If collections become necessary, courteous and straightforward letters and telephone exchanges are the most effective. The goal of all billing and collections is to maintain the relationship with the patient, whereas ensuring good cash flow and payment of accounts receivable in the ambulatory care setting.

STUDY FOR SUCCESS

To reinforce your knowledge and skills of information presented in this chapter:
- ❏ Review the Key Terms
- ❏ Practice any Procedures
- ❏ Consider the Case Studies and discuss your conclusions
- ❏ Answer the Review Questions
  - ❏ Multiple Choice
  - ❏ Critical Thinking
- ❏ Navigate the Internet and complete the Web Activities
- ❏ Practice the StudyWARE activities on the textbook CD
- ❏ Apply your knowledge in the Student Workbook activities
- ❏ Complete the Web Tutor sections
- ❏ View and discuss the DVD situations

REVIEW QUESTIONS

Multiple Choice

1. The Truth-In-Lending Act:
   a. is designed to place limits on the amount of debt for which consumers are liable
   b. is also known as the statute of limitations
   c. is also known as Regulation Z
   d. does not apply to medical facilities
2. Cycle billing is a system of billing:
   a. completed every fourth month
   b. done only by computer
   c. completed by the 25th of the month
   d. in which accounts are divided into sections for billing purposes
3. One of the most common reasons patient bills go unpaid is:
   a. inability to pay because of financial hardship
   b. patients consider the cost of medical care too high
   c. patients think their insurance should cover all medical bills
   d. patients think physicians make too much money
4. Aging accounts:
   a. is a process of identifying overdue patient accounts
   b. describes patients who have a long-term relationship with the ambulatory care center
   c. describes older adult patients with Medicare
   d. applies to accounts considered inactive
5. If an unpaid account goes to small claims court:
   a. the medical office must engage an attorney representative
   b. the medical office is still responsible for collecting even if the court finds in its favor
   c. there is no need to show up at court
   d. a large sum of money must be at issue

6. A collection ratio:
   a. shows status of collections and possible losses
   b. divides the current accounts receivable by the average monthly gross charges
   c. should be 90% or better
   d. a and c
7. A claims register:
   a. identifies how many past-due claims have been collected
   b. may also be called the insurance-pending report
   c. is maintained by each insurance carrier for the physician
   d. is a tickler file that maintains all patients' insurance information
8. Telephone collections:
   a. are best made after 8 PM when patients are home
   b. must abide by the Fair Debt Collection Practice Act
   c. are usually successful after numerous calls at the patient's place of employment
   d. will require overtime pay for the medical office staff
9. A "skip" is defined as:
   a. the time period when legal action cannot be taken
   b. an estate involved in probate
   c. one who moves without a forwarding address and leaves an unpaid bill
   d. one who has paid a portion of a debt
10. For patient accounts, a collection agency:
    a. is better if it handles only medical and dental accounts
    b. creates a bad feeling between patients and physicians
    c. cannot possibly do as good a job as the medical office staff
    d. seldom describes its methods for collections

Critical Thinking

1. Why is prompt and accurate billing important to the success of the ambulatory care setting and to the patient?
2. Describe the procedure used if moving from monthly billing to cycle billing.
3. When the office manager calls a patient regarding a past-due account, she is told by the patient, "I'm not about to pay that bill. The treatment made my pain worse, not better." What steps might be taken now?
4. Seymore Storme's original medical bill is $356. He has no insurance but keeps his account active by paying $25 per month. To date, he has made four payments of $25 in four months. Should a Truth-in-Lending Statement be prepared? Why or why not?
5. With another student, role-play a telephone collections call. One student can be the medical assistant, the other student can be the patient. Have a third student observe and evaluate the call. Discuss.

WEB ACTIVITIES

1. Research the Internet for information on debt collections. Consider keywords such as "credit law," "collections," and "debt recovery." What sources of information are found that might be helpful to an ambulatory care facility?
2. Research the statute of limitations in your state. How much time is allowed for legal action to take place in collecting a past-due account?
3. Go to http://www.whowhere.com and http://www.searchbug.com. Did you find any information that might help you locate a patient who appears to have skipped out on a major bill for elective surgery? What services are free to you? What services require payment? How much is the fee?

REFERENCES/BIBLIOGRAPHY

Fordney, M. T., French, L. L., & Follis, J. J. (2004). *Administrative medical assisting* (5th ed.). Clifton Park, NY: Thomson Delmar Learning.

Lewis, M. A., & Tamparo, C. D. (2002). *Medical law, ethics, and bioethics for ambulatory care* (5th ed.). Philadelphia: F. A. Davis Company.

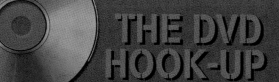

In this chapter, you learned about proper billing and collection procedures.

In the designated scene, you observed Geneva making collection calls.

1. Do you believe that Geneva used a "therapeutic approach" when calling patients about their past-due accounts?
2. How do you feel when you receive collection calls?
3. Why is it important for the office to try and collect the money instead of just turning the patient's account over for collection?

DVD Journal Summary

Write a paragraph that summarizes what you learned from watching the designated scene from today's DVD program. Suppose that you work both sides of the medical office. You know that a patient is deliberately not paying his or her bills but continually frequents your office because of acute illness. Will you be able to deliver clinical care to the patient without being judgmental?

CHAPTER 21

Accounting Practices

OUTLINE

OBJECTIVES

The student should strive to meet the following performance objectives and demonstrate an understanding of the facts and principles presented in this chapter through written and oral communication.

1. Define the key terms as presented in the glossary.
2. Understand the purpose and range of the accounting function in the ambulatory care setting.
3. Describe the four different types of bookkeeping and accounting systems.
4. Recall the importance of the day-end summary and the accounts receivable trial balance.
5. Compare and contrast financial, managerial, and cost accounting.
6. Explain the use and validity of the income statement and the balance sheet.
7. Recall three useful financial ratios and explain.
8. Identify proper steps in accounts payable management.
9. Discuss the impact of utilization review on reimbursement.
10. Discuss legal and ethical guidelines in accounting practices.

KEY TERMS

Accounting
Accounts Payable
Accounts Receivable (A/R)
   Ratio
Accrual Basis
Assets
Balance Sheet
Cash Basis
Check Register
Collection Ratio
Cost Analysis
Cost Ratio
Fixed Cost
Income Statement
Liability
Owner's Equity
Utilization Review (UR)
Variable Cost

SCENARIO

When James Whitney, one of the physician–owners at Inner City Health Care, and Jane O'Hara, CMA, the office manager, decided to add a new medical assistant to the staff, they first reviewed the financial records for the previous year. Although the volume of work in the center generated the need for an additional employee, Whitney and O'Hara had to be sure it was financially feasible. In addition to past records, they also had to make some projections for the upcoming year; with certain new managed care fees, they had to be sure that anticipated revenues would be sufficient to sustain the salary of a new employee.

INTRODUCTION

Medical financial management in the ambulatory care setting is most important in the daily functioning of the office business because it directly affects overall bookkeeping and accounting procedures. Accounting generates financial information for the ambulatory care setting and is defined as a system of monitoring the financial status of a facility and the specific results of its activities. It provides financial information for decision making.

Previous chapters have included the topics of proper daily bookkeeping financial practices (see Chapter 17), the accurate coding and the specific processing of insurance forms (see Chapters 18 and 19), and the efficient management of collecting on accounts (see Chapter 20). All of these functions are essential to obtain maximum reimbursement and create profitability for the practice.

This chapter ties many of these elements together and creates a total picture of their interdependence. Each element is critical to the ambulatory care setting's accurate accounting practices.

BOOKKEEPING AND ACCOUNTING SYSTEMS

Medical offices use a variety of ways to monitor their financial accounts and the total financial operations of the business. A few offices still use the single-entry bookkeeping and pegboard systems, whereas others prefer double-entry or computerized systems, or a combination.

Spotlight on Certification

RMA Content Outline
- Financial bookkeeping

CMA Content Outline
- Computer applications
- Bookkeeping systems
- Accounting and banking procedures
- Employee payroll

CMAS Content Outline
- Fundamental Financial Management
- Patient Accounts

Financial records should provide the following information at all times:

- Amount earned in a given period
- Amount collected in a given period
- Amount owed in a given period
- Where the expenses incurred in a given period

The financial records can show these data as often as you like, usually on a monthly, quarterly, or yearly basis. Comparisons can be made with similar periods. Analysis of the financial data can help to determine if some services are not profitable, whether the practice is experiencing a healthy growth, or why a loss might be realized. The accounts receivable and accounts payable data are vital to this information.

Single-Entry System

The single-entry system has been used in the physician's office for many years. This includes a daily journal or log, patients' statements or accounts, ledgers, checks, and disbursement (expenditure) records. Information is first recorded in the journal, which provides a chronological record of financial transactions. Information from the journal is then transferred to the ledger through the process of posting. All amounts entered in the journal must be posted to the accounts kept in the ledger to summarize the results. This system has been used extensively in ambulatory care settings because of its simplicity and inexpensive nature. However, it is difficult to find errors, for there are no internal controls, and financial analysis information is inadequate.

Pegboard System

As discussed in Chapter 17, the pegboard, or "write-it-once," system is easier to use than the single-entry system and has greater internal controls. The pegboard system provides control over collections, payments, and charges. It uses No Carbon Required (NCR©) forms that are layered or shingled on pegs on the left of the board so that both income and disbursement entries need to be written only once. Many pegboard plans include a charge slip or encounter form, which simplifies third-party payment processing for both the medical office and the patients. The charge slip is used to record the input needed during the patient's visit, while serving as the patient's receipt for services performed and fees charged. An advantage of the pegboard system is its accuracy, because data are entered at the time of service and not recopied, few errors can creep in.

Double-Entry System

The double-entry system is based on the fact that each transaction has two aspects; that is, a dual effect on the accounting elements. This system is based on the accounting principle that assets equal liabilities plus owner's equity. **Assets** are the properties owned by the business (supplies, equipment, accounts receivable, and so on). **Liabilities** include what is owed to creditors. **Owner's equity** is the amount by which the business assets exceed the business liabilities. Net worth, proprietorship, and capital are often used as synonyms for owner's equity.

The double-entry system requires that the two aspects involved in every transaction be recorded on each side of the equation and that the two sides always be in balance. Although this accounting system requires time and skill, it provides a comprehensive financial picture and has built-in accuracy controls. It is orderly, fairly simple, flexible, and accurate, making it impossible for certain types of errors to remain undetected for long. For example, if one aspect of a transaction is properly recorded but the other aspect is overlooked, the records are out of balance. This occurrence may be easily discovered and subsequently corrected.

Computerized Systems

The majority of medical offices rely on accounting software packages to prepare financial records, such as ledgers and reports, and to retrieve patient information. A computerized accounting system is most likely to be based on the principles of either the pegboard (write-it-once) or a double-entry bookkeeping system, or a combination of both.

Just as the pegboard system is customized to the individual ambulatory care setting, a computer system can also be customized to meet the needs of the practice. Most large multispeciality clinics have a computer system designed particularly for their needs. Medical office software packages have the capabilities of including the most common procedure and diagnostic codes within a database to be recalled when completing insurance claim forms. Medical software programs will assist in matching the charges with the appropriate diagnosis codes.

Computers also have the flexibility of assigning codes in other categories to indicate whether a bill has been paid with cash, a check, or by a third-party payer. Codes may also be assigned to place and type of service and the professional performing the service. This facilitates the tracking of payments and also allows for the analysis of specific sources that generate income for the practice. Adjustments to reflect discounts or reduced fees may also be entered into the computer. The computer is used in the preparation of billing statements, insurance forms, collection letters, and a number of financial ratios and statements to assist in monitoring the practice's financial stability.

Computers and Managed Care. Computerization of the medical facility has increased because of the emphasis placed on the importance of accurate documentation of medical records and the increase in managed care plans. As medical facilities realized they needed to monitor more information, most offices opted for computerization.

Computer and Billing Service Bureaus

An option for ambulatory care settings that choose not to purchase accounting software or computers in their practice is to use a computer service bureau for billing purposes and the creation of many financial records. In this case, the ambulatory care setting provides the data and the bureau provides basic billing and accounting services, furnishing financial statements, completed insurance forms, payroll materials, and checks.

Service bureaus handle accounts from the medical facilities in one of three ways:

1. Through the office's own computer terminal, online sharing occurs where the office is tied directly to the bureau's mainframe computer
2. Through online servicing, where the office has its own terminal, which allows direct communication with the service bureau's computer
3. Through off-line batch processing, where the medical assistant or bookkeeper sends daily batches of data to the bureau to process

Many offices, however, prefer to have their own computerized system because dealing with a computer bureau can compromise patient confidentiality and limit control over computer usage. A proper contract should be negotiated and signed with any computer and billing service bureau to ensure confidentiality and strict privacy of all patient information.

DAY-END SUMMARY

The financial summary at the end of the day is a helpful tool for a quick financial analysis. Computer accounting systems automatically create the day-end summaries. Pegboard systems require the administrative medical assistant to total the summaries that are shown at the bottom of the day sheet.

The first section of the day sheet identifies all the financial transactions of the day. The second section includes the month-to-date totals. This is where today's totals are added to the month-to-date totals; this must be in perfect balance. The third section identifies the year-to-date accounts, which includes all accounts to obtain the year-to-date total. A deposit slip is likely included with most systems that enables the assistant to verify the cash receipts with the checks received. This is helpful in preparing the day's bank deposit.

When the totals do not balance at the end of the day, the medical assistant must begin the search for errors. Some tips are helpful in finding errors.

Tips for Finding Errors

Some tips for finding errors are as follows:

- Check the addition of each column, both horizontally and vertically. If a calculator is used, check the tape for entry errors.

- Compute the difference in the totals that are out of balance. Search the day sheet and patient accounts for that exact amount.

- If the amount of the error is divisible by 9, there may be an error in transposition of numbers.

- If the amount of the error is divisible by 2, the amount may have been posted in the wrong column.

- Check your entries when manually carrying forward previous balances. It is quite easy to carry forward an incorrect amount or to place numbers incorrectly. For example, the number $750 might be carried forward as $75.

Anyone who has worked with a manual pegboard system can report horror stories of chasing errors around for several days before finding them. It might be one error in one patient's account that creates the havoc. Also, a search can be made for an error for such length that the assistant keeps seeing and missing the error. Set the problem aside for a bit, or even a day if you are not pressed with month-end billing deadlines. Have another person check for you. Often that individual sees the error in just a few minutes.

ACCOUNTS RECEIVABLE TRIAL BALANCE

Before preparing monthly statements, a trial balance should be done on the accounts receivable in either a pegboard system or a computer system. The trial balance will indicate any problem between the daily journal and the ledger. Use the following steps to create the trial balance:

1. Pull all patient accounts that have a balance.
2. Total the balance of those accounts.
3. Create an accounts receivable total.
   a. Enter the accounts receivable at the first of the month.
   b. Add the total charges for the month and subtotal.
   c. Subtract the total payments for the month and subtotal.
   d. Subtract the total adjustments for the month.
   e. The final total is the accounts receivable at the end of the month.

This final total, the end of the month accounts receivable, must be the same as the figure received when adding all the patient account balances. If they match, the accounts are then in balance. If they do not balance, the error must be found. See Procedure 21-1.

ACCOUNTS PAYABLE

Accounts payable are an unwritten promise to pay a supplier for property or merchandise purchased on credit or for a service rendered. Accounts payable are the most common liability or financial obligation in a physician's office. These include expenses such as medical and office supplies, salaries, equipment, and services. Payments for these expenses are made by check to ensure complete, accurate records of all money received and disbursed.

Supplies and equipment purchased will usually come with a packing slip that describes the items purchased and their cost. An invoice may also be enclosed that serves as a bill for the items ordered; however, another invoice is sent to the business later as well. Take time to note on the invoice if there is a discount for early payment. Some financial managers suggest attaching the invoice and packing slip to the purchase order (see Chapter 17). File in your tickler file or reminder file on the computer so payment is made in a timely fashion to receive any discount. Some vendors prefer that payment not be made until a statement (or request for payment) is received from them. This is particularly the case if the practice may use that vendor more than once a month. When the statement arrives, check with the invoice for accuracy before sending payment. Prepare the check for the accounts payable as appropriate, either monthly or as necessary to receive a discount. Write the check number on the invoice, as well as the amount paid, and place in a file for accounts paid according to the office filing system.

Disbursement Records

Computer accounts payable systems will track the disbursements and post to appropriate established accounts similar to a manual system. Computer accounts payable systems will have a **check register** that records all checks written and categorizes them into separate columns such as rent, insurance, office supplies, utilities, and so forth. These categories can be designed as detailed or general as preferred. The computer system also can create entries for bank deposits and payroll records.

The computer software will have a check-writing file that presents checks on the screen. The information necessary to complete the check is entered at the keyboard; the computer stores it and prints out the check. Printing the checks can be done individually or by batch if several bills are being paid. The amount is automatically subtracted from the account's balance. The computer system also can recall data that need to be entered on the checks each time there is a payment. For example, the name of the company where most supplies are purchased can be recalled from the database, thus the assistant does not have to key in that information again. This feature is a particular time-saver when payroll checks are prepared. See Chapter 22.

The manual or pegboard system uses a check register page to record checks written. The check is aligned on the pegboard over the check register before completion. The pegboard checks have an NCR transfer strip that copies the date, the payee, the check number, and the amount to the check register. The pegboard checks can be designed so the address is entered beneath the payee line and mailed in a window envelope. This check register will have a number of columns to categorize expenses. All entries are totaled on the check register when completed, and these totals carried forward. A balanced check register provides a way to verify the bank statement when it arrives. The check register can also be used for bank deposits and for payroll records.

THE ACCOUNTING FUNCTION

Accounting is a system of monitoring the financial status of a facility and the financial results of its activities. Accounting may be divided into two major categories: financial and managerial. Financial accounting provides information primarily for entities external to the organization such as the government. In contrast, managerial accounting generates financial information that can enable more efficient internal management. Cost accounting helps to determine what it costs the ambulatory care setting to perform particular services and is an integral part of managerial accounting. A hospital cost report for Medicare is essentially part of financial accounting, because the report is generated for an external user—the Center for Medicare and Medicaid Services (CMS), which administers the Medicare program. However, it is also a part of cost accounting because a cost report on Medicare will show what it costs to care for patients on Medicare.

COST ANALYSIS

An important aspect of the practice is the **cost analysis.** The purpose of the analysis is to determine the costs of each service. There are two factors to consider: fixed costs and variable costs.

Fixed Costs

Fixed costs are costs that do not vary in total as the number of patients vary. For example, the annual depreciation cost of the equipment is fixed because it will remain the same regardless of the number of patients who use it.

Variable Costs

Variable costs are those that vary in direct proportion to patient volume such as clinical supplies and laboratory procedures. Average costs to treat patients decline because of fixed costs not variable costs. The greater the volume, the more widely the fixed costs are spread and the less cost any one unit is responsible for.

Patient cost factors include administrative costs, such as the cost of billing and collections, personnel costs for office staff providing patient care, equipment costs, and costs for clinical supplies. The physician cost will include costs for interpreting tests, diagnosing illnesses, and maintaining professional liability insurance.

Calculating and reviewing costs provide the ambulatory care setting with data to set fees, market the practice, determine profit, and monitor the practice's performance.

FINANCIAL RECORDS

Indicators of the financial status of the medical facility include financial statements that reflect the daily operations of the business. These records comprise an accounting information system that is maintained for numerous reasons, one of which is to provide source data for use in the preparation of various reports. Two financial statements common to the ambulatory care setting are the income/expense statement and the balance sheet.

Income Statement

Figure 21-1 shows a sample **income statement,** the most commonly generated year-end report. The sample shows the profit and expenses for a given month. The income

INNER CITY HEALTH CARE
INCOME STATEMENT

	Month of , 20XX	Year-to-Date	Budget for Year	Overhead Percentages
A. Revenue:				
1. Office #1	$	$	$	
2. Office #2	$	$	$	
B. Total Revenue:	$	$	$	100%
C. Expenses:				
1. Non–doctor (staff) salaries—gross	$	$	$	%
2. Staff fringes				
– Payroll taxes	$	$	$	
– Empl. benefits	$	$	$	
– Empl. seminars	$	$	$	
– Uniforms	$	$	$	
– Retirement plan	$	$	$	
	$	$	$	%
3. Occupancy costs:				
– Rent—Off. #1	$	$	$	
– Rent—Off. #2	$	$	$	
– Property taxes	$	$	$	
– Insurance	$	$	$	
– Utilities	$	$	$	
– Janitor/Grounds	$	$	$	
	$	$	$	%
4. Medical expenses:				
– Medications	$	$	$	
– Supplies	$	$	$	
– Lab fees	$	$	$	
	$	$	$	%
5. Office expenses:				
– Office supplies	$	$	$	
– Postage	$	$	$	
– Telephone	$	$	$	
	$	$	$	%
6. Malpractice ins.	$	$	$	%
7. Professional expenses:				
– Auto expenses (Doctors')	$	$	$	
– Dues/subscriptions	$	$	$	
– Books and videos	$	$	$	
– Dues/memberships	$	$	$	
– Entertainment	$	$	$	
– Professional development	$	$	$	
– Travel	$	$	$	
	$	$	$	%

(continues)

Figure 21-1 A sample income statement that shows profit and expenses for one month.

statement shows the cumulative profit and total expenses by reporting patient income, outside revenue sources, and overhead expenses such as office and medical expenses. Physician's compensation and benefits, employees' compensation, benefits, and withholding taxes can be itemized as well.

Balance Sheet

Sometimes called the statement of financial condition or statement of financial position, the **balance sheet** is an itemized statement of the assets, liabilities, and owner's equity of a medical facility as of a specified date. Its

	Month of ___, 20XX	Year-to-Date	Budget for Year	Overhead Percentages
8. Equipment costs:				
– Depreciation/amortization	$	$	$	
– Rent	$	$	$	
– Service/maintenance	$	$	$	
– Interest (if on equipment purchase loans)	$	$	$	
	$	$	$	%
9. Marketing expenses				
– Advertising	$	$	$	
– Other fees	$	$	$	
	$	$	$	%
10. Professional expenses:				
– Accounting	$	$	$	
– Legal	$	$	$	
– Consulting	$	$	$	
– Ret. Plan Admin.	$	$	$	
	$	$	$	%
11.				
12.				
13.				
14.				
D. Total Non–Doctor Expenses:	$	$	$	%
E. Operating New Income Before Doctors' Costs (B minus C)	$	$	$	%
F. Associate Physician's Costs:				
– Salaries—gross:	$	$	$	
– Benefits	$	$	$	
–	$	$	$	
–	$	$	$	
G. Total Non–Owner Doctors' Costs	$	$	$	%
H. New Income Available to Owner–Doctors (E minus G)	$	$	$	%
I. Owner–Doctors' Costs:				
1. Salaries—gross:				
–Dr. A	$	$	$	
–Dr. B	$	$	$	
2. Bonuses—gross:				
–Dr. A	$	$	$	
–Dr. B	$	$	$	
3. Retirement contributions:				
–Dr. A	$	$	$	
–Dr. B	$	$	$	
4. "Semi-personal" expenses:				
–Dr. A	$	$	$	
–Dr. B	$	$	$	
J. Total Owner–Doctors' Costs	$	$	$	
K. Net Income (H minus J)	$	$	$	

Figure 21-1 (continued)

purpose is to provide information regarding the status of these basic accounting elements.

The balance sheet is made possible through the double-entry system of accounting because every transaction is recorded by two sets of entries made in a ledger or journal. Increases in assets are recorded as debits; decreases are recorded as credits. Increases in liabilities and owner's equity are recorded as credits; decreases are recorded as debits.

Debit and credit entries to one or more accounts make up the system. In any recording, the total dollar amount of the debit entries must equal the total dollar amount of the credit entries. Each ledger or journal entry should have the elements:

1. Date of transaction
2. Journal or ledger account names involved
3. Dollar amount of the charges
4. Brief explanation of the transaction

USEFUL FINANCIAL DATA

A business must determine how and when it will report income earned. There are two systems for doing this. The **accrual basis** reports income at the time charges are generated. This is used mainly in commercial environments. The **cash basis** is most often used in medical practices. In the cash basis, income is recognized when money is collected.

There are a few financial ratios that can help evaluate how the practice is doing. Data from the current year and the previous year's financial statements can be converted into ratios to highlight different financial characteristics. Ratios should always be viewed in relation to the total financial picture, however.

Ratios are not difficult to calculate, but they can be time consuming when using a manual system. They are quick to create in a computer system because all the data are readily available, already totaled, and sometimes created automatically. It is helpful to understand the concept, however, and not rely too heavily on computer-generated reports. If data have been entered incorrectly at some point, it will be reflected in reports generated. The user of accounting software also must train his or her mind to think about the sensibility of the report.

Although two of these ratios were discussed in Chapter 20, some elaboration is in order in the context of this chapter.

Accounts Receivable Ratio

The **accounts receivable (A/R) ratio** formula measures the speed in which outstanding accounts are paid. The accounts receivable ratio provides a picture of the state of collections and probable losses. The longer an account is past due, the less the likelihood is of successfully making the collection.

$$\frac{\text{Total Accounts Receivable}}{\text{Monthly Receipts}} = \text{Turnaround Time}$$

Example:

$$\frac{\$120,000}{\$60,000} = \begin{array}{l} \text{2 Months Turnaround Time} \\ \text{for Payment on an Account} \end{array}$$

The goal of an efficient billing and collecting policy should be a turnaround time of two months or less.

Collection Ratio

The **collection ratio** shows the percentage of outstanding debt collected. The goal should be a 90% collection ratio. Total receipts divided by total charges give the unadjusted collection ratio, but adjustments may include federal and state insurance programs (Medicare and Medicaid, Workers' Compensation), managed care adjustments, and any other adjustments as directed by the physician.

Total Receipts	= $40,000
+ Managed Care Adjustments	$3,000
+ Medicare Adjustments	$2,000
TOTAL	$45,000
Total Charges	$52,000

$$\frac{\text{Total Receipts } \$45,000}{\text{Total Charges } \$52,000} = \begin{array}{l} \text{86.5\% Collection Ratio} \\ \text{after Adjustments} \end{array}$$

Cost Ratio

The **cost ratio** formula shows the cost of a procedure or service and can help in determining, for instance, the cost effectiveness of maintaining a laboratory in the ambulatory care setting. The ratio is:

$$\frac{\text{Total Expenses}}{\text{Total Number of Procedures for One Month}}$$

$$\frac{\text{Total Laboratory Expenses for September}}{\text{Total Number of Procedures Performed for September}}$$

$$\frac{\$48,000}{240} = \$200 \text{ per Procedure}$$

A conclusion might be reached that the laboratory is too costly because each procedure is not billed at $200.00.

LEGAL AND ETHICAL GUIDELINES

It is hoped that a careful hiring process (see Chapter 23) results in the best employees whose credentials, ethics, and personal actions are above reproach. However, embezzlement does occur in medical practices, partly because of the way in which the financial aspect of the practice is designed and managed. Following are some steps to decrease the opportunity for embezzlement:

- The accountant and the managing physician should conduct regular and irregular audits of the practice accounts. Seek an accountant who is available at any time, not just when it is time to report wages or compute the yearly taxes. The accountant also becomes a valuable asset to the practice in providing essential information to the office staff.

- Separate duties among several employees. Consider having one employee open the mail and post checks received. A second employee handles all the cash transactions and prepares the deposit slips. A third employee might order the supplies and write all the checks. Many physicians choose to write the checks; however, this is also a task that can be assigned to the office manager.

- Only one person should use the signature stamp; consider not using a signature stamp at all.

- The signature card on file at the bank must include the names of each individual authorized to sign the checks.

- Seek employees whose personal honesty sets a good example for the staff.

Physicians who demonstrate the same personal honesty and integrity expected of their staff are less likely to be victims of embezzlement.

Bonding

There is another step that can be taken and is often recommended. To protect the practice from embezzlement or other financial loss, physicians can purchase fidelity bonds. These bonds reimburse the practice for any monetary loss caused by the practice's employees. There are three types of bonds to consider, and perhaps reason to have more than one type. These bonds include:

1. Position-schedule bond covers the position rather than a specific individual. For instance, the bookkeeper, office manager, and receptionist might be covered.
2. Blanket-position bond covers all employees. If the staff members often share duties, cover for one another when there are absences, or work really well together as a team during busy periods, this type of bond might be most beneficial.
3. Personal bond is designed to cover specific individuals by name and generally requires a personal background investigation. This type of bond may give the most assurance.

Bonding not only protects the physicians and the practice, but it assures employees that they are covered by a bond should there be a problem with the finances during their shift. Bonding service companies will require implementation of certain procedures and security measures as outlined in their contracts. Costs depend on risk levels, but they are well worth the protection.

Payroll

The administrative medical assistant is likely to be involved in making certain the W-4 form, the Employee's Withholding Allowance Certificate, is completed by all employees. However, salary calculations, withholding taxes, and Social Security calculations are the responsibility of the office manager. See Chapter 22.

UTILIZATION REVIEW

In the present health care climate where there are many managed care plans, more attention has been focused on how the billing and financial management process should proceed. Because of the influence of governmental mandates in the practice of medicine, and the growth of the **utilization review (UR)** industry, more accurate recordkeeping and documentation in all facets of the ambulatory care setting have become necessary. There are numerous UR firms throughout the country. These companies aggressively sell their services to employers and to insurance carriers. UR is actually a review of the patient service required

before it may be performed. If the reviewer determines that the procedure or treatment is not needed, then it will not be approved or covered under the patient's insurance plan. Policies that once permitted medical decisions to be made solely by the physician often are now made by other health professionals who are employed by UR firms. Some clinics may find it beneficial to have one medical assistant whose main responsibility is to present procedures to UR for acceptance or denial. Because of the increasing concern for quality of health care at low cost, more physicians also are realizing they need more documentation of both medical and financial information with more accessible means for retrieval.

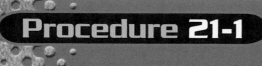

Preparing Accounts Receivable Trial Balance

PURPOSE:
A trial balance will determine if there is any problem between the daily journal and the ledger or patient accounts.

EQUIPMENT/SUPPLIES:
Patient accounts and calculator
Computer and software for computerized systems

PROCEDURE STEPS:
1. Pull all patient accounts that have a balance due. RATIONALE: Provides only amount due information.
2. Enter the balance of those accounts into the calculator. RATIONALE: Makes it possible to add these amounts.
3. Add the balances and total. (A calculator with tape can make it quicker to check for errors.) RATIONALE: Gives you the total amount due to date.

4. Create an accounts receivable total:
   a. Enter the accounts receivable total from the first of the month into the calculator.
   b. Add total charges for this month and subtotal.
   c. Total the amount of all payments received this month.
   d. Subtract the total of payments from subtotal of "b" above and subtotal.
   e. Total the amount of the month's adjustments and subtract from the subtotal in "d" above.
   f. This total is the accounts receivable amount.
   RATIONALE: The end-of-the month accounts receivable total ("f") above must match the total in Step 3 above. If these totals do not match, an error has been made. If they do match, the trial balance is in order.

Case Study 21-1

Because the owners of Inner City Health Care need to make adequate income to pay all overhead and share in a profit, they are instituting new measures to reduce their operating costs. However, they have fixed costs that they cannot change. Therefore, they plan to look at their variable costs to determine where they can reduce expenses without any reduction in quality of service.

CASE STUDY REVIEW

1. What are some fixed costs that Inner City is likely to have?
2. What are some of the variable costs that should be considered when looking at profitability?
3. How may UR procedures affect the profitability of Inner City Health Care?

Case Study 21-2

Richard Saxton is a newly licensed acupuncturist who has been in practice less than a year. He is renting space for his procedures and services with an established doctor of osteopathy. Richard is using a simple pegboard system, makes his own appointments, and collects for most procedures at the time services are rendered unless the patients have medical insurance covering acupuncture. Richard has done fairly well, likes working in the environment the facility offers, and is beginning to show some profit. He would like to purchase a new table, chair, and stool for his acupuncture room.

CASE STUDY REVIEW

1. What facts might Richard want to consider before making the purchases?
2. Consider the variable costs versus the fixed costs of the practice of acupuncture. (You may need to do a little research to determine supplies and other factors.)
3. What information will his pegboard system give him?

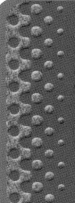

SUMMARY

Medical financial management is crucial to the profitability of the ambulatory care setting. It is necessary for each medical facility to decide on which accounting system best serves the individual practice. Careful monitoring of billing procedures and aging accounts, and accurately documenting both the medical and financial record will help in providing a sound financial analysis and a strong financial foundation for the ambulatory care setting.

STUDY FOR SUCCESS

To reinforce your knowledge and skills of information presented in this chapter:

- ❑ Review the Key Terms
- ❑ Practice any Procedures
- ❑ Consider the Case Studies and discuss your conclusions
- ❑ Answer the Review Questions
  - ❑ Multiple Choice
  - ❑ Critical Thinking
- ❑ Navigate the Internet and complete the Web Activities
- ❑ Practice the StudyWARE activities on the textbook CD
- ❑ Apply your knowledge in the Student Workbook activities
- ❑ Complete the Web Tutor sections

REVIEW QUESTIONS

Multiple Choice

1. If a number has been transposed in financial reports:
   a. the error is divisible by 4
   b. the error is divisible by 2
   c. the error is divisible by 9
   d. none of the above

2. An example of a fixed cost is:
   a. salaries
   b. cost of supplies
   c. depreciation of equipment
   d. cost of treating patients

3. An itemized statement of financial position is the:
   a. income statement
   b. balance sheet
   c. trial balance
   d. collection ratio
4. A check register:
   a. records all checks and categorizes them into separate columns
   b. is used when taking cash from patients
   c. is an accounts receivable record
   d. a and c
5. Utilization review:
   a. looks at the utility of all personnel
   b. examines how useful the ambulatory care center is to patients
   c. is a review of a procedure before it is performed to determine if it is necessary
   d. only affects hospitals
6. Assets include:
   a. equipment and supplies on hand
   b. building or property
   c. accounts receivable
   d. all the above
7. A computer billing and service bureau:
   a. is the service you hire to care for the office computer system
   b. may compromise patient confidentiality
   c. can function through linkage of computers, online servicing, or off-line batch processing
   d. b and c above
8. In a medical facility where the total receipts including any adjustments are $83,500 and the total charges equal $97,750, the collection ratio:
   a. would be great at 94%
   b. would be quite good at 88%
   c. shows a fair return at 85%
   d. shows a modest return at 75%
9. Money can be saved with accounts payable when:
   a. paid promptly
   b. discounts are realized
   c. resisting the urge to buy in bulk
   d. a and b
10. Bonding:
    a. binds physicians to the safe caretaking of their patients
    b. protects medical office staff and physicians if embezzlement occurs
    c. can be purchased in three different types
    d. b and c

Critical Thinking

1. Discuss the pros and cons of an on-site complete computer system and a computer service bureau.
2. Review the importance of financial records and identify and state the differences between the two primary records.
3. The accounting equation can be reported in more than one formula. It may be stated as:

   $$\text{Assets} = \text{Liabilities} + \text{Owner's Equity}$$

   or

   $$\text{Assets} - \text{Liabilities} = \text{Owner's Equity}$$

   Is one easier to interpret? Why or why not? Add some totals of your choice to illustrate.
4. Recall from previous chapters and other studies in which you may be involved some basic guidelines for using computers in the medical facility. Identify these. What is one critical procedure that is done quite regularly, especially at the end of a project or the end of the day?
5. Where and how are financial records and reports kept? Who is responsible for their storage? Is there a length of period that the records might be kept?

WEB ACTIVITIES

1. If you have trouble comprehending the accounting equation, research "The Accounting Equation" on the Internet. What helpful sites did you find? Are there any examples that show how the equation relates to a medical practice? Give an example of what you find.
2. Research "Medical Practice Management" for software packages that would include the accounting reports described in this chapter. Identify at least two that seem to have the broadest coverage of how computers are used in a medical practice. Identify the pieces in the package and what they cover.

REFERENCES/BIBLIOGRAPHY

Droms, W. G. (2003). *Finance and accounting for nonfinancial managers* (2nd ed.). Cambridge, MA: Perseus Publishers.

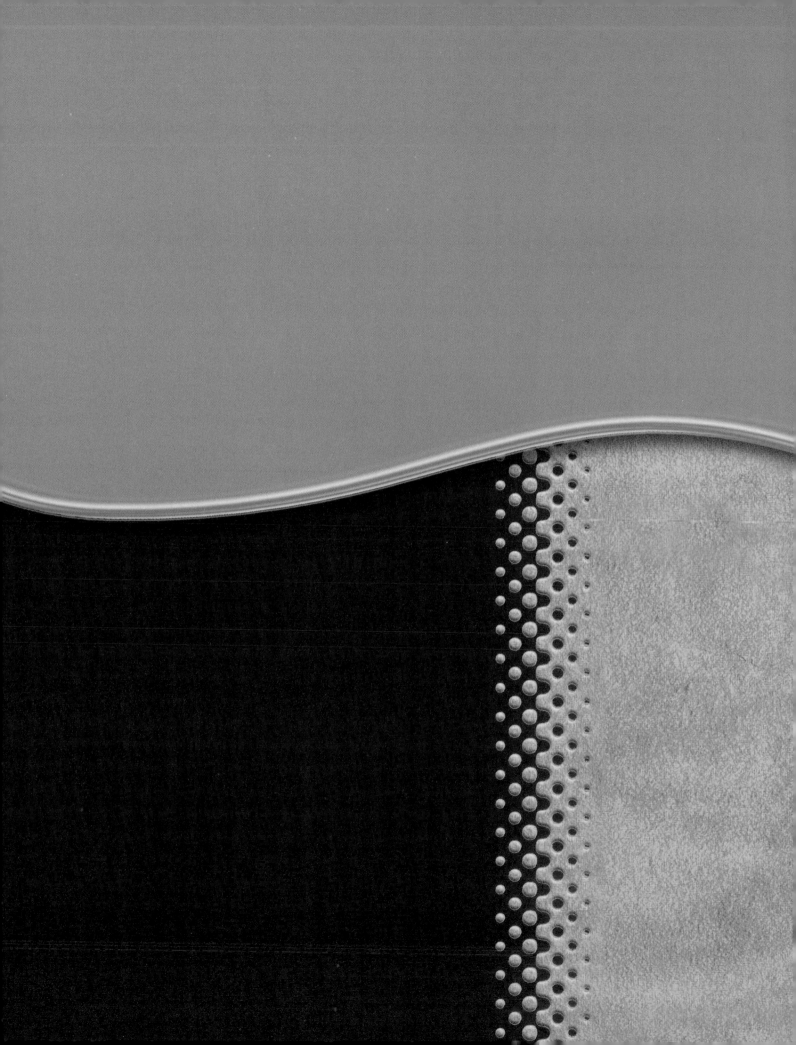

UNIT 6
Office and Human Resources Management

CHAPTER 22

The Medical Assistant as Office Manager

OUTLINE

KEY TERMS

FEATURED COMPETENCIES

CAAHEP—ENTRY-LEVEL COMPETENCIES

Professional Communication

- Respond to and initiate written communications
- Recognize and respond to verbal communications
- Recognize and respond to nonverbal communications

Legal Concepts

- Identify and respond to issues of confidentiality
- Perform within legal and ethical boundaries
- Document appropriately
- Demonstrate knowledge of federal and state health care legislation and regulations

Patient Instruction

- Explain general office policies
- Identify community resources

Operational Function

- Perform an inventory of supplies and equipment
- Perform routine maintenance of administrative and clinical equipment

ABHES—ENTRY-LEVEL COMPETENCIES

Professionalism

- Project a positive attitude
- Maintain confidentiality at all times
- Be a "team player"
- Be cognizant of ethical boundaries

(continues)

438

OBJECTIVES

The student should strive to meet the following performance objectives and demonstrate an understanding of the facts and principles presented in this chapter through written and oral communication.

1. Define the key terms as presented in the glossary.
2. Describe the qualities of a manager.
3. Discuss characteristics of managers and leaders.
4. Differentiate between authoritarian and participatory management styles.
5. Describe management by walking around and its usefulness in ambulatory care settings.
6. Recall a minimum of four common risks and risk-control measures.
7. List three benefits of a teamwork approach.
8. Discuss the importance of a meeting agenda.
9. Describe appropriate evaluation tools for employees.
10. Recall effective methods of resolving conflict.
11. Identify the steps required to make travel arrangements.
12. Define the term itinerary and list important information the itinerary should contain.
13. List three methods of increasing productivity and efficient time management.
14. Describe the purpose of a procedure manual.
15. Discuss the impact of HIPAA's privacy policy in ambulatory care settings.
16. Describe the general concept of marketing and recall at least three marketing tools.
17. Describe the purpose and benefit of marketing.
18. Define records management, financial management, facility and equipment management, and risk management.
19. Describe the steps involved in payroll processing.
20. Describe liability coverage and what bonding means.

SCENARIO

Marilyn Johnson has been employed by Drs. Lewis and King's office for the past eight years. Three years ago, she was promoted to the position of office manager when the facility added the second office for its associates in the next suburb. Marilyn has a baccalaureate degree in business administration. Her responsibilities at Drs. Lewis and King's office include various duties involving personnel, finances, and office efficiency.

- Evidence a responsible attitude
- Be courteous and diplomatic

Communication

- Serve as liaison between physician and others
- Interview effectively
- Recognize and respond to verbal and nonverbal communications
- Professional components

Administrative Duties

- Locate resources and information for patients and employers
- Manage physician's professional schedule and travel

Legal Concepts

- Determine needs for documentation and reporting
- Document accurately
- Use appropriate guidelines when releasing records or information
- Follow established policy in initiating or terminating medical treatment
- Dispose of controlled substances in compliance with government regulations
- Maintain licenses and accreditation
- Monitor legislation related to current healthcare issues and practices
- Perform risk management procedures

(continues)

INTRODUCTION

The drive to improve the productivity of the medical office, precipitated by managed care, Medicare and insurance limits placed on fees, have broadened the scope of employment options and job marketability for medical assistants. This has created an opportunity for medical assistants to advance to the position of office manager.

In small offices, the position of office manager may include the duties of the human resources (HR) representative; in larger clinics, these positions will be independent. This book treats them as separate positions (see Chapter 23). In the larger facilities, the office manager and HR representative must coordinate their personnel-related functions into a seamless organization.

Spotlight on Certification

RMA Content Outline
- Medical law
- Medical ethics
- Human relations

CMA Content Outline
- Basic principles (Psychology)
- Working as a team member to achieve goals
- Evaluating and understanding communication
- Medicolegal guidelines & requirements
- Resource information and community services
- Managing physician's professional schedule and travel
- Managing the office
- Office policies and procedures
- Employee payroll

CMAS Content Outline
- Legal and ethical considerations
- Professionalism
- Patient information and community resources
- Medical records management
- Medical office financial management
- Medical office management

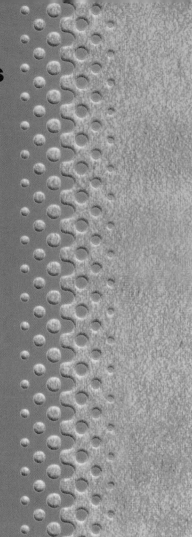

FEATURED COMPETENCIES (continued)

Office Management

- Maintain physical plant
- Operate and maintain facilities and perform routine maintenance of administrative and clinical equipment safely
- Inventory equipment and supplies
- Evaluate and recommend equipment and supplies for practice
- Maintain liability coverage
- Exercise efficient time management

Instruction

- Orient patients to office policies and procedures
- Orient and train personnel

Financial Management

- Process employee payroll

THE MEDICAL ASSISTANT AS OFFICE MANAGER

The office manager of a medical office or ambulatory care facility is a role that can have vast and diverse responsibilities. This chapter covers the following office manager duties:

1. Arrange and maintain practice insurance and develop risk management strategies
2. Supervise office personnel
3. Prepare staff meeting agenda, conduct the meeting, and record minutes
4. Make travel arrangements and prepare an itinerary
5. Assist in improving work flow and office efficiencies (time management)
6. Create and update the office procedure manual, Material Safety Data Sheets (MSDSs), and Health Insurance Portability and Accountability Act (HIPAA) manual.
7. Prepare patient education materials and arrange patient/community education workshops as needed
8. Approve financial transactions and account disposition; generate financial reports as needed

9. Supervise the purchase and storage of office supplies
10. Supervise the purchase, repair, and maintenance of office equipment

QUALITIES OF A MANAGER

An office manager should not feel the need to be superior to employees. The best manager is like an orchestra conductor. He or she constructively blends together the skills and abilities of diverse people to produce a smooth and efficient team. The result is an organization having greater capability than would be achievable by the individuals acting independently.

The office manager should have two overarching goals:

- Get the job done.

- Make the process enjoyable.

This does not mean work should be one big party. It means developing ownership for the work, pride in doing the job well, and a sense of teamwork. There will be times when employees will not like having to stay late to meet important deadlines, but through developed self-actualization, they will take enjoyment from even the most undesirable task.

A good office manager needs to be two persons in one body: leader and manager. The two functions are different, and the good manager will use some of each characteristic in meeting objectives. Table 22-1 illustrates the differences between an authoritarian style manager and a leader/manager.

Good managers are leaders, providing their coworkers with vision, guidance, and a feeling of ownership in the process. They do these things without threats, usually through the power of their personal charisma. It is also important that managers clearly convey their expectations to their employees. Possibly nothing leads to ill feeling between the manager and an employee more than failure to let the employee know what is expected of him or her. Furthermore, a lack of expectations stifles career growth and organizational vitality. Good leaders need to blend many admirable personality traits of leadership to be successful and still control the resources entrusted to them.

Before proceeding with a listing of qualities of a leader/manager, a rule that defines almost all of the ethical qualities needs to be mentioned (Figure 22-1). Some texts call it the Golden Rule; this rule will make the difference between a manager who is successful and one who fails miserably. The rule needs no explanation, and will serve any manager well in any circumstance.

TABLE 22-1	**DIFFERENCES BETWEEN AN AUTHORITARIAN STYLE MANAGER AND A LEADER/ MANAGER**
Manager	**Leader**
• Establishes and adheres to written procedures	• Empower people
• Focused on short-range goals	• Inspires by example
• Authoritarian style of management	• Vision and long range goals
• Bottom line all important	• Consensus or team style of management
• Does things right	• Does the right thing
• Annual raises	• Pay for performance
• Reluctant to change	• Not afraid of change

The following bulleted items list most of the qualities needed by a leader/manager:

• *Effective communication skills.* Communication skills include written and oral methods. The manager must communicate clearly, diplomatically, tactfully, and with respect for the feelings of others.

• *Fairmindedness.* It is important to always be fair with coworkers. Decisions that impact one fellow employee create a ripple effect. That is, you may have to make the same decision for another employee at another time. Decisions should be based, as much as possible, on the assumption that what is granted to one employee will be granted to others in similar situations. This approach will decrease the risk for being accused of playing favorites or being unfair.

• *Objectivity.* The office manager must be able to view challenges without bias or prejudice. For example, when promotions are made, the office manager must be able to focus on the job description criteria and individual qualifications without introducing personal preference.

• *Organizational skills.* Being organized includes being able to prioritize tasks, working efficiently and methodically. Know when and be willing to delegate tasks when others have the expertise and time to complete the task within the time lines.

• *People skills.* The office manager must like people in general and enjoy working with them. Building confidence and self-esteem in others and being interested in promoting constructive relationships are essential qualities of the office manager. The ability to function as an effective team leader provides a role model for other staff members to emulate.

• *Problem-solving skills.* The office manager must be a problem solver. This may include being creative and doing away with old paradigms and traditional approaches to solving a problem. When difficult issues arise, focus on the situation, issue, or behavior, not on the person. A discussion about solving the problem without laying blame is much more productive. Positive solutions may be more readily attained when discussing what was observed rather than what was told by someone else.

• *Technical expertise.* Have a working knowledge of each procedure performed in the office, although it is not necessary to be the acknowledged technical expert. A good office manager is continually learning and encourages **subordinates** to seek opportunities to continue their education and advance their technical skills.

• *Truthfulness.* Lead by example! If an honest mistake is made, be the first to admit to the error and seek the best solution for preventing it from happening again. Respond honestly to requests. For example, two staff members ask for the same day off. The office manager will make the decision that only one member may have the day off and will review the policy manual to determine the appropriate criteria for designating who will have the request granted.

Office Manager Attitude

Many managers share a common enemy—themselves. The part of ourselves that is our enemy is our mind and the outlook we have on the world. People who succeed attribute positive results to their own actions. People who underachieve or fail usually attribute negative results to someone else or to chance, over which they have no control. Because underachievers feel helpless to affect results, psychologists conclude that their motivation to succeed

TREAT OTHERS, AS YOU WOULD LIKE TO BE TREATED!

Figure 22-1 The Golden Rule.

is diminished. A low achiever would be unlikely to have a personal risk management system in place. They would feel they could not affect events. The more positive person could easily take steps to avoid these problems.

The effect of a negative mindset does not stop with failure to accept responsibility for the things that happen to each of us, it continues on. Unless we change our outlook, we lower our expectations and begin accepting the mediocre. Individuals who feel they are helpless to affect events become afraid of success, as well as failure, and subconsciously find a way to fail to avoid the challenges success will bring.

How do you change your mindset? Following are a few suggestions considered helpful:

- Come to terms with what you would have to change if you are to be successful and be ready for the change.
- Identify what you really want to achieve.
- Put your goals in writing using positive terms (say "I will" not "I'll try").
- Begin with small, achievable goals.
- Eliminate poor habits such as procrastination.
- Tune out negative thoughts and focus on positive thoughts.

We are what we think we are. Be careful of your mindset, it can derail you and your job as a manager.

Professionalism

 The medical assistant as office manager must exhibit professional behavior at all times. He or she must be courteous and diplomatic and demonstrate a responsible and positive attitude. All verbal and written communications should be accurate, correct,

 In many offices, the office manager is also designated to fill the role of Security Officer. The responsibilities of the Security Officer include coordinating and overseeing the various impacts of HIPAA on each department and assisting with compliance issues related to HIPAA regulations. The Security Officer must also keep abreast of any changes and rulings and how they may apply to their particular office environment. Some online resources are available at: http://www.cms.hhs.gov; or e-mail questions to askhipaa@cms.hhs.gov.

Critical Thinking

How does the office manager begin to develop good working relationships with other community service organizations to better serve and provide for the patient's health care needs? How would this improve the quality of public relations?

and follow appropriate guidelines. The office manager should demonstrate knowledge of federal and state health care legislation and regulations and must perform within legal and ethical boundaries. All documentation must be performed appropriately.

The office manager serves as a liaison between the physician, patient, and other professionals. Therefore, professional demeanor in all respects must be followed. It is not uncommon to be called on to locate community resources and information for patients and employers. Review Procedure 4-1 for specific information on how this is done. A good working relationship with other community service organizations fosters the sharing of information vital to your patient's health care needs and promotes quality public relations.

MANAGEMENT STYLES

There are many books written on management styles; however, it is possible to break all of them down into only two basic styles, each with an infinite number of variations. Because this is not a management text, we will take a simplistic view and look at only the fundamental styles: authoritarian and participatory. We will also examine a third management style, managing by walking around, which, although not a people interaction style, is an effective management technique for keeping abreast of what is going on in an organization.

Authoritarian Style

Authoritarian managers operate on the premise that most workers cannot make a contribution without being directed, sometimes in the minutest detail, and even if they could, they would not be inclined to do so. This type of manager believes in the carrot and the stick approach to motivate people to work. The carrot is monetary reward, and the stick is docked pay or being reprimanded or fired. The personality of the manager tends to influence natural tendencies of style. Individuals who are task or procedure oriented tend to be authoritarian. Authority control is easily accomplished in the case of simple tasks that can readily be structured and defined. Authoritarian managers try to control work to the maximum extent possible, for example, micro-management. Complex jobs, however, are difficult for the authoritarian manager to control.

Sometimes a manager may need to use the authoritarian style. It should be used quite sparingly, because it may destroy morale and personal incentive. An assumption regarding the character of an employee frequently becomes a self-fulfilling prophecy. Workers with an authoritarian manager either give up and quit, or they become mindless robots asking "how high" when told to jump. As a manager, you will use the authoritarian style in the case of new employees until you have a chance to determine their capabilities, in the case of a worker who has proved to be without self-motivation, or in supervising short-term temporary labor.

Can an authoritarian manager style work in the twenty-first century? Yes. It has worked for a few well-respected, large companies in the United States, but this occurred only because management had unlimited resources to use as a carrot for rewarding employees. Most managers will not have these resources.

Participatory Style

The **participatory management** style is based on the premise that the worker is capable and wants to do a good job. The best known form of participatory management is the use of teams to do work tasks. This type of management is well suited to complex tasks where each member can contribute his specialty to the job at hand. The manager's function in this type of system is to communicate direction and vision to the team and to sell the team on the importance of the task. Managers using this type of style need to be comfortable teaching, coaching, communicating, inspiring, and motivating. Workers engaged in a participatory management style are motivated by much more than monetary reward and develop an ownership for the work in which they are involved. Although the carrot is still important, their reward comes from teamwork, peer recognition, and self-actualization, that is, the pleasure from doing a job well and being recognized for it. Competition between teams is sometimes used as a motivation technique.

Management by Walking Around

Management by walking around (MBWA) is not really a management style, but rather a technique for keeping the manager informed about the health of his or her organization. This style consists of just what the title says, the manager walks around looking at what is going on in the organization and talks with employees to get their opinion on how things could be done better. The manager collects data on new ideas; in a participatory sys-

tem, a team would be assigned to study and come up with a better way of doing the work. The manager must be careful to make sure his or her motives are not to micromanage and to convey this to the workers.

RISK MANAGEMENT

The office manager should formulate a **risk management** procedure that assesses risks to which he or she and the organization is exposed and takes steps to develop contingencies that minimize probable risks. Some common risks and risk-control measures are:

- *Loss of a critical employee.* Have cross training of employees to permit them to assume the duties of an employee who is ill or terminates his or her employment.

- *Failure of a supplier or contractor.* Maintain sufficient inventory to permit contracting with a secondary supplier before having critical shortages. Monitor the status of orders so you are aware of any failures in delivery before they have a negative impact and so supplies can be obtained from a second source. Have a list of secondary sources.

- *Accidental disclosure of confidential information through error or unauthorized entry.* Have protocols in place regarding breach of confidentiality and defining steps to be taken in the event information is compromised. Define protocols to patients alerting them to the unlikely but potential possibility of accidental disclosure. Notify patients immediately if confidential information is compromised, and work with them for resolution.

- *Computer failure.* Back up the system regularly. Have a secondary system that could permit the office to operate until repairs are effected. Have a maintenance contract in place with a reputable firm permitting overnight repair.

- *Injury to a staff member or nonemployee.* Continually review safety procedures and conduct safety surveys. Have adequate liability insurance for the medical office.

Critical Thinking

How would you make the medical office (front- and back-office space) safe for employees and nonemployees (e.g., patients, venders, visitors)? List as many considerations as possible.

- *Managerial position change.* Continuously network with friends and associates to permit you to rapidly seek a new position before experiencing a job loss. It's always easier to get a job while you still have a job.

IMPORTANCE OF TEAMWORK

The use of **teamwork** to improve the efficiency of the office at first may seem incongruent to your desire to improve office efficiency, because it seems that several people are now involved in solving a problem that you as the manager should solve and explain. Teamwork builds morale and actually results in getting more accomplished with the resources you have because the team members develop ownership of the solution to a problem and want to make it work. When it works, it flatters them and builds their esteem.

Efficiency of a team results from the collective working together to plan how to "work smarter" and how to dovetail tasks and support each other so that wasted effort is avoided. To achieve all of these things, a team must not only be given the responsibility and the authority to plan and execute their plan to solve a problem, but they must know your expectations for them. Sometimes this means that you, the office manager, must stick your neck out for them. They will reward you handsomely for doing so.

Getting the Team Started

A successful teamwork approach is not a mysterious event that just happens, it is the result of clear vision, specific goals, and a well-planned strategy on the part of the team leader. For teamwork to be successful, individual team members must understand and support the specifics of the problem they are being asked to solve. This is probably the most significant task of the team leader or the office manager. It is helpful in taking this important step to let the team develop its own **work statement,** for in this way they assume ownership of the goals and objectives you want them to achieve. The work statement frequently outlines specific tasks and their sequential order of accomplishment. Its purpose is to ensure that everyone is working toward the team goals and objectives.

A major pitfall at this stage may be diverse opinions that can lead to a work statement that does not meet the manager's goals and objectives for the team. It is your job as office manager to try to direct the team back to what you want them to work on without undermining their team spirit. Take care at this stage not to begin making assignments or to let team members start solving the problem until the work statement is complete. Under some circumstances, it may be necessary for you, the office manager, to exercise your authority in defining

the work statement, but be careful, because this approach could harm the team's collective spirit.

The next step in team development is to establish a timetable for achieving results and identifying the standards that must be maintained. Without a timetable a team feels no sense of urgency and tends to lose direction. You also have to paint a clear picture of the standards that must be maintained as you attempt to solve the problem. You should let the team develop both the standards and the timetable, but with your leadership and support.

Using a Team to Solve a Problem

Problem solution is the next step in team development. Some people call this stage **brainstorming** a solution. Brainstorming is fun, but unless it is controlled by the leader, it will bog down into needless arguments and hurt feelings. In a successful brainstorming session everyone should feel free to contribute solutions to the problem without any consideration for practicality or flaws in the proposal. Only after everyone has had a chance to speak are the solutions looked at in terms of practicality and for technical correctness. At this point the team should not look at what is wrong with the solution, but what needs to be done to make it a workable solution.

Prioritization of the solutions comes next. To do this, it is helpful to assign scores for impact on solving the problem and for changeability, or the difficulty in implementing a particular solution in your office environment. The result will be a list of solutions to the problem in descending order from the greatest impact on the problem with the least cost or difficulty in implementation. Do a needs assessment, remove oneself from the issue, and look at it from a different perspective. **Benchmark** (compare) your facility to other facilities and organizations to see how they accomplish tasks, compensate employees, and so on.

Planning and Implementing a Solution

The team should work out a detailed plan for implementation of the solution selected, including a schedule. Assignments should be made, resources of equipment and funds available to the team should be defined, and any remaining problems assigned to subteams that will function just as the primary team did in solving them. The team should continue to meet to discuss progress and to resolve additional problems that may occur.

Recognition

A successful team should not be disbanded until it is acknowledged for its efforts and physical recognition is given in the case of an important problem that was solved. In some cases, a dinner or luncheon is in order. This is the most important phase of team development, because it is responsible for developing a team spirit or sense of **self-actualization** within the organization. Once this spirit is implanted into an organization, it becomes infectious.

SUPERVISING PERSONNEL

Creating an atmosphere in which open and honest communication can take place is critical to supervising personnel. This type of communication may be encouraged through the establishment of regular staff meetings, with each staff member sharing ideas for improvement and areas of concern. Eliciting the help of others in problem-solving strategies will promote harmony (Figure 22-2).

Staff and Team Meetings

The office manager usually initiates the staff and team meeting idea and should officiate at such meetings. Failure of the office manager to be present may convey a message that the meeting is an event not worthy of attention. It is important that the office manager be familiar with basic parliamentary procedures. The purchase of books such as *Robert's Rules of Order* or *Parliamentary Procedure at a Glance* is an excellent investment.

Successful staff and team meetings are announced well in advance or on established time lines to enable the majority of office personnel to attend. An **agenda** identifying the subjects to be covered during a given meeting should be issued before the meeting so that each attendee arrives prepared with input or questions relevant to the topics. Procedure 22-1 outlines the procedural steps for creating a meeting agenda. Figure 22-3 is a sample agenda.

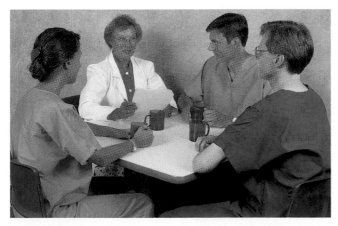

Figure 22-2 Consistently scheduled staff meetings promote communication and harmony among the health care team.

Each meeting should end with opportunity for non-agenda items to be discussed or suggested for inclusion in the next meeting. The meeting should have a fixed time to end.

A written record in the form of **minutes** should be maintained and sent to all team members regardless of whether they attended the meeting. This policy will keep all members informed about policy changes and decisions that impact the office operations. The minutes also trigger a reminder for any new procedures or revisions to be made in the procedure manual. See Chapter 15 for additional information related to agendas and minutes.

The minutes for a staff and team meeting should record action plans under each agenda topic. Summarize all action items agreed to in the meeting in one section of the minutes. This will facilitate easy access to information at a later date should it be required.

The date, time, and place of the next meeting should be included. The person preparing the minutes should always sign them. A copy of the minutes should always be maintained in a book for easy reference.

AGENDA

STAFF MEETING Wednesday, February 16, 20XX
2:00 PM — Conference Room

1. Read and approve minutes of last meeting
2. Reports
   A. Satellite facility — Marilyn Johnson
   B. Patient flow — Joe Guerrero
   C.
3. Discussion of new telephone system
4. Unfinished Business
   A. Review new procedure manual pages
   B.
5. New Business
   A. Appoint committee for design of new marketing brochure
   B.
6. Open discussion and/or topics for next meeting's agenda
7. Set next meeting time
8. Adjourn

Figure 22-3 Sample meeting agenda.

Assimilating New Personnel

The goal in the assimilation of new personnel into the workplace is to make it happen as seamlessly as possible. The office manager and HR representative usually assume this task jointly, with the office manager being responsible for orientation in medical protocols and procedures, and the HR representative handling orientation regarding medical practice rules and regulations and any legal implications.

New Personnel Orientation. The new personnel orientation process consists of orienting and training new employees in the medical protocols and procedures unique to the practice. If the procedure manual is detailed and accurate, this manual now becomes a guide for new employees.

It is important to introduce new employees to other staff members and to assign a **mentor** who can respond to questions that new employees may encounter. Sometimes the individual leaving a position may still be present and is asked to assist in the orientation process. This is especially beneficial if there is a good working relationship between the employee who is leaving and the management of the practice. Depending on the responsibilities of the new employee, a supervisor may be asked to monitor all procedures for a period for accuracy, safety, and patient protection.

The orientation should clearly present what is expected of the new employee and explain that at the end of their probationary period, their performance will be evaluated to determine if full-time employment will be offered. The same procedures followed for new employees should be followed for student practicums, with the exception that expectations and the evaluation process may vary.

Probation and Evaluation. It is common for a new employee to be placed on probation for 60 to 90 days. During this period, both the employee and supervisory personnel determine if the position is a suitable match for both employer and employee. Near the end of the probation period, the employee should be officially evaluated to determine how competently they are performing their assigned tasks/duties. The employee should also be given an opportunity to express their personal thoughts relative to job satisfaction. Figure 22-4 illustrates a sample probationary employee evaluation form. The evaluation becomes part of the employee's personnel record at the end of the probation period.

Supervising Student Practicums. The student **practicum** is a transitional stage that provides opportunity for the student to apply theory learned in the classroom to

---

PROBATIONARY EMPLOYEE EVALUATION FORM

Name _____

Hire Date _____

Job Title _____

Pay Rate_____ Supervisor _____

Do you recommend the employee continue in employment?

_____ Yes _____ No

Please state your reasons for whatever action you recommend. Use the guidelines below to make your decision.

1. Has the employee required more training than is normally needed for the job?

2. Has the employee grasped this job with very little training?

3. Is the employee performing at, above, or below (circle one) the standard for this job?

4. If below, when do you expect the employee to reach the standard?

5. Does the employee get along well with all staff members?

6. Has the employee maintained a good attendance record and a good work attitude?

7. Has the employee expressed any dissatisfactions?

_____ _____
Supervisor's Signature   Date

Figure 22-4 Sample probationary employee evaluation.

---

a health care setting through practical, hands-on experience. Some institutions may use the term **externship** or *internship* and still others may operate through a cooperative education program. The number of hours for the practicum are predetermined together with criteria for site selection and tasks to be performed by the student.

The office manager should schedule an information interview with the student before the practicum begins. During this time, a discussion of the expectations of the office manager and the student may be established. A tour of the facility and introductions to key personnel aid the student in feeling more comfortable the first day of "work."

Because the student will be writing in medical records where correct spelling is mandatory or may be scheduling appointments and must write telephone numbers without transposition, some pretesting may be offered. By giving a spelling test of 10 commonly used medical terms or verbally stating five telephone numbers for the student to write down, an immediate evaluation is attained.

The office manager should directly supervise or identify someone else to supervise the student. During the first few days of the practicum, the student may simply **shadow** the supervisor, learning the routine, physician preference, and protocols for that particular office. As the student begins to feel comfortable in the new environment, minimal tasks should be assigned. Based on the student's ability to follow directions and perform tasks, increased skill-level tasks may be added.

The supervisor will direct and evaluate the student's progress; schedule activities that will provide experience in all aspects of medical assisting, including administrative, clinical, and laboratory procedures; maintain accurate records of attendance and hours "worked"; and communicate the student's progress to the medical assisting supervisor from the educational institution. Procedure 22-2 provides steps for supervising a student practicum.

When working with students, it is important to remember that they still have much to learn and will need lots of reassuring guidance. When you take time to explain each step and to provide the rationale for each, students will learn more quickly. Demonstrating new or different techniques and approaches helps students by providing them with options that they may find more comfortable.

Remember that this type of learning is stressful. The student is not yet accustomed to communication with a "real" patient, let alone working with a physician. Your role as office manager is to reduce as much stress as possible for everyone concerned. Introduce the student to the patient and ask the patient's permission to allow the student to perform a procedure. Many patients will be tolerant when they realize the circumstances and will be quite cooperative.

Employees with Chemical Dependencies or Emotional Problems

Employees with chemical dependencies or emotional problems are ill and are to be treated as such. Approach the situation constructively rather than punitively. Make a commitment to the employee, to the rest of the staff, and to the patients that at no time will patient care be put at risk. Help an employee with a problem to find the support and counseling necessary. No staff member should be permitted to remain on the premise with impaired judgment while under the influence of alcohol or controlled substances. If chemical dependency treatment is necessary, make accommodation as seems appropriate

or is warranted. Everyone occasionally feels discouraged and distressed. Hopefully, the physician–employer and the manager are able to recognize problems before they become too serious.

It has been said that one in four individuals will experience some form of mental health problem during the course of a year. Work-related stress is the base cause of a significant degree of mental ill health. Plan for and create a work environment that reduces as much stress as possible. Actions to consider may include the following:

1. Properly educate and train all employees for their positions.
2. Encourage teamwork and reward those who help each other.
3. Mandate "break periods" in the day for each employee.
4. Create a pleasant work environment (plants, water, music, and so on).
5. Establish a blowing off steam place for when employees are especially frustrated.
6. Take everyone out for lunch at least once a quarter.
7. Have regular staff meetings to discuss employee concerns and office improvements.
8. Celebrate birthdays and special occasions (i.e., length of service).

Keep in mind that a happy employee who feels valued in his or her position will stay much longer than someone who is unhappy and does not feel valued.

Evaluating Employees and Planning Salary Review

It is important that all employees know whether they are performing their job as expected and know how they can improve their performance if necessary.

Performance Evaluation. Not only is evaluation of employees necessary during the probation period, but it is necessary for current employees as well. Evaluations should be performed no less than once a year on the anniversary of the hire date. Some office managers may wish to evaluate an employee more often, especially if a problem has surfaced in an evaluation.

The evaluation may take many forms; it can be formal or informal; it may involve more than one person. The results of the evaluation, however, must be a part of the employee's personnel record. For that reason, a formal evaluation is preferred. Many practices use a written evaluation that requires that the employee evaluate himself before meeting with the office manager (Figure 22-5). The office manager uses the same form for evaluation.

PERFORMANCE REVIEW FORM

_____   _____
Employee Name   Title

_____   _____
Supervisor   Department

TYPE OF REVIEW (Check One)

_____ Quarterly

_____ Annual

_____ Probation

_____ Other _____

Review Period Covered _____ to _____

PERFORMANCE DEFINITIONS

5 = Outstanding	Performance that is clearly superior, beyond the call of duty, or substantially above standard level. Seldom attained level of performance but achievable.
4 = Above Standard	Very commendable performance; exceeds the norm for the job.
3 = Standard	Competent and consistent performance; expected level of activity and performance for the job. Most often rating received.
2 = Below Standard	Performance needs improvement. This level of performance is unacceptable; needs improvement to meet the standards for the job. **Employee new to the job:** Performance might receive below standard rating due to lack of job knowledge and is expected to improve with experience. **Experienced Employee:** Performance is below acceptable level and requires direction and/or counsel.
1 = Unsatisfactory	Performance is unacceptable. Job activity is clearly and substantially lacking in quality, quantity, or timeliness. May also not be meeting cost or budget constraints. Needs much improvement to meet the standards for the job.

(office use only) EVALUATION SUMMARY Total I _____ + Total II _____	FINAL RATING: CHECK ONE (office use only) _____ Merit Increase Recommended _____ No Merit Increase—Satisfactory Performance/No Growth _____ No Merit Increase (Probationary/Special Evaluation) _____ No Merit Increase (Performance Probation) _____ Re-evaluate in 90 Days for Unsatisfactory or in 180 Days for Needed Improvement

GENERAL PERFORMANCE RATING (PART I)

General Criteria	Rating	Comments Supporting Rating
1. **Patient Relations:** How well does the employee communicate a "we care" image to the patients, visitors, physicians, and fellow employees?		
2. **Work Responsibilities:** What is the quality of the employee's work relative to quality, quantity, and timeliness?		
3. **Teamwork:** Does the employee have a team spirit? Does the employee interact well with co-workers/supervisor/manager?		(continues)

Figure 22-5 Sample performance review form.

General Criteria	Rating	Comments Supporting Rating
4. **Adaptability:** Is the employee open to change and new ideas? Does the employee remain flexible to changes in routine, work-load, and assignments?		
5. **Personal Appearance:** How well does the employee maintain appropriate personal appearance, including proper attire, hygiene?		
6. **Communication:** Does the employee communicate well? Is information given and received clearly? Does he/she have good verbal and written skills?		
7. **Dependability:** Can the employee be relied upon for good attendance? Does the employee perform and follow through on work without supervisory intervention or assistance?		

Subtotal I _____ + 7 General Criteria = _____

JOB-SPECIFIC CRITERIA RATING (PART II) (To be used with Job Description attached)

Responsibility and Standard	Rating	Comments Supporting Rating
Complete a section for each responsibility listed on the employee's job description.		

Subtotal II _____ + _____ = _____
job duties

Contributions made since last review:
_____
_____
_____

Education or training received since last review:
_____
_____
_____

Action to be taken based on performance:
_____
_____
_____

Comments:
_____
_____
_____

_____   _____
Employee Signature   Date

_____   _____
Supervisor Signature   Date

_____   _____
Physician Signature   Date

Figure 22-5   (continued)

During the meeting, notes are compared as the evaluation is conducted.

The climate of the performance evaluation should be comfortable and provide privacy (Figure 22-6). The meeting should be friendly, but the employee must sense the importance of the evaluation. Do not allow any disagreements to escalate into arguments during the evaluation. Without reading the employee's self-evaluation, ask the employee to tell about the self-assessment. Acknowledge the employee's point of view and identify when you agree or differ from the self-assessment. Be prepared to describe specific examples of positive performance and negative performance.

When negative performance is identified, ask the employee for possible solutions. Then a plan can be determined to alter the negative performance. In this way, a trusting atmosphere is established in that both of you are working together for a solution that will benefit the medical practice. Always look for and seek a win-win situation whenever possible. The action plan determined should then be evaluated at the next performance evaluation.

At the close of the evaluation, always express your confidence in the individual to make any changes necessary, offer assistance where needed, and thank the employee for participating. End any evaluation with a positive statement about some portion of the employee's performance.

There are occasions when reviews are performed more frequently than annually. A review would occur two to three months after a significant promotion to measure how things are progressing. Reviews occur more often when general performance falls well short of past efforts or a serious error in judgment has been made. This type of review may end with a reprimand, a warning to correct the problem by a given date, or possibly, immediate

dismissal. Document any steps to be taken to correct a problem and any reason that is cause for dismissal.

Salary Review. Although the practice is common in some areas, it may be better not to tie salary increases or bonuses with the annual performance evaluation. Conduct the **salary review** at the beginning of the new year separate from performance evaluations.

Salary review is important. Unfortunately, in smaller medical offices and ambulatory care settings, the review of salary may have to be raised by the employee. Physician–employers tend to forget that their employees have been with them for over a year without a raise or a discussion of financial reimbursement. If this is the case, it is perfectly acceptable for the employee to raise the issue on a yearly basis. However, the best approach is for the office manager to conduct salary reviews at the beginning or end of each calendar year.

Data should be collected before a salary review. The office manager should network with other office managers to determine wages and salaries for comparable individuals with comparable skills. Remember, also, that it is far more cost-effective to reward good employees with a salary increase than it is to train a new employee who commands a lesser salary than current employees. Reward employees well and provide benefits that encourage them to stay with the practice. Employees who stay with the practice for a long time not only fully understand how best to serve their physician–employers, they have established a relationship with patients that is beneficial.

How much of a raise is to be awarded at the time of salary review is difficult to determine and will depend on many factors that might include the profits of the year, the patient load, the workload, and the current cost of living.

The critical shortage of health care employees today is reflected in the shortage of medical assistants across the country. Newspapers advertising for individuals to work in the ambulatory care setting tell the story. A consideration worth mentioning is that often the salary does not match the education, experience, and special training required of someone working in the health care field. Educators often hear, "Why would I spend a year or more in education to be paid what I would make working in a fast food restaurant?" Because it is costly in time and resources to replace employees, it is best to invest that cost into a fair and just salary increase for valued employees.

Conflict Resolution

A good human resources manager will be a master at **conflict resolution,** solving problems between any two parties. The most difficult task is to prevent or solve conflicts that occur between employees or between employees and

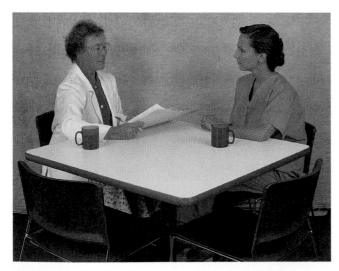

Figure 22-6 A comfortable, private setting encourages discussion during an employee performance review.

supervisors or physician–employers. Most conflict occurs because of poor communication or a misunderstanding, thus effective communication is a goal for any manager.

Volumes of materials have been written about successful conflict management. One can probably never get enough material on the subject. Some guidelines that may be helpful in preventing and resolving conflicts follow:

- Listen to your employees. What do they say? What do they communicate nonverbally?

- Be prepared to temporarily assist an employee having a difficult time.

- Create a safe environment for an employee to admit a mistake.

- Manage by walking around and talking to your employees.

- Acknowledge the stressors of the job and compensate employees.

- Give ample verbal positive comments and pats on the back.

- Be honest with employees at all times.

- Provide office staff meetings in which employees can express their concerns.

- Treat employees fairly.

- Do not tolerate negative comments or actions among employees.

- Remember birthdays and special occasions with cards or small gifts.

- Provide small rewards when possible.

- Expect to work longer and harder than any employee.

- Have the physician–employer host a social lunch every 60 days.

- Keep employees informed of changes impacting them.

- Encourage an open-door policy for concerns and complaints.

- Be a role model for all employees.

- Keep confidences.

- Encourage continuing education through workshops and seminars.

There is no end to such a list. An office manager who cares about each employee, who "carries water for the workers in the trenches," and who administers fairly and honestly creates an environment where conflict will be at a minimum.

Dismissing Employees

Most human resources managers do not enjoy rating the performance of other employees particularly when difficult topics are involved and it may be necessary to dismiss an employee. However, the written performance evaluation actually establishes the format for such a dismissal when necessary and is more likely to remove the emotion from the situation. **Involuntary dismissal** is still difficult when it is necessary.

Involuntary Dismissal. Involuntary dismissal results from two primary causes: poor performance or serious violation of office policies or job descriptions. When it becomes apparent to the office manager that the effectiveness of an employee is dropping well below expectations, it will be known in the review or a performance review may be called. The review allows the employee to be informed of the shortcomings, to explain any reasons for the present situation, and to determine a plan to alleviate the problem. If the problem is a serious one, probation is usually invoked and any lack of significant improvement in the time provided results in immediate dismissal.

When the problem is a violation of either office policy or procedures, both a verbal and a written warning are given to the employee. Involuntary dismissal follows if the situation persists. Dismissal may be immediate if the action is a serious violation of policy. Serious violations will depend on the office practice, but some causes for immediate dismissal include theft, making fraudulent claims against insurance, placing the patient in jeopardy by not practicing safe techniques, and breach of patient confidentiality.

Some key points to keep in mind when dismissal is necessary are:

1. The dismissal should be made in privacy.
2. Take no longer than 10 minutes for the dismissal.
3. Be direct, firm, and to the point in identifying reasons.
4. Do not engage in an in-depth discussion of performance.
5. Explain terms of dismissal (keys, clearing out area of personal items, final paperwork).
6. Listen to employee's opinion and emotions; it is not necessary to agree.
7. Accompany the employee to his or her desk to pack his or her belongings.
8. Escort the employee out of the facility; do not allow him or her to finish the work of the day.

Voluntary Dismissal. Other reasons for dismissal may be more pleasant. Changes in personnel occur for many good reasons and people voluntarily leave their jobs. They may relocate, seek advancement in another facility, or simply have personal reasons for leaving. These employees will give their manager proper notice and will be able to turn their current projects and duties over to their replacements. They have time to say good-bye to their friends and leave with a good feeling about their employment.

PROCEDURE MANUAL

The **procedure manual** provides detailed information relative to the performance of tasks within the facility in which one is employed. Each procedure manual should be designed for that specific office setting and should satisfy its requirements.

The procedure manual serves as a guide to the employee assigned a specific task and may also be useful in evaluating the employee's performance. If a temporary employee is assigned the task, the procedure manual will be invaluable in assuring that each procedure is completed as outlined.

The physician(s) and the office manager should have copies of the procedure manual and it should also be accessible to all employees. Copies of individual sections may be given to the employee responsible for the task; the employee should be instructed to follow these guidelines and told that they may be used as employee evaluation tools.

Organization of the Procedure Manual

It is best to use a loose-leaf binder with separator pages denoting each procedure. Many office managers find it helpful to divide the binder into administrative and clinical sections with subdivisions for each primary task performed (Figure 22-7).

To facilitate using the procedure manual, a consistent format should be developed and used throughout the manual. Each procedure should be a step-by-step outline or list of steps to be taken to complete a task as desired in that facility. Providing the rationale for a step, when appropriate, enhances the learning process, especially for new staff members. Material Safety Data Sheets (MSDSs) are required to be maintained in the clinic and available for personnel to reference at any time. MSDS must be compiled for all chemicals considered hazardous and maintained in an appropriate manual. Some offices opt to maintain these records in a separate tabbed section of the procedure manual. Others choose to maintain a separate MSDS manual. The information must be reviewed and updated on a regular

Administrative Section	Clinical Section
Personnel Management	Physical Examinations
Communication	Infection Control
(oral and written)	Collecting Specimens
Patient Scheduling	Laboratory Procedures
Records Management	Surgical Asepsis
Financial Management	Emergencies
Facility and Equipment	Material Safety Data Sheets
Management	(MSDS)
	OSHA
	CLIA '88

Figure 22-7 Many offices find that dividing the procedure manual into tabbed sections helps organize the material. A table of contents with page numbers helps locate information easily.

basis. Procedure 22-5 provides steps for developing and maintaining a procedure manual.

Updating and Reviewing the Procedure Manual

When new procedures are added to the office routine, a new procedure page should be developed immediately. The new page is then useful as an educational tool or job aid while team members are learning new techniques.

An annual page-by-page review should be done to ascertain if each procedure is still being used and assure that each page is correct in each detail and satisfies all criteria established by the staff personnel. This contributes to an efficient office and gives all employees a sense of pride and satisfaction that they are performing within the scope of their training and to their greatest potential. The procedure manual should be reviewed by personnel performing the various tasks and their suggestions should be evaluated and incorporated into the revisions when appropriate. All new procedure pages and revisions should be dated (Rev. 02/15/XX).

HIPAA IMPLICATIONS

The new HIPAA regulations require each office to develop a separate HIPAA manual that is to be either an electronic form or paper manual. It is to spell out all policies and procedures of the practice and security management measures; identify the security officer; address workforce security issues, information access concerns, security awareness and training, security incidents, and contingency plans; evaluate security effectiveness; and contain copies of all business associate contracts.

The HIPAA manual must be available to all employees and is to be updated on a regular basis. During an audit, the office manager will be asked to produce the HIPAA manual for review and to establish compliance with all regulations. All documentation of policies and procedures are to be kept for six years even though the wording has changed or been eliminated. If an incident is under investigation, this allows an investigator to go back to what a policy said six years ago.

TRAVEL ARRANGEMENTS

The office manager may be asked to make travel arrangements for physicians going on vacation or to conventions, symposiums, or out-of-town seminars and Continuing Medical Education (CME) courses. If the physicians do a fair amount of travel or if they live in a metropolitan area, they may use the services of a travel agent. Attention to detail is extremely important in preventing travel disruptions.

Read carefully the instructions for completing registration forms, complete them, and mail them as quickly as possible to secure reservations to conventions and so forth. Next make hotel and travel arrangements. General information regarding the physician's travel preferences should be maintained in a file folder and be referred to when making travel arrangements. Helpful information to maintain in this file includes:

- Name of travel agents used in the past (ranked by reputation and recommendation)

- Physician's or office credit card numbers

- Car rental preference

- Preferred airline, class of travel, seating choice

- Hotel/motel accommodations (bed size, suite, studio, connecting rooms, price range, amenities)

- Shuttle service

Next, contact the travel agent and identify the destination, date and time for departure and return, number traveling in party, and seating preference. A travel agent can also assist with rental car and hotel accommodations if needed. Take your time and pay attention to details. When tickets are received, always check to see that all departure and arrival times match what is needed and that a confirmation number has been provided for car rentals and hotel arrangements. Procedure 22-3 outlines the procedural steps involved in making travel arrangements through a travel agent.

 The Internet may be used to search for the lowest cost air, auto, and lodging reservations. The procedures do not require extensive knowledge of travel and airline reservation protocols. Searching for information on the **Internet** requires the use of a search engine if you do not already have a list of favorite travel **Web sites.** A **search engine** is a special computer program available through your Internet service provider. With a search engine, you enter only the subject of your search, and the Web will provide a list of Web sites related to your subject. For example, if you are making travel arrangements, you might access a search engine such as Google.com and enter the key words "air fares." The engine will return either a list of Web sites or ask you to further refine your subject with suggestions such as cheap air fares, international travel, and so on. Once you have refined your search, you may have choices such as Travelocity.com, Expedia.com, or Priceline.com. Select the appropriate Web site and follow its instructions.

Priceline.com and similar Web sites are services that allow you to name the price you want to pay; Priceline finds a major airline willing to release seats on flights where they have unsold space. You need to have a reasonable idea of the price of the service you are trying to purchase; unreasonably low bids will just waste your time and effort. Procedure 22-4 outlines the steps for making travel arrangements via the Internet.

Itinerary

If you have used a travel agent in making the travel arrangements, the agency will most likely provide several copies of the **itinerary.** An itinerary is a detailed plan for a proposed trip. The office should maintain one copy of the itinerary in case the physician must be reached for emergencies. The physician should have one copy to carry with him or her and a copy to leave with family members. You may need to develop the itinerary if you have made the travel arrangements via computer. Figure 22-8 shows a sample travel itinerary.

Important information to be included on any itinerary includes:

- *Air travel:* departure and arrival date and time, meals, airline name and telephone number, airport

- *Car rental:* name of provider, telephone number, confirmation number

- *Hotel/motel:* name, confirmation number, dates, telephone number

- *Meeting location:* name, address, room number, telephone number

---

TRAVEL ITINERARY

James Whitney, MD
Inner City Health Care
400 Inner City Way
Seattle, WA 98400

15 Sept 20XX   INVOICE: 880133795

29 Sept Friday
USAIR   630   Coach Class   Equip-Boeing 757 Jet
LV: Seattle   11:55P   Nonstop   Miles-2125   Confirmed
AR: Pittsburgh   7:23A   Elapsed time-4:28   Arrival Date-30Sept
                                              Seat-31C

30 Sept-Saturday
Alamo   1 Compact 2/4 DR   Drop-101CT   Confirmed
Pickup-Pittsburgh   Pittsburgh Airport Chg-USD .00
Rate-   59.98   Baserate   Guaranteed   Extra Hr 10.00-UN
Phone-412-472-5060
                            Confirmation-1870649

01 Oct Sunday
USAIR   1419 Coach Class   Equip-Boeing 737 Jet
LV: Pittsburgh   3:05P   Nonstop   Miles-2125   Confirmed
AR: Seattle   5:27P   Elapsed time-5:22
Lunch   Seat-20A

Ticket Number/s:
Whitney/James   3570933   BA Card $461.00
        Air Transportation $416.36   Tax   44.64   TOTAL $461.00
                                             Sub Total $461.00
                                             Credit Card Payment $461.00-
                                             Amount Due   0.00

TICKET IS NON REFUNDABLE. TRIP INSURANCE IS AVAILABLE. RECONFIRM ALL FLTS 24 HRS PRIOR TO DEPARTURE

Figure 22-8 Sample travel itinerary.

TIME MANAGEMENT

Time management is an item of critical importance to the manager. You may have upward of 20 staff members putting demands on your time, and added to this are vendors, your superiors, business associates, and a host of others. A manager has not a moment to lose in the day, so managing time makes the difference between a normal 8- or 10-hour day and a 15-hour or more day. The following suggestions are some proven means of managing your time:

- *Handle items once.* Once the mail is opened, sorted, and prioritized, try to handle it only once more, when action is taken with it. Picking it up, reading it, and setting it down again without taking action is a real waste of time.

- *Develop a to-do list.* At the end of each day prepare a list of things you plan to complete the next day and try to work down this list. Prioritize the list by importance or by practical order.

- *Guard your time.* Schedule meetings with personnel and vendors so that it does not fragment your time, making you have to restart a task and get up to speed over and over again. Although modern management practice is to have an open-door policy with employees, this does not mean you should allow them to come into your office whenever they think about it. Have them schedule time with you. Make them think about what they want to discuss and do not let them monopolize your time. This is also true of meeting with vendors; require vendors to schedule ahead a time to meet with you.

• *Delegate work.* Assign others or a team to perform some of the functions discussed in this chapter. Having a team prepare weekly work schedules and vacation schedules results in less bickering and feelings of favoritism that you would have to spend time defusing if you made the schedules yourself. This does not mean that you do not have to approve them and, in some instances, make the hard decisions, but it results in your people having ownership in the decisions.

MARKETING FUNCTIONS

Effective communication skills are essential in the management of the ambulatory care setting. These skills are used by the office manager inside the ambulatory care setting to establish friendly, professional relationships with colleagues and patients. Communication is just as critical when relating to external audiences, such as other organizations, potential new patients, and community members. Developing relationships outside the office is often called marketing, a concept that office managers may use to enhance the image and visibility of an ambulatory care setting while also providing benefits to patients, potential patients, and the neighboring community.

In its broadest sense, **marketing** can be defined as the process by which the provider of services makes the consumer aware of the scope and quality of these services. Although marketing is a tool traditionally used by for-profit organizations to promote and sell products and services, it has become increasingly acceptable among health care organizations, whether they are for- or not-for-profit.

Marketing functions and materials are diverse and can include seminars and workshops, patient education brochures, brochures that describe the ambulatory care setting and its scope of services, HIPAA policies, newsletters, press releases, and special events such as open houses or participation in community health care events. Depending on the size and resources of the medical office, the manager may choose to use all or some of these tools (Figure 22-9).

  When producing written material and organizing events, it is essential that ethical guidelines be respected at all times. Marketing tools should be appropriate, in good taste, and designed to quietly enhance the reputation of the office. Cultural issues should always be considered. For example, patient education brochures for a practice with many Spanish-speaking patients should be produced

Marketing Tool	Potential Uses and Value
Seminars	Can educate patients and provide good will in the community. All staff—administrative and clinical—can work as a team to organize, publicize, and deliver the seminars.
Brochures	Brochures are typically of two types: patient education brochures and brochures on office services. Can be simple 8-1/2" x 11" fact sheets, with text only, or more elaborate brochures folded to 4" x 9" that incorporate both text and graphics or photos. Both types of brochures are informative for patients and present a professional image of the ambulatory care setting.
Practice Web site and E-zines	The practice Web site is an excellent means of promoting the practice. Personnel can be introduced, and procedures and technologies can be discussed. The E-zine approach is rapidly catching on as a promotional tool. It can be e-mailed to patients so it saves time and money. The patient may choose to view, delete, or save to read at a later time.
Newsletters	Newsletters can be produced on a biannual or quarterly basis and can form the nucleus of a marketing program. Because they are versatile tools, they can include a wide range of information from health-related articles to staff introductions to insurance updates. They should be sent to individuals on the office's mailing list and be available in the reception area.
Press Releases	Periodic press releases on new equipment, new staff, and expanded or remodeled office space can be a vital link to the local community.
Special Events	Special events are an effective way to join with other community organizations to promote wellness. They can include participation in health fairs, cosponsorship of a charity event, or an open house on the premises to acquaint the community with new services or equipment.

Figure 22-9 Marketing tools and their use in a medical environment.

in bilingual editions, with English on one side and Spanish on the other. Legal issues are important as well; when presenting material of a medical nature, it is extremely important that information be accurate and up to date.

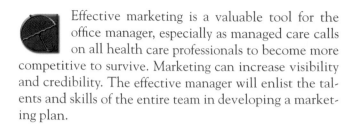

Effective marketing is a valuable tool for the office manager, especially as managed care calls on all health care professionals to become more competitive to survive. Marketing can increase visibility and credibility. The effective manager will enlist the talents and skills of the entire team in developing a marketing plan.

Seminars

As consumers become increasingly aware of lifestyle choices, they look to health care professionals for information and guidance. Seminars and workshops are useful vehicles for presenting health-related information; while expert advice can be given, there is also the opportunity for patients and health care professionals to interact.

Seminars can be organized to meet patient and community needs. Some popular seminar topics include hypertension, diabetes, eating disorders, and exercise and weight management programs.

No matter what the topic area, the content should be oriented to the lay person's level of understanding, with a focused message and a delivery designed to maintain attention. Interactive seminars, which encourage audience participation, can be productive and enjoyable. Audiovisuals, such as projected slides, will provide visual reinforcement. Handouts, either from professional organizations or those produced by office staff, can elaborate on seminar content and help the participant review and remember what was said.

Brochures

Despite the promise of a paperless society, brochures continue to be valuable sources of information. In the health care setting, patients welcome a rack of brochures as a source of current, accurate background on medical issues. New patients also find that a brochure on office services will answer many questions about the practice, its philosophy, and its scope of services, and will provide physician profiles.

Today, it is possible to produce a professional-looking brochure in the office using one of the computer programs that integrate text and graphics. If a brochure is produced in-house, it is important to consider writing, design, and production. Writing should be clear, to the point, and grammatically correct. Always proofread carefully before printing. Design should be kept simple. Avoid the use of too many typefaces; choose a typeface and size for readability, and, if using artwork or photography, consider its reproduction qualities. Black or another dark ink against a light background is best for readability.

Often, a local printer will be able to advise the office manager on how to prepare a brochure or handout for printing. The simplest handouts can be quick-copied (a high-speed photocopy) on a white or lightly colored or textured stock. After printing, brochures should be made accessible to patients and other visitors in a rack or neatly arranged in piles (Figure 22-10). Occasionally, a brochure will be mailed; one that folds to 4×9 inches will fit into a standard #10 business envelope.

Patient Education Brochures. Like seminars, patient education brochures can address a variety of topics, including hypertension, diabetes, eating disorders, and exercise and weight management programs. When writing these brochures, always research material carefully, request permission for copyrighted materials, and present the information in a manner that is accessible to your patient population.

Office Brochures. A brochure on the practice can provide a wide range of information and will orient the new patient to the practice. One way to determine what information to include is to develop a list of frequently asked patient questions. Once this list is compiled, it can serve as the beginning of the brochure outline. Issues to consider might include:

- Brief history of the practice
- Brief résumés or credentials of physicians

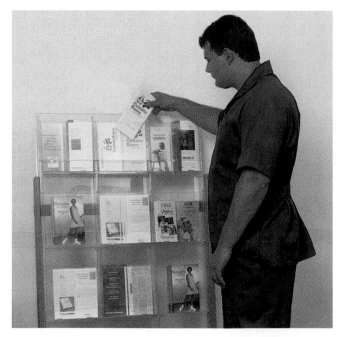

Figure 22-10 Brochures and handouts should be accessible and inviting to patients and office visitors.

- Philosophy of the practice
- Scope of services
- How to reach the practice in case of emergency
- Insurances accepted
- Rights of patients
- Policies regarding the release of information
- Scheduling information: how to schedule an appointment, cancellation policies
- Amenities on the premises such as parking, pharmacy, laboratory
- Location, map if necessary, and location of satellite offices

Newsletters

Newsletters are effective communication tools because they encourage regular contact with patients and other readers. Newsletters are a versatile medium, too; they can contain patient education articles, updates on staff changes, awards, information on insurance carriers, calendars of events, even recipes that are consistent with a healthful lifestyle.

Most newsletters can be written and produced in the office. Like brochures, they should be simple in design and format. An additional factor in newsletter production is mailing; an up-to-date database must be maintained, postal regulations must be followed, and the costs of mailing considered.

Press Releases

Press releases are simple, inexpensive marketing tools. Use them to announce new staff, promote a new service, or publicize a series of seminars. If a professional, courteous relationship is developed with the local press, most will be happy to receive and publish releases. When writing releases, always follow proper format, which includes a date of release, a contact person's name and telephone number, and a short headline. Releases are best kept to one double-spaced typed page. At the end of the release, type "30" or a number sign (#). Maintain an active list of local newspapers and editors' names so that you can mail or fax the release to the appropriate editor.

Special Events

Although they can be time-consuming to organize and participate in, special events are rewarding, for they present an opportunity to interact with the community. They have high visibility, for often a group of community organizations will collaborate to cosponsor an event such as a walk-a-thon, blood pressure clinic, health fair for seniors, or wellness day for children and families. Sponsorship can be as simple as a donation to the cause; other times, staffing a booth or offering a service such as blood pressure checks is appropriate.

Like all marketing efforts, special events require organizational skills and teamwork, but they often result in heightened communication with the community and provide an educational service to patients and their families.

RECORDS AND FINANCIAL MANAGEMENT

Physicians entrust a great deal of responsibility to their medical office managers. The daily payments received through the mail and office visits must be processed and prepared for banking. Office expenses must be processed and paid in a timely fashion to capitalize on any discounts available. Employee requirements and records such as Social Security records, Withholding Allowance Certificates (W-4 forms) (Figure 22-11) indicating the number of exemptions claimed, and Employment Eligibility Verification Forms (I-9) ensuring that all persons employed are either United States citizens, lawfully admitted aliens, or aliens authorized to work in the United States must be completed and filed with the appropriate federal agencies. Also, state and local tax records must be maintained for each employee.

Payroll Processing

In some cases, it is the office manager's responsibility to prepare payroll checks for each employee and record all deductions withheld. A W-2 form (Figure 22-12) summarizing all earnings and deductions for the year must be prepared for each employee by January 31 of each year. The Social Security Administration must receive a summary report of W-2 forms each year.

To comply with all governmental regulations, federal, state, and local, it is important that the office manager who processes payroll maintain complete, up-to-date records on every employee. This information should be gathered from new employees and updated every year and on any change in employee status. For more specific information regarding printed and electronic filing forms, go to the Internal Revenue Service Web site (http://www.irs.gov) for detailed instructions. It is a good idea to have employees update their W-4 form each year in case they want to adjust their deductions or make any other change. To accomplish this, many payroll managers include a new W-4 form with the first paycheck at the beginning of each year. Every employee file should contain Social

Form W-4 (2005)

Purpose. Complete Form W-4 so that your employer can withhold the correct federal income tax from your pay. Because your tax situation may change, you may want to refigure your withholding each year.

Exemption from withholding. If you are exempt, complete only lines 1, 2, 3, 4, and 7 and sign the form to validate it. Your exemption for 2005 expires February 16, 2006. See Pub. 505, Tax Withholding and Estimated Tax.

Note. You cannot claim exemption from withholding if (a) your income exceeds $800 and includes more than $250 of unearned income (for example, interest and dividends) and (b) another person can claim you as a dependent on their tax return.

Basic instructions. If you are not exempt, complete the **Personal Allowances Worksheet** below. The worksheets on page 2 adjust your withholding allowances based on itemized deductions, certain credits, adjustments to income, or two-earner/two-job situations. Complete all worksheets that apply. However, you may claim fewer (or zero) allowances.

Head of household. Generally, you may claim head of household filing status on your tax return only if you are unmarried and pay more than 50% of the costs of keeping up a home for yourself and your dependent(s) or other qualifying individuals. See line **E** below.

Tax credits. You can take projected tax credits into account in figuring your allowable number of withholding allowances. Credits for child or dependent care expenses and the child tax credit may be claimed using the **Personal Allowances Worksheet** below. See Pub. 919, How Do I Adjust My Tax Withholding? for information on converting your other credits into withholding allowances.

Nonwage income. If you have a large amount of nonwage income, such as interest or dividends, consider making estimated tax payments using Form 1040-ES, Estimated Tax for Individuals. Otherwise, you may owe additional tax.

Two earners/two jobs. If you have a working spouse or more than one job, figure the total number of allowances you are entitled to claim on all jobs using worksheets from only one Form W-4. Your withholding usually will be most accurate when all allowances are claimed on the Form W-4 for the highest paying job and zero allowances are claimed on the others.

Nonresident alien. If you are a nonresident alien, see the Instructions for Form 8233 before completing this Form W-4.

Check your withholding. After your Form W-4 takes effect, use Pub. 919 to see how the dollar amount you are having withheld compares to your projected total tax for 2005. See Pub. 919, especially if your earnings exceed $125,000 (Single) or $175,000 (Married).

Recent name change? If your name on line 1 differs from that shown on your social security card, call 1-800-772-1213 to initiate a name change and obtain a social security card showing your correct name.

Personal Allowances Worksheet (Keep for your records.)

A Enter "1" for **yourself** if no one else can claim you as a dependent . . . . A ______

B Enter "1" if: { • You are single and have only one job; or • You are married, have only one job, and your spouse does not work; or • Your wages from a second job or your spouse's wages (or the total of both) are $1,000 or less. } . . B ______

C Enter "1" for your **spouse.** But, you may choose to enter "-0-" if you are married and have either a working spouse or more than one job. (Entering "-0-" may help you avoid having too little tax withheld.) . . . . C ______

D Enter number of **dependents** (other than your spouse or yourself) you will claim on your tax return . . . . . . D ______

E Enter "1" if you will file as **head of household** on your tax return (see conditions under **Head of household** above) . E ______

F Enter "1" if you have at least $1,500 of **child or dependent care expenses** for which you plan to claim a credit . . F ______

(**Note.** Do **not** include child support payments. See **Pub. 503,** Child and Dependent Care Expenses, for details.)

G **Child Tax Credit** (including additional child tax credit):

- If your total income will be less than $54,000 ($79,000 if married), enter "2" for each eligible child.
- If your total income will be between $54,000 and $84,000 ($79,000 and $119,000 if married), enter "1" for each eligible child plus "1" **additional** if you have four or more eligible children. G ______

H Add lines A through G and enter total here. (**Note.** This may be different from the number of exemptions you claim on your tax return.) ▶ H ______

For accuracy, complete all worksheets that apply. {
- If you plan to **itemize or claim adjustments to income** and want to reduce your withholding, see the **Deductions and Adjustments Worksheet** on page 2.
- If you have **more than one job** or are **married and you and your spouse both work** and the combined earnings from all jobs exceed $35,000 ($25,000 if married) see the **Two-Earner/Two-Job Worksheet** on page 2 to avoid having too little tax withheld.
- If **neither** of the above situations applies, **stop here** and enter the number from line H on line 5 of Form W-4 below. }

Cut here and give Form W-4 to your employer. Keep the top part for your records.

Form **W-4** | **Employee's Withholding Allowance Certificate** | OMB No. 1545-0010

Department of the Treasury Internal Revenue Service

▶ **Whether you are entitled to claim a certain number of allowances or exemption from withholding is subject to review by the IRS. Your employer may be required to send a copy of this form to the IRS.**

2005

1 Type or print your first name and middle initial | Last name | 2 Your social security number

Home address (number and street or rural route) | 3 ☐ Single ☐ Married ☐ Married, but withhold at higher Single rate.
Note. If married, but legally separated, or spouse is a nonresident alien, check the "Single" box.

City or town, state, and ZIP code | 4 **If your last name differs from that shown on your social security card, check here. You must call 1-800-772-1213 for a new card.** ▶ ☐

5 Total number of allowances you are claiming (from line **H** above **or** from the applicable worksheet on page 2) 5 ______

6 Additional amount, if any, you want withheld from each paycheck . . . . 6 $ ______

7 I claim exemption from withholding for 2005, and I certify that I meet **both** of the following conditions for exemption.
- Last year I had a right to a refund of **all** federal income tax withheld because I had **no** tax liability **and**
- This year I expect a refund of **all** federal income tax withheld because I expect to have **no** tax liability.

If you meet both conditions, write "Exempt" here . . . . ▶ 7 ______

Under penalties of perjury, I declare that I have examined this certificate and to the best of my knowledge and belief, it is true, correct, and complete.

Employee's signature
(Form is not valid unless you sign it.) ▶ **Date** ▶

8 Employer's name and address (Employer: Complete lines 8 and 10 only if sending to the IRS.) | 9 Office code (optional) | 10 Employer identification number (EIN)

For Privacy Act and Paperwork Reduction Act Notice, see page 2. Cat. No. 10220Q Form **W-4** (2005)

Form W-4 (2005) Page **2**

Deductions and Adjustments Worksheet

Note. Use this worksheet *only* if you plan to itemize deductions, claim certain credits, or claim adjustments to income on your 2005 tax return.

1 Enter an estimate of your 2005 itemized deductions. These include qualifying home mortgage interest, charitable contributions, state and local taxes, medical expenses in excess of 7.5% of your income, and miscellaneous deductions. (For 2005, you may have to reduce your itemized deductions if your income is over $145,950 ($72,975 if married filing separately). See *Worksheet 3* in Pub. 919 for details.) . . . . 1 $ ______

2 Enter: { $10,000 if married filing jointly or qualifying widow(er) / $ 7,300 if head of household / $ 5,000 if single or married filing separately } . . . . 2 $ ______

3 **Subtract** line 2 from line 1. If line 2 is greater than line 1, enter "-0-" . . . . 3 $ ______

4 Enter an estimate of your 2005 adjustments to income, including alimony, deductible IRA contributions, and student loan interest 4 $ ______

5 **Add** lines 3 and 4 and enter the total. (Include any amount for credits from *Worksheet 7* in Pub. 919) . 5 $ ______

6 Enter an estimate of your 2005 nonwage income (such as dividends or interest) . . . . 6 $ ______

7 **Subtract** line 6 from line 5. Enter the result, but not less than "-0-" . . . . 7 $ ______

8 **Divide** the amount on line 7 by $3,200 and enter the result here. Drop any fraction . . . . 8 ______

9 Enter the number from the **Personal Allowances Worksheet,** line H, page 1 . . . . 9 ______

10 **Add** lines 8 and 9 and enter the total here. If you plan to use the **Two-Earner/Two-Job Worksheet,** also enter this total on line 1 below. Otherwise, **stop here** and enter this total on Form W-4, line 5, page 1 . 10 ______

Two-Earner/Two-Job Worksheet (See *Two earners/two jobs* on page 1.)

Note. Use this worksheet *only* if the instructions under line H on page 1 direct you here.

1 Enter the number from line H, page 1 (or from line 10 above if you used the **Deductions and Adjustments Worksheet**) 1 ______

2 Find the number in **Table 1** below that applies to the **LOWEST** paying job and enter it here . . . . 2 ______

3 If line 1 is **more than or equal to** line 2, subtract line 2 from line 1. Enter the result here (if zero, enter "-0-") and on Form W-4, line 5, page 1. **Do not** use the rest of this worksheet . . . . 3 ______

Note. If line 1 is *less than* line 2, enter "-0-" on Form W-4, line 5, page 1. Complete lines 4–9 below to calculate the additional withholding amount necessary to avoid a year-end tax bill.

4 Enter the number from line 2 of this worksheet . . . . 4 ______

5 Enter the number from line 1 of this worksheet . . . . 5 ______

6 **Subtract** line 5 from line 4 . . . . 6 ______

7 Find the amount in **Table 2** below that applies to the **HIGHEST** paying job and enter it here . . . . 7 $ ______

8 **Multiply** line 7 by line 6 and enter the result here. This is the additional annual withholding needed . . 8 $ ______

9 Divide line 8 by the number of pay periods remaining in 2005. For example, divide by 26 if you are paid every two weeks and you complete this form in December 2004. Enter the result here and on Form W-4, line 6, page 1. This is the additional amount to be withheld from each paycheck . . . . 9 $ ______

Table 1: Two-Earner/Two-Job Worksheet

Married Filing Jointly

If wages from **HIGHEST** paying job are—	AND, wages from **LOWEST** paying job are—	Enter on line 2 above
$0 - $40,000	$0 - $4,000	0
	4,001 - 8,000	1
	8,001 - 18,000	2
	18,001 and over	3
$40,001 and over	$0 - $4,000	0
	4,001 - 8,000	1
	8,001 - 18,000	2
	18,001 - 22,000	3
	22,001 - 25,000	4
	25,001 - 30,000	5

If wages from **HIGHEST** paying job are—	AND, wages from **LOWEST** paying job are—	Enter on line 2 above
$40,001 and over	30,001 - 36,000	6
	36,001 - 45,000	7
	45,001 - 50,000	8
	50,001 - 60,000	9
	60,001 - 65,000	10
	65,001 - 75,000	11
	75,001 - 90,000	12
	90,001 - 100,000	13
	100,001 - 115,000	14
	115,001 and over	15

All Others

If wages from **LOWEST** paying job are—	Enter on line 2 above
$0 - $6,000	0
6,001 - 12,000	1
12,001 - 18,000	2
18,001 - 24,000	3
24,001 - 31,000	4
31,001 - 45,000	5
45,001 - 60,000	6
60,001 - 75,000	7
75,001 - 80,000	8
80,001 - 100,000	9
100,001 and over	10

Table 2: Two-Earner/Two-Job Worksheet

Married Filing Jointly		All Others	
If wages from **HIGHEST** paying job are—	Enter on line 7 above	If wages from **HIGHEST** paying job are—	Enter on line 7 above
$0 - $60,000	$480	$0 - $30,000	$480
60,001 - 110,000	800	30,001 - 70,000	800
110,001 - 160,000	900	70,001 - 140,000	900
160,001 - 280,000	1,060	140,001 - 320,000	1,060
280,001 and over	1,120	320,001 and over	1,120

Privacy Act and Paperwork Reduction Act Notice. We ask for the information on this form to carry out the Internal Revenue laws of the United States. The Internal Revenue Code requires this information under sections 3402(f)(2)(A) and 6109 and their regulations. Failure to provide a properly completed form will result in your being treated as a single person who claims no withholding allowances; providing fraudulent information may also subject you to penalties. Routine uses of this information include giving it to the Department of Justice for civil and criminal litigation, to cities, states, and the District of Columbia for use in administering their tax laws, and using it in the National Directory of New Hires. We may also disclose this information to other countries under a tax treaty, to federal and state agencies to enforce federal nontax criminal laws, or to federal law enforcement and intelligence agencies to combat terrorism.

You are not required to provide the information requested on a form that is subject to the Paperwork Reduction Act unless the form displays a valid OMB control number. Books or records relating to a form or its instructions must be retained as long as their contents may become material in the administration of any Internal Revenue law. Generally, tax returns and return information are confidential, as required by Code section 6103.

The time needed to complete this form will vary depending on individual circumstances. The estimated average time is: Recordkeeping, 45 min.; Learning about the law or the form, 12 min.; Preparing the form, 58 min. If you have comments concerning the accuracy of these time estimates or suggestions for making this form simpler, we would be happy to hear from you. You can write to: Internal Revenue Service, Tax Products Coordinating Committee, SE:W:CAR:MP:T:T:SP, 1111 Constitution Ave. NW, IR-6406, Washington, DC 20224. **Do not** send Form W-4 to this address. Instead, give it to your employer.

Figure 22-11 The Form W-4 indicates the number of exemptions claimed by the employee for income tax purposes.

a Control number		OMB No. 1545-0008	Safe, accurate, FAST! Use	IRS e-file	Visit the IRS website at www.irs.gov/efile.

b Employer identification number (EIN)	1 Wages, tips, other compensation	2 Federal income tax withheld

c Employer's name, address, and ZIP code	3 Social security wages	4 Social security tax withheld
	5 Medicare wages and tips	6 Medicare tax withheld
	7 Social security tips	8 Allocated tips

d Employee's social security number	9 Advance EIC payment	10 Dependent care benefits

e Employee's first name and initial Last name	11 Nonqualified plans	12a See instructions for box 12
	13 Statutory employee Retirement plan Third-party sick pay	12b
	14 Other	12c
		12d

f Employee's address and ZIP code				
15 State Employer's state ID number	16 State wages, tips, etc.	17 State income tax	18 Local wages, tips, etc.	19 Local income tax	20 Locality name

Form **W-2** Wage and Tax Statement **2005**   Department of the Treasury—Internal Revenue Service

Copy B—To Be Filed With Employee's FEDERAL Tax Return.
This information is being furnished to the Internal Revenue Service.

Figure 22-12   The Form W-2 summarizes all earnings and deductions for the year and must be prepared for each employee by January 31.

Security number, number of exemptions claimed on the W-4 Form, the employee's gross salary, and all deductions withheld for all taxes, including Social Security, federal, state, local, plus unemployment tax (where applicable), and disability insurance (where applicable).

To process payroll, the physician's office must have a federal tax reporting number, obtained from the Internal Revenue Service. In some states, a state employer number also is needed.

Preparing Payroll Checks. When preparing payroll checks, it is important to keep a record of all tax and insurance amounts deducted from an employee's earnings. Many ambulatory care settings that operate on a manual bookkeeping system find that the write-it-once system is the most efficient way to accurately maintain these records. Payroll records should include:

- Employee name, address, and telephone number
- Social Security number
- Date of employment

Each paycheck stub should contain:

- Number of hours worked, including regular and overtime (if hourly)
- Date of pay periods
- Date of check
- Gross salary
- Itemized deductions for federal income tax, Social Security (FICA) tax, state taxes, city or local taxes
- Itemized deductions for health insurance and disability insurance
- Other deductions such as uniforms, loan payments, and so on
- Net salary (gross earnings minus taxes and deductions)

Figuring Employee Taxes. When figuring federal income taxes and Social Security taxes, use the "Circular E" tables provided by the Internal Revenue Service.

Federal tax is based on amount earned, marital status, number of exemptions claimed, and length of pay period. State and city or local taxes are typically a percentage of the gross earnings.

All federal and state taxes withheld must be paid on a quarterly basis to the appropriate government offices. These monies should be accompanied by the required reporting forms. It is important to observe deposit requirements for withheld income tax and Social Security and Medicare taxes. These requirements, which change frequently, are listed in the Federal Employer's Tax Guide, available from the U.S. Government Printing Office, Internal Revenue Service (or online at: http://www.irs.gov).

Managing Benefits and Other Responsibilities. **Benefits,** or additional remuneration to the salary earned by full-time employees, must also be managed and records maintained for each employee. Examples of benefits may include paid vacation, paid holidays, health/dental insurance, disability, **profit-sharing** options, and complimentary health care. Some ambulatory care settings may refer to all or some of these benefits as **fringe benefits.**

Other responsibilities of the office manager include maintaining a personal file for each employee providing their history with the facility, application for their current position, evaluations, promotions, problems, awards, entitlements, legal forms required by state and federal agencies, and so on. All Occupational Safety and Health Administration (OSHA) data, hazard material training and documentation, HIPAA training documentation, cardiopulmonary resuscitation (CPR) certifications, immunization records, AIDS education, and confidential agreement must be recorded and maintained.

FACILITY AND EQUIPMENT MANAGEMENT

 The physical plant or building must be observed and maintained with safety being a key ingredient. It should be the responsibility of each staff member to report to the office manager any facility repairs that require attention and suggest replacement or recommend new pieces of equipment as required by the practice to support the health care needs of its population.

The office manager is usually responsible for the maintenance of the office and may hire **ancillary services** to provide janitorial and laundry services, dispose of hazardous materials, and maintain aquariums or plants that may enhance the environment of the facility. The office manager must be cognitive of the importance of patient confidentiality when ancillary services are present. Ancillary services must not view confidential material. A signed Business Associate agreement must be on file for each ancillary service contracted.

Magazine subscriptions and health-related literature for the reception area are the responsibility of the office manager. Selections should be made carefully, keeping in mind the interests of the patients and their cultures. These materials should not be kept once they become dog-eared, torn, and outdated. The use of plastic protectors and appropriate storage shelving aid in keeping the area and materials tidy.

The office manager, together with the physician, is also responsible for facility improvements including any necessary repairs, decorating and color scheme, and floor plan suggestions. The wise office manager does not make these decisions independently, but asks for suggestions from staff members. Remember, the team-building approach adds a cohesive element to any office environment.

Inventories

All administrative and clinical equipment in the facility must be inventoried and maintained. Documented files should be maintained for each piece of equipment. These files may be maintained in a separate reference looseleaf binder and may be divided into administrative and clinical categories. The binder may contain pocket pages in which copies of any warranties, service agreements/contracts, and instructions for use and maintenance may be placed. This binder should be accessible to anyone who may need to refer to its pages. It is also important that as new items or updated service agreements/contracts are purchased, the old ones are removed from the binder and replaced with the new items. Equipment must be routinely evaluated and recommendations for new purchases be made to keep the practice efficient.

The office manager is also responsible for overseeing the inventory and storage of controlled substances and sample medications.

Equipment and Supplies Maintenance

The office storage areas should be well maintained, and each item should always be put back in its place with lids replaced properly to prevent any accidents. Medication storage requires special attention. Many medications must be stored at certain temperatures, kept dry, or stored in dark, airtight containers. All medications, including samples, must be kept out of patient access areas. Narcotics should always be stored in a separate locked cabinet. Dispensing requires two individuals to sign off when narcotic supplies are used and maintain a daily inventory.

Laboratory equipment must be maintained and quality-control measures utilized. Calibration checks are required for a number of pieces of equipment: sphygmomanometers and centrifuges to name two. Microscopes and various types of scopes used during physical examinations and specialty procedures contain light sources that must be checked before each use. A replacement supply of bulbs should be available. Assigning a clinical laboratory manager to oversee the equipment is a good idea.

LIABILITY COVERAGE AND BONDING

 Negligence is performing an act that a reasonable and prudent physician would not perform or failure to perform an act that a reasonable and prudent physician would perform. The common term used to describe professional **liability** or legal responsibility today is **malpractice.** It is much easier to prevent malpractice than to defend it in litigation, therefore every effort should be taken to prevent negligence.

Insurance policies specifically designed to protect the physician's assets in the event a liability claim is filed and awarded in the patient's favor are available. Any physician not carrying such insurance is said to be **"going bare"** and would personally be responsible for any court costs, damages, and attorney fees if a malpractice suit were lost.

Practicing medical assistants should carry **professional liability insurance** for protection. Medical assistants who are members of the American Association of Medical Assistants (AAMA) have the option of purchasing personal and professional insurance through the organization at corporate rates.

Some physicians will carry the names of their employees on their policies. If this is the case, always ask to see the policy and verify that your name is printed on the policy—no name indicates no coverage. The manager may need to see that professional liability insurance has been purchased, all appropriate names are listed, and the premiums are paid in a timely fashion.

Professional liability insurance is important if the physician–employer is sued. In this event, the physician and the medical assistant could be named in the suit. If the case were lost, both the physician and the medical assistant could be liable.

Individuals who are responsible for handling financial records and money in the medical office may be bonded. A **bond** is purchased for a cash value in an employee's name that insures that the physician will recover the amount of loss in the event that an employee **embezzles** funds. It is the office manager or the HR manager's responsibility to ask prospective employees if they are bondable. Individuals who are not bondable may not be the best candidates for the position.

LEGAL ISSUES

The office manager must be aware of and follow all State and Federal regulations impacting the practice. Federal regulation for ambulatory/office surgical centers may be found in Chapter 19. The Centers for Medicare and Medicaid Services Web site is also helpful: http://www.cms.hhs.gov/suppliers/acs/.

Procedure 22-1 — Preparing a Meeting Agenda

PURPOSE:
To prepare a meeting agenda, a list of specific items to be discussed or acted on, to maintain the focus of the group and allow business to be transacted in a timely fashion.

EQUIPMENT/SUPPLIES:
List of participants
Order of business
Names of individuals giving reports
Names of any guest speakers
Computer and paper to print agendas

PROCEDURE STEPS:
1. Reserve proposed date, time, and place of meeting. RATIONALE: Ensure that the facilities are available for the meeting.
2. Collect information for meeting agenda by previewing the previous meeting's minutes for old business items, checking with others for report items, and determining any new business items. RATIONALE: Ensure that all old and new business items have been identified.
3. Prepare a hard copy of the agenda and have it approved by chair of the meeting. RATIONALE: Confirmation by the chair of the agenda content ensures that agenda is correct and complete.
4. Send agenda to meeting participants a few days in advance of the meeting. RATIONALE: Permits participants to prepare for the meeting by completing any tasks required and preparing any necessary documentation.

Procedure 22-2 — Supervising a Student Practicum

PURPOSE:
To prepare a training path for a student extern being assigned to the office. To make the involved office personnel aware of their responsibilities. To preplan which jobs the student extern performs and in what sequence they will be assigned. To make the externship successful by providing as much supervision and assistance as necessary.

EQUIPMENT/SUPPLIES:
None needed

PROCEDURE STEPS:
1. Review the clinical externship contract or agreement between your agency and the educational institution. RATIONALE: Guidelines and procedures are reviewed and refreshed in your mind.
2. Determine the amount of supervision the student will require. RATIONALE: Prepares you to speak with the student and site supervisor regarding supervision.
3. Identify the supervisor who will be immediately responsible for the student. RATIONALE: Establishes a person who knows he or she is to supervise the student and be responsible for the externship procedures.
4. Plan what tasks the student will be allowed or encouraged to perform. RATIONALE: The office may or may not permit the student to perform invasive procedures. Determining tasks the student can and can not perform beforehand promotes a better relationship.
5. Create a schedule outlining the time the student will be assigned to each unit. RATIONALE: Establishing a schedule keeps everyone appraised of what is happening and when.
6. Begin orientation for the student as soon as he or she arrives at the office. Include a tour of the office and introduction to the staff. RATIONALE: Orients student and staff to each other and establishes guidelines for procedures.

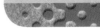

(continues)

Procedure 22-2 (continued)

7. Give the student a copy of the Office Policy Manual and the work schedule for the entire externship. Answer any questions the student might have. RATIONALE: Orients student and staff to each other and establishes guidelines for procedures.

8. Maintain an accurate record of the hours the student works. Also log the date and reason for any missed days, late arrivals, or early dismissals. RATIONALE: Provides necessary documentation for the hours completed by the student.

9. Check with the student frequently to be sure the student is receiving meaningful training from the work experience. RATIONALE: Verifies that necessary training is being provided.

10. Consult physicians and staff members with whom the student has worked for their opinion of the student's capabilities. Follow up on any problems that might be identified. RATIONALE: Verifies that necessary training is being provided.

11. Report the student's progress to the medical assisting supervisor from the educational institution. This person usually visits once or twice each rotation. RATIONALE: Verifies that necessary training is being provided.

12. Prepare the student an evaluation report from comments provided by the supervisor assigned and each employee who worked with the student. RATIONALE: Provides necessary documentation for the externship experience.

Procedure 22-3 Making Travel Arrangements

PURPOSE:
To make travel arrangements for the physician.

EQUIPMENT/SUPPLIES:
Travel plan
Telephone and telephone directory
Computer
Physician's or office credit card to pay for reservations

PROCEDURE STEPS:
1. Confirm the details of the planned trip: dates, time, and place for departure and arrival; preferred mode of transportation (plane, train, bus, car); number of travelers; preferred lodging type and price range; and whether travelers checks are required. RATIONALE: Confirming pertinent travel details ensures that correct arrangements will be made.

2. Make travel and lodging reservations by calling travel agent or using the computer for online ticket services. RATIONALE: Ensure that space for physician is reserved at desired times.

3. Pick up tickets or arrange for their delivery.

4. Check to see that ticket arrangements are accurate (dates, times, places).

5. Check to see that car rental and lodging accommodations are accurate and confirmed. RATIONALE: Avoid inaccuracies and confusion with schedule.

6. Make additional copies of the itinerary or create the itinerary if making arrangements via computer. The itinerary should list date and time of departures and arrivals, including flight numbers and seat assignments. Note mode of transportation to lodging (shuttle, bus, car, taxi). Include name, address, and telephone number of lodgings and meeting places.

7. Maintain one copy of the itinerary in the office file.

8. Give several copies of the itinerary to the physician. RATIONALE: Ensure that a copy is on file with the office and that there are sufficient copies for the traveler(s) and their families.

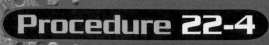

Procedure 22-4 — Making Travel Arrangements via the Internet

PURPOSE:
To make travel arrangements for the physician using the Internet.

EQUIPMENT/SUPPLIES:
Travel plan
Computer
Physician's or office credit card to pay for reservations.

PROCEDURE STEPS:
1. Confirm the details of the planned trip: dates, time, and place for departure and arrival; preferred mode of transportation (plane, train, bus, car); number of travelers; preferred lodging type and price range; and whether travelers checks are required. RATIONALE: Confirming pertinent travel details ensures that correct arrangements will be made.
2. Go to the computer and access the Internet.
3. Select a search engine to locate Web pages using the key term "air fares." Web pages may provide links to air fares, auto reservations, and hotel/motel reservations. Follow Web page instructions for making arrangements. Review and copy confirmation of your transaction. RATIONALE: The Internet can be a time saver and a cost-effective way of securing travel arrangements.
4. Pick up tickets or arrange for their delivery, if necessary. Tickets purchased on the Internet may be mailed or picked up at an airport, or they may be electronic tickets.
5. Make additional copies of the itinerary or create the itinerary. The itinerary should list date and time of departures and arrivals, including flight numbers and seat assignments. Note the mode of transportation to lodging (shuttle, bus, car, taxi). Include name, address, and telephone number of lodgings and meeting places.
6. Maintain one copy of the itinerary in the office file.
7. Give several copies of the itinerary to the physician. RATIONALE: Ensure that a copy is on file with the office and that there are sufficient copies for the traveler(s) and their families.

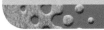

Procedure 22-5 — Developing and Maintaining a Procedure Manual

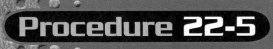

PURPOSE:
To develop and maintain a comprehensive, up-to-date procedure manual covering each medical, technical, and administrative procedure in the office, with step-by-step directions and rationale for performing each task.

EQUIPMENT/SUPPLIES:
Computer or electronic typewriter (electronic storage allows changes and revisions to be made easily)
Binder, such as a three-ring binder
Paper
Standard procedure manual format

PROCEDURE STEPS:
1. Write detailed, step-by-step procedures and rationales for each medical, technical, and administrative function. Each procedure is written by experienced employees close to the function and then reviewed by a supervisor and office manager. Rationales help employees understand *why* something is done. RATIONALE: Establishes consistent guidelines to be followed.
2. Include regular maintenance instructions and a flow sheets for cleaning, servicing, and calibrating of all office equipment, both in the clinical

(continues)

Procedure 22-5 (continued)

area and in the office/business areas. RATIO-NALE: Equipment will need to be cleaned and maintained on a regular basis to assure it is working properly and that it lasts as long as needed. Some manufacturer guarantees and service contracts require regular cleaning and maintenance, especially on new and leased equipment. Instructions are necessary so the task can be performed properly. The flow sheets provide documentation of dates the equipment was cleaned, serviced, and/or calibrated and the person who performed the task.

3. Include step-by-step instruction on how to accomplish each task in the office/clinic in both the clinical area and in the office/business areas. RATIONALE: Clear and concise instructions assure that each task is consistently performed to the clinic standards.

4. Include local and out-of-the-area resources for clinical staff, office/business staff, physicians/providers, and patients. Provide a listing in each area with contact information and services provided. RATIONALE: The procedures and instructions listed in the Procedure Manual should provide supporting documentation needed for accomplishing each task. An example would be if the clinic requires that local public transportation resources be given to each patient who needs transportation, the Procedure Manual would have a listing of all transportation available in the area with numbers and schedules. This document could either be printed from the computer or photocopied from the Manual and provided to the patient.

5. Include basic rules and regulations, state and federal, which are related to processes performed in both clinical and office/business areas. RATIONALE: Having a listing of the rules and regulations will assist in performing those regulated duties correctly and legally.

6. Include the clinic procedures and flow sheets for taking inventory in each of the areas and instructions on ordering procedures. RATIONALE: When a clinic has processes clearly written for managing inventory and ordering of equipment and supplies, the clinic is less likely to run out of needed items and may even be able to take advantage of discounts offered by the manufacturers.

7. Collect the procedures into the Office Procedure Manual. RATIONALE: Provides a reference guide with step-by-step instruction and examples where appropriate.

8. Store one complete manual in a common library area. Provide a completed copy to the physician–employer and the office manager. Distribute appropriate sections to the various departments. RATIONALE: Provides a reference guide with step-by-step instruction and examples where appropriate.

9. Review the procedure manual annually and add any new procedures, delete or modify as necessary, and indicate the revision date (Rev. 10/12/XX). RATIONALE: Maintains current office protocols.

Case Study 22-1

Drs. Lewis and King have requested sigmoidoscopy procedures to be scheduled for two different patients. The patients are scheduled. Both patients are put on a strict diet and pretest protocol for several days to prepare for the procedures. The day of the appointments, it is discovered that the two sigmoidoscopy procedures have been scheduled at the same time. The problem is that the office has only one sigmoidoscope available.

CASE STUDY REVIEW

1. Divide the class into two groups to discuss problem-solving solutions. Assume that rescheduling a patient is not an acceptable solution because of the patient's pretest protocol. The patients would be upset if the procedure could not be performed due to a scheduling problem.

2. How could this problem have been avoided?

3. Both patients have been told about the scheduling problem and one is upset and argumentative. What role should the office manager assume in this predicament?

Case Study 22-2

Anita Juarez, the office receptionist, speaks privately with Jane O'Hara, the office manager and the person responsible for personnel. Anita has a suspicious lump in her breast. She has seen both her internist and a surgeon for evaluation. Next week, she will have the lump removed, perhaps even a complete mastectomy. Anita is concerned about the time she will need to be away from the office.

CASE STUDY REVIEW

1. Identify the first and immediate concerns to be addressed.

2. What action might be taken to help both Anita and the office manager address these concerns?

3. Is it helpful to plan for the best results, the worst results, or both?

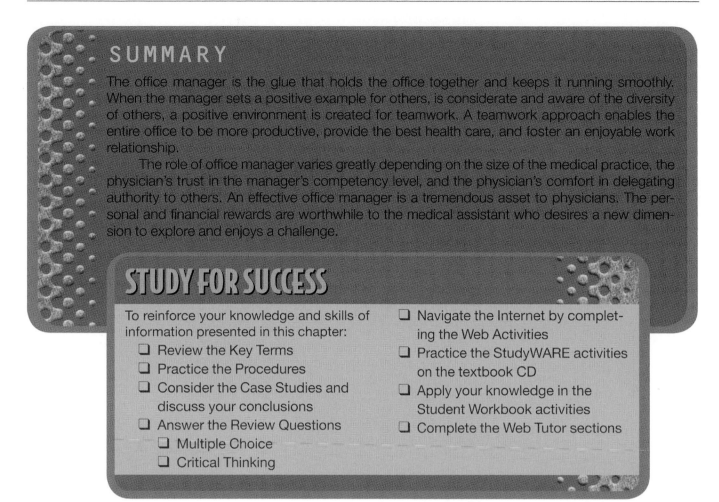

SUMMARY

The office manager is the glue that holds the office together and keeps it running smoothly. When the manager sets a positive example for others, is considerate and aware of the diversity of others, a positive environment is created for teamwork. A teamwork approach enables the entire office to be more productive, provide the best health care, and foster an enjoyable work relationship.

The role of office manager varies greatly depending on the size of the medical practice, the physician's trust in the manager's competency level, and the physician's comfort in delegating authority to others. An effective office manager is a tremendous asset to physicians. The personal and financial rewards are worthwhile to the medical assistant who desires a new dimension to explore and enjoys a challenge.

STUDY FOR SUCCESS

To reinforce your knowledge and skills of information presented in this chapter:
- ❏ Review the Key Terms
- ❏ Practice the Procedures
- ❏ Consider the Case Studies and discuss your conclusions
- ❏ Answer the Review Questions
  - ❏ Multiple Choice
  - ❏ Critical Thinking

- ❏ Navigate the Internet by completing the Web Activities
- ❏ Practice the StudyWARE activities on the textbook CD
- ❏ Apply your knowledge in the Student Workbook activities
- ❏ Complete the Web Tutor sections

REVIEW QUESTIONS

Multiple Choice

1. For teamwork to be successful, individual team members must:
   a. do as they are told by the office manager
   b. not ask why they are doing something a certain way
   c. understand and support the task
   d. think independently and solve the problem on their own

2. Meeting minutes:
   a. should address each agenda topic and include a brief summary of discussions, actions taken, name of each person making a motion, the exact wording of motions, and motion approval or defeat
   b. are a detailed plan for a proposed trip
   c. include information regarding mode of transportation and lodging reservations
   d. must follow parliamentary procedures

3. When working with externship students, it is important to remember that:
   a. they should have expert knowledge about their field
   b. they do not need supervision when working with a patient
   c. they are experienced with working on real patients
   d. they have much to learn

4. Which of the following statements is *not* correct regarding a student practicum?
   a. It is a transitional stage that provides opportunity for students to apply theory learned in the classroom to a health care setting through hands-on experience.
   b. It assumes that the student is an employee who does not need to be introduced to patients.
   c. It may require the student to shadow another medical assistant for a few days.
   d. It involves an evaluation of the student's progress.

5. The procedure manual:
   a. is a detailed plan for a proposed trip
   b. provides detailed information regarding mode of transportation and lodging reservations
   c. provides detailed information relative to the performance of tasks within the health care facility
   d. summarizes action details of staff meetings
6. Developing relationships outside the office is often called:
   a. marketing
   b. benchmarking
   c. advertising
   d. sales
7. Record and financial management involves all of the following *except*:
   a. payroll processing
   b. preparing payroll checks
   c. figuring taxes
   d. equipment and supplies maintenance
8. Controlled substances must:
   a. be kept separate from other drugs
   b. be stored in a double locked cabinet
   c. be recorded in a book that is maintained daily
   d. all of the above

Critical Thinking

1. How would you, as the office manager, handle someone who is spreading a harmful rumor about another employee in the office?
2. How can the office manager promote open and honest communication?
3. The student practicum can be a stressful time for the extern. As an office manager, how can you help the extern feel more at ease the first day of "work"?
4. Describe how a procedure manual for a single-physician practice would differ from a procedure manual for a multiphysician practice.
5. Describe how a procedure manual could become outdated and need revision.

Use the Web sites described in the text, or alternative sites you know about, to plan a trip between two cities within the United States. Compare the fares for Sunday departure and Friday return dates with the fares for low volume days as obtained from the Priceline.com site. Also compare fares on flights purchased within one week of departure with fares on flights purchased a month before departure. Follow the instructor's instructions on completing and turning in your results.

REFERENCES/BIBLIOGRAPHY

Colbert, B. J. (2000). *Workplace readiness for health occupations.* Clifton Park, NY: Thomson Delmar Learning.

ingenix. (2003, December). HIPAA Tool Kit. Salt Lake City, UT: St. Anthony Publishing/Medicode.

Institute for Management Excellence (2004, June). *Linking personality with management style.* Retrieved from http://itstime.com/jun98.htm. Accessed May 16, 2005.

Krager, D., & Krager, C. (2005). *HIPAA for Medical Office Personnel.* Clifton Park, NY: Thomson Delmar Learning.

Pyzdek, T. (2004). *Management styles: Participatory management style.* Retrieved from http://www.qualityamerica.com/knowledgecente/articles/CQMStyle2.html. Accessed May 16, 2005.

CHAPTER 23

The Medical Assistant as Human Resources Manager

OBJECTIVES

The student should strive to meet the following performance objectives and demonstrate an understanding of the facts and principles presented in this chapter through written and oral communication.

1. Define the key terms as presented in the glossary.
2. Describe the role of the human resources manager.
3. Explain the function of the office policy manual.
4. Identify methods of recruiting employees for a medical practice.
5. Discuss the interview process.
6. Identify items to keep in an employee's personnel record.
7. List and define a minimum of four laws related to personnel management.

SCENARIO

Jane O'Hara, CMA, is the officer manager at Inner City Health Care. She also functions in the role of the human resources manager. Part of her responsibilities includes recruiting, hiring, and orienting employees.

In one day Jane may meet with Dr. Rice to update the policy manual; begin the hiring process for a new medical assistant; welcome a new physician to the practice, being sure she completes all of the necessary employment forms; and meet with another staff member to evaluate her continuing education.

INTRODUCTION

The medical assistant's employment responsibilities are many and varied. As you learned in Chapter 22, often they become office managers and assume a quite different function in the medical setting. The size of the ambulatory care setting and the number of employees likely determines if a human resources (HR) manager is a part of the practice. Whether the HR manager heads an HR department in a large, corporate medical setting with the title Human Resources Manager or is a medical assistant/office manager who serves as the HR representative, there are some common tasks assigned as specific HR duties.

TASKS PERFORMED BY THE HUMAN RESOURCES MANAGER

Tasks usually assigned to the HR manager include determining job descriptions, hiring, and orienting employees, and maintaining employee personnel records that include credentials and continuing education units (CEUs). With today's quest for greater office efficiency and the tremendous increase in federal and state regulatory requirements, the skills required of an HR manager have greatly broadened. Former responsibilities have been expanded to include preparing the policy manual, scheduling employee evaluations, preventing and investigating discrimination and harassment claims, and complying with regulatory agencies. The HR manager also assists in providing training and educational opportunities for employees so they are up to date in all aspects of quality patient care.

Increasingly, HR managers are expected to be able to support the organization's efforts that focus on productivity, service, and quality. In a climate in which there are too few persons for the positions to be filled, and the delivery methods for health care are changing almost daily, productivity, service, and quality are essential to a successful practice. It becomes the responsibility of the HR manager to see that every employee's productivity level is high, that the service is A+, and that quality is at the highest level. Today's customers, the patients, often choose their health care provider on the basis of service and quality.

 The position of HR manager now requires a higher level of education and experience to better grasp the legal and regulatory aspects of personnel management. The HR manager also must have excellent people skills, a strong sense of fairness, and the ability to resolve conflicts. None of this is accomplished in a vacuum. It requires working in close cooperation with the office manager and the physician–employer(s).

This chapter discusses these responsibilities in the following separate but overlapping functions:

1. Creating and updating the office policy manual
2. Recruiting and hiring office personnel
3. Orienting new personnel
4. Scheduling salary reviews
5. Conducting exit interviews
6. Maintaining personnel records
7. Complying with all state and federal regulations regarding personnel
8. Planning/providing employee training and education
9. Maintaining records of credentials, CEUs, and certificates such as cardiopulmonary resuscitation (CPR)

THE OFFICE POLICY MANUAL

The procedure manual described in Chapter 22 identifies specific methods of performing tasks. The policy manual provides more general guidelines for office practices.

Possible Content of Policy and Procedure Manual	
Policy Manual	**Procedure Manual**
General practices and policies of an office	Daily guide; step-by-step instructions for procedures

The policy manual will identify clear guidelines and directions required of all employees, as well as define appropriate expectations and boundaries of the employment relationship. Having written policies means not having to determine a policy on a case-by-case basis. Policy manuals will vary by the size of the practice or problems to be addressed, but some topics include the mission statement of the practice, biographic data on each physician, employment policies, wage and salary policies, benefits to be awarded, and employee conduct expectations.

Establishing and stating the mission of the practice clearly identifies for employees the goals and objectives to be sought by each employee. Having biographic data of each physician helps employees to respond to queries from patients about a physician's experience, education, and interests.

Employment policies might include statements on equal employment opportunity, job requirements for particular positions and to whom the person reports, recruitment and selection procedures, orientation of new employees, probation, and dismissal. Wage and salary policies should be in writing. How are employees classified, what are the working hours, how is overtime compensated, how are salary increases determined, what benefits (medical, retirement, vacation, holidays, sick leave, profit sharing) does the practice have? The answers to such questions are part of the policy manual. Employee conduct is another piece of the policy manual. Guidelines should be established about uniforms, dress codes, appearance, and personal hygiene. Can an employee hold a second job outside the practice? Is smoking allowed? Are staff members responsible for housekeeping duties? A statement regarding the confidentiality of all information received in the practice is essential in this area of the policy manual.

Having a policy manual with clearly written directives helps employees understand the expectations and boundaries of the employment relationship. The policy manual should be reviewed with each new employee and updated on a regular basis. See Procedure 23-1 for details on developing and maintaining a policy manual.

RECRUITING AND HIRING OFFICE PERSONNEL

Before recruiting and hiring personnel to fill positions within the medical office, the HR manager and physician–employer must know exactly what the role and responsibilities of the position are by having a current job description for the position and following a recruiting policy that is effective, fair, and observes all appropriate laws and regulations.

Job Descriptions

Before any position is filled, a **job description** must be in place. This usually is created cooperatively by the office manager and the physician–employer. Once the job qualifications are defined, the lead personnel and HR manager can begin efforts to fill the position.

In daily operations most job descriptions are on file, but if the situation involves a new or greatly expanded office, a complete set of job descriptions is needed before recruiting can begin. Even when a written description is on file, it should be reviewed when a new employee is to be hired. The person who is leaving the position is often an excellent resource for the accuracy of the current job description and any changes that should be made.

The job description must include basic qualifications for the position and have enough information to provide both the supervisor and the employee with a clear outline of what the job entails (Figure 23-1). Necessary work experience, skills, education, and any special

---

JOB DESCRIPTION

POSITION TITLE:
Administrative Medical Assistant

REPORTS TO:
Office Manager and Physician–Employer

RESPONSIBILITIES AND DUTIES:
- Being a therapeutic and helpful receptionist
  1. Answer telephone as quickly as possible, hopefully by the second ring
  2. Greet all patients warmly and with a helpful attitude
- Efficiently managing time with appropriate scheduling for patients and professional staff
  1. Schedule patients according to their needs, office scheduling guidelines, staff availability, and equipment readiness
  2. Call to remind patients of their visit the day before appointment
- Responding to patient requests on the telephone and in person
  1. Ascertain reason for request
  2. Satisfy patient request or refer patient to one who can
- Preparing patient charts for professional staff
  1. Print out schedules and encounter forms
  2. Pull patient charts late afternoon on the day before appointment
  3. Check charts for completeness
  4. Attach encounter form when patient arrives to check in

AUTHORITY BOUNDARIES:
The office manager will assist in answering questions. Remember that it is better to ask than to make an error. Triage concerns not identified in a policy/procedure manual also can be directed to the clinical medical assisting staff.

POSITION REQUIREMENTS:
Two years experience and/or graduate of a medical assistant program. CMA, RMA, or CMAS preferred.

Figure 23-1 Sample job description for administrative medical assistant.

certification or licensure that is expected is to be identified in the job description. See Procedure 23-2 for details on preparing job descriptions.

Another important point with respect to the job description is that a review and update of the description should be done every year. Most jobs change constantly whether from a minor shifting of duties or the addition of some new technical procedure or device. Without updating a job description, a person with the wrong qualifications may be recruited to fill a vacancy.

Recruiting

A major challenge facing the HR manager today is recruitment. Medical assistants are listed in the top 10 occupations with the fastest employment growth through 2012 according to the U.S. Department of Labor, Bureau of Labor Statistics. One reason for this demand is the aging of the U.S. population. It is estimated that more than 80% of jobs are in the service industry, and all health care positions fit into that category. When physician–employers have been unsuccessful in recruiting qualified medical assistants, they have turned to contracting out some work, such as transcription and billing.

Once the hiring need is determined, the HR manager begins the recruitment process. Often a process called networking is a highly effective method of finding employees. **Networking** is a process in which people of similar interests exchange information in social, business, or professional relationships. For instance, the HR manager may network with members of the American Association of Medical Assistants and express an interest in a new employee for a position that is open. Current employees are often an excellent resource because they may know of a qualified person who is looking for a position.

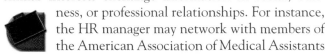

Checking with nearby colleges' medical assistant departments is another good resource. Employing a private or state placement agency is another possibility. Although newspaper advertisements may generate many résumés, they are only marginally effective as a search tool. It is often far too time consuming to review the large volume of applications generated by this approach. Online options may be beneficial. There are a number of medical Web sites that identify positions for medical assistant personnel, often in specific localities.

Preparing to Interview Applicants

Once several applicants have expressed interest in the position, preparation for the interview begins. The HR manager should have a number of résumés to consider. Some may have already filled out a job application when they dropped off a résumé. The résumés and applications can be reviewed together. Some important points to remember in reading résumés and applications follow.

When considering education, look beyond the degree earned. Look for a good performance record at school and the kinds of supplemental education achieved. Does attendance at seminars and short-course training programs relate to your position needs? When reading a person's work history, make note of unexplained gaps in employment. You may want to ask specific questions in the interview. Has advancement been gained in each new position? Are the responsibilities and duties of the applicant's positions explained, or will questions need to be asked of the prospective employee?

Look for information that indicates if this candidate really enjoys the kind of work setting you have. Is the applicant comfortable serving the infirm? Can you truly identify the level of skill from the descriptions, or are the skills vague? The cover letter, if one is included, should address the specifics required of your position. Does the person display a negative or a positive attitude? Do not excuse any errors or unprofessional appearance in the job application or the résumé. Each should be letter perfect. An individual who is careless in this respect is likely to be careless on the job.

Some applications will be discarded after using the preceding guidelines. With the remaining candidates, determine who is to be interviewed and make telephone calls to establish interviews. You may make note of the quality of speaking skills, especially if this person will be using the telephone on the job. Make an interview appointment date with only those who seem truly interested in the position during your telephone conversation.

The Interview

The interview is usually conducted by only one person if second interviews are anticipated. The physician–employer, office manager, or another employee may be present in either the first or the second interview, however (Figure 23-2). The interviewer(s) will want to review the application and résumé before the interview for particular points to ask the candidate. Before the interview, those doing the interviews should establish a set of questions for the applicants. These predetermined questions will help alleviate one applicant being given privileges over another and will help assure continuity throughout

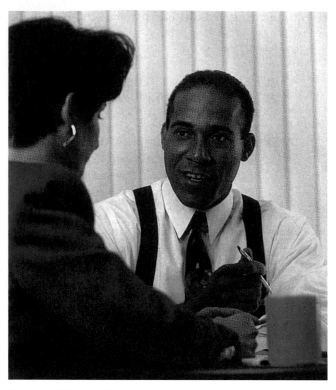

Figure 23-2 The interview can be conducted on a one-to-one basis with only the applicant and one staff member or with several staff members meeting with the applicant at once.

General Questions
- What are your strengths and weaknesses?
- Why did you leave your last job?
- Identify what is most important to you in a job.

Questions Related to Work Relationships
- Describe an individual you have enjoyed working with.
- Explain how a conflict with a coworker was resolved.
- How would a coworker describe you?

Questions Related to Problem Solving
- Describe a work-related decision that made you very proud.
- Identify a task/procedure/assignment you could not do, and explain why.
- How do you approach a task when it seems mundane or boring?

Questions Related to Integrity
- If asked to do something illegal or unethical, what would you do?
- Tell us about a time when you broke a confidence.
- If you saw a coworker put a patient at risk, what would you do?

Figure 23-3 Common interview questions.

---

all the interviews. An interview worksheet is an excellent tool to use to make certain that you are fair and equitable with each candidate. The worksheet should provide enough room for notes taken during the interview.

Suggested items for the interview worksheet are:

- Applicant's name
- Telephone number
- Education and training
- Work experience
- Special skills
- Professional demeanor
- Voice and mannerisms specific to position
- Questions and responses
- Ability to problem solve when given a scenario
- Any health-related or work-related problems applicant discloses
- Interviewer's personal impressions and recommendations

Conduct interviews in a quiet and private setting. Do not schedule interviews back to back without time to collect your thoughts or to allow you to compare notes with others participating in the interview. Ask job-related questions. For example, Describe your last job. What did you like best about it? What did you like least? What is most important to you about a job? Describe your administrative and clinical skills. Figure 23-3 shows some sample questions. Let the applicant do the most of the talking.

 Any questions related to age, sex, race, religion, or national origin are inappropriate. Inquiries about medical history, drug use, or arrest records may not be made. Keep your questions related to performance on the job. If you may want to bond this employee, you may ask candidates if they have been bonded before or are willing to be bonded. It may be best to leave salary discussions for a second interview, but it can also be helpful to determine if applicants' salary expectations are in line with what you can offer. A question such as What salary are you expecting? is appropriate. Do not make a job offer until all the candidates selected for interview have been interviewed, and do not prejudge someone on any factor during or after the interview, except the person's qualifications.

At the close of the interview, let the applicant know when a decision will be made or whether a second interview will be conducted and how notification will be made. A tour of the facility and introduction to key staff members may be offered but are not necessary at the time of the first interview. Finally, thank the applicant for participating in the interview and being interested in the position.

Selecting the Finalists

Shortly after the final interview is completed, the HR manager should compare notes with all the others involved in the interview to select the top candidates. This is done by comparing notes and impressions from the interviews and by taking into consideration the ability of a candidate to work with patients and colleagues who might have a variety of problems and cultural backgrounds. The next step is to check references from former employers, supervisors, coworkers, and instructors. A large corporate medical practice may even have a consent form each candidate is asked to sign that gives permission to check references and call former employers and instructors. You may need to recognize, however, that even with a release from a potential new employee, many organizations and businesses restrict the release of reference information to only name, dates of employment, and title of position served. Telephone checks for references are an excellent strategy before you receive an immediate response. If you stress confidentiality when you make the contact, it will be easier for the person to respond to your questions. Always check with more than one reference and former employer to get an accurate assessment of the candidate. All reference information is to be kept confidential. A sample telephone reference check form is shown in Figure 23-4.

A checklist of questions to ask might include:

1. What were the dates of employment of (name of applicant) in your firm?
2. Describe the job performed.
3. Reason for leaving the job?
4. Strong points of the employee?
5. Limitations of the employee?
6. Can you comment on attendance and dependability?
7. Would you rehire?
8. Anything else we should know about this candidate?

Offer the position when a first-choice candidate has been determined and indicate when a response is needed. Be prepared with a second-choice candidate should the preferred candidate respond negatively. At the time of

TELEPHONE REFERENCE

Name of Applicant _____

Person Contacted _____

Position and Name of Business _____

_____

Telephone Number _____

Relationship to Applicant _____

- May I verify the employment history of (applicant's name) who is applying for a position with our medical clinic?

  _____, 20____ to _____, 20____

- Describe the responsibilities held by this individual.

- Identify the salary _____

- What are this individual's strong points?

- What are this individual's weak points?

- Describe this individual's overall attitude toward the job and toward patients.

- Please comment on dependability and attendance.

- Given the opportunity, would you rehire? Why or why not?

- Why did this individual leave the job?

- Describe personal and professional growth this individual made while in your firm.

- Is there anything else you would like to tell us?

Reference call made by _____

Date _____

Figure 23-4 Sample form to use for telephone references.

the offer, the candidate should understand the salary offered, the starting date, the practice policies, and the benefits. When a candidate has accepted the position, a confirmation letter should be written that clearly spells out details discussed earlier. Give specific instructions on when and where the new employee should report the first day on the job. If practical, the employee should be given the policy and procedure manuals to read.

For the unsuccessful applicants, send a letter explaining that "we have selected another candidate whose qualifications and experience more closely meets our needs at this time. We would like to keep your résumé on file should another suitable position become available." Copies of these letters, as well as the interview checklists, should be kept for a minimum of six months should any questions arise regarding your choice of candidates. See Procedure 23-3 for details on interviewing.

ORIENTING NEW PERSONNEL

Orienting new employees is usually the responsibility of both the office manager and lead personnel who are most likely to work the closest with the new employee. It is common for a new employee to be placed on **probation** for 60 to 90 days during which time both the employee and supervisory personnel may determine if the environment and the position are satisfactory for the employee. Procedure 23-4 outlines how to orient personnel.

Important elements to orientation include the introduction of the new employee to other staff members, assigning a mentor who can respond to questions, and making the employee aware of the procedures to be performed in this new position. If the procedure manual is detailed and accurate, this manual now becomes the daily guide for the new employee. Sometimes the individual leaving a position may still be present and is asked to assist in the orientation process. This is especially beneficial if there is a good working relationship between the employee who is leaving and the management of the practice. Depending on the responsibilities of the new employee, a supervisor may be asked to monitor all procedures for a period for accuracy, safety, and patient protection. During the probation period, the employee should be officially evaluated by the office manager.

DISMISSING EMPLOYEES

The function of employee dismissal falls mostly to the office manager; however, in a large facility with an HR representative, discussing dismissal with that individual can be quite beneficial. Such a discussion assures that all the information necessary is in place before a dismissal. There are voluntary and involuntary dismissals.

Voluntary dismissals usually occur when an employee is relocating, advancing to another position elsewhere, retiring, or leaving for personal reasons. A letter of resignation is usually submitted to both the office manager and the HR representative. These employees will give their manager proper notice and may be able to turn current projects and duties over to their replacement. There is also time to say good-bye to their colleagues and have a good feeling about their employment.

Involuntary dismissals usually occur when an employee's performance is poor or there has been a serious violation of the office policies or job description. The office manager is aware of poor performance through the probationary reviews. Verbal and written warnings must be given to the employee and be well documented. Dismissal can be immediate if there is a serious breach of office policy. The HR director can provide necessary detail to the office manager regarding when and if immediate dismissal is recommended. If an office manager expects any serious difficulties with an employee during an immediate dismissal, the HR director should be present when the employee is notified. See Chapter 22 for a more detailed discussion.

Exit Interview

An **exit interview** is an excellent opportunity for the employee who voluntarily leaves a practice and the HR manager to discuss the positive and negative aspects of the job and what changes might be made for a new person coming into the facility. A sample exit interview form is shown in Figure 23-5. It also allows the opportunity for the employee to ask for a **letter of reference** or to view the personnel file before leaving. In a voluntary dismissal, a **letter of resignation** for the personnel file is necessary.

Any dismissal process, voluntary or involuntary, must include a statement in the personnel file. For involuntary dismissal, be certain that the reasons for the dismissal are well documented in an honest, nonjudgmental statement. State only the facts in the personnel file; do not state opinion. Remember that employees have the right to view their personnel file at any time.

The physician–employer should always be informed of any dismissal as quickly as possible. Some may be involved in the actual dismissal process.

MAINTAINING PERSONNEL RECORDS

An important aspect of the responsibilities of the HR manager is maintaining personnel records. All documentation and correspondence related to each employee from 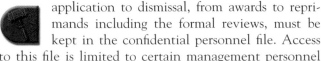 application to dismissal, from awards to reprimands including the formal reviews, must be kept in the confidential personnel file. Access to this file is limited to certain management personnel and the employee. Not all of these people are allowed to

---

EXIT INTERVIEW FORM

1. What did you like and dislike about the work you have been doing?

    (Including: support on the job; opportunity for personal growth; recognition and rewards)

2. What kind of people have you found the doctors, your immediate supervisor, and co-workers to be?

    (Including: attitude; fairness; scheduling and assignment of work; work expectations; technical competence; assistance and guidance available; team spirit)

3. What is your view of our management practices and policies?

    (Including: clarity and fairness of practice policies; communications; management and staff)

4. How have you felt about performance appraisals, your salary and benefits?

    (Including: adequacy of salary; regularity and fairness of appraisals)

5. What are your principal reasons for leaving the practice?

    (Including: primary dissatisfactions; job or personal changes)

6. In what areas do you feel we need to improve?

Interviewer signature: _____ Date _____

Employee signature: _____ Date _____

Figure 23-5 Sample exit interview form. (From *Personnel Management Handbook,* 2nd ed., by Maryann Ricardo, The McGraw-Hill Companies, Inc. Copyright 1992. Reprinted with permission.)

see the entire file. These files are usually kept for a period of three to five years after employees leave the practice.

This file also includes the kind of information normally maintained for payroll and business practices. That information includes name, address, and sex of employee. The position title, date of beginning employment, rate of pay (hourly or otherwise), total overtime pay, deductions or additions to wages, wages paid each pay period, and date employee leaves the practice also are included.

COMPLYING WITH PERSONNEL LAWS

This text is not meant to be a legal guide for an HR manager. The practice attorney should always be contacted if there is any question regarding personnel laws, which may vary in some states depending on the size of the practice. Only a brief introduction of the laws related to the ambulatory care setting are given.

Overtime must be addressed in each practice. Who is reimbursed for overtime and how is that reimbursement determined? Typically, medical receptionists and secretaries, insurance billers, medical transcriptionists, and medical assistants are likely to be paid overtime. Overtime pay at a rate of not less than one and one-half times the regular rate of pay after a 40-hour work week is standard. Each week stands alone and one week cannot compensate for another. If the practice does not want to be involved in overtime situations, require that any overtime be preauthorized in advance.

The Equal Pay Act of 1963 prevents wage discrimination for jobs that require equal skill, effort, and responsibility. The Civil Rights Act of 1964 prevents employers from discriminating against individuals on the basis of race, color, religion, sex, age, or national origin.

Sexual harassment violates Title VII of the Civil Rights Act. Steps must be taken to ensure that all employees are working in an atmosphere that is not hostile, where sexual gestures, the presence of pornographic or offensive materials, or obscene language are not allowed.

Employees have a right to expect safe working conditions. The Occupational Safety and Health Act (OSHA) was established to prevent injuries and illnesses resulting from unsafe or unhealthy working conditions. Compliance with this law requires that each employee be aware of possible risks associated with chemical hazards and how to protect themselves. Because there are many of these hazards in a medical practice, compliance and protection for employees are extremely important, and training sessions should be held in this area.

The Immigration Reform Act requires employers to verify the right of employees to work in the United States. Documentation acceptable for verification is a Social Security card or birth certificate. The U.S. Department of Justice Immigration and Naturalization Service will provide instructions and a form for employees and employers to complete, commonly referred to as the I-9 or Employment Eligibility Verification form.

Employers cannot discriminate or condemn any full-time employee for jury duty. Although the employer does not have to continue pay during jury duty, the employee cannot lose seniority, insurance, or other benefits. Many employers continue an employee's full pay during the time of service on a jury because the reimbursement for jury service is so small. This is a way to benefit your employees and encourage good citizenship.

This list is by no means comprehensive but does include personnel regulations most likely to affect the medical practice. Any concerns should be directed to the practice's attorney.

SPECIAL POLICY CONSIDERATIONS

There are several other managerial issues that may arise in a medical setting for which the office manager and the HR manager will have to plan. These can include policies for temporary employees, smoking, avoiding discrimination, and having a support system in place for employees who need physical or emotional help.

Temporary Employees

Temporary employees who may be employed for 90 days or less include students who are serving an internship or externship from a local college practicing their skills for when they will be on the job. They should be reviewed on a regular basis in cooperation with their college supervisor. Give them as much actual hands-on experience as possible; they are your future employees. Accommodating students in the practice is a two-way benefit. Students learn what reality is in the ambulatory care setting and are able to practice newly developed skills. Current staff members in the facility are "sharpened" by the students' presence. Teaching and monitoring someone's actions always results in sharpening and rethinking the skills of the current staff. Many HR directors and managers depend on these programs for future job applicants.

Smoking Policy

Smoking on the premises has become a greater concern in the last decade or so. Many places of employment do not allow smoking at all. Some states and cities have laws that may govern this issue for you. When a policy is established, it should cover everyone—employers, employees, and patients. The objective is to have a policy that is workable and enforceable, promotes health, encourages employee morale and productivity, and sets examples for patients. A designated place for smoking may be considered.

Discrimination

The Americans with Disabilities Act (ADA) prohibits discrimination by all private employers with 15 or more employees. Some states may further prohibit discrimination in facilities regardless of the size of their workforce. *All* public entities are prohibited from discrimination against qualified individuals with disabilities. The ADA establishes guidelines prohibiting discrimination against a "qualified individual with a disability" in regard to employment. Someone with a disability who satisfies the skills necessary for the job; has the experience, education, and any other job requirements; and who, with reasonable accommodation, can perform the job cannot be discriminated against. Employers often find that persons with disabilities are their finest employees.

Persons who are HIV-positive or have AIDS are included in the guidelines set forth by the ADA. Persons with HIV/AIDS cannot be discriminated against. It can be assumed that if you are providing a safe working environment and all employees follow the rules for Standard Precautions then reasonable accommodation has been made for the person with HIV or AIDS.

An employer cannot refuse the job to a qualified person on the belief that in the future the employee may become too ill to work. The hiring decision must be based on the individual's ability to perform the functions of the position at the present time. If a current employee reveals to the manager that he or she is HIV positive or has AIDS, that information must be kept confidential and must be kept apart from the general personnel file. The manager may choose to hold a discussion at that time of what accommodations might be needed in the future.

PROVIDING/PLANNING EMPLOYEE TRAINING AND EDUCATION

Health care changes daily; new procedures are established, a better technique is discovered for performing a particular task. Major changes regularly occur in medical insurance. Computer systems are updated or new software is added. A more sophisticated telephone system is installed to make certain patients are responded to promptly. New state or federal regulations mandate additional training or compliance in safety. New medications become available that physicians may prescribe and employees must understand. All this demands that employees receive a continuing and constant update in their area of employment.

Training and education may be accomplished within the practice or outside the practice. When an employee is a member of a professional organization such as the American Association of Medical Assistants, many monthly meetings will include continuing education opportunities. Numerous seminars and conferences held throughout the country may be beneficial to employees. Local hospitals often have continuing education opportunities that might be beneficial. Managers will keep abreast of these opportunities and encourage employees to attend. Any continuing education opportunity that may benefit the employee on the job and the medical practice itself should ideally be paid for by the physician–employer(s). Credentialed employees will always need to update skills and earn CEUs to maintain their credentials in active status. An important function of HR is to make opportunities available to employees for CEUs.

It is often best to provide training and education within the facility when the training necessary is specific to the medical practice. For instance, training on new computer software is apt to be specific to the particular setting. When sophisticated new equipment is purchased, companies often provide in-house training for the individuals who will be using the equipment. Take advantage of as many of those opportunities as are available and for as many of your employees as possible. When the training is quite expensive or time consuming, make certain one person receives the training. Then have that individual train others. Whenever possible, provide training outside of regular hours when patients are not being seen—before or after the office closes or during a lunch period. Always pay employees for any time served over their regular working hours. Offer certificates for any inservices.

Careful attention to continuing education and training for employees will pay for itself many times over again. The more confident and secure employees feel in the skills they are expected to perform, the more satisfied the practice's patients will be.

Procedure 23-1 Develop and Maintain a Policy Manual

PURPOSE:
To develop and maintain a comprehensive, up-to-date policy manual of all office policies relating to employee practices, benefits, office conduct, and so on.

EQUIPMENT/SUPPLIES:
Computer
Binder, such as a three-ring binder
Paper
Standard policy manual format

PROCEDURE STEPS:
1. Following office format, develop precise, written office policies detailing all necessary information pertaining to the staff and their positions. The information should include benefits, vacation, sick leave, hours, dress codes, evaluations, rules of-conduct, and grounds for dismissal. RATIONALE: Well-defined policies clearly outlined for each employee are necessary for efficient and effective staff operations.
2. Identify procedures for reimbursing overtime, preventing discrimination and harassment, creating a safe working environment, and allowing for jury duty.
3. Include a policy statement related to smoking.
4. Identify steps to follow should an employee become disabled during employment.
5. Determine what employee opportunities for continuing education, if any, will be reimbursed; include requirements for recertification or licensure.
6. Provide a copy of the policy manual for each employee.
7. Review and update the policy manual regularly. Add or delete items as necessary, dating each revised page.

Procedure 23-2 — Prepare a Job Description

PURPOSE:
To provide a precise definition of the tasks assigned to a job, to determine the expectations and level of competency required, and to specify the experience, training, and education needed to perform the job for purposes of recruiting and performance evaluation.

EQUIPMENT/SUPPLIES:
Computer
Paper
Standard job description format

PROCEDURE STEPS:
1. Detail each task that creates the job. RATIONALE: A detailed job description identifies clear expectations for each employee.
2. List special medical, technical, or clerical skills required.
3. Determine the level of education, training, and experience required for the position.
4. Determine where the job fits in the overall structure of the office.
5. Specify any unusual working conditions (hours, locations, and so on) that may apply.
6. Describe career path opportunities.

Procedure 23-3 — Conduct Interviews

PURPOSE:
To screen applicants for training, experience, and characteristics to select the best candidate to fill the position vacancy.

PROCEDURE STEPS:
1. Review résumés and applications received.
2. Select candidates who most closely match the education and experience being sought.
3. Create an interview worksheet for each candidate listing points to cover.
4. Select an interview team; this team should always include the HR or office manager and the immediate supervisor to whom the candidate will report.
5. Call personally to schedule interviews; this allows you to judge the applicant's telephone manners and voice.
6. Remind the interviewers of various legal restrictions concerning questions to be asked.
7. Conduct interviews in a private, quiet setting. RATIONALE: Careful interviewing of potential employees is an important step in hiring the best candidate for the position.
8. Put the applicant at ease by beginning with an overview about the practice and staff, briefly describing the job, and answering preliminary questions.
9. Ask questions about the applicant's work experience and educational background using the résumé and interview worksheet as a guide.
10. Provide the most promising applicants additional information on benefits and a tour of the office if practical.
11. Applicant's general salary requirements may be discussed, but avoid discussion of a specific salary until a formal offer is tendered.
12. Inform the applicants when a decision will be made and thank each for participating in the interview.
13. Do not make a job offer until all the candidates have been interviewed.
14. Check references of all prospective employees.
15. Establish a second interview between the physician–employer(s) and the qualified candidate if necessary.
16. Confirm accepted job offers in writing, specifying details of the offer and acceptance.
17. Notify all unsuccessful applicants by letter when the position has been filled.

Procedure 23-4 Orient Personnel

PURPOSE:
To acquaint new employees with office policies, staff, what the job encompasses, procedures to be performed, and job performance expectations.

PROCEDURE STEPS:
1. Tour the facilities and introduce the office staff.
2. Complete employee-related documents and explain their purpose.
3. Explain the benefits programs.
4. Present the office policy manual and discuss its key elements.
5. Review federal and state regulatory precautions for medical facilities.
6. Review the job description.
7. Explain and demonstrate procedures to be performed and the use of procedure manuals supporting these procedures.
8. Demonstrate the use of any specialized equipment.
9. Assign a mentor from the staff to help with the orientation. RATIONALE: Without proper orientation and training, the best new employee can fail.

Case Study 23-1

Daly Jacobsen, RMA, is an administrative medical assistant at Inner City Health Care. The HR manager has suggested that she might expand her skills and learn some of the procedures in the hiring process. A new medical assistant who specializes in nutrition is coming on board. Daly has been asked to make certain the I-9 form is completed appropriately. The HR manager tells Daly that she will need to download the latest form before completion.

CASE STUDY REVIEW

1. Daly knows that the I-9 is a government form verifying employment eligibility. What keywords might she use in her Inernet search to find the form?
2. Once the form has been located, identify the specific rules necessary in completion of the form. What document in List A might a number of prospective employees likely have?
3. In what area of the office might you post the lists of acceptable documents for the I-9 form?
4. With what agency is the form filed on successful completion?

Case Study 23-2

Charles Kensington has just been hired as the HR manager in a large metropolitan clinic. In studying the policy manual, he notes that there is no defined policy for sick leave or bereavement leave. Describe the steps he might take to write such a policy.

CASE STUDY REVIEW

1. To whom should he speak regarding what currently occurs when an employee is ill or when there is a death in the family?
2. What might Charles consider in writing this policy?
3. How should a policy be approved once it is written?
4. What parameters would you suggest for the policy?

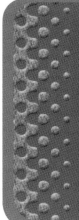

SUMMARY

As shown in this discussion, HR management is a challenge. It is, however, a rewarding one. While physician–employers are responsible for patients' physical care, the management team is responsible for hiring and maintaining the employees in the organization. The HR manager who is successful will hire the right people for the jobs and monitor employees in a way that enables and encourages them to give the best patient care possible. The medical assistant who has good communication skills and acquires additional training in HR management will always have variety on the job and will have the satisfaction of watching a health care team run smoothly and efficiently.

STUDY FOR SUCCESS

To reinforce your knowledge and skills of information presented in this chapter:
- ❏ Review the Key Terms
- ❏ Practice the Procedures
- ❏ Consider the Case Studies and discuss your conclusions
- ❏ Answer the Review Questions
  - ❏ Multiple Choice
  - ❏ Critical Thinking
- ❏ Navigate the Internet and complete the Web Activities
- ❏ Practice the StudyWARE activities on the textbook CD
- ❏ Apply your knowledge in the Student Workbook activities
- ❏ Complete the Web Tutor sections

REVIEW QUESTIONS

Multiple Choice

1. HR managers:
   a. need no special training for the job
   b. are responsible for hiring and orienting personnel
   c. usually work harder and longer hours than other employees
   d. both b and c

2. The following questions may be asked in an interview:
   a. How old are you?
   b. Have you ever been arrested?
   c. Can you supply a birth certificate or a Social Security card?
   d. Do you plan to start a family soon?

3. When a candidate has been accepted for a position, the HR manager should:
   a. call the candidate to determine what salary is preferred
   b. write a letter defining the position details
   c. check references listed by the candidate
   d. notify patients of a staff change

4. Overtime hours in the medical setting:
   a. are to be expected as part of the job
   b. do not require prior authorization
   c. are usually paid at no less than one and one-half times the regular pay rate
   d. are paid only to managers

5. The HR manager will work closely with:
   a. the physician–employer
   b. the office manager
   c. all employees
   d. all the above

6. OSHA:
   a. requires employers to verify an employee's right to work in the United States
   b. protects employees who have disabilities from employment discrimination
   c. protects employees with chemical dependencies or emotional problems
   d. protects employees from unsafe or unhealthy working conditions

7. The best area for hiring medical employees comes from:
   a. students in a business college
   b. newspaper advertisements
   c. networking sources
   d. the state's unemployment office
8. Employees receiving training or education necessary to the job:
   a. will seek that training after hours and not expect reimbursement
   b. will be continuous and constant in the health care field
   c. should always be paid for any time served over regular working hours
   d. both b and c
9. Personnel records:
   a. are usually kept for three to five years after employment ends and may include payroll data
   b. are not available for everyone to view and must be kept confidential
   c. include all papers related to employment and personal data
   d. all the above
10. Dismissal:
    a. may be voluntary or involuntary
    b. should always be documented
    c. is a good time for an exit interview
    d. all the above

Critical Thinking

1. You have just accepted a position to work in a larger, more specialized clinic where you will be able to use skills you are not currently able to exercise. Identify two or three main points for a letter of resignation you will prepare.
2. An employee approaches you, the HR manager, identifying that he or she has just become responsible for the care of an aging parent and may require occasional time away from work. You have no policy about how this absence should be treated. What kind of policy might be helpful? Where would you look for suggestions?
3. An exit interview form has been introduced in this chapter. Another simple form for an exit interview is to use the ABCs. A stands for "awesome." What do we do that is really good? B stands for "better." What could we do better in our organization? C stands for "change." What would you recommend we change? Discuss the merits of both forms for an exit interview.
4. Do a simple comparison of salaries in your community. Compare the hourly wages of a secretary, a medical assistant, a plumber, your automobile mechanic, and a person working in a fast-food restaurant. How might you use this material when seeking salary increases?
5. What might physician–employers and HR managers do to make certain they keep valued employees? Is salary really the most important issue?

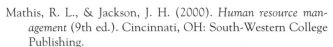

WEB ACTIVITIES

1. Research the Centers for Medicare & Medicaid Services Web site (http://www.cms.hhs.gov) for information related to the prohibition of discrimination on the basis of sexual orientation. What do you find? Are there other sources on this subject that are helpful? Can the manager choose not to hire a person who is otherwise qualified on the basis that he or she is gay? Why or why not?
2. "NOLO Law for All" has a helpful Web site with many topics in their encyclopedia. Research the area related to personnel policies and practices. What suggestions do they make for establishing goals and standards for employee evaluations? Do they identify any helpful evaluation tips? If so, outline them for your instructor.
3. Research the ADA Web site to determine if there are any examples of accommodations made in the medical setting. If yes, describe them. Are all physician–employers covered by the ADA? If not, how might discrimination be prevented?

REFERENCES/BIBLIOGRAPHY

Mathis, R. L., & Jackson, J. H. (2000). *Human resource management* (9th ed.). Cincinnati, OH: South-Western College Publishing.

Ricardo, M. (1992). *Personnel management handbook* (2nd ed.). New York: McGraw-Hill, Inc.

UNIT 7
Entry into the Profession

Preparing for Medical Assisting Credentials

OUTLINE

OBJECTIVES

The student should strive to meet the following performance objectives and demonstrate an understanding of the facts and principles presented in this chapter through written and oral communication.

1. Define the key terms as presented in the glossary.
2. List the necessary qualifications to sit for the CMA certification examination.
3. State when the CMA certification examination is offered and the registration deadlines.
4. List the necessary qualifications to sit for the RMA examination.
5. State when the RMA examination is offered and the registration protocols.
6. Differentiate between being certified and being registered.
7. Identify the benefits of certification and registration.
8. Describe several methods for continuing education opportunities.
9. Explain when recertification must take place for the CMA.
10. Describe the procedure for recertification for the RMA.

KEY TERMS

Accrediting Bureau of
    Health Education
    Schools (ABHES)
American Association of
    Medical Assistants
    (AAMA)
American Medical
    Technologists (AMT)
Certification Examination
Certified Medical Assistant
    (CMA)
Commission on Accredita-
    tion of Allied Health
    Education Programs
    (CAAHEP)
Continuing Education Units
    (CEUs)
Recertification
Registered Medical
    Assistant (RMA)
Task Force for Test
    Construction (TFTC)

FEATURED COMPETENCIES

CAAHEP—ENTRY-LEVEL COMPETENCIES

Legal Concepts

- Perform within legal and ethical boundaries
- Demonstrate knowledge of federal and state health care legislation and regulations

ABHES—ENTRY-LEVEL COMPETENCIES

Professionalism

- Allied health professions and credentialing

SCENARIO

Dr. Ray Reynolds currently is the senior physician at Inner City Health Care, a multi-physician urgent care center. When he began his practice 32 years ago, however, he had a private practice and employed one full-time and two part-time medical assistants. Dr. Reynolds felt the office ran smoothly, except when an assistant had to be replaced. Retraining a new person consumed a great deal of valuable time. Even if the new employee came with experience from another medical office, the procedures still required retraining.

Dr. Reynolds finds that when he needs to replace a medical assistant now, he looks at the applicants' résumés and interviews only those candidates who are Certified Medical Assistants or Registered Medical Assistants. The office is too busy to spend time training and retraining new people.

INTRODUCTION

Thirty years ago, medical assistants were trained on the job by the practitioner with whom they were employed. Quality control of training varied because there were no established criteria for evaluating such training.

Hence, the **Certified Medical Assistant (CMA)** *certification examination was developed by the* **American Association of Medical Assistants (AAMA),** *and the* **Registered Medical Assistant (RMA)** *examination was developed by the* **American Medical Technologists (AMT).** *Both examinations, together with methods of continuing education and recertification establish criteria for evaluating training.*

PURPOSE OF CERTIFICATION

Certification is intended to set a consistent minimum standard for evaluating an individual's professional competence as a medical assistant. The CMA is awarded to those candidates who successfully pass the **certification examination** offered by the Certifying Board of the AAMA or administered by the National Board of Medical Examiners. Only graduates of **Commission on Accreditation of Allied Health Education Programs (CAAHEP)** and **Accrediting Bureau of Health Education Schools (ABHES)** accredited

medical assistant (MA) programs may sit for the CMA and RMA examinations.

The American Medical Technologists (AMT), a national certifying body for health professionals, established the Registered Medical Assistant (RMA) credential for those students graduating from schools accredited by the ABHES. To be eligible for the RMA examination, on-the-job training with five years' experience may qualify, or a student must graduate from an approved training program. Approved programs include either a CAAHEP- or ABHES-accredited MA program, a postsecondary MA program with regional accreditation, or medical training from the armed forces.

Hiring physicians view these credentials as professional and an indication of proficiency in entry-level skills. Maintaining the credential demonstrates a lifelong commitment to continuing education. The graduate medical assistant has a goal and challenge to which to aspire, first by earning the credential, and second by maintaining the credential through recertification.

Critical Thinking

Take time to think through your personal medical assisting career goals. Will credentialing be an important consideration? Why or why not?

Spotlight on Certification

RMA Content Outline
• Medical law
• Oral and written communication

CMA Content Outline
• Displaying a professional attitude
• Professional communication and behavior

CMAS Content Outline
• Legal and ethical considerations
• Communication

Formal medical assistant programs are offered throughout the country in vocation-technical colleges, proprietary schools, postsecondary vocational schools, community and junior colleges, and four-year colleges. Medical assistants may be trained on the job; however, physicians recognize that their offices operate more efficiently with professionally educated personnel.

PREPARING FOR THE EXAMINATION

Preparation for the examination requires planning, scheduling, and discipline. It is important to plan well in advance to ensure confidence and a passing score to earn your credential. If you are sitting for the examination immediately on graduation, your preparation time for the examination may only allow two to three months. If you have been out of school for some time or your work experience has been very specialized, you may need longer to prepare for the examination.

During the planning stage, determine the date you want to sit for the examination. Check with the appropriate Web site or call the appropriate examination department to obtain the current application form. The application form will contain information such as dates, times, and locations of test sites; policies regarding deadlines; incomplete applications; examination verification information; and information regarding study guides.

It is also important to consider looking for a study group or partner. The right study environment can be invaluable to your success for several reasons. First, it is important to select a study partner or group who shares your commitment to a successful outcome and who plans to sit for the examination on or near the same date you have selected. A study partner can also give you some accountability for keeping to the planned schedule.

Once it has been determined when and where you will sit for the examination and who your study partner(s), if any, will be, a meeting should be scheduled to discuss the review/study approach. It may be that your group will decide to review/study each subject provided in the Curriculum Content Outline accompanying the application. Other groups review/study only those areas in which they feel less confident. A plan that meets the needs of each group member and that all can agree to works best.

Meeting once or twice a week helps the group stay focused and on task. Independent study should be done throughout the week. During the independent study time, each group member may be asked to write 10 multiple choice questions relevant to the weeks' study topic. Answers to these questions should be on a separate page. Some find it helpful to also provide the rationale or textbook page number that supports their answer. When the group meets, a discussion of the study topic could take place and copies of the questions could be distributed for answering. The questions could then be corrected and discussion of any questionable or missed answers could take place.

Once a schedule has been established and agreed on, discipline is required. It is critical that each group member spend time individually preparing for the next group meeting. Someone should be put in charge of each group meeting to keep the event from turning into a social time. To help with this, it is a good idea to set a specific time limit for the study/review session. If individuals want to visit after the session, they are free to do that without disrupting the purpose of the session. All members should be committed to being prepared and attending each scheduled review/study session.

CMA

The AAMA offers the CMA certification examination. After successfully passing the certification examination, the CMA credential is awarded. The credential appears after your name and distinguishes you as a professional signifying achievement in a demanding career field.

CMAs are recognized by peers for their commitment to continued professional development. Survey results indicate that many employers recognize the value of this credential by paying higher salaries and offering more benefits to CMAs. Broader career advancement opportunities and enhanced job security represent other benefits of certification. The CMA credential is a national credential, and therefore is valid wherever the practitioner is employed within the United States.

The AAMA requires current CMA status for MAs to use the CMA registered trademarked credentials after their name in their place of employment. CEU requirements must be satisfied to qualify and apply for **recertification.** Individuals not having current status as a CMA can be charged with fraudulent use and be denied access to recertification. For more information, contact the AAMA at 1-800-228-2262.

Examination Format and Content

The CMA certification examination is a comprehensive test of the knowledge actually used in today's medical office. The content is drawn from an in-depth analysis of the numerous tasks medical assistants perform on a daily basis.

Examination questions are formulated by the Certifying Board's **Task Force for Test Construction (TFTC).** This group is composed of practicing medical assistants, physicians, and medical assisting educators from across the United States. The TFTC updates the CMA examination annually to reflect changes in medical assistants' day-to-day responsibilities, as well as the latest developments in medical knowledge and technology.

The three major areas tested include:

1. *General (Transdisciplinary):* anatomy and physiology, medical terminology, medical law and ethics, psychology, and communication.
2. *Administrative:* data entry, equipment, computer concepts, records management, screening and processing mail, scheduling and monitoring appointments, resource information and community services, managing physician's professional schedule and travel, managing the office, office policies, and procedures, and managing practice finances.
3. *Clinical:* principles of infection control, treatment area, patient preparation and assisting the physician, patient history interview, collecting and processing specimens, diagnostic tests, preparing and administering medications, emergencies, and nutrition.

Students must enroll as an AAMA member before their graduation date to be eligible for the reduced student rate. Once they are a student member they may stay at the student rate for one year after graduation if they do not choose to be an active or associate member and pay the higher dues amount. The additional year of membership at the reduced rate helps the recent graduate maintain membership while finding a job and getting established in a career.

Application Process

Candidates should read all instructions carefully before completing the application form. Incomplete or incorrect applications will not be processed and will be returned to the candidate. Postmark deadlines for applications, cancellations, and examination location changes are strictly enforced.

The examination is offered at more than 260 test sites nationwide and in Guam. A complete listing of the locations is included in the application. Applications are available from the AAMA Certification Department, 20 North Wacker Drive, Suite 1575, Chicago, IL 60606-2903; telephone: 312-424-3100; or e-mail: certification@aama.ntl.org. The application may also be downloaded from the AAMA Web site (http://www.aama-ntl.org.)

The appropriate application form must be completed and postmarked by October 1 for the January examination and by March 1 for the June examination.

The certification examination is scheduled from 9:00 AM to 1:00 PM the last Friday of January and the last Saturday in June. An admission card will be mailed to the applicant on verification of information and approval by the AAMA approximately one to two weeks before the examination date. Photo identification is required for admission to the examination and candidates are not permitted to use any supplies other than #2 soft-leaded pencils and erasers. No electronic devices (e.g., cellular phones, pagers, and calculators) are allowed in the examination area.

It is recommended that the application be sent by certified mail, return receipt requested to verify delivery. The application must be typewritten or printed using black ink only. Be sure the application is signed and dated properly and the eligibility category section is completed appropriately.

Tear off the application page from the instruction pamphlet. Do not mail the instructions back with the application. Keep this information for future reference together with a copy of everything submitted, including a copy of your completed payment check or money order.

Critical Thinking

You will graduate from a CAAHEP-accredited program in June and want to sit for the CMA examination the last Saturday of June (the same month in which you graduate). When must your application be postmarked for acceptance for this test date?

If you are paying by VISA or MasterCard, provide the requested information at the top of the application.

A guide for the certification examination entitled *A Candidate's Guide to the AAMA Certification Examination* provides explanations of how to approach the types of questions used on the examination and tips on how to study for the content that will be tested. A sample 120-question examination is included to help assess your knowledge of the categories tested and the format used to formulate the questions.

Eligibility Categories and Requirements

You must fulfill one of the four eligibility categories to apply for the CMA examination.

Grounds for Denial of Eligibility

The following are grounds for denial of eligibility for the CMA credential, or for discipline of CMAs:

- Obtaining or attempting to obtain certification, or recertification of the CMA credential, by fraud or deception

- Knowingly assisting another to obtain or attempt to obtain certification or recertification by fraud or deception

- Misstatement of material fact or failure to make a statement of material fact in application for certification or recertification

- Falsifying information required for admission to the CMA examination, inpersonating another examinee, or falsifying education or credentials

- Copying answers, permitting another to copy answers, or providing or receiving unauthorized advice about examination content during the CMA examination

- Unauthorized possession or distribution of examination materials, including copying and reproducing examination questions and problems

Individuals who have been found guilty of a felony, or pleaded guilty to a felony, are not eligible to take the CMA examination. However, the Certifying Board may grant a waiver based on mitigating circumstances, which may include, but need not be limited to the following:

- The age at which the crime was committed
- The circumstances surrounding the crime

- The nature of the crime committed
- The length of time since the conviction
- The individual's criminal history since the conviction
- The individual's current employment references
- The individual's character references
- Other evidence demonstrating the ability of the individual to perform the professional responsibilities competently, and evidence that the individual does not pose a threat to the health or safety of patients

How to Recertify

Effective January 2005, all newly certified and recertifying CMAs will be current through the last day of their birth month in the 6th calendar year following their last certification/recertification. In other words, if you were born on August 6th and certified in June 2000, you would be due to recertify by the end of August 2006.

This process may be achieved by either reexamination or by the continuing education method. Recertification credits are evaluated on supportive documentation and on their relevancy to medical assisting as defined by the AAMA Medical Assistant Role Delineation Study or the Content Outline for the Certification/Recertification Examination.

A total of 60 points is necessary to recertify the CMA credential. A minimum of 15 points is required in each category: general, administrative, and clinical. The remaining 15 points may be accumulated in any of the three content areas or from any combination of the three categories. At least 20 of the required 60 recertification points must be accumulated from AAMA-approved **continuing education units (CEUs).** If desired, all 60 points may be AAMA CEUs.

On successfully passing the Certification Examination and earning the CMA credential, one should begin to document all CEUs earned. It is important to have the following information for CEU documentation:
- Complete date of the activity
- Sponsor (group or organization issuing the credit for the continuing education activity)
- Program title
- Amount and type of credit earned (e.g., CEU, CME, contact hour or college credit)
- Recertification points (AAMA CEUs or other credit)
- Points per content area (general, administrative, clinical)

CMAs applying for recertification must also provide documentation of current cardiopulmonary resuscitation (CPR) certification for health care professionals or providers. Acceptable courses of CPR include the American Red Cross, the American Heart Association, or the National Safety Council. The components of certification must include adult and pediatric CPR and obstructed airway training and Automated External Defibrillator (AED) instruction.

Applicants who accumulate all 60 points through AAMA CEUs, and in the correct content areas, may order a recertification over the telephone. Application fees still apply, however an application form is not required. All CMAs employed or seeking employment must have current certified status to use the CMA credential.

Continuing education courses are offered by local, state, and national AAMA groups. Guided study programs are also available through AAMA's "Quest for Excellence" program. CMA *Today*, the official bimonthly publication of AAMA, provides articles designated for CEUs.

A CMA need not be a member of the AAMA, nor currently employed, to recertify. The entire recertification by continuing education instructions and application can be downloaded from AAMA's Web site (http://www.aama-ntl.org). Review of recertification applications can take up to 90 days. If all criteria are met, recertification is granted. The date that the application is postmarked to the AAMA Executive Office will be the date of recertification.

On meeting recertification requirements, the applicant receives a seal to affix to the original certificate. A Recertification Certificate is also available for purchase.

RMA

The AMT, a national certifying body for health professionals, established the RMA credential in 1976. The RMA/AMT has its own bylaws, officers, local, state, and national organizations. Applicants for the RMA examination may have graduated from an accredited program, an accredited school, a U.S. Armed Forces program, or have 5 years employment in the field of medical assisting. Currently, there are more then 52,000 RMAs certified by AMT.

Examination Format and Content

AMT certification examinations are intended to evaluate the competence of entry-level practitioners. The Education, Qualifications, and Standards Committee of American Medical Technologists develop RMA examinations. The MA committee writes test questions and reviews questions submitted from other sources (e.g., instructors, experts, practitioners, and other individuals associated with the MA profession). The MA committee also determines certification requirements and addresses standard-setting issues related to the credential. Once test construction has been completed, the examination is reviewed and approved by the AMT Board of Directors.

The AMT registration examination consists of 200 to 210 four-option multiple-choice questions. Examinees are required to select the single best answer; multiple answers for a single item are scored as incorrect. Test questions may require examinees to recall facts, interpret graphic illustrations, interpret information presented in case studies, analyze situations, or solve problems. The approximate percentages of questions in content areas are as follows:

1. General Medical Assisting Knowledge—42.5%
   - anatomy and physiology
   - medical terminology
   - medical law
   - medical ethics
   - human relations
   - patient education

2. Administrative Medical Assisting—22.5%
   - insurance
   - financial bookkeeping
   - medical secretarial-receptionist

3. Clinical Medical Assisting—35.0%
   - asepsis
   - sterilization
   - instruments
   - vital signs
   - physical examinations
   - clinical pharmacology
   - minor surgery
   - therapeutic modalities
   - laboratory procedures
   - electrocardiography
   - first aid

All AMT registration examination tests are available in paper-and-pencil format or computerized formats at over 200 locations in the United States, its territories, and Canada. Tests may be scheduled daily except Sundays and holidays. Both formats are identical in length; however, experience has shown the computerized test takes less time to complete. Your computerized test score is displayed moments after completing your test. A paper copy of your result letter is provided to you before leaving the testing center.

Application Process

The following criteria have been established for applicants sitting for the RMA examination:

1. Applicant shall be of good moral character and at least 18 years of age.
2. Applicant shall be a graduate of an accredited high school or acceptable equivalent.
3. Applicant must meet one of the following requirements:
   a. Applicant shall be a graduate of a(n):
      - MA program that holds programmatic accreditation by (or is in a post-secondary school or college that holds institutional accredition by) the ABHES or the CAAHEP.
      - MA program in a postsecondary school or college that has institutional accreditation by a Regional Accrediting Commission or by a national accrediting organization approved by the U.S. Department of Education. That program must include a minimum of 720 clock hours (or equivalent) of training in medical assisting skills (including a clinical externship).
      - Formal medical services training program of the U.S. Armed Forces.
   b. Applicant shall have been employed in the profession of medical assisting for a minimum of five years, no more than two years of which may have been as an instructor in a postsecondary MA program.
4. Applicants applying under 3 A or B *must* take and pass the AMT certification examination for RMA.
5. The AMT Board of Directors has further determined that applicants who have passed generalist MA certification examination offered by another medical assisting certification body (provided that examination has been approved for this purpose by the AMT Board of Directors), who have been working in the medical assisting field for the past three of five years, and who meet all other AMT training and experience requirements may be considered for the RMA (AMT) certification without further examination.

Applications may be downloaded from AMT's Web site (http://www.amt1.com) either in print and fill-in format or as online fill-in format.

Application Completion and Test Administration Scheduling

All applications must be completed online or printed clearly except for the signatures required. All ancillary documentation must also be submitted (e.g., application fee; proof of high school graduation or equivalent; official final transcripts stating graduation from MA school, college, or training program [with school seal affixed or notarized]).

When the AMT Registrar has received the application and all required information, an authorization letter containing a toll-free number is mailed to you. You may then contact Prometric, through AMT, to schedule a date and time to take the examination. Two forms of valid identification are required both bearing your signature and at least one bearing your photo. Photo identification is limited to a driver's license, state-issued identification card, military identification, or passport.

The RMA credential is granted in conjunction with other indicators of training and experience because test results provide only one source of information regarding examinee competence. The credential remains current as long as membership is maintained in the AMT organization. Recertification of the RMA credential requires an annual fee of $48 every December.

PROFESSIONAL ORGANIZATIONS

Professional organizations have evolved to establish standards by which MAs and MA programs may be evaluated. Programs accredited by agencies must meet criterion, and students must pass national examinations to become certified. MAs are not licensed and need not be certified to meet employment requirements; however, those certified are viewed as professionals with entry-level skills and a commitment to continued education.

AAMA

The AAMA was recognized by the U.S. Department of Education in 1978 working solely for the profession of medical assisting. They were instrumental in defining the scope of training required for the profession and developed standards and guidelines by which programs could become accredited and MA credentialed.

The AAMA Endowment is a not-for-profit corporation that provides funding for two purposes:

- Awarding of scholarships to students in CAAHEP-accredited medical assisting education programs
- Accreditation of medical assisting education programs through CAAHEP

The Curriculum Review Board (CRB) operates under the authority of the endowment and evaluates medical assisting programs according to standards adopted by the endowment and the CAAHEP. The CRB recommends programs to CAAHEP for accreditation. The CRB also reviews standards for medical assisting curricula, conducts accreditation workshops for educators, and provides medical assisting educators with current information about CAAHEP, accreditation laws, policies, and practices. CAAHEP's purpose is to accredit entry-level, allied health education programs.

Some of the benefits of AAMA membership include:

- Medical assisting news and health care information through the bimonthly magazine CMA *Today*

- CEUs for AAMA activities entered in the Continuing Education Registry and access to your transcript online

- Educational events provided by local chapters, state societies, and national meetings

- Answers to legal questions regarding job-related issues

- If eligible, application for the prestigious CMA examination at a reduced fee

- Discounts on car rentals, conventions, workshop and seminar fees, and self-study courses

- Opportunity to network with other practicing MAs

AMT

The AMT is another nonprofit certification agency and professional membership association representing allied health care individuals. It began in the 1970s and certifies MAs by awarding the RMA national credential to those candidates successfully satisfying requirements. AMT has many local chapters, 38 State Societies, and a Uniform Services Committee. Each of these societies meets regularly and annually for a national convention.

AMT benefits and services include:

- Continuing education through the *Journal of Continuing Education Topics & Issues* published three times a year

- AMT's Institute for Education (AMTIE), which monitors your continued education credits and sends a "report card" to you each year

- Four scholarships available to members who want to return to school, and five scholarships for current students enrolled in allied health care programs

- State Societies that offer opportunities for continued education, activities, and networking

- Peer recognition through AMT's prestigious RMA credential

- Personal discount programs

Case Study 24-1

It is February, and Juan Estaban is beginning to research the procedures and requirements for taking the CMA examination. Juan is enrolled in a CAAHEP-accredited program.

CASE STUDY REVIEW

1. If Juan wants to take the examination in June, what is the procedure for applying?
2. Juan is setting up a study schedule. He plans to review course textbooks and tests, purchase a certification review study guide, and set up a study group. Set up a sample study schedule.
3. What criteria should Juan use when asking people to join his study group?

Case Study 24-2

It is May, and Nancy McFarland, who graduated from an ABHES-accredited program four-and-a-half years ago, is beginning to research the procedures and requirements for taking the RMA examination. Nancy completed her internship at Inner City Health Care and was hired to work there full-time (35 hours per week) when she graduated.

CASE STUDY REVIEW

1. If Nancy wants to take the examination in January, what is the procedure for applying?
2. Nancy is setting up a study schedule. She plans to review course textbooks and tests, purchase a study guide, and set up a study group. Develop a simple study schedule.
3. What criteria should Nancy use when asking people to join her study group?

SUMMARY

Many advantages for certification/recertification and registration have been discussed in this chapter. Although certification examinations are not legally required for practicing MAs, it is the goal of CAAHEP-accredited and ABHES-accredited institutions to encourage graduates to sit for and maintain their credentials. Membership in the AAMA or in the AMT is also encouraged.

With nearly 400 local AAMA chapters and 51 affiliate state societies, there is the benefit of networking with others in the profession. As an information source for both professional and association issues, the executive staff at the AAMA's national headquarters is available to answer questions at a toll-free number (1-800-228-2262).

AMT currently has 38 chapters that meet regularly and allow networking with other RMAs plus other allied health professionals registered through the AMT, including phlebotomists, medical laboratory technicians, and dental assistants.

STUDY FOR SUCCESS

To reinforce your knowledge and skills of information presented in this chapter:

- ❏ Review the Key Terms
- ❏ Consider the Case Studies and discuss your conclusions
- ❏ Answer the Review Questions
  - ❏ Multiple Choice
  - ❏ Critical Thinking
- ❏ Navigate the Internet and complete the Web Activities
- ❏ Practice the StudyWARE activities on the textbook CD
- ❏ Apply your knowledge in the Student Workbook activities
- ❏ Complete the Web Tutor sections
- ❏ View and discuss the DVD situations

REVIEW QUESTIONS

1. The goal and challenge of each graduating medical assistant should be to:
   a. find employment
   b. have a good benefit package
   c. possess entry-level skills
   d. earn the CMA/RMA credential and maintain it
2. The certification examination is:
   a. a comprehensive test based on tasks medical assistants perform daily
   b. all true/false questions
   c. developed by the AMTIE
   d. developed by the NBME
3. Benefits from membership in a professional organization such as AAMA or AMT include all of the following *except*:
   a. discounted rates on legal representation
   b. legal advice
   c. nationwide networking opportunities
   d. professional journal publications
4. Recertification of the CMA credential options include:
   a. submit work experience
   b. reexamination or CEU method
   c. submit on-the-job training
   d. submit military training
5. Applications for the CMA examination must be postmarked by:
   a. October 1 for January examination and March 1 for June examination
   b. October 31 for January examination and March 31 for June examination
   c. September 30 for January exam and April 30 for June examination
   d. September 1 for January examination and April 1 for June examination
6. The RMA was established by the:
   a. ABHES
   b. CAAHEP
   c. AMT
   d. AAMA
7. Candidates who graduate from a medical assisting program that is not CAAHEP-accredited on the date of graduation, but is accredited by CAAHEP within 36 months of that date, are eligible to apply for the CMA examination under which category(ies)?
   a. Category 1
   b. Category 4
   c. Categories 3 or 4
   d. Categories 1 or 2
8. RMA examinations:
   a. are offered at Prometric testing center locations
   b. are offered twice a year
   c. are offered three times a year
   d. are offered six times a year

Critical Thinking

1. You are a recent high school graduate and have decided to pursue medical assisting as a career. What will you do to find a school offering an accredited program? Is accreditation important? How might your school selection impact your future as a professional MA?
2. After graduation you plan to sit for the certification examination. How will you prepare for the examination to assure a positive outcome and earn your CMA/RMA credential?
3. After graduating from an accredited program, you immediately went to work as an MA. Now that you have been working several years you decide to become credentialed. How will you achieve this?

WEB ACTIVITIES

Using the World Wide Web, search your local and state AAMA or AMT Web sites. Print and turn in to your instructor the location, meeting schedules, and any upcoming events planned for your state. Review the certification process that applies to your program.

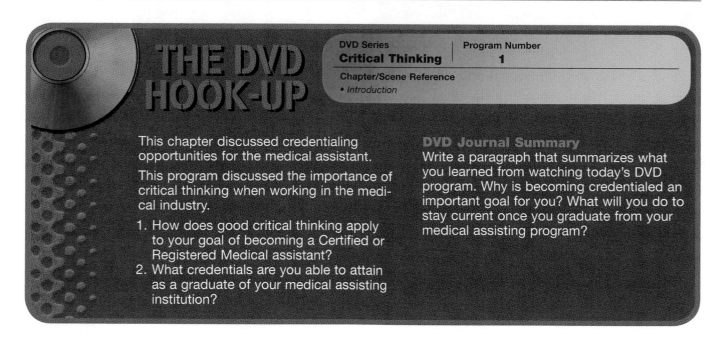

THE DVD HOOK-UP

DVD Series
Critical Thinking

Program Number
1

Chapter/Scene Reference
• *Introduction*

This chapter discussed credentialing opportunities for the medical assistant.

This program discussed the importance of critical thinking when working in the medical industry.

1. How does good critical thinking apply to your goal of becoming a Certified or Registered Medical assistant?
2. What credentials are you able to attain as a graduate of your medical assisting institution?

DVD Journal Summary
Write a paragraph that summarizes what you learned from watching today's DVD program. Why is becoming credentialed an important goal for you? What will you do to stay current once you graduate from your medical assisting program?

REFERENCES/BIBLIOGRAPHY

American Association of Medical Assistants. (2004–2005). *AAMA certification/recertification examination for medical assistants;* January and June 2005 application instructions. Retrieved from http://www.aama-ntl.org. Accessed May 16, 2005.

American Medical Technologists. Retrieved from http://www.amt1.com. Accessed May 16, 2005.

Fordney, M.T., French, L.L., Follis, J.J. (2004). *Administrative medical assisting* (5th ed.). Clifton Park, NY: Thomson Delmar Learning.

CHAPTER 25

Employment Strategies

OUTLINE

Developing a Strategy
  Attitude and Mindset
  Self-Assessment
Job Search Analysis and
Research
Résumé Preparation
  Résumé Specifications
  Clear and Concise Résumés
  Accomplishments
  References
  Accuracy
  Résumé Styles
  Vital Résumé Information

Application/Cover Letters
Completing the Application
Form
The Interview Process
  The Look of Success
  Preparing for the Interview
  The Actual Interview
  Closing the Interview
Interview Follow-Up
  Follow-Up Letter
  Follow Up by Telephone
Professionalism and
Employment Strategies

KEY TERMS

Accomplishment
  Statements
Application/Cover Letter
Application Form
Benefits
Bullet Point
Career Objective
Chronologic Résumé
Contact Tracker
Direct Skills
E-résumé
Functional Résumé
Interview
Keywords
Power Verbs
References
Résumé
Targeted Résumé
Transferable Skills

OBJECTIVES

The student should strive to meet the following performance objectives and demonstrate an understanding of the facts and principles presented in this chapter through written and oral communication.

1. Define the key terms as presented in the glossary.
2. List the steps involved in job analysis and research.
3. Describe a contact tracker and its usefulness.
4. Give three examples of accomplishment statements.
5. Differentiate chronologic, functional, and targeted résumés.
6. Identify the purpose and content of a cover letter.
7. Demonstrate effective ways to anticipate and respond to an interviewer's questions.
8. Describe appropriate overall appearance and dress for an interview.
9. Identify the benefits of writing a follow-up letter.
10. Discuss professionalism as it relates to employment strategies.

SCENARIO

Eun Mee Soo is a graduate of an accredited medical assisting program and recently passed the certification examination. She is now preparing her résumé and beginning her job search. Eun Mee plans to move out of state (she always dreamed of moving north), so she will also be looking for a new apartment. All of these changes are a bit unsettling for Eun Mee. She is beginning to wonder if she should defer relocating at this time and stay close to home until she feels more secure.

INTRODUCTION

So you are about to graduate from the medical assistant program! This time is often unsettling because many changes are occurring; the loss of security the classroom environment provided, loss of contact with fellow classmates, and loss of a structured schedule are just a few changes. Questions such as: Am I ready for my first job? How do I find a job? What do I say at the interview? begin to surface.

The focus on employment may represent apprehension and doubt or be sparked with anticipation and a sense of fulfillment. This chapter has been included to provide direction and to help answer some of the questions related to the job search.

DEVELOPING A STRATEGY

It is best to begin developing your job search strategy early in your training as a medical assistant. If you have not started this phase, determine to begin today.

497

Spotlight on Certification

Content Outline
- Medical law
- Human relations
- Oral and written communications

CMA Content Outline
- Displaying professional attitude
- Job readiness and seeking employment

CMAS Content Outline
- Legal and ethical considerations
- Professionalism
- Communication

Attitude and Mindset

One important quality an employer will look for in employees is their attitude. Your attitude is not something you turn on and off or learn in school. It is the result of your innate personality combined with the events that mold you during your life. Your instructors and acquaintances have a significant impact over who you are. Your attitude is reflected by how you react to:

1. taking direction
2. seeking excellence or doing just enough to get by
3. meeting employer's needs, not just looking forward to payday
4. assuming responsibility for your actions and considering your problems to be someone else's fault

If you find yourself having a negative attitude in any of the ways mentioned in the preceding list, you need to make an effort to change while you are still in training. An employer will zero in on a negative attitude and eliminate you as a candidate almost immediately. Your formal training is important and you can be retrained to do things the way a new employer desires, but your attitude takes time to change and requires a willingness to make the change. Develop a strategy to evolve a positive attitude while you are still in school because this is a time when you will have professional guidance and resources, as well as excellent models.

Beyond a positive attitude, being successful in your search for a job requires positive thinking on your part. There is a good position out there for you. Finding it is your first job. Those individuals who are successful at finding that first job devote many hours per week at job strategy tactics. You should not become discouraged by rejection, but rather seek to learn from it and apply what you have learned to the next interview opportunity.

Self-Assessment

As you begin your job search campaign, you should identify what you want in a job. It is always better to do work you enjoy in the type of practice you find most interesting. Take a moment now to complete the self-evaluation worksheet in Figure 25-1. When you have finished, you will have some idea of the type of practice you would like to work in and what position you would find most satisfying.

As part of the self-assessment you should also evaluate what direct and transferable skills you have that will make you a contributing member of the medical team. **Direct skills** are the medical procedures you have acquired in school and in which you are proficient. **Transferable skills** are those skills that would be useful in a wide variety of professions and may have been perfected during the education process or learned in other employment settings. Leadership, communication, writing, computer literacy, keyboarding, linguistics, and spelling are some examples of transferable skills.

When you have completed this portion of the self-assessment, you will be in a better position to determining what type of job to seek. You will also have identified the skills that you can highlight as you prepare your application/cover letter and résumé.

The final part of your self-assessment is conducting a budgetary need analysis to determine how much income you need to make per month to meet your living expenses.

The budgetary analysis should include listing the **benefits** you will find necessary; that is, medical, dental, and vision insurance, 401K program, stock options, and so forth. You might also need to consider work schedule, location/travel, medical benefits, childcare leave policies, and so on.

To accomplish this, begin to keep a diary of all purchases and payments. By reviewing your checkbook register, you should be able to itemize basic expenditures; that is, rent, utilities, payments (car, credit card), food, clothing, insurance, taxes, and so on. Once a monthly expenditure record is established, an estimate of the money required to live on may be calculated.

JOB SEARCH ANALYSIS AND RESEARCH

The job analysis and research phase of your job search should also start before graduation. Telephoning or visiting various clinics and asking questions to determine what the duties of a medical assistant are in different types

---

SELF-EVALUATION WORK SHEET

Respond to the following questions honestly and sincerely. They are meant to assist you in self-assessment.

1. List your three strongest attributes as related to people, data, or things.

   i.e., Interpersonal skills related to people

      Accuracy related to data

      Mechanical ability related to things

   _____ related to _____

   _____ related to _____

   _____ related to _____

2. List your three weakest attributes as related to people, data, or things.

   _____ related to _____

   _____ related to _____

   _____ related to _____

3. How do you express yourself? Excellent, Good, Fair, Poor

   Orally _____ In writing _____

4. Do you work well as a leader of a group or team? Yes _____ No _____

5. Do you prefer to work alone? Yes _____ No _____

6. Can you work under stress/pressure? Yes _____ No _____

7. Do you enjoy new ideas and situations? Yes _____ No _____

8. Are you comfortable with routines/schedules? Yes _____ No _____

9. Which work environment do you prefer?

   Single-physician setting _____   Multiple-physician setting _____

   Small clinic setting _____   Large clinic setting _____

10. Which type of practice do you prefer?

    Pediatrics _____   Obstetrics/Gynecology _____

    Geriatrics _____   General Medicine _____

    Internal Medicine _____   Other _____

11. Which work setting do you prefer?

    Front office, (reception) _____   Back office, (assisting physician) _____

    Laboratory (phlebotomy) _____   Administrative (coding/billing) _____

Figure 25-1 Self-evaluation work sheets can help determine a person's strengths, weaknesses, and preferences before the job search begins.

of practices will help to further clarify where you would like to work and will help you become acquainted with a potential employer or identify a possible site for externship. If you visit the facility, dress appropriately just as you would for an interview. You want to impress the clinic personnel just as if it were a formal interview. Remember to send a letter thanking the person taking time on the telephone or authorizing the visit.

Based on the self-assessment you have completed and preliminary job analysis, you know what type of clinic or practice you want to work in, so now is the time to compile a list of potential employers in the geographic area where you want to work. Compile a list from the Yellow Pages, Job Expositions, the Internet, Want Ads for your specialty in the local papers, American Association of Medical Assistants/American Medical Technologists

(AAMA/AMT) publications, and contacts acquired through attending state and local meetings. Other sources include your program director and instructors and the network of contacts at the site where you did your externship. An externship site is frequently your best prospect because they will know your capabilities and your attitude and have expended time and resources in your training. If the site is hiring and you performed well, experience has shown that most sites will frequently hire the extern.

Candidate job sites can also be found through employment agencies. These agencies usually charge a fee, although sometimes the employer will pay the fee. Extreme caution should be exercised in dealing with agencies because fees are sometimes excessive. Fees should only be paid after successfully obtaining a job and never for getting an interview.

Prioritize the list based on your assessment of chances of employment. Sites where you have personal contacts or where you have done your externship should be at the top of the list, with sites advertising for help wanted next. Further down the list should be sites that, in sales parlance, would be called cold prospecting. You can further prioritize the list by putting your personal choices at the top each category.

Now is the time to complete detailed homework or research on each prospective employer. Start collecting information on each prospective site, identifying their services, policies, fees and insurance protocol, hours of service, number of physicians, and very importantly their mission statement and philosophy of practice criteria. Brochures may be available in their offices, on the Internet, and in wellness publications for patients. Pamphlets

> Copy or design your own contact tracker form and document all pertinent information regarding your job search contacts.

on new procedures are also sources of this information. You can use this information in preparation of the cover letter for your résumé and to brief yourself should you be invited for an interview.

As part of a serious job search, you should contact many individuals and will need some means of recording the contacts, their responses, and your actions. The table presented in Figure 25-2 is a helpful sample **contact tracker.** It should be used to prevent confusion and to keep track of valuable information and action items.

RÉSUMÉ PREPARATION

A **résumé** is a summary data sheet or a brief account of your qualifications and progress in the career you have chosen and should include both direct and transferable skills. The purpose of your résumé is to sell you. It provides opportunity to describe your education, what you have done, and what you can do, and lists those who can vouch for your integrity and experience. A résumé that is well thought out and written in such a way as to create interest in what you have to contribute to the employer may reward you with many interviews. During the interview your résumé serves as a reference from which the interviewer may be prompted to ask questions.

CONTACT TRACKER

	Company Name/Address	Telephone Number	Contact's Name	Resume Sent	Application/ Cover Letter	Application Form Sent	Follow-Up Phone	Follow-Up Letter	Result
1.									
2.									
3.									
4.									
5.									
6.									

Figure 25-2 A simple contact tracker such as this can help organize all communication you may have with potential employers.

Résumé Specifications

The résumé should be limited to one page in length whenever possible. Each page should contain your name and the page number. Keep a 1- to 1½-inch margin on all four sides of the page to create a picture-like frame. Capitalize major headings and single space between lines. Double space between sections. The use of **bullet point** lists instead of paragraphs aids the interviewer in gleaning key points quickly.

Select a high-quality bond stationery that is standard 8½ × 11 inches with a weight of between 16 and 25 pounds. This paper weight provides aesthetic benefit and will also accept the ink better resulting in a clean, sharp print resolution. Buff or ivory paper with matching envelope has great eye appeal and helps distinguish your résumé from others.

Use a word processing program to produce your résumé. It allows you the freedom to experiment with placement to create a picture-perfect résumé or to individualize the résumé for a particular position or facility.

Clear and Concise Résumés

Your résumé must be concise and easy to read and understand. Use statements that are positive, reflect confidence, and portray you as a problem solver. Be sure that any information given within your résumé or application form is not misleading or exaggerated. Leave out the word *I* when writing your résumé. This is your personal résumé and it is understood that you are referring to yourself.

Accomplishments

Use **accomplishment statements** if you have them from your externship or work experience. Accomplishment statements begin with **power verbs** and give a brief description of what you did, and the demonstrable results that were produced. Figure 25-3 provides a list of sample power verbs. Some accomplishment statement examples are: "Utilized computer skills to schedule and reschedule patient appointments" and "Demonstrated skills in setting up sterile trays and assisting with sterile procedures."

Accompanied	Changed	Corrected	Entertained	Implemented	Listed
Accumulated	Charged	Corresponded	Enumerated	Improved	Listened
Achieved	Charted	Counseled	Established	Improvised	Loaded
Acquired	Classified	Created	Estimated	Increased	Located
Administered	Cleaned	Debated	Evaluated	Indexed	Logged
Admitted	Cleared	Decided	Examined	Indicated	Mailed
Advised	Closed	Delegated	Exchanged	Influenced	Maintained
Allowed	Coded	Delivered	Exhibited	Informed	Managed
Analyzed	Collated	Demonstrated	Expanded	Initiated	Manufactured
Answered	Collected	Deposited	Expedited	Inspected	Marked
Applied	Commanded	Described	Experienced	Installed	Marketed
Appointed	Communicated	Detailed	Fabricated	Instructed	Measured
Appraised	Compiled	Determined	Facilitated	Insured	Met
Arranged	Completed	Developed	Figured	Integrated	Modified
Assembled	Composed	Devised	Filled	Interpreted	Monitored
Assessed	Computed	Diagnosed	Financed	Interviewed	Motivated
Assigned	Conducted	Directed	Finished	Introduced	Negotiated
Attached	Conferred	Discovered	Fitted	Inspected	Nominated
Attained	Constructed	Dismantled	Fixed	Inventoried	Noted
Attended	Consulted	Dispatched	Formalized	Investigated	Notified
Authorized	Contacted	Distributed	Formulated	Invoiced	Observed
Balanced	Contracted	Documented	Fulfilled	Issued	Obtained
Billed	Contrasted	Drew	Generated	Judged	Opened
Bought	Contributed	Drove	Graded	Justified	Operated
Budgeted	Controlled	Earned	Graphed	Kept	Ordered
Built	Converted	Educated	Greeted	Learned	Organized
Calculated	Convinced	Employed	Headed	Lectured	Outlined
Cashed	Coordinated	Encouraged	Hired	Led	
Catalogued	Copied	Engineered	Identified	Licensed	(continues)

Figure 25-3   These sample power verbs may help you define your previous job responsibilities.

Overcame	Priced	Ran	Related	Secured	Summarized
Packaged	Printed	Rated	Relayed	Selected	Supervised
Packed	Processed	Read	Renewed	Sent	Supplied
Paid	Procured	Rearranged	Reorganized	Separated	Taught
Participated	Produced	Rebuilt	Repaired	Served as	Telephoned
Patrolled	Programmed	Recalled	Replaced	Serviced	Tested
Perfected	Promoted	Received	Reported	Set up	Trained
Piloted	Prompted	Recommended	Requested	Showed	Transferred
Placed	Proofread	Reconciled	Researched	Sold	Transported
Planned	Proposed	Recorded	Responsible for	Solicited	Typed
Posted	Proved	Reduced	Retrieved	Sorted	Verified
Prepared	Provided	Referred	Revised	Stocked	
Prescribed	Published	Registered	Routed	Stored	
Presented	Purchased	Regulated	Scheduled	Straightened	

Figure 25-3 (continued)

References

Select a variety of **references** to be included with your résumé. References should be listed on a separate sheet of paper that matches your résumé. Remember to include the same letterhead as on your résumé on the references page. An individual who knows you or has worked with you long enough to make an honest assessment and recommendation regarding your background history is an excellent reference person. Use only nonrelated persons as references unless the work relationship has been formalized.

Choose references who are well-respected and are clear speakers and writers. No matter how much someone likes you and your work, they may not be helpful to you if they cannot convey the information in a business-like manner. Professional references such as a former instructor, physician, externship supervisor, or fellow coworkers are excellent reference choices.

Always ask permission to use someone as a reference *before* the name is printed on the reference list. You will want to verify the correct spelling of the reference's name, title, place of employment and position, and telephone number for prospective employers.

Help your references aid you in obtaining an interview and employment. A personal visit or telephone call to discuss your career objectives and how you plan to conduct your job search will be helpful. Ask for any suggestions they may have to offer. Provide them with a copy of your résumé and cover letter. This helps them visualize the position for which you are applying and picture how you may benefit that employer.

Keep in touch with references. Check back to see who has called and how things went. Knowing what employers ask may produce some valuable pointers for your next letter, résumé, or interview.

Finally, thank your references. They will appreciate knowing how you are doing and that you value their assistance.

Leave out "References Upon Request" if necessary to shorten your résumé to save space. Employers know they can ask for references at a later date.

Accuracy

Proofread, proofread, and proofread your résumé. Ask someone who is a good speller or your references to edit your résumé. Then proofread it again yourself. Do not rely on your computer spell check; it does not differentiate between words such as to, too, two or here and hear. Eliminate repetition of information such as task descriptions. Summarize employment before 10 years ago or leave it off entirely if not relevant to the position you are seeking.

Résumé Styles

Various résumé styles have been developed, each having specific résumé and disadvantages. You will want to choose the style or combination of styles that best describes your strengths and ability to do the job. It may be to your advantage to check with the human resources department of the facility to which you are applying to see if there is a résumé style preference.

Chronologic Résumé. Your **chronologic résumé** should be organized so the most important information you want to share is the first thing the reader sees. If your job experience is your greatest asset and may set you apart from other applicants, put your work history and job skills first. If your education and training is your best professional feature, put your education and training first. Some medical managers and human resources directors only take 10 seconds to scan

---

ASHLEY JACKSON, CMA
2031 Craig Street ~ Renton, Washington 98055

Work: 206-878-1545   Cell: 206-835-9879
Home: 253-838-6690   e-mail: asjack@pinetree.com

WORK EXPERIENCE

September, 1999-Present   GROUP HEALTH COOPERATIVE
    Directed support for a dermatology/surgery practice.
    Patient preparation.
    Medical and surgical asepsis.
    Assist with sterile procedures.
    Patient follow-up.

June, 1997-August, 1999   VALLEY INTERNAL MEDICINE
    Clinical responsibilities.
    Assisted with surgeries in ambulatory care setting.
    Patient preparation.
    Medical and surgical asepsis.
    Assisted with sterile procedures.

March, 1997-June, 1997   VALLEY INTERNAL MEDICINE
    Medical Assistant Externship
        Administrative duties and clinical responsibilities utilizing all medi-
        cal assisting skills, including patient induction, chief complaint, vital
        signs, patient preparation, EKGs, medical and surgical asepsis, and
        sterile procedures.

EDUCATION/CERTIFICATION

    Associate in Applied Science degree, June, 1997, Highline Community College,
    Des Moines, Washington, 98198-9800.

    Certified Medical Assistant, June, 1997.

Figure 25-4   Sample chronological résumé.

a résumé. You want them to see clearly and quickly what you have to offer.

The chronologic résumé is advantageous when:

- The position is in a highly traditional field, such as teaching, law, or health care, where specific employers are of paramount interest
- You are staying in the same field as prior jobs
- Job history shows real growth and development
- Prior titles are impressive

The chronologic résumé is *not* advantageous when:

- Your work history is spotty
- You are changing career goals

- You have been in the same job for many years
- You are looking for your first job

Figure 25-4 is an illustration of a chronologic résumé.

Functional Résumé. The **functional résumé** highlights specialty areas of accomplishment and strengths. It allows you to organize these in an order that supports your work objective.

The functional résumé is advantageous when:

- Your experience can be sorted into areas of function; i.e., administrative, clinical, supervisory
- You are changing careers

- You are reentering the job market after an absence

- Your career path or growth is not clear from a chronologic listing

- You have had a variety of different, apparently unconnected work experiences

- Much of your work has been volunteer, freelance, or temporary

- You want to eliminate repetition of descriptions of job duties

- You have extensive specialized experience

The functional résumé is *not* advantageous when:

- You want to emphasize a management growth pattern

- Your most recent employers have been highly prestigious and the specific employers are of paramount interest

A sample of a functional résumé for a person reentering the job market is shown in Figure 25-5.

Targeted Résumé. The **targeted résumé** is best for focusing on a clear, specific job target. It should contain a

---

JOAN BISHOP, RMA
4320 Sprig Street
Renton, Washington 98055

Work: 206-878-1545   Cell: 206-835-9879
Home: 253-838-6690   e-mail: jbishop@abc.net

TEACHING:

Instructed community groups on issues related to child abuse.

Taught volunteers how to set up community program for victims of domestic violence.

Conducted workshops for parents of abused children.

Instructed public school teachers on signs and symptoms of potential and actual child abuse.

COUNSELING:

Consulted with parents for probable child abuse and suggested courses of action.

Worked with social workers on individual cases, in both urban and suburban settings.

Counseled single parents on appropriate coping behaviors.

Handled pre-take interviewing of many individual abused children.

ORGANIZATION/COORDINATION:

Coordinated transition of children between original home and foster home.

Served as liaison between community health agencies and schools.

Wrote proposal to state for county funds to educate single parents and teachers.

WORK HISTORY:

| 1998–2000 | Community Mental Health Center, Tacoma, Washington Volunteer Coordinator—Child Abuse Program |
| 2000–2003 | C.A.R.E.—Child-Abuse Rescue-Education, Trenton, New Jersey County Representative |

EDUCATION:

| 1998 | B.S. Sociology, Douglass College, New Brunswick, New Jersey |

Figure 25-5 Sample functional résumé; this style is useful for a person reentering the job market.

career objective and list your skills, capabilities, and any supporting accomplishments related to that objective. Graduating students will find this résumé style enables them to list classes related to their career objective, grade point average, student awards, and achievements. This information adds substance to a résumé when work experience is minimal and should be at the beginning of the résumé because it is your most significant asset.

The targeted résumé is advantageous when:

- You are very clear about your job target

- You have had a variety of experiences that appear unrelated to each other, but that include skills that you can use in a skills list related to your job target

- You can go in several directions and want a different résumé for each

- You are just starting your career and have little experience, but know what you want and are clear about your capabilities

- You are able to keep your résumé on a computer disk

The targeted résumé is *not* advantageous when:

- You want to use one résumé for several different applications

- You are not clear about your abilities and accomplishments

Figure 25-6 provides a sample of a targeted résumé.

ASHLEY JACKSON, CMA
2031 Craig Street ~ Renton, Washington 98055

Work: 206-878-1545   Cell: 206-835-9879
Home: 253-838-6690   e-mail: asjack@pinetree.com

CAREER OBJECTIVES: To obtain a challenging position as a medical assistant in an ambulatory care/surgery facility.

ACHIEVEMENTS:
Certified Medical Assistant.
Graduate of an Accredited Medical Assistant Program.
Experienced in providing assistance with surgeries in an ambulatory care setting.
Excellent communication and interpersonal skills.

SKILLS AND CAPABILITIES:
Post-surgery patient follow-up.
Patient induction.
Vital Signs.
Patient preparation.
EKGs.
Medical and surgical asepsis.
Sterile procedures.

WORK HISTORY:

September, 1996 to present	Group Health Cooperative, Seattle, WA Surgical Medical Assistant.
June, 1994-August, 1996	Valley Internal Medicine, Renton, WA Clinical Medical Assistant.
March 1994-June, 1994	Valley Internal Medicine, Renton, WA Externship Student/Trainee.

EDUCATION/CERTIFICATION:
Associate in Applied Science Degree, Highline Community College.
Certified Medical Assistant.

AFFILIATIONS:
American Association of Medical Assistants.

Figure 25-6   Sample targeted résumé; this style is useful when focusing on a specific job target.

E-Résumé. An electronic résumé, also known as an **e-résumé,** may be electronically delivered via e-mail, submitted to Internet job boards, or placed on Web pages. When employers post jobs on their own Web sites, they generally expect job seekers to respond electronically.

Special care must be taken when preparing the e-résumé because many employers place résumés directly into searchable databases. The following are some points to consider:

- Formatting must be removed before the résumé can be placed in a database. Submitting a formatted résumé may cause it to be eliminated.

- Submit a text résumé, also known as a text-based résumé, plain-text résumé, or ASCII text résumé. These variations are preferred when submitting résumés electronically.

- The e-résumé is not visually appealing. Eye appeal is not required because its main purpose is to be placed into one of the keyword-searchable databases.

- The text résumé is not vulnerable to viruses and is compatible across computer programs and platforms.

- The text résumé is versatile and may be used for:
  - Posting on job boards
  - Pasting piece-by-piece into the profile forms of job boards, such as Monster.com
  - Pasting into the body of an e-mail to be sent to prospective employers
  - Converting to a Web-based HTML résumé
  - Sending as an attachment to prospective employers
  - Conversion to a scannable résumé

Employers are often inundated with résumés from job seekers each time they advertise a position opening. Therefore, in an effort to save time and to determine the best-qualified candidates for the position, employers digitize the résumés to create an electronic résumé. Using software to search for specific **keywords** that relate to the position, the numbers of candidates can quickly be narrowed. If you apply for a job with a company that searches databases for keywords and your résumé does not conform, you may not be considered for the position.

How do you determine keywords? Begin scrutinizing employment ads and list keywords repeatedly mentioned in association with jobs that interest you. Nouns that relate to the skills and experience the employer is looking for will quickly surface. Keywords may include:

- Job specific skills/profession-specific words (e.g., specialty experience, bilingual, scheduling, data entry, insurance verification, telephone and communication skills, laboratory/X-ray experience)

- Technologic terms and descriptions of technical expertise (including hardware and software in which you are proficient; e.g., PRISM, DEXA experience)

- Job titles, certifications (e.g., MA, CMA, RMA, CMAS, Biller, Coder)

- Types of degrees, names of colleges (e.g., AAS, BA)

- Awards received, professional organization memberships (e.g., Dean's list, scholarships, certificates, AAMA or AMT member)

Keywords should be used throughout the résumé, however it should be front loaded. Front loaded means to use as many keywords as possible in the first 100 words of the résumé. A good goal is to aim for 25 to 35 keywords. This may be achieved by using synonyms, various forms of the keyword, and using both the spelled-out and acronym versions of common terms. If a person reviews the résumé, he or she will see enough keywords to process it through the software search.

Vital Résumé Information

All résumé styles must contain certain vital information about the job applicant. Essential information includes:

- Your full name and credential, address including street number, city, state, and zip code.

- Your telephone number or a number where a message may be left. The telephone selected should be one you are confident will be answered in a professional manner. Always include the area code with the number.

- Your e-mail address.

- Your education. Begin with the most recent school attended and include the name, address, and graduation date with the diploma, certificate, or degree earned.

- Work experience. List company name and address. Do not underestimate the value of any job; relate transferable skills to your career objective.

- Skills that are necessary for the job. The list may be completed from your program curriculum. Be careful not to list course titles that have no meaning to the reader. It is much better to list the skills obtained in courses.

APPLICATION/COVER LETTERS

The **application/cover letter** is a means of introducing yourself and submitting your résumé to a potential employer with the goal of obtaining an interview. A well-written cover letter will highlight your qualifications and experience for employment and will enhance the information contained within your résumé. The letter should follow a standard business style and should not be more than one page in length. It should be printed on the same paper as the résumé.

Because this may be your first contact with a potential employer, the letter should sell you and describe your intentions regarding employment, display your personality, and create an interest in reading your enclosed résumé.

Some guidelines to follow in writing the application/cover letter include:

1. Address your letter to a specific individual whenever possible. You may need to make a telephone call to obtain the name, title, and correct spelling.
2. Keep the letter concise, use correct grammar and spelling, and follow standard business letter format.
3. The first paragraph should state your reason for writing and focus the reader's attention. It should not give as a reason "in response to a help wanted ad."
4. The second paragraph should identify how your education, experience, and qualifications relate to the job and refer to the enclosed résumé.
5. The last paragraph should close with a request for an interview.
6. Do not reproduce cover letters. An original letter should be sent to each individual.
7. The cover letter should be placed on top of the résumé and mailed in a business size envelope that matches its contents or in an 8½ × 11 manila envelope containing your return address.
8. Do not staple the cover letter to the résumé.

A sample of an application/cover letter is shown in Figure 25-7A.

An alternate example of an application/cover letter using Information Mapping® to highlight and draw attention to specific information in your letter is shown in Figure 25-7B. This format is considered easier to read because the focus is on specific blocks of information. In addition, its uniqueness draws attention to your letter and may result in your being selected when competition is keen.

COMPLETING THE APPLICATION FORM

Sooner or later during the job search you will be asked to complete an **application form.** How well you complete this task may be a key factor in obtaining an interview and that first job.

Reading through the application form questions, you may be tempted to write in "See résumé" rather than repeat pertinent information already contained within your résumé. Do not fall into this pitfall. Answer every item completely. The application is organized in the manner that suites the clinic, whereas individual résumés are organized in a variety of ways. Finding specific information on a résumé is more time consuming for the clinic, whereas finding the same information on the job application is easy and quick because they know where to look for it. Read all the directions carefully. Look for seemingly insignificant directions placed at the top or-bottom of the page that state "Print Carefully," "Complete in Your Own Handwriting," or "Please Type." Employers may use this to assess your ability to read and follow directions and pay attention to detail.

If the application is to be handwritten, use black ink to complete the form. Black ink is considered legal and often is an indelible (permanent) ink and is more legible if the form must be duplicated. Concentrate when completing the form and be sure to print clearly and make no errors. When possible, copy the application before beginning in case an error is made.

The current trend is toward on-line application forms. These forms are prepared by keying information into the appropriate spaces or blocks by using a computer. The completed forms may then be printed and mailed to the perspective employer or sent electronically. Sending electronically is increasingly the preferred method. All of the concerns relative to care in following instructions, providing complete and accurate information, and proofing the application for any errors before sending are applicable.

If you are asked to list experience but the application does not specify "paid experience," be sure to list any volunteer or externship experience that relates to the position you are seeking. Part-time employment can be important as an indicator of your willingness to work, your ability to serve the public, and your organizational skills.

You may be asked to complete the application form "on the spot." Plan ahead for this event and

2031 Craig Street
Renton, Washington 98055
August 22, 20XX

Sarah Molles, Manager
Seattle Group Health Cooperative
304 Fourth Avenue
Seattle, Washington 98124-1716

Dear Ms. Molles:

I am interested in the medical assistant position to assist in a dermatology surgery practice. I meet the qualifications and would like to be considered for the position.

I am currently a certified medical assistant graduated from a two-year accredited program. I have experience as a clinical assistant in an internal medicine clinic and have excellent communication and interpersonal skills.

I will be available Tuesday and Thursday afternoon from 1:00 p.m. to 4:00 p.m. I will call you next Thursday to set up an appointment for an interview.

Yours truly,

Ashley Jackson, CMA

Enclosure, Résumé

Figure 25-7A Sample application/cover letter.

carry a completed copy of your résumé, reference list, and application/cover letter with you. Information not included in your résumé, such as which years you attended high school and your salary history, should also be carried with you. These documents should provide all the information needed to complete the application form and may be submitted with the application form. This demonstrates to the potential employer your seriousness and preparedness for finding a job.

THE INTERVIEW PROCESS

If your application/cover letter, résumé, and application have made a favorable impression with the organization, you may be invited for an interview. An **interview** is a meeting in which you and the interviewer discuss the employment opportunities within that particular organization. It will be the interviewer's responsibility to determine if you have the personality, education, and skills to perform the job. The interviewer will use the interview process to access appearance, attitude, and dependability. They will also try to verify that you have been honest in the skills you claim to have mastered. You, on the other hand, will be selling your qualifications and assessing if this is an organization in which you want to be employed.

Being well prepared for the interview will increase your self-confidence and ability to focus during the actual interview. Knowing that your application/cover letter, résumé, and references all support your career goal and objectives allows you time to concentrate on interview preparation and presentation.

2031 Craig Street
Renton, Washington 98055
August 22, 2005

Sarah Molles, Manager
Seattle Group Health Cooperative
304 Fourth Avenue
Seattle, Washington 98124-1716

SUBJECT: SURGICAL MEDICAL ASSISTANT POSITION

Background	I am interested in the medical assistant position to assist in a dermatology surgery practice. I meet the qualifications and would like to be considered for the position.
Qualifications	I am currently a certified medical assistant graduated from a two-year accredited program. I have experience as a clinical assistant in an internal medicine clinic and have excellent communication and interpersonal skills.
Requested Action	I will be available Tuesday and Thursday afternoon from 1:00 p.m. to 4:00 p.m. I will call you next Thursday to set up an appointment for an interview.

Yours truly,

Ashley Jackson, CMA

Enclosure, Résumé

Figure 25-7B   Sample information mapped letter.

The Look of Success

 The look of success begins with the outward appearance. First impressions are lasting, so strive for a favorable, professional look from head to toe. Appropriate conservative attire is important. Remember, your goal is to sell your professional abilities.

Hair should be clean, and healthy looking, and worn in an appropriate style for the ambulatory care setting. Long hair should be worn off the collar in perhaps a French braid or twist. Strive for a neat, professional style.

The skin should have a healthy glow. Consultation with a cosmetician may prove helpful in solving skin problems or provide opportunity for trying new products. A basic understanding of your personal skin type and selection of cosmetics that complement your skin tone aid in the presentation of a professional appearance. The natural look is most appropriate for the medical office.

A daily shower and use of personal hygiene products is advised. Remember to use caution where perfumes and scents are concerned because many magnify when the body is under stress and the scent may be offensive or cause allergic reactions in others. Smokers should be aware that smoke odor carries in their hair, skin, and clothing. This odor may not be accaptable in health care settings.

Fingernails should be short and oval shaped or have rounded corners. Only clear nail polish should be worn in the ambulatory care setting if you are not working in the clinical area. Nail polish that is chipped or cracked must be removed or replaced immediately because it creates crevices in which pathogens may hide, multiply, and spread.

First impressions are lasting, so make yours professional in all respects. Conservative business attire is appropriate. A tailored suit for both men and women is effective in portraying a professional image. Pay attention to details such as your accessories and shoe selection. Accessories should be small and tasteful. Shoes should be clean, polished, and in good repair. They should fit properly and be comfortable and easy to walk in (Figure 25-8).

The purse should be neat and small; the briefcase should be of a slip-in type that does not require a flat surface to open. Both should be in good repair. A portfolio is recommended in which to keep an extra copy of your résumé, reference list, application, and cover letter. A pen

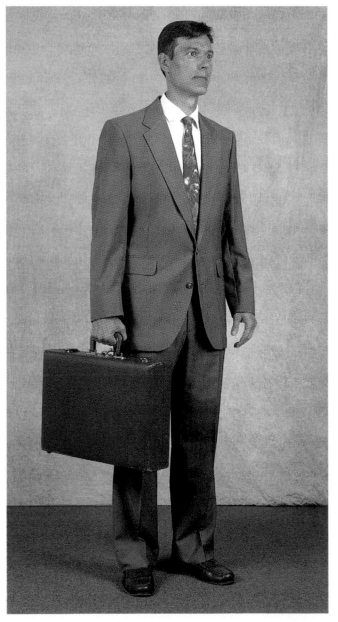

Figure 25-8 Medical assistant appropriately dressed and prepared for the interview.

Critical Thinking

If you are a smoker, how can you minimize the smoke odor carried on your person before you go on a job interview? Make a list and prioritize each suggestion into a plan of action.

should be handy. Do not plan to search in either a purse or a briefcase for a pen or papers, keys, and so forth. Also, be sure that your cell phone has been turned off before entering the clinic.

When you feel well and know that you look good, you project a confident and professional appearance. In other words, you are professionally poised. Webster's dictionary defines *poise* as balance and stability; ease and dignity of manner. Personal poise combines all of the previously mentioned body appearances plus smoothness of movement and physical flexibility.

Preparing for the Interview

Before the interview takes place, you will want to study carefully the organization for which you are interviewing. Be prepared to relate your skills and interests to the needs of this organization. In other words, what can you contribute and why should they hire you? The interview is your opportunity to sell yourself and identify ways in which you can benefit the employer.

A copy of your résumé and cover letter should be brought to the interview just in case the interviewer can not locate the original or wants another copy. You should also have copies of letters of recommendation, a list of references, a copy of your transcript from the schools you attended, and copies of any certificates such as AIDS training, First Aid, and CPR. These items should not be presented unless dictated by events that take place during the interview. You might also have with you the name of the interviewer and a copy of any questions you plan to ask the interviewer. A last-minute review will refocus your thoughts before you go into the interview. You could also keep your list available for quick reference in the event that your mind goes blank when you are asked if you have questions.

To arrive 5 to 10 minutes early, you may need to check a map for directions or make a trip the day before your interview. Try to travel about the same time as you would for the interview so you have an idea of the time it takes, traffic flow, construction areas encountered, and parking availability. Plan for inclement weather (raincoat, umbrella, shoes, and so forth). It is a good idea to make a quick trip to the restroom on arrival to change shoes or recheck your appearance.

Introduce yourself confidently to the receptionist and identify by name the person you wish to see and the time of your appointment. Always arrive alone. The employer wants to see you and sense your self-reliance and responsibility. While you wait, try to relax and observe the office setting, other employees, what they are wearing, and their manner of conducting business. This may be helpful to you during the interview and in making a decision to work there.

Review Figure 25-9 for reasons employers do not hire applicants.

The Actual Interview

When you enter an interviewer's office, think of yourself as a guest and take your cues from him or her. Most interviewers will introduce themselves and extend a hand. A firm handshake, responding by introducing yourself, and smiling confidently convey a positive professional image. Remain standing until you are invited to be seated. Keep your personal items on your lap or place them on the floor near your chair. Do not invade the interviewer's territory by placing your things on the desk.

Sit erect in the chair with your feet flat on the floor or cross only your ankles. Avoid nervous mannerisms while you speak and maintain good eye contact, but do not stare the interviewer down. Be natural and positive about the position, organization, and yourself. Present a professional image by using medical terminology when responding to questions or providing information. Observe the interviewer carefully for cues. Respond to questions completely, trying not to repeat yourself or give more information than was requested.

Be prepared for the kinds of questions that may be asked during the interview process. Ask yourself, "If I were the employer, what would I want to know about the applicant?" Figure 25-10 contains examples of standard questions asked by most employers. Consider how you would respond to each question.

Remember that the interviewer is asking questions to determine if you are qualified for the position and if

---

REASONS FOR EMPLOYERS NOT HIRING

Employers in business were asked to list reasons for not hiring a job seeker. Given in rank order (from most unwanted to least unwanted), the 15 biggest gripes are as follows:

1. Poor appearance (not dressed properly, poorly groomed).
2. Acting like a know-it-all.
3. Cannot express self clearly; poor voice, diction, grammar.
4. Lack of planning for work—no purpose or goals.
5. Lack of confidence or poise.
6. No interest in or enthusiasm for the job.
7. Not active in school extracurricular programs.
8. Interested only in the best dollar offer.
9. Poor school record (academic, attendance).
10. Unwilling to start at the bottom.
11. Making excuses, hedges on unfavorable record.
12. No tact.
13. Not mature.
14. No curiosity about the job.
15. Critical of past employers.

Figure 25-9 Reasons for employers not hiring.
(Courtesy of Highline Community College, Counseling/Career Center, Des Moines, WA).

TYPICAL QUESTIONS ASKED DURING AN INTERVIEW

1. I see from your résumé you graduated from _____ college. What did that college have to offer that others didn't?
2. What subjects did you enjoy the most and why?
3. What do you see yourself doing five years from now?
4. What salary do you expect and what do you think it will be in five or ten years?
5. What do you consider to be your greatest strengths and weaknesses?
6. How do you think a friend or professor who knows you well would describe you?
7. What qualifications do you have that make you think you would be successful in this position?
8. In what ways do you think you can make a contribution to our organization?
9. What two or three accomplishments have given you the most satisfaction?
10. What didn't you like about your last employer?
11. How well do you work under pressure?
12. Will you be able to work overtime occasionally?
13. How do you respond to criticism?
14. How would you respond if a patient or co-worker made advances toward you?
15. How would you handle following procedures with which you do not agree?
16. Describe a specific medical procedure.
17. Do you have any questions you would like to ask?

Figure 25-10 Knowing how you would answer some of these typical questions can prepare you for your interview.

you are the kind of person that will fit into the organization. *Think* before answering questions; try to provide the information requested in a positive and professional manner. *Listen* carefully so that you understand what information the question is requesting. *Ask* for clarification if you are uncertain. This demonstrates your ability to be open enough to ask questions when in doubt.

Closing the Interview

By observing the interviewer and listening carefully, you will be able to determine when the interviewer feels he or she has enough information about you to make a decision. Usually during the closing the interviewer will ask if you have any additional questions. This is your opportunity to collect information helpful in making a decision to accept or decline an offer. Your questions provide another opportunity to sell yourself, show that you have done your homework about the organization, and have listened carefully during the interview. Select three or four questions that will help you the most.

Questions about the organization are excellent choices. Examples might be:

- "What are the opportunities for advancement with this organization?"

- "I read that your organization has educational benefits. Could you explain briefly how that program works?"

- "You mentioned in-house training programs for employees. Could you give one or two examples?"

You may also have some questions about the job itself. Examples of these types of questions are:

- "Is this a newly created position? If so, what results are you hoping to see?"

- "Was the last person in this position promoted? What contributed to their advancement?"

- "What do you consider the most difficult task on this job?"

- "What are the lines of authority for this position?"

Do not use this question time to ask about salary, sick leave, vacations, or retirement benefits. At this point, your focus should be on the value and skills you can contribute to the organization. These questions may be asked during a second interview or when a position is offered.

Before you leave, thank the interviewer for taking time to discuss the position with you. If you definitely are interested in the position, ask to be considered as a candidate for the position. If follow-up procedures have not been explained, now is the time to ask when the final selection will be made and how you will be notified. A firm handshake as you leave, a pleasant smile, and confidence as you exit will leave a professional picture in the interviewer's mind.

INTERVIEW FOLLOW-UP

Following up after the interview is essential. This is the time to telephone your references to let them know the name of the organization and the person's name with whom you interviewed, something about the position, and your qualifications. Share any information that will help your references support you in obtaining the position.

Follow-Up Letter

Take time to write a follow-up letter or handwritten note to the interviewer a day or two after your interview to thank them for the time spent interviewing you. The letter should be written in standard business format and printed on the same paper as your application/cover letter and résumé. Be sure that all spelling and grammar are correct.

The follow-up letter provides another opportunity to express your interest in the organization and the position. You can briefly emphasize the experience and skills you have to offer and again request being considered a candidate for the position.

Record the mailing date on your contact tracker and keep a copy of the letter in a file with other information about the organization. Figure 25-11 is a sample follow-up letter.

Follow Up by Telephone

Allow a few days for your follow-up letter to reach the interviewer. If you do not hear from the interviewer within a week or by the designated time established during the interview, you may telephone to ask if you are still being considered for the position or if a decision has been made.

Speak directly into the mouthpiece of the telephone using good diction and voice volume. Identify yourself and provide some information to aid the interviewer in recalling who you are. Perhaps mentioning the date you interviewed will suffice. Be polite and professional and remember to thank the individual for speaking with you. At the end of the conversation say good-bye and wait until the other person hangs up before you break the connection. Log the telephone call and its response on your contact tracker for future reference.

2031 Craig Street
Renton, Washington 98055
August 28, 20XX

Sarah Molles, Manager
Seattle Group Health Cooperative
304 Fourth Avenue
Seattle, Washington 98124-1716

Dear Ms. Molles,

Thank you for scheduling a personal interview with me last Wednesday, August 26, at 9:45 AM. I enjoyed discussing the medical assistant position open in one of your dermatology surgery practices. I would like to be considered for the position.

After talking with you, I feel my qualifications match closely with those you requested. My communication and interpersonal skills are excellent and a necessary ingredient for any medical assistant.

I look forward to hearing from you September 5 as you mentioned during the interview. If there are any questions I may answer, please telephone me.

Sincerely,

Ashley Jackson

Ashley Jackson, CMA
(206) 255-1365

Figure 25-11   Sample follow-up letter.

PROFESSIONALISM AND EMPLOYMENT STRATEGIES

 Areas of professionalism directly related to the medical office may include:

- Display a professional manner and image. The chapter content stresses the importance of having a positive attitude, taking pride in doing the best you can, being prepared, and dressing appropriately for job interviews.

- Promote your CMA/RMA or CMAS credential. On graduation from an accredited school, you will be ready to sit for the national certification examination. On notification of passing the exami-

nation, you will be awarded the appropriate credential. When signing your name, include your credential as well and educate others regarding its significance.

Critical Thinking

As you begin to prepare for a job interview, how can you prepare yourself to reflect a professional image, attitude, demeanor, verbal and nonverbal communication skills, as well as articulately describe your skills and abilities to fit the position to which you are applying? Develop a complete written checklist and review it before an interview.

Case Study 25-1

Eun Mee Soo is a recent graduate of an accredited medical assisting program and has no medical work experience except her externship at Inner City Health Care. Eun Mee has been employed part-time as a sales representative (clerk) in one of the city's prestigious clothing stores while she attended school.

CASE STUDY REVIEW

1. Which résumé style would represent Eun Mee best and why?
2. What information should Eun Mee provide in the vital information section of the résumé?
3. What is the purpose of an accomplishment statement? Provide an example of one that Eun Mee might use.

Case Study 25-2

Drs. Lewis and King maintain a two-doctor family physicians' office. They are in need of a new medical assistant to take the place of one who will be leaving at the end of the month. They have established interviews with five applicants. Eun Mee Soo is the first candidate to be interviewed.

CASE STUDY REVIEW

1. Eun Mee enters the interview with some papers in her hand. What paperwork should she have brought with her?
2. Why should Eun Mee arrive 5 to 10 minutes early for the interview?
3. How should Eun Mee enter the room?

SUMMARY

Finding your first job is your first job. How well you research, plan, prepare, and implement your tasks will make the difference between being hired or not being hired. Learn from each interview session. Listen to the questions that were asked and formulate answers that you feel would be appropriate for your next interview. Tell everyone you are looking for a job and solicit their help. Follow up on all leads and do not become discouraged.

Once you have been hired at that first job, continue your learning experience. Ask appropriate questions and try not to ask the same question a second or third time. Pay attention to details and learn individual preferences. Become a team player and look for ways you can help others. Carry your share of responsibility and do not be afraid to admit you are unfamiliar with certain aspects of the office. Employers need to know you can be trusted to work within the scope of your education and not beyond. Practice being an asset to your employer.

STUDY FOR SUCCESS

To reinforce your knowledge and skills of information presented in this chapter:

- ❏ Review the Key Terms
- ❏ Consider the Case Studies and discuss your conclusions
- ❏ Answer the Review Questions
  - ❏ Multiple Choice
  - ❏ Critical Thinking
- ❏ Navigate the Internet by completing the Web Activities

- ❏ Practice the StudyWARE activities on the textbook CD
- ❏ Apply your knowledge in the Student Workbook activities
- ❏ Complete the Web Tutor sections
- ❏ View and discuss the DVD situations

REVIEW QUESTIONS

Multiple Choice

1. The résumé:
   a. is a summary data sheet or brief account of your qualifications and progress in your career
   b. is also known as a contact tracker
   c. always includes references
   d. is used to introduce yourself and identify qualifications

2. References:
   a. must always be listed on the résumé
   b. should be a relative
   c. should be someone who likes you and your work but may not be a good communicator
   d. should be someone who knows you or has worked with you long enough to make an honest assessment of your capabilities and integrity

3. The targeted résumé is advantageous:
   a. when prior titles are impressive
   b. when reentering the job market after an absence
   c. when you are just starting your career and have little experience
   d. when you have extensive specialized experience

4. The application/cover letter is:
   a. a detailed data sheet describing your vital information, education, and experience
   b. introduces you to a prospective employer and captures their interest in you as a candidate for the position
   c. lists individuals who can vouch for you
   d. should be lengthy and detailed

5. The interview:
   a. does not require much thought or preparation
   b. requires you to think before answering questions, listen carefully, and ask for clarification if uncertain of the question
   c. provides time to ask questions about salary, vacation, and benefits
   d. does not require any follow-up
6. Preparing for the interview:
   a. bathe yourself, groom your hair and fingernails, and wear clean and pressed conservative business attire
   b. allow adequate time to get to the interview
   c. prepare a packet to give the interviewer containing certificates, letters of recommendation, a list of references, and your list of questions
   d. a, b, and c
7. Job analysis should include:
   a. compiling a list of potential employers
   b. gathering information about employers in whom you have interest
   c. preparing a budgetary needs analysis
   d. all of the above
8. The best source for job search data is:
   a. the Internet
   b. friends and acquaintances
   c. the yellow pages and classified ads
   d. all of the above

Critical Thinking

1. Discuss the various résumé styles with a classmate and how to determine which style will best present your knowledge and skills to a prospective employer?
2. After reading the section discussing methods of researching a prospective employer, how will you proceed with your research?
3. Review Figure 25-9, which lists reasons for employers not hiring, with a classmate. How will you prevent the 15 biggest gripes from being an employment stumbling block for you personally?
4. How will you prepare a budget for living expenses to determine job salary requirements?
5. Sometimes employers may ask illegal or inappropriate questions during an interview in true innocence, or true ignorance. Give a legal reason why

an employer might need the following information once you have been hired.
   a. Are you married?
   b. How many kids do you have?
   c. How old are you?
   d. Where were you born?

1. Being prepared to answer and discuss interview questions is critical in the selection for the position opening. Using Google.com, or your favorite search engine, search job interview questions. Many sites will provide sample questions and appropriate answers. Study these and prepare a list of questions with personal responses you feel are appropriate.
2. There are some illegal interview questions based on Federal Discrimination Laws enforced by the Equal Employment Opportunity Commission. They are questions that specifically discriminate against you on the basis of:
   - Age
   - Color
   - Disability
   - Sex
   - National origin
   - Race, religion, or creed

Using your favorite search engine, research these inappropriate questions and ways in which you might handle them appropriately. Compile a list of questions and your personal appropriate response to each. Discuss these with a classmate and role-play responding to the questions.

REFERENCES/BIBLIOGRAPHY

Farr, M. (2000). *Quick resume & cover letter book.* Indianapolis, IN: JIST Works, Inc.

Noble, D. F. (2000). *Gallery of best resumes for people without a four-year degree.* Indianapolis, IN: JIST Works, Inc.

Washington, T. (2000). *Resume power selling yourself on paper in the new millennium.* Indianapolis, IN: JIST Works, Inc.

THE DVD HOOK-UP

DVD Series	Program Number
Critical Thinking	1

Chapter/Scene Reference
• *Preparing for a Job*

This chapter discusses strategies that you can use to help gain employment.

One of the first testimonials in this scene showed Paula talking about the fact that she can determine a person's professionalism within five minutes of the interview.

1. Do you really think that it is possible to gauge a person's professionalism within five minutes of an interview?
2. What do you think about the outfit that Dee was wearing for her interview? Do you think it was professional?
3. What will you wear for your interviews when you apply for a medical assisting position?

DVD Journal Summary

Write a paragraph that summarizes what you learned from watching the selected scenes from today's DVD program. Using a scale of 1 to 10, how would you have rated your professionalism skills when you started the program? How would you rate your professional skills now that you have almost completed with the program? What improvements do you need to make to be the best possible medical assistant you can be?

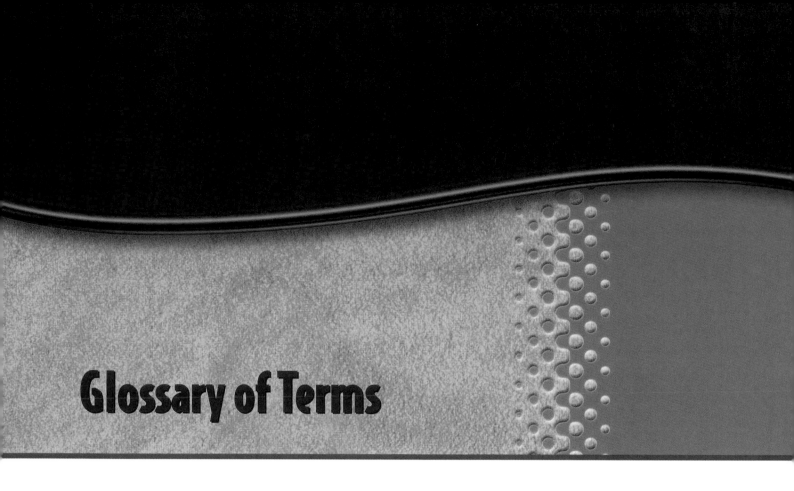

Glossary of Terms

abuse misuse; excessive or improper use, especially of narcotics or psychoactive drugs (Ch. 18).

accession record (numeric system) logbook used to assign numbers to correspondence or patients (Ch. 14).

accomplishment statements statements that begin with a power verb and give a brief description of what you did, and the demonstrable results that were produced (Ch. 25).

accounting system of monitoring the financial status of a facility and the financial results of its activities, providing information for decision making (Ch. 21).

accounts payable sum owed by a business for services or goods received (Ch. 17); also unwritten promise to pay a supplier for property or merchandise purchased on credit or for a service rendered (Ch. 21).

accounts receivable amount owed to a business for services or goods supplied (Ch. 17).

accounts receivable (A/R) ratio assets outstanding accounts receivable divided by the average monthly gross income for the past 12 months (Ch. 20, 21).

accreditation process whereby recognition is granted to an educational program for maintaining standards that qualify its graduates for professional practice; to provide with credentials (Ch. 1).

Accrediting Bureau of Health Education Schools (ABHES) entity accrediting institutions for the American Medical Technologists (Ch. 24).

accrual basis accounting reports income at the time charges are generated (Ch. 21).

acquired immunodeficiency syndrome (AIDS) disorder of the immune system caused by a human immunodeficiency virus (HIV), a retrovirus that destroys the body's ability to fight infection. As the disease progresses, the individual becomes overcome by disorders, including cancers and opportunistic infections. There is no known cure for AIDS (Ch. 22).

active listening received message is paraphrased back to the sender to verify the correct message was decoded (Ch. 4).

acupuncture treatment to relieve pain and disease by puncturing the skin with thin needles at specific points (Ch. 2).

adjustments increases or decreases to patient accounts not due to charges incurred or payments received (Ch. 17).

administer to give a medication (Ch. 7).

administrative law establishes agencies that are given the power to make laws and enact regulations (Ch. 7).

agenda printed list of topics to be discussed during a meeting, sometimes giving time allocation (Ch. 15, 22).

agent person representing another (Ch. 7).

algorithm a special method for solving a specific kind of problem (Ch. 11).

allopathic method of treating disease with remedies that produce effects different from those caused by the disease itself. Most traditional physicians today are considered allopathic physicians (Ch. 3).

alternative dispute resolution (ADR) an alternative to trial that encourages the parties to settle their differences out of court (Ch. 7).

Ambu Bag™ a brand name for a bag placed over nose and mouth to assist in providing artificial ventilation to the lungs (Ch. 9).

ambulatory care setting health care environment where services are provided on an outpatient basis. Ambulatory is from the Latin and means "capable of walking." Examples include the solo-physician's office, the group practice, the urgent care center, and the health maintenance organization (Ch. 1, 2).

American Association for Medical Transcription (AAMT) nonprofit organization founded by medical transcriptionists to promote the profession (Ch. 16).

American Association of Medical Assistants (AAMA) professional organization dedicated to serving the interests of Certified Medical Assistants (Ch. 24).

American Medical Technologists (AMT) national organization which certifies health care professionals, including Registered Medical Assistants and Certified Medical Administrative Specialists (Ch. 24).

anaphylaxis hypersensitive state of the body to a foreign protein or drug (Ch. 9).

ancillary services professional occupational companies hired to complete a specific job (Ch. 22).

answering services services employed to answer the calls of an ambulatory care setting after hours; unlike an answering machine, a live operator answers the call and forwards it appropriately (Ch. 12).

antiglare screen a filter put over the screen of a computer monitor to reduce glare (Ch. 11).

application/cover letter letter used to introduce yourself and your résumé to a prospective employer with the goal of obtaining an interview (Ch. 25).

application form form devised by a prospective employer to collect information relative to qualifications, education, and experience in employment (Ch. 25).

application software software that performs a specific data-processing function (Ch. 11).

arbitration a form of dispute resolution that allows a neutral party to settle the dispute (Ch. 7).

articulating expressing oneself clearly and distinctly (Ch. 12).

asepsis protecting against infection caused by pathogenic microorganisms (Ch. 3).

assets properties of value that are owned by a business entity (Ch. 21).

assignment of benefits signing over of benefits by the beneficiary to another party (Ch. 18).

attribute inherent characteristic (Ch. 1).

authentication dictates physician signs or authenticates the document indicating that the information was accurate and complete at the time of signing (Ch. 16).

authoritarian manager operates on the premise that most workers cannot make a contribution without being directed (Ch. 22).

automated external defibrillator (AED) portable, self-contained, automatic device with voice instructions on use for individuals in cardiac arrest. It is used externally to electronically "shock" the myocardium into contracting again. Same as cardioversion (Ch. 9).

automated routing unit (ARU) telephone system that answers a call and uses a recorded voice to identify departments or services (Ch. 12).

autopsy report also called an autopsy protocol, a necropsy report, or a medical examiner report. Autopsies are performed to determine the cause of death or to ascertain and confirm disease presence (Ch. 16).

bachelor's degree degree of bachelor conferred by colleges and universities (Ch. 1).

backup copying or saving data to a secure location to prevent loss of data in the event of a disaster (Ch. 11).

balance amount owed (N); to verify posting accuracy (V); records difference between debit and credit columns (Ch. 17).

balance sheet itemized statement of assets, liabilities, and equity; a statement of financial condition (Ch. 21).

bandage nonsterile gauze or other material applied over a sterile dressing to protect and immobilize (Ch. 9).

benchmark making a comparison among different organizations relative to how they accomplish tasks, such as office computerization, organizing file systems, and employee remuneration (Ch. 11, 22).

beneficiary person under a policy eligible to receive benefits (Ch. 18).

benefit remuneration that is in addition to the salary (Ch. 22, 25).

bias slant toward a particular belief (Ch. 4).

bioethics branch of medical ethics concerned with moral issues resulting from high technology and sophisticated medical research. Social issues such as genetic engineering, abortion, and fetal tissue research raise important bioethical questions (Ch. 8).

biometric a type of electronic signature that may use alphanumeric computer key entries as identification, an electronic writing device, or a biometric system using voice, fingerprints, or the retina of the eye (Ch. 16).

birthday rule method to determine which of two or more policies covering a dependent child will be primary; that parent with the birthday falling first in the calendar year has the primary policy (Ch. 18).

blind copy protects the privacy of e-mail. Other recipients cannot identify who else may have received the transmitted message (Ch. 15).

body language nonverbal communication that includes unconscious body movements, gestures, and facial expressions that accompany verbal messages (Ch. 4).

bond binding agreement with an employee ensuring recovery of financial loss should funds be stolen or embezzled (Ch. 22).

bond paper durable, strong paper usually used for correspondence (Ch. 15).

booting everything that happens between the time a computer is turned on to when it is ready to accept input (Ch. 11).

brainstorming process of developing ideas through a synergistic interaction among participants in an environment free of criticism (Ch. 22).

bubonic plague infectious disease with a high fatality rate transmitted to humans from infected rats and ground squirrels by the bite of the rat flea (Ch. 3).

buffer words expendable words used while answering the telephone (Ch. 4, 12).

bullet point asterisk or dot followed by a descriptive phrase; helps the reader identify important points easily (Ch. 25).

bundled codes a grouping of several services are directly related to a specific procedure and are paid as one (Ch. 19).

burnout a state of fatigue or frustration brought about by a devotion to a cause, a way of life, or a relationship that failed to produce the expected reward (Ch. 5).

capitation use of the number of members enrolled in a plan to determine salary of the physician; the physician is paid a fixed fee for each member no matter how many times that member is seen by the physician (Ch. 18).

caption method of designation used on file guides (Ch. 14).

cardiopulmonary resuscitation (CPR) combination of rescue breathing and chest compressions performed by a trained individual on a patient experiencing cardiac arrest (Ch. 9).

cardioversion conversion of a pathological cardiac rhythm (arrhythmia), such as ventricular fibrillation, to normal sinus rhythm (Ch. 9).

career objective expresses your career goal and the position for which you are applying (Ch. 25).

cash basis accounting reports income at the time money is collected (Ch. 21).

cashier's check bank's own check drawn against the bank's account (Ch. 17).

cauterized to destroy tissue through application of a caustic agent, a hot instrument, an electric current, or other agent (Ch. 9).

cellular telephones battery-operated portable telephones that are typically found in automobiles and other unfixed locations. One can receive and send messages from cellular phones (Ch. 12).

Centers for Medicare and Medicaid Services (CMS) formerly known as HCFA. CMS is a Federal agency within the U.S. Department of Health and Human Services (DHHS). The agency administers Medicare, Medicaid, and the State Children's Health Insurance Program (SCHIP). CMS also administers the Health Insurance Portability and Accountability Act of 1996 (HIPAA) and Clinical Laboratory Improvement Act of 1988 (CLIA '88) (Ch. 18).

central processing unit (CPU) brain of the computer that performs instructions defined by software (Ch. 11).

certification guarantees as being true or as represented by or as meeting a standard (Ch. 1).

certification examination standardized means of evaluating medical assistant competency (Ch. 24).

certified check depositor's own check that the bank has indicated with a date and signature to be good for the amount written (Ch. 17).

Certified Medical Assistant (CMA) a medical assistant who has successfully completed the AAMA's national certification examination (Ch. 1, 24).

Certified Medical Transcriptionist (CMT) recognized professional credential obtained through successful completion of both parts of the core certification examination administered by the MTCC at AAMT (Ch. 16).

chart notes (also called progress notes) physician's formal or informal notes about presenting problem, physical findings, and plan for treatment for a patient examined in the office, clinic, acute care center, or emergency department (Ch. 16).

check register record of checks written; categorized into separate and identified columns (Ch. 21).

chief complaint (CC) specific symptom or problem for which the patient is seeing the physician today (Ch. 16).

chronologic résumé résumé format used when you have employment experience (Ch. 25).

civil law law related to actions between individuals (Ch. 7).

claim register diary or register of claims submitted to each insurance carrier. When payment is received, the date and amount of payment is entered in the register (Ch. 19).

clinical e-mail electronic messages sent to or by the physician's office regarding medical questions or advice (Ch. 15).

closed questions questions answered with a yes or no (Ch. 4).

clustering a grouping together of nonverbal messages into statements or conclusions. Can also be used to describe a scheduling system where patients with similar complaint/conditions are scheduled consecutively (example is scheduling all the allergy injections for 3:00 PM to 4:00 PM every Tuesday and Thursday) (Ch. 4).

CMS 1500 formerly known as the HCFA 1500 form that is the office health insurance claim form for Medicare and Medicaid (Ch. 19).

CMS-1500 (12-90) the insurance claim form used to submit claims for reimbursement. Formerly known as the HCFA-1500 (Ch. 19).

coinsurance that percentage paid by the company or that paid by the insured (Ch. 18).

collection ratio gross income divided by the amount that could have been collected less disallowances (Ch. 20, 21).

Commission on Accreditation of Allied Health Education Programs (CAAHEP) entity accrediting institutions for the American Association of Medical Assistants (Ch. 24).

common law refers to laws developed in England and France and brought to the United States by the early settlers; sometimes referred to as judge-made law (Ch. 7).

compact disk (CD) see **optical disk** (Ch. 11).

compensation overemphasizing of characteristics to make up for a real or imagined failure or handicap (Ch. 4).

competency legally qualified or adequate (Ch. 1).

compliance conformity in fulfilling official requirements (Ch. 1).

confidentiality ethical and legal rules in regard to patient privacy (Ch. 16).

confidentiality agreement when signed, the agreement signifies that the medical transcriptionist is committed to keep all patient information confidential (Ch. 16).

conflict resolution solving problems between coworkers or any two parties (Ch. 22).

congruency the verbal message and the nonverbal message must agree (Ch. 4).

consecutive or serial filing numeric filing method where numbers are considered in ascending order using the entire set of figures (Ch. 14).

constitutional law consists of laws that are made by constitutions of the United States or individual states (Ch. 7).

constriction band term used to replace tourniquet (no longer used) in emergencies. A band of material used to control severe bleeding in an extremity that has been injured due to trauma. The band is applied above the source of bleeding, but not so tight that it restricts the flow of blood completely. Some slight trickling of blood should be evident. This action avoids loss of an extremity because of complete blood flow restriction. Complete blood flow restriction results in no blood flow to the extremity's cells and tissues; therefore, the cells, tissues and body part receive no oxygen and die (Ch. 9).

consultation report document that reports the findings and advice of another physician requested to see a patient by the attending physician (Ch. 16).

contact tracker form used to keep track of employment contact information such as name of employer, name of contact person, address and telephone number, date of first contact, résumé sent, interview date, follow-up information, and dates (Ch. 25).

continuing education (CE) method of recertification of the certified medical transcriptionist credential (Ch. 16).

continuing education units (CEU) method for earning points toward recertification (Ch. 24).

contract law law that refers to agreements between individuals and entities that are binding (Ch. 7).

coordination of benefits (COB) the provision of an insurance contract that limits benefits to 100% of the cost (Ch. 18).

co-payment payment required when seen by the physician (Ch. 18).

cost analysis procedure that determines the costs of each service (Ch. 21).

cost ratio formula that shows the cost of a procedure or service and helps determine the financial value of maintaining certain services (Ch. 21).

crash tray or cart tray or portable cart that contains medications and supplies needed for emergency and first aid procedures (Ch. 9).

credentialed testimonials showing that a person is entitled to credit or has a right to exercise official power (Ch. 1).

credit decreases balance due; column used for entering payments (Ch. 17).

crepitation grating sound heard on movement of ends of a broken bone (Ch. 9).

criminal law law related to wrongs committed against the welfare and safety of society as a whole (Ch. 7).

cross-reference notation in a file to direct the reader to a specific record that may be filed under more than one name/subject (e.g., married name/maiden name or foreign names) where the surname is not easily recognizable (Ch. 14).

cryopreservation storage of biologic materials (sperm, embryo, tissue, plasma) at extremely cold temperature for use at a later time (Ch. 8).

cultivate to foster the growth of (Ch. 1).

cultural brokering the act of bridging, linking, or mediating between groups or persons through the process of reducing conflict or producing change (Ch. 4).

Current Procedural Terminology (CPT) standard codes for procedures and services. Used by most ambulatory care settings in encoding the claim form and recognized by most insurance carriers (Ch. 19).

current reports reports such as history and physical examinations that should be complete within 24 hours (Ch. 16).

cyberspace reference to the nonphysical space of binary computer communication (Ch. 11).

database management software (DBMS) computer applications software designed for the manipulation of data within a database. This software allows for creation and editing capabilities, sorting capabilities, and comparing and summarizing activities (Ch. 11).

data storage device device capable of permanently or temporarily storing digital data (Ch. 11).

data storage memory permanent memory not part of the motherboard. Uses any suitable data storage device. Can be read-only or read-write type of memory (Ch. 11).

day sheet form used with pegboard system to record daily patient transactions (Ch. 17).

debit used for entering charges and description of services; column is on the left (Ch. 17).

decode to translate into language that is easily understood; to interpret (Ch. 4).

deductible that amount of incurred medical expenses that must be met before the insurance policy will begin to pay (Ch. 18).

defendant person who defends action brought in litigation (Ch. 7).

defense mechanism behavior that protects the psyche from guilt, anxiety, or shame (Ch. 4).

defragmentation reorganization of information on a hard disk to store files as continuous units rather than as small packets. A computer with little fragmentation of files will operate at a higher speed (Ch. 11).

denial rejection of or refusal to acknowledge (Ch. 4).

deposition oral testimony given by an individual with a court reporter and attorneys for both sides present; often used as part of the discovery process (Ch. 7).

dexterity skill and ease in using the hands (Ch. 1).

digital speech standard (DSS) format standard used to compress and store digital audio data (Ch. 16).

digital video disk/digital versatile disk (DVD) an optical disk that holds 4.7 to 9.0 gigabytes of data depending on format (Ch. 11).

digitally processed dictation process of converting audio sound into a string of 0s and 1s, the language of the computer. The data are stored on a data storage device by the computer (Ch. 16).

diploma a document bearing record of graduation from or of a degree conferred by an educational institution (Ch. 1).

direct skills skills that are job specific. Skill in taking a blood pressure reading would be specific to the medical field (Ch. 25).

discharge summary (DS) medical reports that document the hospitalization history of a patient (Ch. 16).

discovery the time in which both parties are allowed access to all information and evidence related to a case; follows the subpoena process (Ch. 7).

dispense prepare and give out a medication to be taken at a later time (Ch. 7).

displacement   displacing negative feelings onto something or someone else with no significance to the situation (Ch. 4).

disposition   temperament, character, personality (Ch. 1).

doctrine   principle of law established through past decisions (Ch. 7).

documentation   written material that accompanies purchased software containing the information necessary for using the software appropriately; sometimes known as the manual (Ch. 11).

down-coding   insurance carriers down-code if documentation or codes are ambiguous and reimburse for the lowest possible fee (Ch. 19).

dressing   sterile gauze or other material applied directly to a wound to absorb secretions and to protect (Ch. 9).

driver   computer program designed to convert data output from one device to a format compatible with another device (Ch. 11).

durable power of attorney for health care   legal form that allows a designated person to act on another's behalf in regard to health care choices (Ch. 6, 7).

E codes   ICD-9-CM codes for the external causes of injury, poisoning, or other adverse reactions that explain how the injury occurred (Ch. 19).

e-résumé   electronic résumés may be delivered electronically via e-mail, submitted to Internet job boards, or placed on Web pages (Ch. 25).

editing   the process of manipulating text to avoid inaccuracies and inconsistencies within a document (Ch. 16).

electronic mail (e-mail)   communications that are sent, received, stored, and forwarded online from computer to computer by means of a modem (Ch. 12, 15).

emancipated minor   persons under age 18 years who are financially responsible for themselves and free of parental care (Ch. 7).

embezzle   to appropriate fraudulently to one's own use (Ch. 22).

Emergency Medical Services (EMS)   Emergency Medical Services (EMS) system is a local network of police, fire, and medical personnel trained to respond to emergency situations. In many communities, the system is activated by calling 911 (Ch. 9).

empathy   ability to be objectively aware of and have insight into another's feelings, emotions, and behaviors, and to be aware of the significance and meaning of these to the other person (Ch. 1).

encode (encoding)   creating a message to be sent (Ch. 4).

encounter form   formerly known as a charge slip or superbill. A copy of the encounter form is given to the patient after seeing the physician. It identifies the procedures performed, diagnoses, charges, and when to return (Ch. 17, 19).

encryption technology   converts information into code; used to protect privacy and confidentiality of individuals in computer software (Ch. 13).

enunciation   speaking clearly; articulating (Ch. 12).

ergonomics   scientific study of work and space, including factors that influence worker productivity and that affect workers' health (Ch. 11).

ethernet   references the networking of computers using metallic conductors or hard wires (Ch. 11).

ethics   defined in terms of what is morally right and wrong; ethics will differ from person to person; often defined by a code or creed as in the Code of Ethics from the American Association of Medical Assistants (AAMA) (Ch. 8).

etiquette   manners, politeness, proper behavior (Ch. 12).

evaluation   assessment of an employee's job performance (Ch. 23).

exclusion   specific disease or condition listed in an insurance policy for which the policy will not pay (Ch. 18).

exclusive provider organization (EPO)   a closed-panel PPO plan where enrollees receive no beneifts if they opt to receive care from a provider who is not in the EPO (Ch. 18).

exit interview   opportunity for departing employees to provide their positive and negative opinions of the position and facility (Ch. 23).

expert witness   individual with highly specialized knowledge and skills in a particular area who testifies to a standard of care (Ch. 7).

explanation of benefits (EOB)   insurance report that is sent with claim payments explaining the reimbursement of the insurance carrier (Ch. 19).

explicit   fully revealed or expressed without ambiguity or vagueness, leaving no question as to intent (Ch. 9).

expressed contract   written or verbal contract that specifically describes what each party in the contract will do (Ch. 7).

externship   transition stage between the classroom and actual employment; may also be referred to as internship or practicum (Ch. 1, 22).

facilitate   to make an action or process easier (Ch. 1).

Fair Debt Collection Practice Act   1977 federal law that outlines collection practices (Ch. 20).

fax (facsimile)   machine that sends documents from one location to another by way of telephone lines (Ch. 12).

felony   a serious crime such as murder, larceny, or thefts of large sums of money, assault, and rape (Ch. 7).

field   basic data category within the database. Fields can be either numeric (numerals), alphanumeric (letters and numerals), logical, or memo (Ch. 11).

firewall   hardware device or software program designed to prevent unauthorized access to a computer system (Ch. 11).

first aid   immediate (or first) care provided to persons who are suddenly ill or injured; first aid is typically followed by more comprehensive care and treatment (Ch. 9).

fiscal intermediary   local administrator for Medicare (Ch. 18).

fixed cost   cost that does not vary in total as the number of patients vary (Ch. 21).

flag   method of identifying a blank space or a question regarding dictator's meaning by attaching a note or marker to indicate the question (Ch. 16).

flash drive   solid-state data storage device (Ch. 11).

floppy drive   portable read-write data storage device. It is storable and transferable between computers. Capacity is approximately 1.4 megabytes of data. Data are stored permanently until overwritten. Floppy drive unit is required to read-write data from disk (Ch. 11).

fluent   facility in the use of a language (Ch. 12).

footer   page formatting feature that allows for the bottom of all pages to be marked with keyed-in data. Although the data are keyed in only once, it appears on every page in the document (Ch. 11).

form letter   letter containing the same content in the body but sent to different individuals (Ch. 15).

fracture   break in a bone. There are several types of fractures, but all are classified as either open or closed fractures (Ch. 9).

fraud   deliberate misrepresentation of facts (Ch. 18).

freelance MTs   self-employed medical transcriptionists (Ch. 16).

fringe benefit   benefit above and beyond salary to which an employee may be entitled. Examples include health and life insurance, paid vacation, sick days, personal days, and tuition reimbursement for courses related to employment (Ch. 2, 22).

full block letter   major letter style in which all lines begin flush with the left margin. This style is suggested for offices desiring a contemporary-looking, efficient letter (Ch. 15).

functional résumé   résumé format used to highlight specialty areas of accomplishment and strengths (Ch. 25).

G-Hz range   refers to computer operational speed of computations per second (Ch. 11).

genetic engineering   alteration, manipulation, replacement, or repair of genetic material (Ch. 8).

gestures/mannerisms   movement of various body parts while communicating (Ch. 4).

gigabyte   approximately one billion bytes of computer data (Ch. 11).

goal   result or achievement toward which effort is directed (Ch. 5).

"going bare"   said of a physician who does not carry professional liability insurance (Ch. 22).

Good Samaritan laws   laws designed to protect individuals from legal action when rendering emergency medical aid, without compensation, within the areas of their training and expertise (Ch. 12).

graphics software   applications software used to create pictorial representations or to create new digital imaging data (Ch. 11).

gross examination   viewing specimens with the naked eye (Ch. 16).

guarantor   the person identified as responsible for payment of the bill (Ch. 17).

hacker   person who uses sophisticated software to gain unauthorized access to computer systems and files. Hacker gains access through use of a linked computer or a computer connected to the Internet (Ch. 11).

hard drive   read-write data storage device permanently attached to the computer cabinet containing the CPU. Data are stored permanently until overwritten. Capacity is approximately 20 gigabytes or more of data (Ch. 11).

hardware   physical equipment used by the computer system to process data (Ch. 11).

hard-wired networks   networks connected by metallic conductors or cables; under some circumstances, optical cables could be used (Ch. 11).

header   page formatting feature that allows the top of a page to be printed with identifying information. The data are only keyed in once but appear on all pages in the document (Ch. 11).

Health Insurance Portability and Accountability Act (HIPAA)   government rules, regulations, and procedures resulting from legislation designed to protect the confidentiality of patient information (Ch. 16).

health maintenance organization (HMO)   type of managed care operation that is typically set up as a for-profit corporation with salaried employees. HMOs "with walls" offer a range of medical services under one roof; HMOs "without walls" typically contract with physicians in the community to provide patient services for an agreed-upon fee (Ch. 2, 18).

Healthcare Common Procedure Coding System (HCPCS)   a coding system consisting of the CPT, national codes (level II), and local codes (level III); previously known as HCFA Common Procedure Coding System (Ch. 19).

Heimlich maneuver   abdominal thrusts designed to overcome breathing difficulties in patients who are choking (Ch. 9).

hierarchy of needs   needs that are arranged in a specific order or rank; sequential arrangement. Associated with Abraham Maslow (Ch. 4).

history and physical examination report (H&P)   report of patient's history and physical examination to document reason for visit (Ch. 16).

history of present illness (HPI)   the chronologic description of the development of the patient's illness (Ch. 16).

home-based MTs   medical transcriptionists employed by transcription services (Ch. 16).

homeopathy   a healing modality that uses diluted doses of certain substances to create an "energy imprint" in the body to bring about a cure (Ch. 2).

hypothermia   extremely dangerous cold-related condition that can result in death if the individual does not receive care and if the progression of hypothermia is not reversed. Symptoms include shivering, cold skin, and confusion (Ch. 9).

implicit   capable of being understood from something else though unexpressed; implied (Ch. 9).

implied consent   consent assumed by the health care provider, typically in an emergency that threatens the patient's life. Implied consent also occurs in more subtle ways in the health care environment; for example, when a patient willingly rolls up the sleeve to receive an injection (Ch. 7).

implied contract   contract indicated by actions rather than words (Ch. 7).

improvise   to make, invent, or arrange in an unplanned or spontaneous manner (Ch. 1).

income statement   financial statement showing net profit or loss (Ch. 21).

incompetence   legally, a person who is insane, inadequate, or not an adult (Ch. 7).

independent physician association (IPA)   independent network of physicians in private practice who contract with the association to treat patients for an agreed-upon fee (Ch. 2).

indexing   selecting the name, subject, or number under which to file a record and determining the order in which the units should be considered (Ch. 14).

indirect statements means of eliciting a response from a patient by turning a question into a statement of interest (Ch. 4).

informatics the science of how information is produced and stored; that is, electronic medical records (Ch. 10).

information retrieval system system that allows electronic access to large databases for the retrieval of information; for example, Medlais and Medline (Ch. 11).

informed consent consent given by the patient who is made aware of any procedure to be performed, its risks, expected outcomes, and alternatives (Ch. 7).

inner-directed people people who decide for themselves what they want to do with their lives (Ch. 5).

input device a device used to input data into a computer (Ch. 11).

instant messaging (IM) electronic text communication between persons who are online at the same time (Ch. 12).

integrate to incorporate into a larger unit; to form or blend into a whole (Ch. 1).

integrated delivery system (IDS) a health care organization of affiliated provider sites combined under a single ownership that offers the full spectrum of managed health care (Ch. 18).

integrative medicine bringing together of two or more treatment modalities so they function as a harmonious whole; as seen in alternative forms of health care (Ch. 2).

***International Classification of Diseases, 9th Revision, Clinical Modification* (ICD-9-CM)** standard diagnosis codes used to identify a patient's medical problem. Used by most ambulatory care settings in encoding the claim form and recognized by most insurance carriers (Ch. 19).

Internet worldwide computer network available via modem that connects universities, government laboratories, companies, and individuals around the world (Ch. 11, 22).

internship transition stage between classroom and employment (Ch. 1).

interrogatory a written set of questions that must be answered, under oath, within a specific time period; part of the discovery process (Ch. 7).

interview meeting in which you and the interviewer discuss employment opportunities and strengths you can contribute to the organization (Ch. 25).

interview techniques methods of encouraging the best communication between the applicant and the interviewer (Ch. 4).

involuntary dismissal termination of employment based on poor job performance or violation of office policies (Ch. 22, 23).

itinerary detailed written plan of a proposed trip (Ch. 22).

jargon words, phrases, or terminology specific to a profession (Ch. 12).

Jaz® drive read-write data storage device. It is storable and transferable between computers. Capacity is approximately 1 to 2 gigabytes of data. Data are stored permanently until overwritten. Jaz drive unit is required to read-write data from the disk (Ch. 11).

job description outline of tasks, duties, and responsibilities for every position in the office (Ch. 23).

Joint Commission on Accreditation of Healthcare Organizations (JCAHO) commission established to improve the quality of care and services provided in organized health care setting through a voluntary accreditation process (Ch. 16).

key (keyed) to input data by keystrokes on a computer, word processor, or typewriter (Ch. 15).

key unit first indexing unit of the filing segment (Ch. 14).

keywords words that relate to a job specific position. Keywords may be job-specific skills or profession-specific words (Ch. 25).

kinesics study of body language (Ch. 4).

lackluster dull, lacking in sheen (Ch. 9).

ledger record of charges, payments, and adjustments for individual patient or family (Ch. 17).

letter of reference letter usually written by an employee's past employer describing the employee's performance, attitude, or qualifications. This letter is presented to a potential employer when applying for a new job (Ch. 23).

letter of resignation letter informing the current employer of the employee's decision to resign from a current position (Ch. 23).

liability debts and financial obligations for which one is responsible (Ch. 21); legal responsibility (Ch. 22).

libel false and malicious writing about another constituting a defamation of character (Ch. 7).

license permission by competent authority (the state) to engage in a profession; permission to act (Ch. 1); permission statement authorizing the use of copyrighted computer software (Ch. 11).

licensure granting of licenses to practice a profession (Ch. 1).

litigation court action (Ch. 7).

litigious prone to engage in lawsuits (Ch. 1).

living will document allowing a person to make choices related to treatment in a life-threatening illness (Ch. 6).

local area network (LAN) network of computers usually in one office or building (Ch. 11).

long-range goals achievements that may take three to five years to accomplish (Ch. 5).

M codes (morphology codes) used primarily with cancer registries. M codes further identify behavior and the cell type of a neoplasm (Ch. 19).

macro a series of keystrokes that has been saved under a separate file name to be used and inserted repeatedly into a document or documents (Ch. 11).

macroallocation of scarce medical resources; decisions are made by congress, health systems agencies, and insurance companies (Ch. 8).

magnetic tape plastic tape coated with magnetic material used to store analog or digital data (Ch. 16).

mainframe computer large computer system capable of processing massive volumes of data (Ch. 11).

malaria acute infectious disease caused by the presence of protozoan parasites within the red blood cells; usually comes from the bite of a female mosquito (Ch. 3).

malfeasance conduct that is illegal or contrary to an official's obligations (Ch. 7).

malpractice professional negligence (Ch. 7, 22).

managed care operation any health care setting or delivery system that is designed to reduce the cost of care while still providing access to care (Ch. 2).

managed care organization (MCO) a health insurance organization that adheres to the principles of strong dependence on selective contracting with providers, the use of primary care physicians, prospective and retrospective utilization management, use of treatment guidelines for high cost chronic disorders, and an emphasis on preventive care, education, and patient compliance with treatment plans (Ch. 18).

management by walking around (MBWA) a technique for keeping managers informed about the health of their organization (Ch. 22).

marketing process by which the provider of services makes the consumer aware of the scope and quality of those services. Marketing tools might include public relations, brochures, patient education seminars, and newsletters (Ch. 22).

masking attempt to conceal or repress true feelings or the message (Ch. 4).

matrix to establish an appointment matrix, a physician's unavailable time slots are marked with an X. Patients are not scheduled during those times (Ch. 13).

mature minor a person, usually younger than 18 years, who is able to understand and appreciate the consequences of treatment despite their young age (Ch. 7).

mediation dispute resolution that allows a facilitator to help the two parties settle their differences and come to an acceptable solution (Ch. 7).

Medical Transcriptionist Certification Commission (MTCC) credentialing program of the American Association for Medical Transcription (Ch. 16).

Medical Transcriptionist (MT) one who transcribes dictation into written documents (Ch. 16).

medically indigent refers to those individuals unable to pay for their own medical coverage (Ch. 7).

Medicare Part A benefits covering inpatient hospital and skilled nursing facilities, hospice care, and blood transfusion (Ch. 18).

Medicare Part B benefits covering outpatient hospital and health care provider services (Ch. 18).

Medigap policy an individual plan covering the patient's Medicare deductible and copay obligations that fulfills the federal government standards for Medicare supplemental insurance (Ch. 18).

megabyte one million bytes of data (Ch. 11).

memorandum interoffice correspondence, usually referred to as a memo (Ch. 15).

memory refers to storage of computer data. Memory can be volatile (lost when computer is turned off) or nonvolatile (permanently written to storage device) (Ch. 11).

mentor person assigned or requested to assist in training, guiding, or coaching another (Ch. 22).

merge operation word-processing operation designed to produce form letters (Ch. 11).

microallocation of scarce medical resources; decisions are made by physicians and individual members of the health care team (Ch. 8).

microcomputer personal or desktop computer. Also, a handheld or laptop model (Ch. 11).

microscopic examination viewing a specimen with the aid of a microscope (Ch. 16).

minicomputer one of the four categories of computers based on size: larger than a microcomputer and smaller than a mainframe (Ch. 11).

minor person who has not reached the age of majority, usually 18 years (Ch. 7).

minutes written record of topics discussed and actions taken during meeting sessions (Ch. 15, 22).

misdemeanor a lesser crime; misdemeanors vary from state to state in their definition. Punishment is usually probation or a time of public service and a fine (Ch. 7).

misfeasance is a civil law term referring to a lawful act that is improperly or unlawfully executed (Ch. 7).

modified block letter, indented modified letter style with indented paragraphs. Paragraphs in this style of letter may be indented five spaces (Ch. 15).

modified block letter, standard major letter style where all lines begin at the left margin with the exception of the date line, complimentary closure, and keyed signature. The exceptions usually begin at the center position or a few spaces to the right of center (Ch. 15).

modified wave scheduling system where multiple patients are scheduled at the beginning of each hour, followed by single appointments every 10 to 20 minutes the rest of the hour (Ch. 13).

modulated speech that varies in pitch and intensity (Ch. 12).

money market savings accounts bank accounts that pay the highest interest rate (money-market rate) and permit writing a limited number of checks (Ch. 17).

motherboard printed circuit board on which the CPU, ROM, and RAM chips and other electronic circuit elements of a digital computer are frequently located (Ch. 11).

moxibustion ancient Chinese method of treatment that uses a powdered plant substance on the skin to raise a blister (Ch. 3).

negligence failure to exercise a certain standard of care (Ch. 7, 22).

network interface software, servers, and cable connections used to link computers (Ch. 11).

networking connecting two or more computers together to share files and hardware. The system is called a network (Ch. 11); process in which people of similar interests exchange information in social, business, or professional relationships (Ch. 23).

noncompliant failure to follow a required command or instruction (Ch. 7).

nonconsecutive filing numeric filing method where numbers are considered in ascending order using subsets of figures within a number; for example, in the number 574 19 2863: 2863 is unit 1, 19 is unit 2, 574 is unit 3 (Ch. 14).

nonfeasance a civil law term referring to the failure to perform an act, official duty, or legal requirement (Ch. 7).

normal saline a solution of sodium chloride (salt) and distilled water. It has the same osmotic pressure as blood serum. It is also known as isotonic or physiologic saline (Ch. 9).

notary (notary public) someone with the legal capacity to witness and certify documents; can take depositions (Ch. 17).

obfuscation making things clouded or confused (Ch. 12).

occlusion closure of a passage (Ch. 9).

old reports reports such as a discharge summary that should be completed within 71 hours (Ch. 16).

open-ended questions questions that encourage verbalization and response; questions that seek a response beyond a simple yes or no (Ch. 4).

operating system (OS) Software used to control the computer and its peripheral equipment. Referred to as system software and is abbreviated OS (Ch. 11).

operative report (OR) medical reports that chronicle the details of a surgical procedure (Ch. 16).

optical character reader (OCR) U.S. Postal Service's computerized scanner that reads addresses printed on letter mail. If the information is properly formatted, then the OCR will find a match in its address files and print a bar code on the lower right edge of the envelope (Ch. 15).

optical disk portable and transferable read-write or read-only data storage device. Sometimes called a CD-ROM, CD-RW, or compact disk. Capacity is 1 to 8 gigabytes of data. Optical drive unit is required to read-write data from the disk (Ch. 11).

orphan in typesetting, a term describing the situation in which a new paragraph begins on the last line of a printed page or column (Ch. 11).

outer-directed people people who let events, other people, or environmental factors dictate their behavior (Ch. 5).

out guide or sheet card, folder, or slip of paper inserted temporarily in the files to replace a record that has been retrieved from the files (Ch. 14).

output device a device used to output data from a computer. Includes printers, faxes, data storage drivers, and so on (Ch. 11).

overtime money paid at a rate of not less than one and one-half times the regular rate of pay after a 40-hour work week is completed (Ch. 23).

owner's equity amount by which business assets exceed business liabilities. Also called net worth, proprietorship, and capital (Ch. 21).

pagers also known as beepers. One-way paging systems often used inside hospitals and by physicians on call. Pagers only receive signals (Ch. 12).

parasympathetic nervous system part of the autonomic nervous system that returns the body to its normal state after stress has subsided (Ch. 5).

participatory manager operates on the premise that the worker is capable and wants to do a good job (Ch. 22).

patch modification to software to fix deficiencies in the software. Frequently downloaded from the software supplier's Web site or from floppy disks provided by the supplier (Ch. 11).

pathology report medical reports generated to describe the gross and microscopic examinations performed during a surgical procedure (Ch. 16).

Patient Self-Determination Act (PSDA) the Act that includes the Advance Directive giving patients the rights to be involved in their health care decisions (Ch. 7).

payee person named on check who is to receive the amount indicated (Ch. 17).

pegboard system most commonly used manual medical accounts receivable system (Ch. 17).

perception conscious awareness of one's own feelings and the feelings of others (Ch. 4).

personal computer (PC) also known as microcomputer (Ch. 11).

Personal Digital Assistant (PDA) an electronic tool for organizing data, a handheld computerized personal organizer device (Ch. 11).

petty cash small sum kept on hand for minor or unexpected expenses (Ch. 17).

pharmacopoeia book describing drugs and their preparation or a collection or stock of drugs (Ch. 3).

physician's directive another name for a living will (Ch. 6).

plaintiff person bringing charges in litigation (Ch. 7).

pluralistic (pluralism) society where there are several distinct ethnic, religious, or cultural groups that coexist with one another (Ch. 3).

point-of-service (POS) device device allowing direct communication between a medical office and the health care plan's computer (Ch. 19).

point-of-service (POS) plan a plan that allows direct communication between a medical office and the health insurance company (Ch. 18).

portfolio notebook or file containing examples of materials commonly used (Ch. 15).

posting recording financial transactions into a bookkeeping or accounting system (Ch. 17).

power verbs action words used to describe your attributes and strengths (Ch. 25).

practicum transitional stage providing opportunity to apply theory learned in the classroom to a health care setting through practical, hands-on experience (Ch. 1, 22).

preauthorization obtaining an insurance carrier's consent to proceed with patient care and treatment. Unless authorization is obtained, insurance carriers may not pay benefits for specific problems (Ch. 18).

precedents refers to rulings made at an earlier time and include decisions made in a court, interpretations of a constitution, and statutory law decisions (Ch. 7).

preferred provider organization (PPO) organization of physicians who network together to offer discounts to purchasers of heath care insurance (Ch. 2, 18).

prejudice opinion or judgment that is formed before all the facts are known (Ch. 4).

prescribe to order or recommend the use of a drug, diet, or other form of therapy (Ch. 7).

primary care physician (PCP) primary care physician for a patient; all care is coordinated through the PCP (Ch. 18).

privileged confidential information that may only be communicated with the patient's permission or by court order (Ch. 16).

probate court court that administers estates and validates wills (Ch. 20).

probation period during which the employee and supervisory personnel may determine if both the environment and the position are satisfactory for the employee (Ch. 23).

problem-oriented medical record (POMR) a type of patient chart recordkeeping that uses a sheet at a prominent location in the chart to list vital identification data. Patient medical problems are identified by a number that corresponds to the charting; for example, bronchitis is #1, a broken wrist is #2, and so forth (Ch. 14).

procedure manual manual providing detailed information relative to the performance of tasks within the job description (Ch. 22).

professional liability insurance insurance policy designed to protect assets in the event a claim for damages resulting from negligence is filed and awarded (Ch. 22).

professionalism the qualities that characterize or distinguish a professional person who conforms to the technical and ethical standards of the profession (Ch. 1).

profit sharing sharing in the financial profits, gains, and benefits of an organization (Ch. 22).

progress notes also called chart notes. Physician's formal or informal notes about presenting problem, physical findings, and plan for treatment for a patient examined in the office, clinic, acute care center, or emergency department (Ch. 16).

projection act of placing one's own feelings on another (Ch. 4).

pronunciation saying words correctly (Ch. 12).

proofread to read a document to verify the accuracy of content and that correct grammar, spelling, punctuation, and capitalization were used (Ch. 15, 16).

proprietary privately owned and managed facility, a profit-making organization (Ch. 1).

psychomotor retardation slowing of physical and mental responses; may be seen in depression (Ch. 6).

purging method of maintaining order in the files by separating active from inactive and closed files (Ch. 14).

quality assurance (QA) process to provide accurate, complete, consistent health care documentation in a timely manner while making every reasonable effort to resolve inconsistencies, inaccuracies, risk management issues, and other problems (Ch. 16).

radiology and imaging reports medical reports that describe the findings and interpretations of the radiologist (Ch. 16).

random access memory (RAM) a type of computer memory that can be written to and read from. The word *random* means that any one location can be read at any time. RAM commonly refers to the internal memory of a computer. RAM is usually a fast, temporary memory area where data and programs reside until saved or until the power is turned off (Ch. 11).

rationalization act of justification, usually illogically, that one uses to keep from facing the truth of the situation (Ch. 4).

read-only memory (ROM) permanently stored computer data that cannot be overwritten without special devices. Stores instructions required to start up the computer. Located on the motherboard (Ch. 11).

recertification documentation admitted to support continued education for maintaining a professional credential (Ch. 24).

references individuals who have known or worked with a person long enough to make an honest assessment and recommendation regarding your background history (Ch. 25).

referral term used by managed care facilities for authorization for someone other than the patient's primary care physician to treat the patient (Ch. 18).

Registered Medical Assistant (RMA) credential awarded for successfully passing the AMT examination (Ch. 1, 24).

regression moving back to a former stage to escape conflict or fear (Ch. 4).

repression coping with an overwhelming situation by temporarily forgetting it; temporary amnesia (Ch. 4).

rescue breathing performed on individuals in respiratory arrest, rescue breathing is a mouth-to-mouth (using appropriate protective equipment) or mouth-to-nose procedure that provides oxygen to the patient until emergency personnel arrive (Ch. 9).

resource-based relative value scale (RBRVS) basis for the Medicare fee schedule (Ch. 18).

résumé written summary data sheet or brief account of qualifications and progress in your chosen career (Ch. 25).

review of systems (ROS) inquires about the system directly related to the problems identified in the history of the present illness (Ch. 16).

risk management techniques adhered to in the ambulatory care setting that keep the practice, its environment, and its procedures as safe for the patient as possible. Proper risk management also reduces the possibility of negligence that leads to torts and malpractice suits (Ch. 7, 9, 16, 22).

roadblocks verbal or nonverbal messages that block communication (Ch. 4).

salary review informing the employee of their revised base pay rate (Ch. 22).

scope of practice the range of clinical procedures and activities that are allowed by law for a profession (Ch. 1).

search engine specialized computer program designed to find specific information on the Internet (Ch. 22).

self-actualization being all that you can be; developing your full potential and experiencing fulfillment (Ch. 5, 22).

self-insurance insurance carried by large companies, nonprofit organizations, and government to reduce costs and gain more control of their finances. Each plan differs in coverage and claim filing requirements (Ch. 18).

septicemia invasion of pathogenic bacteria into the bloodstream (Ch. 3).

server computer with massive hard drive capacity that is used to link other computers together so that data can be shared by multiple users. A computer system in an ambulatory care facility is likely to be linked or networked with a central server (Ch. 11).

shadow follow a supervisor or delegated subordinate to learn facility protocol (Ch. 22).

shingling method of arranging charts in which sheets of paper are "shingled" up or across the page, with the most recent report placed on top of the previous one, giving access to the most current information first (Ch. 14).

shock potentially serious condition in which the circulatory system is not providing enough blood to all parts of the body, causing the body's organs to fail to function properly (Ch. 9).

short-range goals long-range goals are dissected and reassembled into smaller, more manageable time segments (Ch. 5).

simplified letter major letter style recommended by the Administrative Management Society that omits the salutation and complimentary closure. All lines are keyed flush with the left margin. In medical offices, this style is most often used when sending a form letter (Ch. 15).

slander false and malicious words about another constituting a defamation of character (Ch. 7).

SOAP acronym for patient progress notes based on subjective impressions (S), objective clinical evidence (O), assessment or diagnosis (A), and plans for further studies (P) (Ch. 14).

software equivalent of a computer program or programs (Ch. 11).

sort frequently used data processing operation that arranges data in a particular sequence or order (Ch. 11).

source-oriented medical record (SOMR) a type of patient chart record keeping that includes separate sections for different sources of patient information, such as laboratory reports, pathology reports, and progress notes (Ch. 14).

splint any device used to immobilize a body part. Often used by EMS personnel (Ch. 9).

sprain injury to a joint, often an ankle, knee, or wrist, that involves a tearing of the ligaments. Most sprains are minor and heal quickly; others are more severe, include swelling, and may not heal properly if the patient continues to put stress on the sprained joint (Ch. 9).

spreadsheet software computer applications packages that act as "number crunchers" because of their mathematic processing capabilities (Ch. 11).

Standard Precautions precautions developed in 1996 by the Centers for Disease Control and Prevention (CDC) that augment universal precautions and body substance isolation practices. They provide a wider range of protection and are used any time there is contact with blood, moist body fluid (except perspiration), mucous membranes, or nonintact skin. They are designed to protect all health care providers, patients, and visitors (Ch. 9).

STAT abbreviation for the Latin *statim*, meaning immediate (Ch. 16).

statute of limitations statute that defines the period in which legal action can take place (Ch. 20).

statutory law refers to the body of laws established by states (Ch. 7).

strain injury to the soft tissue between joints that involves the tearing of muscles or tendons. Strains often occur in the neck, back, or thigh muscles (Ch. 9).

stream scheduling system where patients are seen on a continuous basis throughout the day; for example, at 15-, 30-, or 60-minute intervals, each patient having a distinct appointment time (Ch. 13).

stress body's response to change; can be manifested in a variety of ways, including changes in blood pressure, heart rate, and onset of headache (Ch. 5).

stressors demands to change that cause stress (Ch. 5).

sublimation redirecting a socially unacceptable impulse into one that is socially acceptable (Ch. 4).

subordinate in an organization, a person under the direction of (reporting to) a person of greater authority (Ch. 22).

subpoena written command designating a person to appear in court under penalty for failure to appear (Ch. 7).

supercomputer fastest, largest, and most expensive of the four classes of computers currently being manufactured (Ch. 11).

surge protection protection of the fragile electronics from spikes in electrical voltage that occur on electric distribution lines (Ch. 11).

surrogate substitute; someone who substitutes for another (Ch. 8).

sympathetic nervous system large part of the autonomic nervous system that prepares the body for fight-or-flight (Ch. 5).

syncope fainting (Ch. 9).

systemic pertaining to the whole body (Ch. 9).

system software see **operating system** (Ch. 11).

tape drive data storage device that uses magnetic tape as the storage media (Ch. 11).

targeted résumé résumé format utilized when focusing on a clear, specific job target (Ch. 25).

Task Force for Test Construction (TFTC) committee of professionals whose responsibility is to update the CMA examination annually to reflect changes in medical assistants' responsibilities and to include new developments in medical knowledge and technology (Ch. 24).

teamwork persons synergistically working together (Ch. 22).

therapeutic communication use of specific and well-defined professional communication skills to create a feeling of comfort for patients even when difficult or unpleasant information must be exchanged (Ch. 4).

tickler file system to remind of action to be taken on a certain date (Ch. 14).

tort wrongful act that results in injury to one person by another (Ch. 7).

tort law laws that stem from torts, or wrongful acts that cause harm to one person, by another (Ch. 7).

transcriber device that makes it possible to transform voice recordings into a transcript or printed documents (Ch. 16).

transferable skills skills that would be used in a host of different and unrelated occupations. Keyboarding skill is an example of a

transferable skill. It could be used by a secretary, data entry clerk, medical assistant, or clothing manufacturer (Ch. 25).

traveler's check often used in place of cash when traveling; available in denominations of $10 to $100; requires a signature at place of purchase as well as signature at the time the check is used (Ch. 17).

triage process to determine and prioritize patients' needs and the likely benefit from immediate medical attention. From the French *trier*, meaning "to sort" (Ch. 2, 9, 12, 13).

TRICARE formerly the Civilian Health and Medical Program for Uniformed Services (CHAMPUS). TRICARE offers HMO, PPO, and fee-for-service medical insurance for dependents of active duty and retired military personnel, and dependents of personnel who died while on active duty (Ch. 18).

triple option plan a managed care model allowing enrollees the option of traditional, HMO, or PPO health plans (Ch. 18).

Truth-in-Lending Act also known as the Consumer Credit Protection Act of 1968; an act requiring providers of installment credit to state the charges in writing and to express the interest as an annual rate (Ch. 20).

turnaround time specific time limits established for completion of medical reports (Ch. 16).

typhus (typhoid) acute infectious disease that causes severe headache, rash, high fever, and progressive neurologic involvement. Prevalent where conditions are unsanitary and congested (Ch. 3).

unbundling codes refers to separating the components of a procedure and reporting them as billable codes with charges to increase reimbursement rates (Ch. 19).

undoing actions designed to make amends to cancel out inappropriate behavior (Ch. 4).

Uniform Bill 92 (UB92) unique billing form used extensively by acute care facilities for processing inpatient and outpatient claims (Ch. 19).

uniform resource locator (URL) Web address that identifies and displays a particular Web page (Ch. 15).

unit each part of a name (business or person), words, or numbers that will be indexed and coded for filing (Ch. 14).

universal emergency medical identification symbol identification sometimes carried by individuals to identify health problems they may have (Ch. 9).

universal system bus (USB) port a type of data entry portal or bus for computer data (Ch. 11).

up-coding also known as code creep, overcoding, and overbilling. Up-coding occurs when the insurance carrier deliberately bills a higher rate service than what was performed to obtain greater reimbursements (Ch. 19).

usual, customary, and reasonable (UCR) fee schedule often used by Medicare and some insurance carriers. *Usual* refers to the fee typically charged by a physician for certain procedures; *customary* is based on the average charge for a specific procedure by all physicians practicing the same specialty in a defined geographic region; and *reasonable* refers to the midrange of fees charged for this procedure (Ch. 18).

utilization review (UR) review of medical services before they can be performed (Ch. 21).

V codes ICD-9-CM codes representing either factors that influence a person's health status or legitimate reasons for contacting the health facility when the patient has no definitive diagnosis or active symptom of any disorder (Ch. 19).

variable cost cost that varies in direct proportion to volume (Ch. 21).

voucher check check with detachable form used to detail reason check is drawn; commonly used in payroll checks (Ch. 17).

watermark design incorporated in paper during the papermaking process that is visible when the paper is held up to the light (Ch. 15).

wave scheduling system where patients are scheduled for the first half hour of every hour, and then seen throughout the hour (Ch. 13).

waveform audio (WAV) format standard used to compress and store digital audio data (Ch. 16).

Web site a remote computer that stores World Wide Web documents consisting of Web pages (Ch. 22).

wide area network (WAN) connecting together of computers on a large area for the purpose of sharing data (Ch. 11).

widow in typesetting, a term describing the situation in which a line of text that is the end of a paragraph ends on a new page or column of printed text (Ch. 11).

WiFi standards industry standards for wireless computer devices that are designed to guarantee interoperability (Ch. 11).

wireless network a joining of two or more computers and peripheral equipment using wireless elements (Ch. 11).

word processing software computer application that allows the user to format and edit documents before printing (Ch. 11).

work statement concise description of the work you plan to accomplish (Ch. 22).

Workers' Compensation insurance medical and paycheck insurance for workers who sustain injuries associated with their employment (Ch. 18).

wound a break in the continuity of soft parts of body structures caused by violence or trauma to tissues. In an open wound, skin is broken as in a laceration, abrasion, avulsion, or incision. In a closed wound, skin is not broken as in contusion, ecchymosis, or hematoma (Ch. 9).

yellow fever acute infectious disease where a person develops jaundice, vomits, hemorrhages, and has a fever; caused mostly by mosquitoes (Ch. 3).

ZIP+4 standard Zip code including four additional digits that identify a postal delivery area. Mail will be processed more efficiently and effectively with the use of the ZIP+4 code in the address (Ch. 15).

Zip® drive portable read-write data storage device. It is storable and transferable between computers. Capacity is approximately 250 megabytes of data. Data are stored permanently until overwritten. Zip drive unit is required to read-write data from disk (Ch. 11).

APPENDIX A

Common Medical Abbreviations and Symbols

a̅a̅	of each
AAMA	American Association of Medical Assistants
AAMT	American Association of Medical Transcription
AAPC	American Academy of Professional Coders
ab	abortion
abd	abdomen
ABE	acute bacterial endocarditis
ABG	arterial blood gases
ABHES	Accrediting Bureau of Health Education Schools
ABO	blood groups
abs	absent
ac	before meals (ante cibum)
ac	acute
ACAP	Alliance of Claims Assistance Professionals
ACTH	adrenocorticotropic hormone
ADA	Americans with Disabilities Act
ADL	activities of daily living
ad lib	as desired
adm	admission
AED	automated electronic defibrillator
AFP	alpha fetal protein
AHD	arteriosclerotic heart disease
	atherosclerotic heart disease
AHIMA	American Health Information Management Association
AIDS	acquired immunodeficiency syndrome
alb	albumin
AM	before noon (ante meridiem)
AMA	against medical advice
	American Medical Association
AMI	acute myocardial infarction
amt	amount
AMT	American Medical Technologists

AMTIE	American Medical Technologists Institute for Education
ant	anterior
ante	before
A&P	anterior and posterior
	auscultation and palpation
	auscultation and percussion
APC	ambulatory payment classifications
aq	water
A/R	accounts receivable
ARDS	acute (or adult) respiratory disease syndrome
ARU	automated routing unit
ASA	acetylsalicylic acid
ASAP	as soon as possible
ASCAD	arteriosclerotic coronary artery disease
ASCVD	arteriosclerotic cardiovascular disease
	atherosclerotic cardiovascular disease
A&W	alive and well
Ba	barium
BaE	barium enema
BBB	bundle branch block
BC	birth control
BCP	birth control pills
BC/BS	Blue Cross/Blue Shield
BE	bacterial endocarditis
bid	twice a day
bil	bilateral
BM	basal metabolism
	bowel movement
BMR	basal metabolism rate
BP	blood pressure
BPH	benign prostatic hypertrophy

BS	blood sugar
	bowel sounds
	breath sounds
BSA	body surface area
BSL	blood sugar level
BSN	bowel sounds normal
BSO	bilateral salpingo-oophorectomy
BSR	blood sedimentation rate
BUN	blood urea nitrogen
BW	below waist
	birth weight
	body weight
Bx	biopsy
C	Celsius
	centigrade
c̄	with
C1	first cervical vertebra
CA	cancer
	carcinoma
Ca	calcium
CAAHEP	Commission on Accreditation of Allied Health Education Programs
CAD	coronary artery disease
CAHD	coronary arteriosclerotic heart disease
caps	capsules
CAT	computerized axial tomography
CBC	complete blood count
CC	chief complaint
CCA	Certified Coding Associate
CCR	continuity of care record
CCS	Certified Coding Specialist
CCS-P	Certified Coding Specialist-Physician-Based
CCU	coronary care unit
C&D	cystoscopy and dilation
CDC	U.S. Centers for Disease Control and Prevention
CE	continuing education
cerv	cervical
	cervix
CEU	continuing education unit
CF	conversion factor
CHAMPVA	Civilian Health and Medical Program of the Veterans Administration
CHD	childhood disease
	congenital heart disease
	congestive heart disease
	coronary heart disease
CHF	congestive heart failure
CHO	carbohydrate
CIN	cervical intraepithelial neoplasia
ck	check
Cl	chlorine
cldy	cloudy
CLIA	Clinical Laboratory Improvement Amendments
cm	centimeter
CMA	Certified Medical Assistant
CMAS	Certified Medical Administrative Specialist
CME	continuing medical education
CMS	Centers for Medicare and Medicaid Services
CMT	Certified Medical Transcriptionist

CNS	central nervous system
C/O	complains of
CO_2	carbon dioxide
COB	coordination of benefits
COPD	chronic obstructive pulmonary disease
CPC	Certified Professional Coders
CPC-A	Certified Professional Coders-Apprentice
CPC-H	Certified Professional Coders-Hospital
CPC-HA	Certified Professional Coders-Hospital Apprentice
CPR	cardiopulmonary resuscitation
CPT	Current Procedural Code
CPU	central processing unit
CRB	Curriculum Review Board
crit	hematocrit
CS	cerebrospinal
	cesarean section
C&S	culture and sensitivity
CSF	cerebrospinal fluid
CT	computerized tomography
CVA	cerebrovascular accident
CVP	central venous pressure
CVS	chorionic villus sampling
cx	cervix
CXR	chest X-ray
cysto	cystoscopic examination
	cystoscopy
DACUM	developing a curriculum
DC	doctor of chiropracty
D&C	dilation and curettage
DDS	doctor of dentistry
DEA	U.S. Drug Enforcement Agency
dec	decrease
del	delivery
DHHS	U.S. Department of Health and Human Services
diab	diabetic
diag	diagnosis
diff	differential white blood cell count
dil	dilute
disc	discontinue
disp	dispense
DM	diabetes mellitus
DNA	deoxyribonucleic acid
	does not apply
DNR	do not resuscitate
DO	doctor of osteopathy
DOA	dead on arrival
DOB	date of birth
DOD	date of death
DOE	dyspnea on exertion
dos	dosage
DPM	doctor of podiatric medicine
DPT	diphtheria, pertussis, and tetanus
DR	delivery room
Dr	doctor
dr	dram
DRGs	diagnosis-related groups
DS	discharge summary
DSD	dry sterile dressing
dsg	dressing

DSS	digital speech standard
DT	delirium tremens
DTR	deep tendon reflex
D&V	diarrhea and vomiting
DW	distilled water
D/W	dextrose in water
dx	diagnosis
ea	each
EBV	Epstein–Barr virus
ECG	electrocardiogram
Echo	echocardiogram
	echoencephalogram
E. coli	*Escherichia coli*
ECT	electroconvulsive therapy
	electronic claims transmission
EDC	estimated date of confinement or expected date of confinement
EDD	estimated date of delivery or expected date of delivery
EEG	electroencephalogram
EENT	eyes, ears, nose, and throat
e.g.	for example
EKG	electrocardiogram
elix	elixir
e-mail	electronic mail
EMG	electromyography
EMR	electronic medical record
EMS	emergency medical service
ENT	ear, nose, and throat
EOB	explanation of benefits
eos	eosinophil
EPA	Environmental Protection Agency
EPO	exclusive provider organization
eq	equivalent
ER	emergency room
ERT	estrogen replacement therapy
ESR	erythrocyte sedimentation rate
EST	electroshock therapy
exam	examination
ext	extract
F	Fahrenheit
	female
fax	facsimile
FBS	fasting blood sugar
FDA	U.S. Food and Drug Administration
FECA	Federal Employees Compensation Act Program
FH	family history
FHR	fetal heart rate
FHS	fetal heart sound
fl	fluid
fl dr	fluid dram
fl oz	fluid ounce
FMP	first menstrual period
FP	family practice
freq	frequent
FSH	follicle-stimulating hormone
ft	foot

FTA	fluorescent treponemal antibody
FTP	file transfer protocol
fx	fracture
G	gravida
g	gram
GB	gallbladder
GC	gonococcus
	gonorrhea
GI	gastrointestinal
gm	gram
GP	general practice
GPCI	Geographic Practice Cost Index
gr	grain
grav	pregnancy
GTH	gonadotropic hormone
GTT	glucose tolerance test
gtt(s)	drop (drops)
GU	genitourinary
GYN	gynecology
h	hour
HBP	high blood pressure
HCFA	U.S. Health Care Financing Administration
hCG	human chorionic gonadotropin
HCl	hydrochloric acid
HCPCS	Healthcare Common Procedure Coding System
Hct	hematocrit
HCVD	hypertensive cardiovascular disease
HEENT	head, eyes, ears, nose, and throat
Hgb	hemoglobin
H&H	hemoglobin and hematocrit
HIPAA	Health Insurance Portability and Accountability Act
HMO	health maintenance organization
H/O	history of
H_2O	water
H&P	history and physical
HPI	history of present illness
HPV	human papillomavirus
HR	human resources
HRS	Healthcare Reimbursement Specialist
HRT	hormone replacement therapy
ht	height
hx	history
Hz	hertz
ICCU	intensive coronary care unit
ICD	International Classification of Diseases, Adapted
ICD-9-CM	International Classification of Diseases, 9th revision, Clinical Modification
ICU	intensive care unit
ID	intradermal
I&D	incision and drainage
IM	instant messaging
	internal medicine
	intramuscular
imp	impression
inf	infusion

inj	injection
I&O	intake and output
IPPB	intermittent positive pressure breathing
IPPS	inpatient prospective payment systems
ISP	Internet service provider
IUD	intrauterine device
IV	intravenous
IVP	intravenous pyelogram
JAAMT	*Journal of the American Association for Medical Transcription*
JAMA	*Journal of the American Medical Association*
JCAHO	Joint Commission on Accreditation of Healthcare Organizations
jt	joint
K	potassium
kg	kilogram
KOH	potassium hydroxide
KUB	kidney, ureter, and bladder
kV	kilovolt
L	left
	liter
l	length
LA	left atrium
	lactic acid
L&A	light and accommodation
lab	laboratory
lac	laceration
LAN	local area network
lap	laparotomy
lat	lateral
lb	pound
LBBB	left bundle branch block
LDL	low-density lipoprotein
LE	lupus erythematosus
liq	liquid
LLQ	lower left quadrant
LMP	last menstrual period
LP	lumbar puncture
LRQ	lower right quadrant
LUQ	left upper quadrant
L&W	living and well
lymphs	lymphocytes
M	male
m	meter
℥	minim
MBCD	management by coaching and development
MBCE	management by competitive edge
MBDM	management by decision models
MBP	management by performance
MBS	management by styles
MBWA	management by wandering around
MBWS	management by work simplification
MCHC	mean corpuscular hemoglobin and red cell indices
MCO	managed care organization
MCV	mean corpuscular volume and red cell indices

MD	doctor of medicine
	muscular dystrophy
MDR	minimum daily requirement
med	medicine
mEq/L	milliequivalents per liter
MFS	Medicare fee schedule
mg	milligram
MH	marital history
	medical history
	menstrual history
MHx	medical history
MI	maturation index
	myocardial infarction
ml	milliliter
mm	millimeter
mm^3	cubic millimeter
mm Hg	millimeters of mercury
MMR	measles, mumps, and rubella
MOM	milk of magnesia
mono	mononucleosis
MP	menstrual period
MRI	magnetic resonance imaging
MS	mitral stenosis
	multiple sclerosis
MSDS	material safety data sheets
MSHA	Mine Safety and Health Administration
MT	medical technologist
	medical transcriptionist
MTCC	Medical Transcriptionist Certification Commission
multip	multipara
MVP	mitral valve prolapse
NA	not applicable
NaCl	sodium chloride
narc	narcotic
NB	newborn
N/C	no complaints
ND	doctor of naturopathy
NEBA	National Electronic Billers Alliance
NEC	not elsewhere classified
neg	negative
NG	nasogastric
NGU	nongonococcal urethritis
NL	normal limits
NMP	normal menstrual period
noct	at night
Non-PAR	nonparticipating provider
non rep	do not repeat
NOS	not otherwise specified
NPI	national provider number
NPO	nothing by mouth
NR	no refill
	nonreactive
	normal range
NS	nonspecific
	normal saline
	not significant
	not sufficient
N&T	nose and throat

N&V	nausea and vomiting	peds	pediatrics
NVD	nausea, vomiting, and diarrhea	PEG	pneumoencephalography
		PERRLA	pupils equal, round, regular, react to light, and accommodation
O	oral		
	oxygen	PET	positron emission transmission or tomography
O₂	oxygen	PH	past history
OB	obstetrics		personal history
OB-GYN	obstetrics-gynecology		public health
OC	office call	pH	hydrogen in concentration
	on call	PHI	protected health information
	oral contraceptive	PHO	physician-hospital organization
occ	occasionally	PI	present illness
OCR	Office of Civil Rights		pulmonary infarction
	optical character reader	PID	pelvic inflammatory disease
OGTT	oral glucose tolerance test	PKU	phenylketonuria
OM	office manager	PM	after noon (post meridiem)
OOB	out of bed		post mortem (after death)
OP	outpatient	PMN	polymorphonuclear neutrophils
O&P	ova and parasites	PMP	past menstrual period
OPIM	other potentially infectious material	PMS	premenstrual syndrome
OPPS	outpatient prospective payment systems	PNC	penicillin
OPV	oral poliovaccine	PO	postoperative
OR	operating room	po	by mouth
	operative report	POB	place of birth
ortho	orthopedics	POMR	problem-oriented medical record
os	mouth	POS	point-of-service plan
OSHA	U.S. Occupational Safety and Health Administration	pos	positive
		poss	possible
OT	occupational therapist	postop	postoperative
	occupational therapy	PP	postprandial
OTC	over the counter	PPB	positive pressure breathing
OURQ	outer upper right quadrant	PPBS	postprandial blood sugar
OV	office visit	PPD	purified protein derivative
OWCP	Office Workers' Compensation Programs	PPO	preferred provider organization
oz	ounce	PPT	partial prothrombin time
		preop	preoperative
P	phosphorus	PRERLA	pupils round, equal, react to light and accommodation
	pulse		
P&A	percussion and auscultation	primip	woman bearing first child
PA	physician's assistant	prn	as the occasion arises, as necessary
	posteroanterior	procto	proctoscopy
PAC	phenacetin, aspirin, and codeine	prog	prognosis
	premature atrial contraction	PROM	premature rupture of membranes
Pap	Papanicolaou (smear, test)	pro-time	prothrombin time
PAR	participating provider	PSA	prostate-specific antigen
para	number of pregnancies	PSRO	Professional Standards Review Organization
para I	primipara	PT	physical therapy
PAT	paroxysmal atrial tachycardia		prothrombin time
path	pathology	pt	patient
PBI	protein-bound iodine	PTA	prior to admission
pc	after meals	pulv	powder
PC	personal computer	PVC	premature ventricular contraction
PCA	patient-controlled analgesic	px	physical examination
PCC	Poison Control Center		prognosis
PCN	penicillin		
PCP	primary care physician	q	each; every
PCV	packed cell volume	q AM	every morning
PDA	personal digital assistant	QA	quality assurance
PDR	*Physician's Desk Reference*	qh	every hour
PE	physical examination	q (2, 3, 4)h	every 2, 3, or 4 hours

qid	four times a day		SOP	standard operating procedure
QISMC	Quality Improvement System for Managed Care		SOS	if necessary
qn	every night		spec	specimen
qns	quantity not sufficient		sp gr	secific gravity
qs	of sufficient quantity		spont ab	spontaneous abortion
qt	quart		SR	sedimentation rate
			SS	signs and symptoms
R	registration		$\overline{ss}$	one-half
	right		SSI	Supplemental Security Income
RAM	random access memory		Staph	Staphylococcus
RBC	red blood cell		stat	immediately
RBC/hpf	red blood cells per high power field		STD	sexually transmitted disease
RBCM	red blood cell mass		Strep	Streptococcus
RBCV	red blood cell volume		subcut	subcutaneous
RBRVS	Resource-Based Relative Value Scale		supp	suppository
REM	rapid eye movement		surg	surgery
resp	respiration		sx	signs
Rh	rhesus (factor)			symptoms
Rh-	rhesus negative		sym	symptoms
Rh+	rhesus positive		syr	syrup
RHD	rheumatic heart disease			
RLQ	right lower quadrant		T	temperature
RMA	Registered Medical Assistant		T_3	tri-iodothyronine
RNA	ribonucleic acid		T_4	thyroxine
R/O	rule out		T&A	tonsillectomy and adenoidectomy
ROA	received on account		tab	tablet
ROM	range of motion		TB	tuberculin
	read-only memory			tuberculosis
ROS	review of systems		tbs	tablespoon
RT	radiation therapy		TC	throat culture
RUQ	right upper quadrant			tissue culture
RVUs	relative value units			total capacity
Rx	prescription			total cholesterol
			TFTC	Task Force for Test Construction
S	subjective data (POMR)		ther	therapy
$\overline{s}$	without		therap	therapeutic
S&A	sugar and acetone (urine)		TIA	transient ischemic attack
SA	sinoatrial		tid	three times a day
SARS	severe acute respiratory syndrome		tinct	tincture
SBE	shortness of breath on exertion		TLC	tender loving care
	subacute bacterial endocarditis		TMJ	temporomandibular joint
SE	standard error		top	topically
sed rate	sedimentation rate		TOPV	trivalent oral poliovirus vaccine
segs	segmented neutrophils		TP	total protein
seq	sequela		TPI	treponema pallidum immobilization test
SF	scarlet fever		TPR	temperature, pulse, and respiration
	spinal fluid		tr	tincture
SG	specific gravity		trig	triglycerides
SH	social history		TSH	thyroid-stimulating hormone
SIDS	sudden infant death syndrome		tsp	teaspoon
sig	instructions, directions		TUR	transurethral resection
sigmoid	sigmoidoscopy		tus	cough
SMA 12/60	Sequential Multiple Analyzer (12-test serum profile)		T&X	type and cross match
SOAP	subjective data, objective data, assessment, and plan		UA	urinalysis
			UB92	Uniform Bill 92
SOB	shortness of breath		UCG	urinary chorionic gonadotropin
SOF	signature on file		UCHD	usual childhood diseases
sol	solution		UCR	usual, customary, reasonable
solv	solvent		ULQ	upper left quadrant

ung	ointment
UR	utilization review
urg	urgent
URI	upper respiratory infection
URL	Uniform Resource Locator
urol	urology
URQ	upper right quadrant
URT	upper respiratory tract
URTI	upper respiratory tract infection
USB	universal system bus port
USP	United States Pharmacopoeia
UT	urinary tract
UTI	urinary tract infection
UV	ultraviolet
vac	vaccine
vag	vagina
	vaginal
VD	venereal disease
VDRL	Venereal Disease Research Laboratory
vit	vitamin
vit cap	vital capacity
vol	volume
VS	vital signs
WAN	wide area network
WAV	waveform audio
WBC	white blood cell
WC	white cell
WDWN	well developed, well nourished
WHO	World Health Organization
WN	well nourished
WNF	well-nourished female
WNL	within normal limits

WNM	well-nourished male
WO	written order
w/o	without
wt	weight
x	multiply by
XR	X-ray
YOB	year of birth
yr	year

Symbols

*	birth
†	death
♂	male
♀	female
+	positive
−	negative
±	positive or negative, indefinite
÷	divide by
=	equal to
>	greater than
<	less than
×	multiply by
#	number, pound
′	foot, minute
″	inch, second
ℨ	dram
℥	ounce
μ	micron
@	at

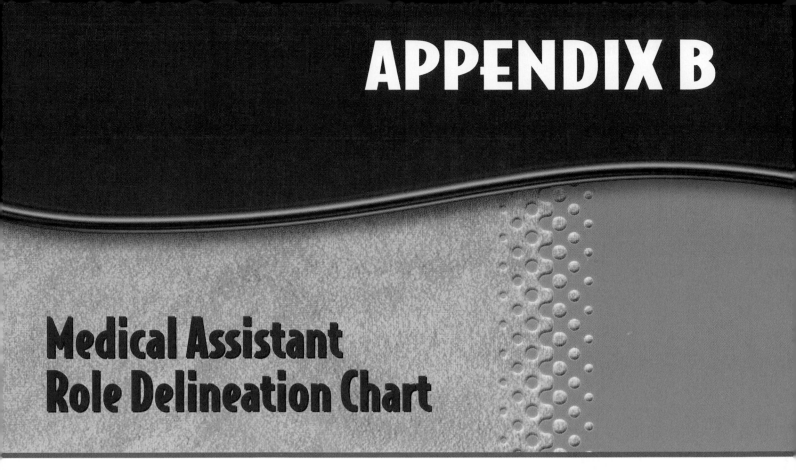

APPENDIX B

Medical Assistant Role Delineation Chart

ADMINISTRATIVE

Administrative Procedures

- Perform basic administrative medical assisting functions
- Schedule, coordinate, and monitor appointments
- Schedule inpatient/outpatient admissions and procedures
- Understand and apply third-party guidelines
- Obtain reimbursement through accurate claims submission
- Monitor third-party reimbursement
- Understand and adhere to managed care policies and procedures
- * Negotiate managed care contracts

Practice Finances

- Perform procedural and diagnostic coding
- Apply bookeeping principles

- Manage accounts receivable
- * Manage accounts payable
- * Process payroll
- * Document and maintain accounting and banking records
- * Develop and maintain fee schedules
- * Manage renewals of business and professional insurance policies
- * Manage personnel benefits and maintain records
- * Perform marketing, financial, and strategic planning

CLINICAL

Fundamental Principles

- Apply principles of aseptic technique and infection control
- Comply with quality assurance practices
- Screen and follow up patient test results

Reprinted with permission of the American Association of Medical Assistants.

*Asterisk denotes advanced skill.

Diagnostic Orders

- Collect and process specimens
- Perform diagnostic tests

Patient Care

- Adhere to established patient screening procedures
- Obtain patient history and vital signs
- Prepare and maintain examination and treatment areas
- Prepare patient for examinations, procedures, and treatments
- Assist with examinations, procedures, and treatments
- Prepare and administer medications and immunizations
- Maintain medication and immunization records
- Recognize and respond to emergencies
- Coordinate patient care information with other health care providers
- Initiate IV and administer IV medications with appropriate training as permitted by state law

GENERAL

Professionalism

- Display a professional manner and image
- Demonstrate initiative and responsibility
- Work as a member of the health care team
- Prioritize and perform multiple tasks
- Adapt to change
- Promote the CMA credential
- Enhance skills through continuing education
- Treat all patients with compassion and empathy
- Promote the practice through positive public relations

Communication Skills

- Recognize and respect cultural diversity
- Adapt communications to individual's ability to understand

- Use professional telephone technique
- Recognize and respond to verbal, nonverbal, and written communications
- Use medical terminology appropriately
- Use electronic technology to receive, organize, prioritize, and transmit information
- Serve as liaison

Legal Concepts

- Perform within legal and ethical boundaries
- Prepare and maintain medical records
- Document accurately
- Follow employer's established policies dealing with the health care contract
- Implement and maintain federal and state health care legislation and regulations
- Comply with established risk management and safety procedures
- Recognize professional credentialing criteria
- *Develop and maintain personnel, policy and procedure manuals*

Instruction

- Instruct individuals according to their needs
- Explain office policies and procedures
- Teach methods of health promotion and disease prevention
- Locate community resources and disseminate information
- *Develop educational materials*
- *Conduct continuing education activities*

Operational Functions

- Perform inventory of supplies and equipment
- Perform routine maintenance of administative and clinical equipment
- Apply computer techniques to support office operations
- *Perform personnel management functions*
- *Negotiate leases and prices for equipment and supply contracts*

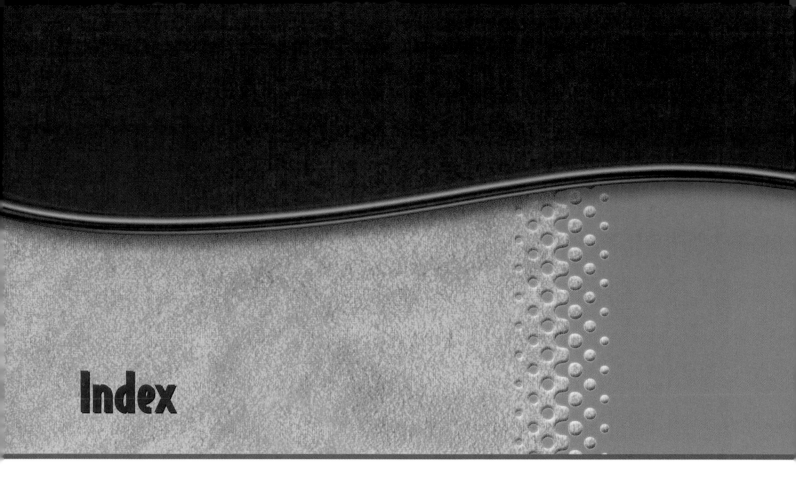

Index

Note: Page references in **bold type** refer to boxes, procedures, figures, and tables.

Minimum System Requirements for Student Software CD

Operating System: Microsoft Windows (98 SE, 2000 or XP)
Processor: Pentium PC 500 MHz or higher (750Mhz recommended)
RAM: 64 MB of RAM (128 MB recommended)
Free Drive Space: 120 MB • Screen Resolution: 800 x 600 pixels
Color Depth: 16-bit color (thousands of colors)
Sound Card: Yes • Macromedia Flash Player V7.x.
Free Macromedia Flash Player can be downloaded from http://www.macromedia.com

Installation Instructions for Student Software CD

1. Insert disc into CD-ROM player. The installation program should start up automatically. It will prompt you to install program on your hard drive. Follow each step. Leave the box for "Install icon on desktop" unchecked. Program should launch automatically. If program does not install, go to step 2.
2. From My Computer, double click the icon for the CD drive. Double click the setup.exe file to start the program.
3. When program is launched, a menu page will appear.
4. Click icon of program you want to open (Audio Library, Critical Thinking Challenge, or StudyWARE™) and it should launch immediately.

Technical Support

Telephone: 1-800-477-3692, 8:30 A.M.-5:30 P.M. Eastern Time
Fax: 1-518-881-1247 E-mail: delmarhelp@thomson.com

StudyWARE™ is a trademark used herein under license. Microsoft® and Windows® are registered trademarks of the Microsoft Corporation. Pentium® is a registered trademark of the Intel® Corporation.

Thomson Delmar Learning End User License Agreement

IMPORTANT! READ CAREFULLY: This End User License Agreement ("Agreement") sets forth the conditions by which Thomson Delmar Learning, a division of Thomson Learning Inc. ("Thomson") will make electronic access to the Thomson Delmar Learning-owned licensed content and associated media, software, documentation, printed materials, and electronic documentation contained in this package and/or made available to you via this product (the "Licensed Content"), available to you (the "End User"). BY CLICKING THE "I ACCEPT" BUTTON AND/OR OPENING THIS PACKAGE, YOU ACKNOWLEDGE THAT YOU HAVE READ ALL OF THE TERMS AND CONDITIONS, AND THAT YOU AGREE TO BE BOUND BY ITS TERMS, CONDITIONS, AND ALL APPLICABLE LAWS AND REGULATIONS GOVERNING THE USE OF THE LICENSED CONTENT. **1.0 SCOPE OF LICENSE** 1.1 Licensed Content. The Licensed Content may contain portions of modifiable content ("Modifiable Content") and content which may not be modified or otherwise altered by the End User ("Non-Modifiable Content"). For purposes of this Agreement, Modifiable Content and Non-Modifiable Content may be collectively referred to herein as the "Licensed Content." All Licensed Content shall be considered Non-Modifiable Content, unless such Licensed Content is presented to the End User in a modifiable format and it is clearly indicated that modification of the Licensed Content is permitted. 1.2 Subject to the End User's compliance with the terms and conditions of this Agreement, Thomson Delmar Learning hereby grants the End User, a nontransferable, nonexclusive, limited right to access and view a single copy of the Licensed Content on a single personal computer system for noncommercial, internal, personal use only. The End User shall not (i) reproduce, copy, modify (except in the case of Modifiable Content), distribute, display, transfer, sublicense, prepare derivative work(s) based on, sell, exchange, barter or transfer, rent, lease, loan, resell, or in any other manner exploit the Licensed Content; (ii) remove, obscure, or alter any notice of Thomson Delmar Learning's intellectual property rights present on or in the Licensed Content, including, but not limited to, copyright, trademark, and/or patent notices; or (iii) disassemble, decompile, translate, reverse engineer, or otherwise reduce the Licensed Content. **2.0 TERMINATION** 2.1 Thomson Delmar Learning may at any time (without prejudice to its other rights or remedies) immediately terminate this Agreement and/or suspend access to some or all of the Licensed Content, in the event that the End User does not comply with any of the terms and conditions of this Agreement. In the event of such termination by Thomson Delmar Learning, the End User shall immediately return any and all copies of the Licensed Content to Thomson Delmar Learning. **3.0 PROPRIETARY RIGHTS** 3.1 The End User acknowledges that Thomson Delmar Learning owns all rights, title and interest, including, but not limited to all copyright rights therein, in and to the Licensed Content, and that the End User shall not take any action inconsistent with such ownership. The Licensed Content is protected by U.S., Canadian and other applicable copyright laws and by international treaties, including the Berne Convention and the Universal Copyright Convention. Nothing contained in this Agreement shall be construed as granting the End User any ownership rights in or to the Licensed Content. 3.2 Thomson Delmar Learning reserves the right at any time to withdraw from the Licensed Content any item or part of an item for which it no longer retains the

right to publish, or which it has reasonable grounds to believe infringes copyright or is defamatory, unlawful, or otherwise objectionable. **4.0 PROTECTION AND SECURITY** 4.1 The End User shall use its best efforts and take all reasonable steps to safeguard its copy of the Licensed Content to ensure that no unauthorized reproduction, publication, disclosure, modification, or distribution of the Licensed Content, in whole or in part, is made. To the extent that the End User becomes aware of any such unauthorized use of the Licensed Content, the End User shall immediately notify Thomson Delmar Learning. Notification of such violations may be made by sending an e-mail to delmarhelp@thomson.com. **5.0 MISUSE OF THE LICENSED PRODUCT** 5.1 In the event that the End User uses the Licensed Content in violation of this Agreement, Thomson Delmar Learning shall have the option of electing liquidated damages, which shall include all profits generated by the End User's use of the Licensed Content plus interest computed at the maximum rate permitted by law and all legal fees and other expenses incurred by Thomson Delmar Learning in enforcing its rights, plus penalties. **6.0 FEDERAL GOVERNMENT CLIENTS** 6.1 Except as expressly authorized by Thomson Delmar Learning, Federal Government clients obtain only the rights specified in this Agreement and no other rights. The Government acknowledges that (i) all software and related documentation incorporated in the Licensed Content is existing commercial computer software within the meaning of FAR 27.405(b)(2); and (2) all other data delivered in whatever form, is limited rights data within the meaning of FAR 27.401. The restrictions in this section are acceptable as consistent with the Government's need for software and other data under this Agreement. **7.0 DISCLAIMER OF WARRANTIES AND LIABILITIES** 7.1 Although Thomson Delmar Learning believes the Licensed Content to be reliable, Thomson Delmar Learning does not guarantee or warrant (i) any information or materials contained in or produced by the Licensed Content, (ii) the accuracy, completeness or reliability of the Licensed Content, or (iii) that the Licensed Content is free from errors or other material defects. THE LICENSED PRODUCT IS PROVIDED "AS IS," WITHOUT ANY WARRANTY OF ANY KIND AND THOMSON DELMAR LEARNING DISCLAIMS ANY AND ALL WARRANTIES, EXPRESSED OR IMPLIED, INCLUDING, WITHOUT LIMITATION, WARRANTIES OF MERCHANTABILITY OR FITNESS OR A PARTICULAR PURPOSE. IN NO EVENT SHALL THOMSON DELMAR LEARNING BE LIABLE FOR: INDIRECT, SPECIAL, PUNITIVE OR CONSEQUENTIAL DAMAGES INCLUDING FOR LOST PROFITS, LOST DATA, OR OTHERWISE. IN NO EVENT SHALL THOMSON DELMAR LEARNING'S AGGREGATE LIABILITY HEREUNDER, WHETHER ARISING IN CONTRACT, TORT, STRICT LIABILITY OR OTHERWISE, EXCEED THE AMOUNT OF FEES PAID BY THE END USER HEREUNDER FOR THE LICENSE OF THE LICENSED CONTENT. **8.0 GENERAL** 8.1 <u>Entire Agreement</u>. This Agreement shall constitute the entire Agreement between the Parties and supercedes all prior Agreements and understandings oral or written relating to the subject matter hereof. 8.2 <u>Enhancements/Modifications of Licensed Content</u>. From time to time, and in Thomson Delmar Learning's sole discretion, Thomson Delmar Learning may advise the End User of updates, upgrades, enhancements and/or improvements to the Licensed Content, and may permit the End User to access and use, subject to the terms and conditions of this Agreement, such modifications, upon payment of prices as may be established by Thomson Delmar Learning. 8.3 <u>No Export</u>. The End User shall use the Licensed Content solely in the United States and shall not transfer or export, directly or indirectly, the Licensed Content outside the United States. 8.4 <u>Severability</u>. If any provision of this Agreement is invalid, illegal, or unenforceable under any applicable statute or rule of law, the provision shall be deemed omitted to the extent that it is invalid, illegal, or unenforceable. In such a case, the remainder of the Agreement shall be construed in a manner as to give greatest effect to the original intention of the parties hereto. 8.5 <u>Waiver</u>. The waiver of any right or failure of either party to exercise in any respect any right provided in this Agreement in any instance shall not be deemed to be a waiver of such right in the future or a waiver of any other right under this Agreement. 8.6 <u>Choice of Law/Venue</u>. This Agreement shall be interpreted, construed, and governed by and in accordance with the laws of the State of New York, applicable to contracts executed and to be wholly preformed therein, without regard to its principles governing conflicts of law. Each party agrees that any proceeding arising out of or relating to this Agreement or the breach or threatened breach of this Agreement may be commenced and prosecuted in a court in the State and County of New York. Each party consents and submits to the nonexclusive personal jurisdiction of any court in the State and County of New York in respect of any such proceeding. 8.7 <u>Acknowledgment</u>. By opening this package and/or by accessing the Licensed Content on this Web site, THE END USER ACKNOWLEDGES THAT IT HAS READ THIS AGREEMENT, UNDERSTANDS IT, AND AGREES TO BE BOUND BY ITS TERMS AND CONDITIONS. IF YOU DO NOT ACCEPT THESE TERMS AND CONDITIONS, YOU MUST NOT ACCESS THE LICENSED CONTENT AND RETURN THE LICENSED PRODUCT TO DELMAR LEARNING (WITHIN 30 CALENDAR DAYS OF THE END USER'S PURCHASE) WITH PROOF OF PAYMENT ACCEPTABLE TO THOMSON DELMAR LEARNING, FOR A CREDIT OR A REFUND. Should the End User have any questions/comments regarding this Agreement, please contact Thomson Delmar Learning at delmarhelp@thomson.com.